CARING FOR THE RENAL PATIENT

CARING FOR THE
RENAL PATIENT

THIRD EDITION

David Z. Levine, MD

Professor of Medicine and Head, Division of Nephrology
University of Ottawa and Ottawa General Hospital
Ottawa, Ontario, Canada

W.B. SAUNDERS COMPANY
A Division of Harcourt Brace & Company
Philadelphia   London   Toronto   Montreal   Sydney   Tokyo

W.B. SAUNDERS COMPANY
A Division of Harcourt Brace & Company

The Curtis Center
Independence Square West
Philadelphia, Pennsylvania 19106

Library of Congress Cataloging-in-Publication Data

Caring for the renal patient / [edited by] David Z. Levine.—3rd ed.

p.   cm.

Includes bibliographical references and index.

ISBN 0–7216–6243–9

1. Kidneys—Diseases—Treatment.   I. Levine, David Z.   [DNLM: 1. Kidney
    Diseases—diagnosis.   2. Kidney Diseases—therapy.   WJ 300 C271 1997]

RC902.A2C37 1997   616.6′106—dc20

DNLM/DLC   96–26583

CARING FOR THE RENAL PATIENT, Third Edition   ISBN 0–7216–6243–9

Last digit is the print number: 9   8   7   6   5   4   3   2   1

To Alfred Coll,
my patient and friend,
who sustained me
through the most
difficult times.

CONTRIBUTORS

Sharon G. Adler, MD
Professor of Medicine, University of California, Los Angeles, School of Medicine, Los Angeles; Associate Chief, Division of Nephrology and Hypertension, Harbor-UCLA Medical Center, Torrance, California
Diabetic Nephropathy

Robert J. Alpern, MD
Professor, Internal Medicine, Ruth W. and Milton P. Levy, Sr. Chair in Molecular Nephrology, and Chief, Division of Nephrology, University of Texas Southwestern Medical Center, Dallas, Texas
Sodium and Potassium Disturbances in Renal Patients

Nicholas B. Argent, MB, ChB, FRCP(C)
Assistant Professor of Medicine, University of Ottawa; Assistant Professor and Active Staff, Ottawa General Hospital, Ottawa, Ontario, Canada
Urgent Problems in the Renal Patient

James L. Bailey, MD
Assistant Professor of Medicine, Emory University School of Medicine, Atlanta, Georgia
Nutritional Concerns for Patients with Kidney Disease

Robert C. Bell, MD, FRCP(C)
Associate Professor, University of Ottawa; Active Staff, Ottawa General Hospital, Ottawa, Ontario, Canada
Urgent Problems in the Renal Patient

William M. Bennett, MD
Professor of Medicine and Pharmacology, Oregon Health Sciences University, Portland, Oregon
Drug Use in Renal Patients and the Extracorporeal Treatment of Poisonings

Kevin D. Burns, MD, FRCP(C)
Assistant Professor of Medicine, University of Ottawa; Assistant Professor and Active Staff, Ottawa General Hospital, Ottawa, Ontario, Canada
Acid-Base Disorders in Azotemic Patients; Urgent Problems in the Renal Patient

Daniel C. Cattran, MD, FRCP(C), FACP
Professor of Medicine, University of Toronto; Associate Director, Division of Nephrology, Toronto Hospital, Toronto, Ontario, Canada
Acute Nephritic Syndrome

Jack W. Coburn, MD, FACP
Professor of Medicine, University of California, Los Angeles, School of Medicine; Staff Physician, West Los Angeles VA Medical Center (Wadsworth Division), Los Angeles, California
Renal Bone Diseases and Aluminum Toxicity in Renal Patients

Cecil H. Coggins, MD
Associate Professor of Medicine, Harvard Medical School; Physician and Clinical Director, Renal Unit, Massachusetts General Hospital, Boston, Massachusetts
Hematuria, Proteinuria, and Nephrotic Syndrome

George E. Digenis, MD
Staff, Therapeutic Clinic, University of Athens, Medical School; Staff, Renal Unit, Alexandra Hospital, Athens, Greece
Peritoneal Dialysis

Nicholas V. Dombros, MD, FRCP(C), FACP
Assistant Professor of Medicine, Aristotle University of Thessaloniki Medical School; Staff, First Department of Medicine, and Director, Peritoneal Dialysis Unit, Ahepa University Hospital, Thessaloniki, Greece
Peritoneal Dialysis

Thomas D. DuBose, Jr., MD
Professor, Departments of Internal Medicine and Integrative Biology and Director, Division of Renal Diseases and Hypertension, University of Texas Medical School–Houston; Medical Director, University Kidney Center, and Medical Director, Acute Hemodialysis Unit, Hermann Hospital, Houston, Texas
Chronic Renal Failure

Stella Feld, MD
Nephrology Research Fellow, Harbor-UCLA Medical Center, Torrance, California
Diabetic Nephropathy

Kevin W. Finkel, MD
Assistant Professor of Internal Medicine, Division of Renal Diseases and Hypertension, University of Texas Medical School–Houston; Attending Physician, Hermann Hospital, Houston, Texas
Chronic Renal Failure

Richard J. Glassock, MD
Professor and Chair, Department of Internal Medicine, University of Kentucky College of Medicine, Lexington, Kentucky
Diabetic Nephropathy

William G. Goodman, MD
Professor of Radiology and Medicine, University of California, Los Angeles, School of Medicine; Attending Physician, UCLA Medical Center, Los Angeles, California
Renal Bone Diseases and Aluminum Toxicity in Renal Patients

Simin Goral, MD
Instructor, Department of Medicine, Vanderbilt University Medical Center, Nashville, Tennessee
Renal Transplantation: Approaches to Graft Dysfunction and the Consequences of Immunosuppression

Raymond M. Hakim, MD, PhD
Professor of Medicine, Vanderbilt University School of Medicine, Nashville, Tennessee
Hemodialysis

John T. Harrington, MD
Professor of Medicine and Dean ad Interim, Tufts University School of Medicine; Consulting Nephrologist, Tufts-New England Medical Center, Boston, Massachusetts
Assessment of the Patient with Renal Disease

J. Harold Helderman, MD
Professor of Medicine, Microbiology, and Immunology, Vanderbilt University; Medical Director, Vanderbilt Transplant Center, Vanderbilt University, Nashville, Tennessee
Renal Transplantation: Approaches to Graft Dysfunction and the Consequences of Immunosuppression

Nuhad Ismail, MD
Associate Professor of Medicine and Director, ESRD Program, Vanderbilt University School of Medicine, Nashville, Tennessee
Hemodialysis

Saulo Klahr, MD
John and Adaline Simon Professor and Co-Chairman, Department of Medicine, Washington University School of Medicine; Physician, Barnes-Jewish Hospital, St. Louis, Missouri
Obstructive Uropathy

David Z. Levine, MD, FRCP(C)
Professor of Medicine and Head, Division of Nephrology, University of Ottawa and Ottawa General Hospital, Ottawa, Ontario, Canada
Acid-Base Disorders in Azotemic Patients

Mortimer Levy, MD, FRCP(C)
Professor of Medicine and Physiology, McGill University Faculty of Medicine; Director of Nephrology and Senior Physician, Royal Victoria Hospital Nephrology Division, Montreal, Quebec, Canada
Edematous States and Hepatorenal Syndrome

Norman B. Levy, MD
Clinical Professor of Psychiatry and Adjunct Professor of Medicine, State University of New York, Health Science Center at Brooklyn; Director of Consultation-Liaison Psychiatry and Emergency Services, Coney Island Hospital, Brooklyn, New York
Psychiatric Aspects of Renal Care

Marshall D. Lindheimer, MD
Professor of Medicine, Obstetrics, and Gynecology and Clinical Pharmacology, University of Chicago Pritzker School of Medicine, Division of Biological Sciences; Head, Medical High Risk Clinic, University of Chicago Hospital, Chicago Lying-in Hospital, Chicago, Illinois
Renal Disease and Hypertension in Pregnancy

Ronald Baker Miller, MD
Clinical Professor of Medicine and Director of Program in Medical Ethics, University of California, Irvine, Irvine; Attending Physician and Vice-Chair of Medical Ethics Committee, University of California, Irvine, Medical Center, Orange; Consultant and Chairman, Scientific Advisory Board, Spectra Laboratories (a national laboratory devoted to the care of patients with end stage renal disease), Fremont, California
Selected Ethical Issues in Caring for the Renal Patient

William E. Mitch, MD
Garland Herndon Professor of Medicine, Emory University School of Medicine, Atlanta, Georgia
Nutritional Concerns for Patients with Kidney Disease

Dimitrios G. Oreopoulos, MD
Professor of Medicine, University of Toronto; Staff, Division of Nephrology, and Director, Peritoneal Dialysis Program, The Toronto Hospital, Toronto, Ontario, Canada
Peritoneal Dialysis

Biff F. Palmer, MD
Associate Professor of Internal Medicine, University of Texas Southwestern Medical Center; Director of Chronic Dialysis Unit and Peritoneal Dialysis Program, Parkland Memorial Hospital, Dallas, Texas
Sodium and Potassium Disturbances in Renal Patients

Linda Panther, BScN, CNeph(C)
Nursing Unit Manager, Artificial Kidney Unit, Ottawa General Hospital, Ottawa, Ontario, Canada
The Role of the Nurse in Caring for the Renal Patient

Isidro B. Salusky, MD
Professor of Pediatrics, University of California, Los Angeles, School of Medicine; Director, Pediatric Dialysis Program, and Program Director, General Clinical Research Center, UCLA Center for Health Sciences, Los Angeles, California
Renal Bone Diseases and Aluminum Toxicity in Renal Patients

Roger A. L. Sutton, DM
Professor and Chairman, Department of Medicine, Aga Khan University, Karachi, Pakistan
Stone Disease

Suzanne K. Swan, MD
Assistant Professor of Medicine, University of Minnesota; Staff, Hennepin County Medical Center, Minneapolis, Minnesota
Drug Use in Renal Patients and the Extracorporeal Treatment of Poisonings

Robert D. Toto, MD
Professor of Medicine, University of Texas Southwestern Medical Center at Dallas, Dallas, Texas
Sodium and Potassium Disturbances in Renal Patients

Jason G. Umans, MD, PhD
Associate Professor of Medicine and Clinical Pharmacology, and Director, Renal Outpatient Clinic, University of Chicago, Chicago, Illinois
Renal Disease and Hypertension in Pregnancy

Norman M. Wolfish, BSc (Hon), MD, FRCP(C), FAAP
Professor of Pediatrics, Faculty of Medicine, University of Ottawa; Head, Nephrology Service, Children's Hospital of Eastern Ontario, Ottawa, Ontario, Canada
Pediatric Nephrology

PREFACE

Learning from One Hundred People with Kidney Illnesses

Three new elements have been introduced in this edition: it is problem oriented, it is patient oriented, and it brings to the trainee the most current advances in patient management.

First, the presentation of the ill person steers the discussion. Each chapter consists of several cases, followed by diagnostic and management issues. Indeed, this is problem-based learning (PBL). One of our distinguished contributors at first wondered if this wasn't too novel or too awkward. I replied this wasn't really new. Remember Grand Rounds in the past when patients were routinely presented? Besides, I thought, if there were no ill person to whom one could refer in the text, then maybe that part of the discussion should be outside of the scope of our practical approach.

Second, we have tried not to forget that those of us afflicted with kidney disease are people with illnesses, often bewildered and broken-hearted. Folks with siblings, and spouses, and stories to tell. Those small, poorly functioning kidneys are only part of an engulfing *illness* with long psychosocial shadows. In addition to Norman Levy's Chapter 16 on psychiatric aspects of renal care, we now have two new chapters. In Chapter 17 Ron Miller deals extensively with ethical issues in nephrology, and in Chapter 18 Linda Panther provides detailed planning for nursing care. These chapters emphasize the tough situations we share with our patients. Moreover, taking instruction from Francis Peabody's 1927 comment, ". . . the secret of the care of the patient is in caring for the patient," I changed the title of the book to emphasize the immutable importance of *caring* for our patients.

Third, this new edition has brought us up to date: our trainees will be able to apply to daily management regimens the newest nephrology advances of the past six years.

I am indebted, first and foremost, to my many dialysis patients—dear understanding people who have taught me so much and showed such courage in the face of devastating illness. Second, I thank my colleagues and contributors who have gone out of their way to make this problem-oriented text both compassionate and up to date. Last, Ray Kersey and David Kilmer of the W.B. Saunders Company have my gratitude for their encouragement and for allowing me to put a more human face on this edition of *Caring for the Renal Patient*.

DAVID Z. LEVINE, MD

CONTENTS

1 | ASSESSMENT OF THE PATIENT WITH

RENAL DISEASE

John T. Harrington

Assessment of patients with known or suspected renal disease embraces the traditional triad of methods used by clinicians in their evaluation of patients with any medical problem—namely, history taking, physical examination, and judicious use of laboratory studies. The objective of this introductory chapter is to demonstrate the importance of critical questions in assessing patients with renal disease; these questions are applied to a select series of case discussions. The answers to the questions obtained by history, physical examination, and laboratory studies enable clinicians to acquire relevant data. In addition to emphasizing the history and physical examination, we focus on three fundamental nephrologic laboratory tests: (1) serum creatinine concentration as an estimation of renal function, (2) the urinalysis and in particular examination of the urinary sediment by the clinician, and (3) quantitation of proteinuria either by 24-hour urine protein testing or by use of the urine protein-to-creatinine ratio. Discussion of more sophisticated serologic, radiologic, and pathologic testing, including interpretation of urinary electrolyte values, can be found in subsequent chapters.

Patients with intrinsic renal disease present most often with (1) acute renal failure, (2) chronic renal failure, (3) edema with proteinuria, or (4) hematuria. Hypertension and urinary tract infections, also important renal problems, are not addressed here. We assume that readers are well versed in the fundamentals of renal physiology, pathology, and pathophysiology.

Acute Renal Failure

PATIENT NUMBER 1

Rosie, a 24-year-old graduate student, collapsed after finishing the Boston marathon. She had noted muscle cramps and had vomited just before crossing the finish line in a time of approximately 4 hours, 35 minutes. She drank a few cups of bouillon and felt somewhat better. Because of continued leg cramps and pain, however, she came to the emergency room, where she passed a small volume of red urine.

Results of physical examination were normal (with no orthostatic change in blood pressure or pulse), except for a slight decrease in skin turgor and tender calves. Initial laboratory studies:

BUN	21 mg/dl
Serum creatinine	3.2 mg/dl
Sodium	142 mEq/L
Potassium	6.1 mEq/L
Chloride	108 mEq/L
Bicarbonate	18 mEq/L
Calcium	6.1 mg/dl
Phosphate	8.6 mg/dl
Hematocrit	54%

Urinalysis revealed pink urine (the plasma was clear) with a specific gravity of 1.012, 2+ protein, and 4+ heme by dipstick; light microscopic examination by the intern in the emergency room revealed 2 to 5 RBCs and 1 to 3 WBCs per high-power field (hpf); also seen were many renal tubular cells, renal tubular cell casts, and muddy-brown casts.

The diagnosis in this classic case is straightforward (especially in Boston)—rhabdomyolysis with consequent acute tubular necrosis (ATN). As is often the case, the history makes the diagnosis, and this patient's diagnosis was made in the emergency room by the medical intern on duty on the basis of history alone. Suppose, however, we did not have the history, rather the laboratory data alone (*not* the way to treat patients). The elevated serum creatinine concentration of 3.2 mg/dl clearly indicates the presence of moderate to severe renal failure.

The critical questions in the setting of newly discovered renal failure are

1. **Is the renal failure acute or chronic?**
2. **Assuming it is acute (which always should be assumed unless incontrovertible evidence for chronic renal failure exists), is the renal dysfunction due to prerenal factors? postrenal factors? or intrinsic renal disease?**
3. **Assuming that intrinsic renal disease is the cause of the renal failure, is the renal disease a primary renal disease or a systemic disease with renal involvement (e.g., diabetes mellitus, lupus erythematosus, Wegener's granulomatosis, and so on)?**

Let's answer these questions for our patient, Rosie.

First, is the renal failure acute or chronic? The history certainly indicates an acute illness, and the urine sediment examination is consistent with ATN. Moreover, rhabdomyolysis is not a recurrent problem, save in rare patients with inherited muscle disorders, such as McArdle's syndrome. In an ideal setting, one would like to have results of previous renal function tests (BUN, serum creatinine) or urinalyses, but most often such information is not available. Renal sonography, not indicated in our patient, provides a close estimate of renal size and cortical thickness and rules out obstruction with hydronephrosis. If a renal sonogram had been performed on our patient, the results likely would have been normal or perhaps would have shown some mild enlargement of the kidneys (as is often found with ATN). Normal-size kidneys suggest an acute process (with exceptions such as polycystic kidney disease), whereas small shrunken kidneys are found in patients with chronic renal failure. The elevated hematocrit (54%) in our patient Rosie also suggests an acute process. In general, patients with advanced chronic renal failure present with anemia whereas patients with acute renal failure present with a normal hematocrit. There are many exceptions to this rule, however, such as systemic lupus erythematosus with acute nephritis and simultaneous hemolytic anemia.

Second, is the renal dysfunction due to prerenal factors, postrenal factors, or intrinsic renal disease? Prerenal factors include both volume depletion (e.g., severe diarrhea) and volume overload (e.g., congestive heart failure). The volume status of a patient *cannot* be determined by the laboratory! History and especially physical examination are crucial. One must search for fluid losses both to the "outside world" (e.g., severe diarrhea, copious vomiting, hypotonic fluid losses via sweating) and to the "inside world" (e.g., "third spacing," such as due to loss of salt and water into the peritoneal cavity in a patient with acute peritonitis). Measurement of pulmonary capillary wedge pressure often is required in critically ill patients. It is clear that our patient Rosie is hemoconcentrated (hematocrit is 54%; she has just finished a marathon), but her blood pressure was normal without a significant orthostatic fall and her skin turgor over the anterior thighs was only slightly decreased. The diagnosis of congestive heart failure doesn't make sense in a marathoner, and no rales or edema was found on physical examination. The possibility of urinary tract obstruction, highly unlikely in a 24-year-old woman, was dismissed on clinical grounds. The urine sediment in both prerenal failure and postrenal failure is bland.

How do we really know this patient had rhabdomyolysis with consequent ATN? First, one piece of information, withheld until now, is that Rosie's CPK level was >10,000 U/L. Second, as noted earlier, the urinary sediment revealed renal tubular cells (Color Fig. 1–1), renal tubular cell casts (Color Fig. 1–2) and muddy-brown casts (Color Fig. 1–3). These sediment findings alone indicate the presence of ATN in our patient. **Examination of the urine sediment remains the most useful simple screening test for detection and initial classification of renal disease.**

Examining the Urine Sediment

I have several rules.

1. The urine should be examined by the clinician caring for the patient.
2. Collect and look at the sediment as soon as possible, preferably within 1 hour.

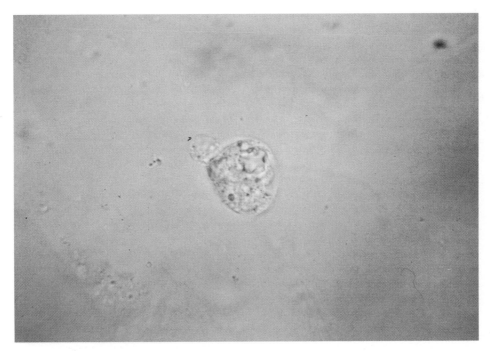

Figure 1-1. Renal tubular cell (×430).

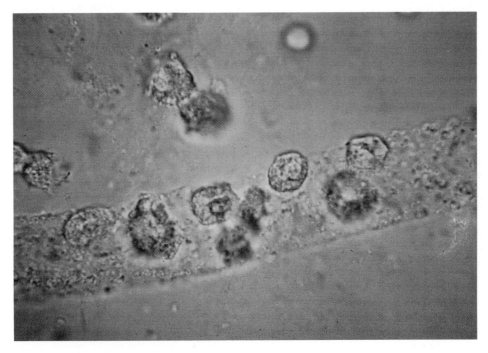

Figure 1-2. Renal tubular cell cast (×430).

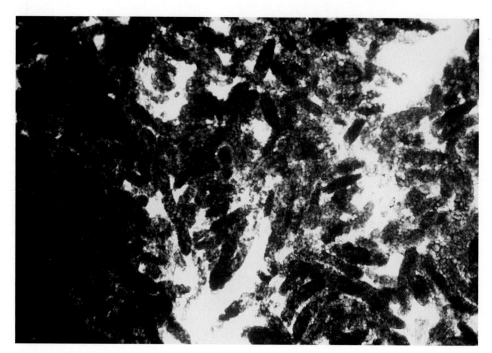

Figure 1-3. Muddy-brown casts in a patient with ATN (×100).

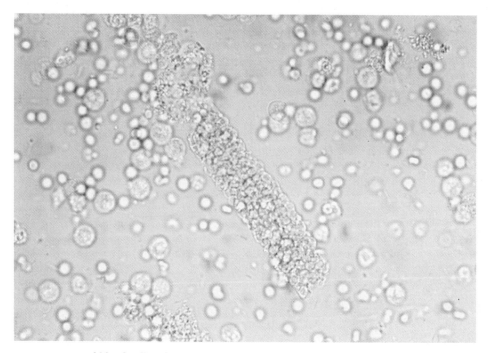

Figure 1-4. Red blood cell cast in a patient with acute nephritis (×430).

3. Spin the urine in a conical centrifuge tube (12 ml) for 5 minutes at 1500 rpm (establish a standard for your own practice).

4. Decant the supernatant, leaving only 0.1 ml or so in the tip of the tube. Using a sharp-tipped disposable Pasteur pipette, "pick the button" of sediment and transfer it onto a microscope slide.

5. Using the 10× objective, the "uroscopist" (the physician caring for the patient) should systematically scan the coverslip looking for cells, casts of various types, and other elements such as crystals and yeast. Examination of unstained sediment by routine light microscopy usually is all that is required.

Normal urine sediment has an average of less than 2 to 3 RBCs and 3 WBCs per hpf. Nonglomerular RBCs are nearly uniform in size and shape, whereas RBCs of glomerular origin are small and dystrophic, presumably because of cleavage of small portions of the RBCs as they course through the glomerular capillary wall. I prefer to search for RBC casts because they are virtually pathognomonic of glomerulonephritis or vasculitis of the kidneys. Hemoglobin or blood casts are degenerated RBC casts with blurred or indistinct margins of the cells; the casts appear granular and have an orange to red-brick hemoglobin color. WBC casts (along with WBCs) are seen in acute and chronic interstitial nephritis but may also be found in patients with acute exudative glomerulonephritis. In patients with acute urinary tract infection, the finding of leukocyte casts identifies the kidneys as the site of infection.

Renal tubular cells, renal tubular cell casts, and muddy-brown casts are seen in approximately 80% of patients with ATN; these sediment abnormalities, noted in our patient Rosie, confirmed the clinical diagnosis of ATN. I believe that the appropriate clinical setting and the urine sediment abnormalities just described are more useful in making a diagnosis of ATN than other methods, such as measurement of the fractional excretion of sodium. Finally, the urine should be examined for crystals, particularly in patients with stones (looking for cystine, uric acid, or calcium oxalate crystals) and in patients with the combination of high anion gap metabolic acidosis and suspected intoxication, looking for the numerous calcium oxalate ("envelope") crystals excreted in the urine of patients with ATN secondary to ethylene glycol intoxication.

Third, is the intrinsic renal disease a primary renal disease or is it part of a systemic disease such as Wegener's granulomatosis, diabetes mellitus, or systemic lupus erythematosus? In our patient, Rosie, the acute nature of the illness, the ready identification of the acute renal insult (i.e., the marathon, with muscle damage and release of intracellular constituents), and the diagnostic urinary sediment abnormalities establish the diagnosis of ATN, a *primary* renal disorder. In situations that are not as clear-cut, searching for evidence of disease in other organ systems is mandatory. The possibilities are myriad, but classic examples include diabetic retinopathy in patients with diabetes, otorhinolaryngologic and pulmonary abnormalities in patients with Wegener's, a butterfly rash in patients with lupus, hemolytic anemia in hemolytic-uremic syndrome, and cardiac conduction defects in patients with amyloidosis. Diagnosis of these systemic diseases obviously *cannot* be made using only the serum creatinine value, urine sediment examination, and quantitative urine protein testing. Discussion of the diagnostic workup of systemic diseases with an important renal component can be found in Chapter 3.

PATIENT NUMBER 1 (continued)

Rosie had only one critical question that she asked the day after admission: "Will I get better?" Given the preceding information, I said yes. Four months later, she was running again, but only in 10-mile races!

Chronic Renal Failure

PATIENT NUMBER 2

Frank, a 45-year-old anxious office worker, was transferred to our hospital with pruritus, leg cramps, numbness and tingling of both lower extremities, insomnia, and intermittent episodes of confusion. He stated that he had had frequent sore throats in childhood, and he was known to have had proteinuria for nearly 25 years. Four years before the present admission, he was seen because of dark urine and severe headache 3 to 4 days after a severe sore throat (no culture had been done). His blood pressure then was 160/100 mm Hg. The urinary sediment revealed 10 to 15 RBCs/hpf, 0 to 2 WBCs/hpf, rare granular and hyaline casts, and 2 definite RBC casts. His serum creatinine value was 2.5 mg/dl, BUN was 60 mg/dl, and hematocrit was 30%. A renal sonogram showed both kidneys to be equal but slightly diminished in size; 24-hour urine protein excretion was 2.4 g. One year before admission, his serum creatinine level was 6 mg/dl, BUN was 80 mg/dl, and hematocrit was 25%. He struggled with fatigue, inability to do his job, and impotence, but **most of all, he was afraid he would die and not see his young children grow up.** Despite treatment with a low-protein diet and antihypertensive agents, his renal function continued to deteriorate and his serum creatinine level rose to 12 mg/dl and BUN to 180 mg/dl on admission.

Frank obviously has chronic renal failure secondary to chronic glomerulonephritis. He had had proteinuria for 2 to 3 decades, and RBC casts (Color Fig. 1–4) had been found in his urine sediment 4 years before the final admission. No kidney biopsy was performed on this patient, but on statistical grounds, the likely histopathologic diagnoses are either IgA nephropathy or poststreptococcal glomerulonephritis. For the balance of the discussion of this patient, we assume that a specific diagnosis had been made.

The two critical questions in patients with established chronic renal failure are

1. **What is the present level of renal function?**
2. **Is there a "reversible" component to the patient's present level of renal function?**

First, what is the level of renal function? Direct or indirect measurements of the GFR are most often used clinically to estimate the overall function of the kidneys. Classically, inulin clearance was used to establish normal values in men and women, corrected for differences in body surface area and for age. More recently, the GFR has been measured by various isotopic markers, most commonly ^{125}I-sodium iothalamate. One carefully described set of iothalamite clearance data revealed a GFR at birth of 122 ml/min/1.73 m², falling to 89 ml/min/1.73 m² (a loss of 27%) at age 60 years and to 68 ml/min/1.73 m² (a loss of 44%) at age 80 years. Despite the accuracy and validity of direct GFR measurements using either inulin, iothalamate, or other markers, the costs and difficulties of directly measuring the GFR have led clinicians nearly always to use indirect estimates of GFR both in hospitalized patients and in out-of-hospital settings. The two most pragmatic methods available at present are creatinine clearance (measured directly or estimated by formula) and serum creatinine determination. Measurement of serum creatinine

concentration remains the most widely used laboratory test for estimation of renal function. Most laboratories use the Jaffé picrate reaction, which is based on creation of a complex between creatinine and picrate; this method detects real or true creatinine and a small amount of noncreatinine chromagens. Creatinine, the breakdown product of creatine in muscle, appears in the urine of healthy adults in the range of 15 to 20 mg/kg/day in women and 20 to 25 mg/kg/day in men. Normal serum values for males are up to 1.4 to 1.5 mg/dl and for females up to 1.1 to 1.2 mg/dl. The coefficient of variation is approximately 10%, leading to potential interlaboratory differences of as much as 1 to 1.5 mg/dl in the abnormal range. Significant levels of acetone, ascorbic acid, acetoacetate, and some cephalosporins (e.g., cefoxitin) can falsely elevate the serum creatinine value. True creatinine can be measured by newer automated enzymatic slide-based techniques; using these methods, the upper limit of the normal serum creatinine level is approximately 1.1 to 1.2 mg/dl.

Unfortunately, creatinine is not handled by the kidneys in a fashion identical to inulin. First, a small degree of extrarenal (gastrointestinal) clearance occurs. Second and more important, a variable degree of tubular secretion occurs, ranging from 5% in normal persons to 50% in patients with near end-stage renal disease. Third, several careful clinical studies have shown that the serum creatinine level may not rise above the normal range until more than a 50% reduction in GFR has occurred. In patients with established renal failure, changes in serum creatinine values do parallel changes in inulin clearance, especially in the range of 1.5 to 4.0 mg/dl. Clinicians accordingly must use age, gender, weight, muscle mass, catabolic state, and so forth to interpret the serum creatinine concentration most accurately. Using this information, clinicians caring for our patient Frank could roughly estimate his overall renal function to be definitely less than 50% of normal 4 years before the present admission (serum creatinine value then was 2.5 mg/dl); that GFR had fallen to less than 15% to 20% of normal when his serum creatinine level was 6.0 mg/dl 1 year before admission; and that the serum creatinine level of 12 mg/dl reflected a GFR of approximately 5% to 10% of normal. If greater precision is required, an iothalamate test of GFR can be carried out.

Second, is there a reversible component to this patient's present level of renal impairment? The answer in Frank's case, unfortunately, was no, and hemodialysis was instituted soon after admission. Common, potentially reversible factors causing worsening of renal function include sodium and water depletion, urinary tract obstruction, severe urinary tract infection, congestive heart failure, hypercalcemia, severe or malignant hypertension, and drug-induced renal dysfunction (Table 1–1). To have significant sodium and water depletion cause worsening of renal function, the history should include excess fluid loss (e.g., nausea with vomiting; diarrhea; or pancreatitis with loss of extracellular fluid into the peritoneum). In addition, the patient usually has a greater than 20 mm Hg decline in blood pressure and greater than 20 beats per minute rise in pulse on standing. Urinary tract obstruction (usually benign prostatic hypertrophy in men and pelvic cancers in women; rarely retroperitoneal fibrosis) usually can be readily diagnosed or eliminated from consideration. The bladder should be carefully palpated and rectal/pelvic examination carried out routinely. If bladder outlet obstruction is suspected in a man, a bladder catheter should be inserted *after* the patient has attempted to void. Renal sonogram virtually always detects obstruction; the one rare exception is patients with a solitary kidney, in whom acute *total* obstruction has resulted in an acute decline in GFR to zero, thereby resulting in no increase in intraureteral pressure and thus no hydronephrosis. Urinary tract infection causes worsening of renal function only when severe and bilateral; this diagnosis is made on clinical grounds and by finding pyuria and WBC casts in the urinary sediment. Congestive heart failure results in impaired renal perfusion in most patients. In patients with preexisting normal renal function, the development of severe congestive heart failure is likely to result in a rise of serum creatinine to a level no higher than 2 to 2.5 mg/dl. Patients who have congestive heart failure and who present with a serum creatinine level of 4 to 5 mg/dl thus clearly have underlying renal disease as well as an element of renal dysfunction due to the superimposed congestive heart failure itself. Treatment of the congestive heart failure in conventional fashion by salt and water restriction, digoxin, diuretics, and angiotensin-converting en-

zyme (ACE) inhibitors usually results in restoration of the preexisting level of renal function. Obviously, if the patient has had excessive diuresis, the resulting salt and water depletion could cause a decline in renal function after an initial improvement. In complex situations, particularly in patients with diastolic dysfunction, the use of a Swan-Ganz catheter to measure pulmonary capillary wedge pressure is required. Hypercalcemia causes renal dysfunction because of renal vasoconstriction and a direct toxic effect on the renal tubules as well as salt and water depletion. Drug-induced renal dysfunction in hospitalized patients usually is related to aminoglycosides, contrast media, or nonsteroidal antiinflammatory agents. In outpatients with a decline in renal function, *all* medications should be reviewed while seeking the possibility of drug-induced allergic interstitial nephritis or a reduction in renal perfusion (e.g., as in some patients with bilateral renal artery stenosis and in patients with severe congestive heart failure when both types of patients are treated with ACE inhibitors). Only after thorough review of these issues should the clinician conclude that there is no reversible component to the patient's renal dysfunction.

PATIENT NUMBER 2 (continued)

In our patient Frank, as noted, hemodialysis was begun the day he was transferred. No reversible component of renal failure was identified. To Frank's question "Will I get better?" I responded that he would but that his kidneys would not, but his luck changed soon thereafter. Three of his four siblings were found to be HLA identical to him, and all were ready, willing, and able to give him a kidney. Five years later, Frank is fine, as is his brother who donated the kidney.

Proteinuria

TABLE 1–1. Reversible Causes of Acute Renal Failure

Sodium and water depletion
Urinary tract obstruction
Urinary tract infection (severe)
Congestive heart failure
Hypercalcemia
Malignant hypertension
Drug-induced renal dysfunction

PATIENT NUMBER 3

Gary, a 25-year-old man, was admitted to the hospital for evaluation of the nephrotic syndrome. He had been in good health until proteinuria was first detected approximately 12 months before admission. Urinary protein excretion remained in the range of 5 to 10 g/day throughout the year, serum albumin concentration varied between 2.0 and 3.1 g/dl, and serum creatinine concentration had been normal on several occasions. Gary had no history of previous renal disease, previous streptococcal infection, genitourinary symptoms, or allergies and was taking no medications.

Physical examination revealed a blood pressure of 124/76 mm Hg and a pulse of 80 without postural changes. The general examination was unremarkable except for 2 to 3 + pitting edema from the knees to the ankles. Laboratory data included normal findings on a complete blood count, a serum creatinine level of 0.9 mg/dl, BUN of 15 mg/dl, normal serum electrolytes, a total protein value of 5.7 g/dl, a serum albumin level of 2.6 g/dl, and serum cholesterol value of 350 mg/dl. Urinalysis revealed a specific gravity of 1.020, pH of 5.5, 3 + proteinuria by dipstick, 5 to 10 WBCs/hpf, and 2 to 3 RBCs/hpf; 24-hour urine protein excretion was 5.5 g. Renal sonogram revealed kidneys of normal size with no evidence of obstruction. Results of serologic testing including ANA, rheumatoid factor, complement, and antineutrophilic cytoplasmic antibody were unremarkable. Renal biopsy revealed membranous glomerulopathy. Diffuse thickening of peripheral capillary walls and mild mesangial hypercellularity were identified. A typical spike pattern of the glomerular capillary wall was noted in silver methenamine preparations. Immunofluorescent findings revealed a 3 + IgG coarse granular pattern with less intense staining for complement and IgM. Electron microscopy disclosed diffuse subepithelial electrodense deposits and foot process fusion. No mesangial or subendothelial deposits were found.

Our patient Gary obviously has the nephrotic syndrome, defined as proteinuria greater than 3.5 to 5 g/day, hypoalbuminemia, edema, and a variable degree of hypercholesterolemia. Proteinuria can present either in the nephrotic range, as in this patient, or as asymptomatic proteinuria.

The critical questions in patients with proteinuria are

1. **Is the proteinuria albuminuria or globulinuria?**
2. **What is the quantitative magnitude of the proteinuria?**
3. **Is a kidney biopsy required for diagnosis and optimal management of the patient?**

First, is the proteinuria albuminuria or globulinuria? The standard qualitative tests for proteinuria usually use dipstick technology. Reagent strips (impregnated with the indicator tetrobromphenol blue) change color with increasing protein concentrations at a stable pH; citrate buffer fixes the pH of the tetrobromphenol blue indicator near 3.0. Protein concentrations from approximately 20 to more than 500 mg/dl can be determined. Highly buffered alkaline urine, gross hematuria, or medications such as phenazopyridine can cause false-positive results. Low-molecular-weight proteins such as immunoglobulin light chains, present in the urine of some patients with multiple myeloma, often are not detected by this method. Older testing methods, such as use of sulfosalicylic acid, are no longer widely used and have no practical advantage over reagent strips. The only clinical clue to the presence of globulinuria frequently is the finding of 4 + proteinuria with a normal serum albumin level, suggesting that the protein being lost in the urine is not albumin but globulin. Urinary immunoelectrophoresis ultimately is required to make a definitive diagnosis of globulinuria. Globulinuria should be suspected in patients with a normal serum albumin level and proteinuria, as just noted, and in patients with suspected multiple myeloma or Waldenstrom's macroglobulinemia.

Second, what is the quantitative magnitude of the proteinuria? In our patient Gary, we are given the answer, and it was 5.5 g/day—that is, he has nephrotic-range proteinuria. Normal urine protein excretion is less than 100 to 150 mg/day. Filtered serum proteins account for 60% of the normal urinary protein excretion, and 40% is composed of albumin (<30 mg/day, or 20 μg/min). The remaining 40% of the daily normal urinary protein excretion is composed for the most part of Tamm-Horsfall protein secreted by the thick ascending limb of Henle's loop. Small amounts of urokinase and secretory IgA also are found in normal urine. Upright posture, fever, and exercise all can cause a transient rise in filtration of serum proteins. Because urine volume varies widely in response to wide variations in water intake, the concentration of protein in a single random urine specimen has no precise relationship to the 24-hour urine protein excretion. Thus, some standardization is required, and during the past 30 years or so, the 24-hour urine protein excretion value has been used as the gold standard. Standard laboratory assays for quantitative proteinuria testing have an interassay variability of 10% even with the Coomassie blue dye binding method, one of the more precise techniques available. The major problem with the measurement of 24-hour urine protein excretion is that patients often bring in an incomplete collection. Measurement of urinary creatinine value can help to identify this problem. Daily creatinine excretion is approximately 1000 to 2000 mg for men (20 to 25 mg/kg/day) and 750 to 1500 (15 to 20 mg/kg/day) for women. Because of the progressive loss in muscle mass with aging, creatinine production progressively declines, and thus 24-hour creatinine excretion also declines (up to 40% to 50% by 80 years of age). This phenomenon underlies the stability of serum creatinine levels between ages 50 and 90 or more despite the progressive decline in GFR.

Multiple studies in various clinical circumstances during the past decade have demonstrated a close correlation between the 24-hour urine protein excretion and the urine protein-to-creatinine ratio in random urine specimens. The normal ratio is near 0.1 (100 to 150 mg of protein per 24 hours and 1000 to 1500 mg of creatinine per 24 hours). A urine protein-to-creatinine ratio of 1.0 correlates well with quantitative proteinuria of approximately 1 g/24 hr, a ratio of 2.0 with 2g/24 hr, a ratio of 3 with 3 g/24 hr, and so on (Fig. 1–5). Given this strong correlation, this test provides a physician with information sufficient to classify proteinuria as mild (<1 g/day), moderate (1 to 3 g/day), or heavy (i.e., nephrotic, >3.5 to 5 g/day).

Third, is a kidney biopsy necessary for diagnosis and optimal management? Obviously, a precise histopathologic diagnosis cannot be made in the absence of a kidney biopsy. The real question centers around management. In patient Gary, who clearly was in end-stage renal failure with a serum creatinine level of 12 mg/dl,

there was no indication for biopsy. **In patients with normal blood pressure, normal renal function, and no hematuria and in whom 24-hour urine protein excretion is less than 2 g, information obtained from the renal biopsy is unlikely to alter the treatment of the patient, and thus biopsy usually is not indicated.** In patients with the nephrotic syndrome, such as Gary, the usual practice is to perform a kidney biopsy and base treatment on the results of that biopsy, although not all nephrologists agree with this approach.

Kidney biopsy is sometimes contraindicated. Before biopsy is carried out, the clinician caring for the patient must be sure that the patient is able to comply with the instructions necessary during the biopsy procedure, that there is no bleeding diathesis, that two functioning kidneys are present, and that the kidneys are not very small (6 to 8 cm). Other contraindications such as severe hypertension, renal abscesses, multiple cysts, and a potential renal tumor often preclude percutaneous biopsy. Complications using either the disposable Tru-Cut needle or an automated biopsy instrument are quite uncommon. Hematuria is the most common complication of percutaneous biopsy, usually resolving within a few days; however, in approximately 0.5% of patients, hematuria can persist for as long as 2 to 3 weeks. Transfusions are required in less than 1% of patients, and surgery for massive bleeding in only

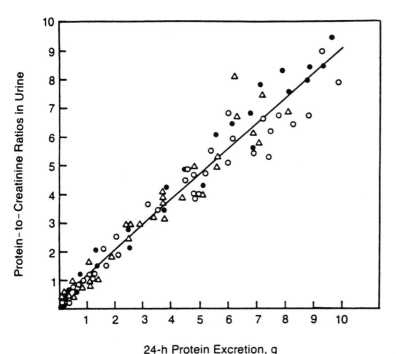

Figure 1–5. Relation between urine protein-to-creatinine ratio (vertical axis) and 24-hour urine protein excretion (horizontal axis) in random, single-voided specimens. (From Schwab SJ, Christensen RL, Daugherty RN, et al: Arch Intern Med 147:943–947. Copyright 1987, American Medical Association.)

0.1% to 0.2% of patients. If a renal sonogram or renal computed tomography scan is carried out 1 day after the biopsy procedure, perinephric hematomas can be detected in 50% to 80% of patients. Most of them are clinically silent, however, and rarely require any treatment. Arteriovenous fistulas also are common and have been claimed to be present in as many as 10% to 20% of patients if arteriography is routinely carried out shortly after the procedure. Virtually all of these fistulas resolve spontaneously over 2 years, and surgical treatment rarely is required. The risk of nephrectomy is between 1 in 2000 and 1 in 5000 after renal biopsy; the risk of surgery to repair a laceration due to biopsy is approximately 1 in 500 to 1 in 1000.

In patients with asymptomatic proteinuria, although renal biopsy may identify a specific morphologic type of glomerular disease, management usually is not altered because no well-defined treatment for glomerular diseases with less than nephrotic-range proteinuria exists. In patients with heavy proteinuria or nephrotic syndrome, renal biopsy aids in distinguishing between primary (or "idiopathic") nephrotic syndrome and a systemic disease affecting the kidneys while simultaneously resulting in nephrotic syndrome.

Approximately 80% of patients with primary nephrotic syndrome are found to have one of four well-described primary renal diseases: membranous nephropathy (as in our patient Gary), minimal change disease, focal and segmental glomerulosclerosis, or membranoproliferative glomerulonephritis; in as many as 20% of cases, diseases other than these four primary renal diseases are found. **In essence, the decision for biopsy in patients with idiopathic nephrotic syndrome rests between therapy based on the biopsy findings and empiric treatment with high-dose, alternate-day steroids.** The information obtained from the biopsy, even if it does not directly affect therapy, might be beneficial in overall treatment of the patient. The histologic severity of disease can be judged and information obtained that might be useful, should transplantation be required and if the question of the possibility of recurrent disease in a transplanted kidney is raised. Finally, in a small percentage of patients with apparent primary renal disease, evidence of a systemic disease (e.g., subendothelial deposits in patients with systemic lupus erythematosus) may be found, thus changing the overall management of the patient.

PATIENT NUMBER 3 (continued)

Interestingly, Gary was most concerned about the need for dialysis or transplantation, despite his normal kidney function. He said that all he read in the papers about patients with kidney disease centered around those two topics. He was reassured, and later after treatment with prednisone, he underwent a complete remission. His fatigue, more bothersome to him than his edema, disappeared when his serum albumin rose to >3.0 g/dl.

Hematuria

PATIENT NUMBER 4

Wally, a 23-year-old man, was referred because of recurrent episodes of gross hematuria occurring simultaneously or within 1 to 2 days after an upper respiratory tract infection. Several urinalyses during the past 3 to 4 years had revealed microscopic hematuria without proteinuria. When seen because of gross hematuria, he also complained of a severe sore throat. No genitourinary symptoms other than the hematuria were present. Physical examination revealed a temperature of 39°C and a blood pressure of 120/80 mm Hg. The general examination was unremarkable, except for severe pharyngitis. Laboratory data included a BUN of 15 mg/dl, serum creatinine value of 1.1 mg/dl, normal blood sugar level, normal serum electrolyte values, urine specific gravity of 1.020, urine pH of 5, and urine findings of 4+ blood and 1+ protein. Microscopic examination of the urinary sediment revealed RBCs too numerous to count; careful examination revealed 3 to 4 RBC casts per coverslip. Urine culture results were negative, as were results of a renal sonogram. A renal biopsy was carried out and is discussed later.

The single critical question in a patient with either microscopic or gross hematuria is, is the urinary bleeding secondary to glomerular disease, stones, infection, or a malignancy? (One should also realize that hypercalciuria can be associated with hematuria, especially in children and adolescents, but also in adults). Although stones, urinary tract infections, and malignancy (of the kidney, ureter, or bladder) obviously far outweigh the likelihood of glomerular disease, glomerular disease must be considered. This question is answered by an analysis of the clinical presentation, by careful review of renal imaging studies, and most importantly by examination of the urine sediment.

> In elderly individuals with sudden onset of painless hematuria, statistically the more likely diagnosis is either bladder cell cancer or renal cell carcinoma. On the other hand, in younger patients with repeated bouts of gross hematuria in conjunction with repeated upper respiratory tract infections, the likely diagnosis is IgA nephropathy, the single most common glomerular disease worldwide.

Unfortunately, too often a full battery of renal imaging testing including renal sonography, intravenous pyelography, computed tomography scanning, and cystoscopy (with or without retrograde pyelography) is carried out in all patients with hematuria before a simple examination of the urine sediment is performed. Patients in whom dysmorphic RBCs and particularly RBC casts are found require no such tests. Instead, one needs to discuss just as with patients with proteinuria, whether or not a renal biopsy is required.

PATIENT NUMBER 4 (continued)

Renal biopsy was carried out in Wally and revealed IgA nephropathy, as predicted by the clinicians caring for the patient before obtaining the biopsy.

Does a renal biopsy need to be performed on all such patients? Just as in patients with proteinuria, nephrologists argue strenuously over this issue. If management will not be altered by the results of the biopsy, obviously no biopsy is indicated. Some nephrologists use this argument for conservative management, and this is my own practice in patients who have hematuria and RBC casts and no evidence of systemic disease, little or no proteinuria, normal blood pressure, and a normal, stable serum creatinine level. On the other hand, if kidney function deteriorates, as measured by a rise in serum creatinine concentration, for example, renal biopsy is indicated. Biopsy was carried out in our patient Wally to arrive at a specific diagnosis to reassure him that he had no malignancy, his major worry.

SELECTED READINGS

Bauer JH, Brooks CS, Burch RN: Clinical appraisal of creatinine clearance as a measure of glomerular filtration rate. Am J Kidney Dis 3:337–346, 1982.

Cockcroft DW, Gault MH: Prediction of creatinine clearance from serum creatinine. Nephron 16:31–41, 1976.

Haber MH, Corwin HL (eds): Urinalysis. Clin Lab Med 8:415–621, 1988.

Levey AS: Nephrology forum. Measurement of renal function in chronic renal disease. Kidney Int 38:167–184, 1990.

Madaio MP: Nephrology forum. Renal biopsy. Kidney Int 38:529–543, 1990.

Parrish AE: Complications of percutaneous renal biopsy: A review of 37 years experience. Clin Nephrol 38:135–141, 1992.

Rolin HA, Hall PM: Evaluation of glomerular filtration rate and renal plasma flow. *In* Jacobson HR, Striker GE, Klahr S (eds): The Principles and Practice of Nephrology, 2nd ed. St. Louis, CV Mosby, 1995.

Schwab SJ, Christensen RL, Daugherty RN, et al: Quantitation of proteinuria by use of protein-to-creatinine ratios in single urine samples. Arch Intern Med 147:943–944, 1987.

Sox HC Jr (ed): Common Diagnostic Tests: Use and Interpretation, 2nd ed. Philadelphia, American College of Physicians, 1990.

Tomita M, Kitamoto Y, Nakayama M, et al: A new morphologic classification of erythrocytes for differential diagnosis of glomerular hematuria. Clin Nephrol 37:84–89, 1992.

2 | HEMATURIA, PROTEINURIA, AND NEPHROTIC SYNDROME

Cecil H. Coggins

DETECTION OF HEMATURIA OR PROTEINURIA

Hematuria or proteinuria is generally detected through urinalysis. The dipsticks most frequently used for this purpose detect blood by a pseudo-peroxidase reaction. A positive reaction reflects the presence of the heme structure and does not differentiate clearly among RBCs, free hemoglobin, and myoglobin. Examination of the urine sediment detects the presence of abnormal numbers of RBCs. Variability in a patient's urine flow rate, the volume centrifuged, the time and speed of the centrifugation, the volume used to suspend the sediment, and the magnification of the microscope objective and eyepiece make the measurement imprecise, but the presence of more than 3 to 4 RBCs per high-power field (hpf) is considered abnormal.

The proteinuria test square on the dipstick contains a pH color indicator dye buffered by citric acid at pH 3.5. Albumin influences the dye to show a color, falsely indicating a higher pH, which can be read as 1+, 2+, or 3+ proteinuria. Errors are possible in this measurement. Globulins and light chains have a much weaker effect in changing the indicator color and may not be detected by dipstick measurement.

Prolonged immersion of the dipstick in the urine sample or its use in strongly alkaline urine might overcome the buffering ability of the citric acid. An alkaline color would register on the dipstick and be erroneously interpreted as proteinuria. The dipstick should be dipped just long enough to wet it thoroughly.

Hematuria

PATIENT NUMBER 1

Barney, a 32-year-old orthopedist, had been a track athlete in high school but did not run seriously in college or medical school. Now having just started practice and after 3 months of running, he unofficially entered the Boston marathon. He is unusually muscular for a distance runner and finishes well back in the pack. The day is rather warm. He comes to the aid station reporting that he has just passed dark red urine. You are the aid station physician. How will you investigate his problem?

Gross and Microscopic Hematuria

Gross hematuria may appear pink, red, or the color of tea or cola. A few drops of blood color a liter of urine distinctly red, and hematuria ordinarily does not represent serious blood loss. With smaller quantities of RBCs, the urine looks normal grossly, and only microscopic hematuria is present. Urine may also occasionally appear reddish from precipitated urate crystals, from the ingestion of beets, from porphyria, or from certain drug metabolites. The urinalysis dipstick registers positive for blood, hemoglobin, or myoglobin.

Approach to the Patient

When the dipstick examination is positive for blood, it is first necessary to differentiate among hematuria, hemoglobinuria, and myoglobinuria. The presence of large numbers of RBCs in the urine sediment establishes the diagnosis of hematuria. If only small numbers are present or if the dipstick is more strongly positive than would be expected from the number of RBCs per high-power field, then the possibility of hemoglobinuria or myoglobinuria should be considered.

Hemoglobinuria

Free hemoglobin results from rupture or leakage of RBCs. This may happen in the urinary tract when bleeding occurs into very dilute urine and the cells rupture osmotically. The hemolysis may occur intravascularly from trauma (e.g., aortic valve replacement), immunologic factors, or other causes. A low serum haptoglobin level and the presence of free serum hemoglobin aid in the diagnosis of hemolysis. Although the intact hemoglobin tetramer is too large to be easily filtered at the glomeruli, the dimer and monomer components are filtered and reassembled in the urine.

Myoglobinuria

Myoglobin is released into the blood after muscle damage. Comparable in size to the hemoglobin monomer, myoglobin is quickly filtered and is not found circulating in the blood, even with massive rhabdomyolysis. Serum elevations of muscle enzymes such as creatine phosphokinase and aldolase serve as clues to the diagnosis. Differentiating myoglobin from hemoglobin in the urine is difficult but can be done by radioimmunoassay or enzyme-linked immunoassay.

Glomerular Versus Nonglomerular Hematuria

When the presence of RBCs in the urine has been established, it is extremely useful to distinguish glomerular from nonglomerular sources. If the origin can confidently be assigned to the glomeruli or to a location high in the renal tubules, lower tract workup (e.g., cystoscopy, intravenous urogram, computed tomography [CT] scans, ultrasonography studies, arteriography) need not be performed. Four clues help in this determination. A physician must look at the urine sediment and be skillful in its interpretation. Laboratory technicians are generally unable to give to a single specimen the time and attention necessary to search for RBC casts (Table 2–1).

Red Blood Cell Casts. The presence of RBCs in casts formed in the renal tubules establishes a glomerular or proximal tubular source. The significance of the finding is so great that the observer must be absolutely sure that (1) the structure seen is a cast, not a clump or streak of mucus and (2) that the RBCs are within the cast and not simply stuck on its surface. Although not as specific as RBC casts, epithelial cell or WBC casts or numerous granular casts would suggest renal disease and a probable renal source for the RBCs.

Dysmorphic Red Blood Cells. When hematuria results from glomerular disease, a large fraction of the cells in the urine are smaller than circulating RBCs and have visible defects in their membranes, often with irregular protrusions. These are visible under high power by light microscopy but are more clearly evident by phase-contrast microscopy. The passage of such cells through the glomerular membrane and through the changes in osmolarity, pH, and enzymatic environment in different portions of the nephron apparently produces these effects, which are not seen when the bleeding source is the prostate, bladder, ureter, or renal pelvis.

Accompanying Proteinuria. If a dipstick shows more than trace or 1+ proteinuria, renal disease is probably present and is the source of the hematuria.

Three-Glass Test (particularly for males). Three urine collection containers are labeled "1," "2," and "3." A patient is asked to collect during a single continuous voiding the first few milliliters

TABLE 2–1. Investigating Hematuria Flow Sheet

If positive "blood" on urinalysis dipstick test, then centrifuge with examination of sediment by physician.
If numerous RBCs appear in the sediment, then hematuria is present. Check for RBC casts, other cellular casts, dysmorphic RBCs, and accompanying proteinuria. Consider performing the three-glass test.
If cells are of renal origin, check glomerular diseases in the following section. Although less likely, interstitial diseases (Table 2–4) are also possible causes.
If cells are of lower urinary tract origin, check for infection, stone, tumor.
If few or no RBCs are present in the sediment, then consider hemoglobinuria, myoglobinuria, or the hemolysis of RBCs in dilute urine (look for RBC ghosts). Differentiate hemoglobinuria from myoglobinuria by history, physical examination, serum creatine phosphokinase, aldolase, haptoglobin, and free hemoglobin, or request urine radioimmunoassay for myoglobin.

in container 1, then the bulk in 2, and the last few milliliters in 3. If the concentration of RBCs in glass 1 or 3 is considerably higher than in 2, a bleeding source in the urethra or prostate is suspected.

NONGLOMERULAR HEMATURIA

If the careful urinalysis just described suggests a nonglomerular source of the RBCs, the causes listed in Table 2–2 should be considered.

Approach to the Patient. Obtain a urine culture. If history and physical examination do not strongly suggest the cause, obtain renal imaging. Although ultrasonography and abdominal CT can be helpful, in patients with normal renal function an intravenous urogram is likely to give more useful information about structure *and* function. Urologic consultation may be required for further diagnosis and therapy. A careful search for malignancies is particularly important for patients older than 50 years.

Massive Hematuria. Massive hematuria occasionally produces anemia or shock due to blood loss. The urine registers significant hemoglobin or hematocrit levels and usually contains clots. The cause is found in the lower tract (often tumor) or in a vascular malformation in the kidney. An immediate urologic consultation is usually indicated. Patients sometimes have recurrent massive bleeding that stops suddenly before the source can be found. In such cases, prearranging for immediate renal arteriography to be done at the time of the next bleeding episode is wise.

GLOMERULAR HEMATURIA

With Accompanying Proteinuria. If proteinuria accompanies the hematuria, the diseases listed in Table 2–5 should be considered; investigation and treatment are discussed in the section on proteinuria.

TABLE 2–2. Sources of Nonglomerular Hematuria

Infection: cystitis, pyelonephritis (including tuberculosis), urethritis, prostatitis. Pyuria is usually present.
Tumor: of bladder, ureter, renal pelvis, prostate, or kidney.
Stone: of kidney or bladder.
Kidney disease: polycystic kidney or sickle cell nephropathy.
Trauma to kidney or bladder.
Loin pain, hematuria syndrome.
Bleeding diathesis; disease or iatrogenic. Note that anticoagulation may provoke bleeding from an organic lesion in the urinary tract.
Vascular malformation/arteriovenous aneurysm of kidney or collecting system.

With Little or No Proteinuria. The following types of glomerular disease should be considered:

IgA nephropathy (Berger's disease)
Hereditary nephritis (including Alport's disease, with associated nerve deafness and cataract formation)
Thin basement membrane syndrome
Poststreptococcal or other postinfectious glomerulonephritis
Systemic vasculitis, infection, or connective tissue disease such as lupus, Henoch-Schönlein purpura, bacterial endocarditis, hepatitis B

These diseases can also present in more severe forms with substantial proteinuria.

Approach to the Patient. A carefully taken history should include inquiries about streptococcal or other infection and family history of hematuria, renal disease, cataracts, or deafness. Physical examination should devote particular attention to the eyes and ears, nails, patellae, rashes, and spots. Laboratory studies might include, as appropriate, antinuclear antibody, anti-DNase B, hepatitis B surface antigen, blood culture, complement, circulating immune complexes, and antineutrophil cytoplasmic antibodies.

Management. In general, when both hematuria and proteinuria are present, the prognosis of the glomerular disease correlates most closely with the quantity of proteinuria. Thus, patients with normal serum creatinine levels and with hematuria and 0, trace, or 1+ proteinuria (corresponding to <1 g/day), no matter which underlying pathology is present, tend to remain stable for long periods. No specific therapy is generally recommended for this group.

Periodic urinalysis for hematuria and proteinuria, blood pressure assessment, and serum creatinine determinations provide warning of advancing disease. (Note that minimal change nephrotic syndrome may have a favorable prognosis despite large quantities of proteinuria. It rarely has much hematuria, however.)

Despite careful examination, a significant fraction of cases of hematuria remain unexplained.

PATIENT NUMBER 1 (continued)

As you examine Barney, you consider myoglobinuria from anterior tibial compartment ischemia or rhabdomyolysis from heat stroke; hemoglobinuria from traumatic hemolysis of RBCs in the feet; and hematuria from the anterior and posterior bladder walls' rubbing against each other during the run, among other causes. Investigation discloses no fever, positive dipstick for blood, no RBCs in the sediment, normal serum muscle enzymes, and abnormally low levels of serum haptoglobin. You diagnose hemolysis and prescribe running shoes with more generous metatarsal and heel padding.

At a follow-up appointment, Barney has cut down his mileage and is using new, well-padded shoes. The hematuria has subsided, and he is delighted with the "orthopedic approach" to curing his hematuria.

PROTEINURIA AND THE NEPHROTIC SYNDROME

PATIENT NUMBER 2

Helen is a 65-year-old hairdresser who returns before her regularly scheduled visit, describing 2 months of fatigue and discomfort in her shoulders and arms when cutting or washing hair. She reports that both ankles swell at the end of the day in the beauty salon and is proud that she has finally managed to lose 22 lb (10 kg) of weight. On examination, Helen is pale, with 2 + bilateral ankle and foot edema. Her urinalysis dipstick result is strongly positive for protein. How will you proceed?

When proteinuria is detected on dipstick urinalysis (see the earlier section on urinalysis), it is wise to check the finding with a heat and acetic acid test or a sulfosalicylic acid test for protein. These tests are better in estimating quantities of proteinuria and detect Bence Jones protein more accurately. The sulfosalicylic acid test may give false-positive results with metabolites of the penicillins, aspirin, oral hypoglycemia agents, or other drugs.

Glomerular Proteinuria

Glomerular proteinuria occurs when glomerular capillary walls are damaged and become permeable to serum proteins. In some types of glomerulonephritis, the membrane disruption allows albumin, serum globulins, and even RBCs to pass into the urine. In others, a more limited and specific loss of fixed negative electrical charges on membrane surfaces allows a more selective loss of negatively charged albumin molecules. (When proteinuria consists almost exclusively of albumin, it is called *highly selective* and is particularly characteristic of minimal change nephropathy.)

Nephrotic Syndrome

Nephrotic syndrome (or nephrosis) is a term used to describe clinical situations in which large amounts of albumin are lost. The loss of albumin leads to hypoalbuminemia, which is followed by edema, hyperlipidemia, and lipiduria. The combination of these elements constitutes nephrotic syndrome. The presence of the entire syndrome probably has no more diagnostic specificity than that of massive albuminuria itself. Proteinuria (predominantly albumin) of >3 or 3.5 g/day (or 2 g/day/m^2) suffices for the diagnosis.

Tubular Proteinuria

Tubular proteinuria describes a pattern frequently found in tubular and interstitial renal disease. Many small proteins and peptides circulating in the blood are filtered by normal glomeruli. β_2-Microglobulin and amylase are two examples. These proteins are not normally found in urine because they are actively reabsorbed during their passage through the nephron. With tubular disease, they escape reabsorption and appear in the urine as one component of tubular proteinuria. A second component consists of brush border and cellular enzymes and other cellular proteins released from damaged renal tubular cells. A third component is the very high-molecular-weight Tamm-Horsfall protein. This polymer is secreted by cells of the ascending limb of Henle's loop and distal nephron and forms the matrix of most urinary casts. It appears to be secreted in larger quantities in renal disease. Thus, tubular proteinuria is a mix of heterogeneous large and small proteins and does not consist predominantly of albumin. Tubular proteinuria is most frequently found in the range of 0.5 to 1.5 g/day, although it may occasionally reach 2 g. When 3 g/day or more protein is found, the type almost certainly is albumin from glomerular disease (nephrotic) or monoclonal Bence Jones proteinuria.

Monoclonal Overflow Proteinuria

In monoclonal overflow proteinuria, kidneys may be normal, but an abnormal small protein circulates in the blood and is filtered by the glomeruli in quantities exceeding the tubules' capacity for reabsorption. This occurs when myeloma or other hematologic malignancies produce monoclonal globulin fragments. These usually consist of light chains and in the urine are called *Bence Jones proteins*. As noted earlier, they may not be sensitively detected by dipstick urinalysis. Heat and acetic or sulfosalicylic acid tests are more accurate in their detection. Bence Jones proteinuria may be present in quantities ranging from <1 g to 30 or 40 g or more per day.

Approach to Patients with Proteinuria

The objective of the initial evaluation of a proteinuric patient is to identify the quantity, the type, and the reproducibility of the proteinuria.

Quantity of Proteinuria. The quantity of proteinuria can most directly be determined by collecting all the urine produced during a 24-hour period. Provide patients with a suitable bottle (at least 2 L). A preservative such as a cup of vinegar may be used if refrigeration is not possible. Pick a time, such as on arising in the morning, to begin the collection period.

At that time, patients should empty the bladder and *discard* the urine. All urine output during the next 24 hours should be added to the bottle, and the next morning, at precisely the same time, patients should again empty their bladder, adding the urine to the collection. Starting and finishing times and dates should be recorded on the bottle.

Another method to approximate the quantity of proteinuria is to collect a single voiding specimen (preferably the first morning void) and measure both total protein and creatinine in the sample. Assuming that protein and creatinine are excreted in parallel during the day (not an entirely correct assumption) and that daily creatinine excretion remains relatively constant in an individual (also not entirely correct), the ratio of protein to creatinine is an index of proteinuria that can be monitored to mark changes with treatment or disease progression.

Type of Proteinuria. Proteinuria can most easily be categorized as glomerular, tubular, and monoclonal overflow types by sending urine samples for protein electrophoresis and immunoelectrophoresis. Standard protein electrophoresis (e.g., agarose gel or cellulose acetate) shows a predominant albumin peak or band in glomerular proteinurias, a broad grouping of nonalbumin proteins in tubular disease, and often an M spike demonstrating Bence Jones proteins in myeloma. Immunoelectrophoresis is more sensitive in picking up monoclonal light chains and proteins in serum and urine.

Reproducibility of Proteinuria. Small amounts of proteinuria normally follow severe exertion or accompany high fever without indicating any serious renal abnormality. In those settings, workup might only include repeating the dipstick test on a later occasion. Proteinuria occasionally occurs only in the erect position and disappears completely with recumbency. This *orthostatic proteinuria* has a generally benign prognosis. It is best evaluated with 24-hour urine collection as described earlier but divided into daytime ambulatory and nighttime recumbent portions. The bedtime void completes the daytime collection. Patients then remain recumbent until morning. The morning urine sample (plus any urine that may have been voided during the night) constitutes the nighttime specimen. If the nighttime collection has no more than 50 mg/8 hr (or is completely negative by dipstick test) and the day's sample has more than 150 mg/16 hr (or is positive by the dipstick test), orthostatic proteinuria may be diagnosed. It is important to remember that proteinuria of *any* origin is excreted at higher rates during standing and ambulation, so a *completely* normal nighttime protein level is necessary for this diagnosis. The investigation of proteinuria is summarized in Table 2–3.

Management of Monoclonal Overflow Proteinuria

Management involves the evaluation and treatment of myeloma or occasionally lymphoma and

TABLE 2–3. Investigating Proteinuria Flow Sheet

If urine is Bence Jones positive, consider myeloma or lymphoproliferative disease. If it is negative on Bence Jones testing, then proceed as follows:

  If 24-hour collection contains <3 g/day, check protein electrophoresis.

  If a tubular pattern is noted, consider interstitial disease (see Table 2–4).

  If a glomerular pattern (mostly albumin) is noted, check for orthostatic proteinuria and consider mild forms of nephrotic disease (see Table 2–5).

  If 24-hour collection contains more than 3 g/day and is not Bence Jones (light chains), consider nephrotic diseases (see Table 2–5). Check for infections, offending drugs, glucose, antinuclear antibody; perform other pertinent laboratory studies and consider biopsy.

Be alert for renal vein thrombosis, particularly if symptoms suggest pulmonary emboli or if histology shows membranous nephropathy.

Consider searching for malignancy if the histology is membranous and the patient is elderly and has weight loss or other signs suggesting underlying malignancy.

often begins with bone marrow examination including a search for clones of plasma cells expressing exclusively kappa or lambda immunoglobulins. It should be noted that monoclonal "gammopathies" may be associated with amyloid, a cause of nephrotic syndrome. Thus, large amounts of albuminuria together with evidence of a monoclonal serum or urine protein may suggest renal amyloid.

Management of Tubular Proteinuria

A wide variety of tubular and interstitial renal diseases may demonstrate tubular proteinuria. They may be divided into toxic, congenital, immunologic, infectious, metabolic, and vascular categories (Table 2–4).

Diagnostic workup includes taking a careful history of familial renal disease, polyuria, headaches, backaches, or other chronic pain requiring analgesics, and exposure to any of the drugs or substances listed in Table 2–4. Physical findings might include band keratopathy or Kayser-Fleischer rings, lead line on the gums, enlarged kidneys, or gouty arthritis. Laboratory studies might include determinations of serum calcium, potassium, bicarbonate, phosphate, and uric acid, and hemoglobin electrophoresis. Hypercalcemia may be a cause, and Fanconi's syndrome, renal tubular acidosis, or nephrogenic diabetes insipidus may result from tubulointerstitial nephritis. Blood and urine samples may be evaluated for heavy metals as appropriate, and if lead poisoning is a strong possibility, lead excretion after EDTA injection may help establish the diagnosis.

The urine sediment usually contains increased numbers of WBCs and often tubular epithelial cells as well. Granular and cellular casts (neutrophils or epithelial cells) are frequent. Staining for urinary eosinophils may help in the diagnosis of allergic interstitial nephritis, usually due to drugs such as the penicillins. If a high percentage of numerous WBCs in the sediment are eosinophils, the test has fair diagnostic specificity. If only small absolute numbers of eosinophils are present, it is much less specific.

The urine should be cultured whether or not bacteria are visible in the sediment. If pyuria is marked but routine culture is negative, a culture for mycobacteria should be considered. An acute infection can cause interstitial nephritis, and chronic or repeated infections when combined with reflux, obstruction, diabetes, or sickle cell disease can cause severe renal damage.

TABLE 2–4. Causes of Interstitial Nephritis

Drug Toxicity

Analgesic abuse
Nonsteriodal antiinflammatory drugs
Lithium
Cyclosporine
Cisplatin

Heavy Metal Toxicity

Lead (may present as gouty nephropathy)
Cadmium, uranium, mercury

Hereditary/Developmental

Polycystic kidney disease
Medullary cystic disease
Medullary sponge kidney
Wilson's disease
Cystinosis

Immune Diseases

Drug allergy (penicillins, sulfonamides, rifampin, others) (These are more likely to cause acute interstitial nephritis)
Collagen/vasculitis group (lupus, Sjögren's)
IgA nephropathy
Transplant rejection
Sarcoid

Infection, "Pyelonephritis"

Bacterial infection: especially in a kidney with obstruction, reflux, diabetes mellitus, sickle disease
Tuberculosis, leprosy, viral, fungal, parasitic infection

Metabolic

Hyperuricemia, uricosuria
Hypercalcemia
Oxalosis
Amyloid

Vascular

Diabetes mellitus
Hypertension and nephrosclerosis
Atheroemboli
Sickle cell disease
Radiation nephritis

Obstruction/Reflux, especially if combined with infection

Management of Glomerular Proteinuria (Table 2–5)

If the proteinuria is relatively mild, the first investigations should be done to show whether it is reproducible and whether it is orthostatic, as described earlier. **Transient mild proteinuria is generally of little significance and need not be intensively investigated.** Proteinuria that is truly orthostatic generally also has no symptoms and a favorable prognosis and need not be pursued to the point of kidney biopsy or treatment.

TABLE 2–5. Causes of Nephrotic Syndrome

	Approx. Relative Incidence	
	Adults (%)	*Children (%)*
Primary Glomerular Disease	(75)	(90)
Membranous nephropathy	30	
Minimal change (lipoid) nephrosis	15	80–90
Primary and secondary focal glomerular sclerosis	15	
Membranoproliferative GN, including dense deposit disease	7	
Mesangial proliferative GN, including IgA nephropathy	5	
Rapidly progressive GN	3	
Acute poststreptococcal GN	—	
Systemic Conditions	(25)	
Relatively common		
Diabetes mellitus		
Systemic lupus erythematosus (SLE)		
Amyloid (including multiple myeloma)		
Less common causes		
Other immunologic diseases (in addition to SLE): polyarteritis (small-vessel form), Wegener's, dermatomyositis, scleroderma, Takayasu's disease, Sjögren's disease, Henoch-Schönlein purpura, serum sickness, transplant rejection, sarcoid, mixed cryoglobulinemia		
Associated with malignancy		
Hodgkin's lymphoma (usually minimal change)		
Other tumors (usually membranous)		
Heavy metals, drugs, allergens: gold, mercury, probenecid, penicillamine, angiotensin-converting enzyme inhibitors, "street" heroin, nonsteroidal antiinflammatory drugs		
Infections		
Bacterial endocarditis and shunt infections, acquired immunodeficiency syndrome, malaria, hepatitis, secondary and congenital syphilis, schistosomiasis		
Congenital or familial: including Fabry's, Alport's, nail-patella		
Pregnancy associated		

GN, glomerulonephritis.

Asymptomatic Proteinuria. Mild glomerular proteinuria that is reproducible, not orthostatic, and in the range of 1 to 2 g/day usually occurs without accompanying symptoms, although edema may occasionally occur. Investigation of underlying systemic disease is appropriate as described later for nephrotic syndrome. Because the prognosis of asymptomatic proteinuria is often favorable, it is reasonable to monitor patients without biopsy or specific treatment until the proteinuria becomes nephrotic or evidence of deterioration in overall renal function (rise in serum creatinine level) occurs. Nonspecific use of angiotensin-converting enzyme (ACE) inhibitors as described later may reduce the level of proteinuria.

Pathophysiology of Nephrotic Syndrome. Nephrotic levels of proteinuria may occur in many different glomerular diseases, with different histologic appearances (see Table 2–5). They all share, however, an abnormality of the glomer-ular capillary wall, allowing increased passage of plasma proteins.

The urinary loss of protein together with increased rates of catabolism of albumin in the body (including the renal tubular reabsorption and degradation of filtered protein) leads to hypoproteinemia. Renal retention of salt and water leading to edema is caused in some nephrotic patients by the hypoproteinemia and reduced plasma volume. In others, the plasma volume is normal and the glomerular change appears to lead directly to fluid retention.

Hyperlipidemia results largely from overproduction of apolipoproteins by the liver. This synthesis, like that of albumin, appears to be stimulated by reductions in plasma oncotic pressure. Lipiduria follows from the hyperlipidemia and increased glomerular permeability.

Nephrotic patients have varying degrees of hypoalbuminemia and lipid abnormalities, not always proportional to the amount of proteinuria. These differences no doubt reflect differences in nutrition, in the hepatic capacity to synthesize albumin and apolipoproteins, and in genetic predisposition.

General Management of Patients with Nephrotic Syndrome

Edema and Hypoproteinemia

Management of edema is considered in detail in Chapter 11. Nephrotic patients with hypoalbuminemia treated with diuretics generally have contracted plasma volumes. Further attempts to reduce edema with powerful diuretics or diuretic combinations may reduce plasma volume to the point of circulatory impairment, prerenal azotemia, and intractable diuretic resistance. Temporary use of albumin infusions may be considered to reestablish the circulation in such cases. Although albumin administration is fruitless in the long run because of its short life in the circulation of nephrotic patients, it may help in alleviating anasarca (especially in patients without really massive proteinuria). Infusing perhaps 50 g of albumin followed by a large dose of a diuretic combination each day for 2 or 3 days may temporarily provide relief for patients in whom edema and ascites are truly threatening.

The use of ACE inhibitor drugs, especially when combined with diuretics, often reduces the level of proteinuria, sometimes dramatically. Although this effect is no doubt related to reduction of intraglomerular blood pressure and flow, it takes 4 to 6 weeks to develop fully and so probably involves a structural change in the glomerular capillary walls. The physician should start cautiously and be alert for hyperkalemia and rise in serum creatinine level. A diuretic can help prevent excessive K+ rise, and a small rise in serum creatinine level may be acceptable, indicating that the desired glomerular hemodynamic change had in fact occurred. Similar reduction in proteinuria has been described with the use of nonsteroidal antiinflammatory drugs (NSAIDs) such as indomethacin or meclofenamate combined with diuretic. The effect of this NSAID combination, if it occurs, should be evident within a week. These attempts can be monitored by serial measurements of protein-to-creatinine ratio on spot urine samples (best all obtained at the same time of day).

It is important that nephrotic patients have adequate dietary protein to allow for hepatic synthesis of albumin. Raising protein intake above normal, however, seems only to increase the proteinuria without raising serum albumin levels, whereas lowering protein intake reduces protein and may even *raise* serum albumin levels. Protein intakes of 0.8 g of lean body weight supplemented 1 g for each gram of proteinuria would seem appropriate. Proteins of high biologic value should be emphasized. A management summary is provided in Table 2–6.

Hyperlipidemia

When the nephrotic syndrome is responsive to therapy and lasts only a few weeks or months, treatment of hyperlipidemia is probably not indicated. Even when nephrotic hyperlipidemia is of longer duration, its risk of causing atherogenesis is controversial. It seems likely, however, that sustained extreme elevations of low-density lipoprotein cholesterol such as occur in many nephrotic patients merit attempts at treatment. Clofibrate frequently leads to muscle injury in nephrotic individuals, perhaps because of reduced binding to plasma proteins. Lovastatin is better tolerated but may also have to be used in reduced doses to avoid creatine phosphokinase elevations from skeletal muscle. Lovastatin most frequently is insufficient by itself, and even when combined with a bile acid-binding resin or with gemfibrozil, it accomplishes only moderate lipid reductions.

Treatment of Specific Glomerular Diseases

This chapter provides only a brief outline (see also Chapter 3). Referral to a nephrologist is appropriate.

TABLE 2–6. Summary of Management of Nephrotic Syndrome

1. Treat the underlying glomerular disease if effective specific treatment is available.
2. Prescribe a low-sodium, liberal-potassium, low-saturated-fat diet. The protein content should not be high but about 0.8 g/kg/day, emphasizing high-biologic quality protein. Meals should be small and frequent if ascites is present. If hyponatremia occurs, fluid may be restricted; but if there is a sudden diuresis, more salt and water may be needed.
3. Provide a multivitamin supplement with vitamin D and iron (e.g., prenatal formula).
4. Diuretics should be cautiously administered with or without temporary albumin infusion when hypoalbuminemia is severe. Watch for serious reduction in plasma volume with "prerenal" or acute renal failure.
5. Be alert for thromboses and infection.
6. Try cautious use of angiotensin-converting enzyme inhibitor/diuretic or nonsteroidal antiinflammatory drug/diuretic combinations to reduce proteinuria.
7. Treat hyperlipidemia if it is severe and prolonged.

Minimal Change Disease. Minimal change disease (lipoid nephrosis) responds to 4 to 6 weeks of corticosteroid therapy in at least 80% to 90% of cases. One regimen is to give prednisone, 2 mg/kg/day (maximum 80 mg/day). If no response occurs, stop at 4 weeks. If a patient responds with diuresis and almost complete disappearance of proteinuria by dipstick test, then continue for 2 additional weeks, followed by a slow taper (ideally with alternate-day dosage) for 4 to 6 months. Relapses can be treated the same way or with a more prolonged taper. Cyclophosphamide and chlorambucil can prolong remissions but have considerable toxicity, which may not be justified unless the disease is severe. Cyclosporin can induce remissions that almost invariably relapse with drug taper.

Focal Segmental Glomerular Sclerosis. Focal segmental glomerular sclerosis is less likely to respond than minimal change disease. Responses do occur on occasion, however, particularly in children and especially when therapy with prednisone is combined with cyclophosphamide or chlorambucil. Although treatment is controversial, in patients with fairly severe edema and proteinuria but without marked elevation of serum creatinine levels, a vigorous trial of corticosteroid or combined therapy might be undertaken. If no marked improvement occurs, one would then stop treatment to avoid the toxicity, which is much greater with prolonged therapy. Cyclosporin-induced remissions are less frequent than in minimal change disease and usually relapse when the drug is stopped.

IgA Nephropathy. IgA nephropathy (Berger's disease) has not been convincingly shown to respond to any therapy.

Membranoproliferative Glomerulonephritis. The treatment of membranoproliferative glomerulonephritis (MPGN, mesangiocapillary GN) is controversial, and no present treatment leads to clear-cut total remission. Fish oil therapy has been reported to slow progression, and some patients with type I MPGN benefit from prolonged courses of alternate-day prednisone (40 mg/m² every other day). If serious hypertension results, prolonged daily aspirin and dipyridamole treatment is an alternative.

Membranous Nephropathy. Many patients fare well without treatment. For those with risk factors for progressive disease (very high levels of proteinuria, serum creatinine levels beginning to rise above normal, male gender, resistant hypertension), prednisone therapy may help, par-

ticularly when combined with cyclophosphamide or chlorambucil in a prolonged program.

Role of Renal Biopsy in Management of Nephrotic Syndrome

In childhood nephrotic syndrome, the cause in 90% of cases is minimal change disease, so prednisone treatment is often appropriate without a biopsy-proven diagnosis. In adults, however, various underlying diseases requiring specific treatments occur. It has been argued that a uniform 2-month alternate-day prednisone treatment given to all adult nephrotic patients would be helpful to many and harmful to few. In the author's opinion, however, the small risk of percutaneous renal biopsy is outweighed by the guidance for specific treatment, general management, and knowledge of prognosis that a histologic diagnosis provides.

PATIENT NUMBER 2 (continued)

You initially consider myeloma but are puzzled about how Bence Jones proteinuria might be associated with edema and surprised that it registers so strongly on the dipstick test. Further study shows hypoalbuminemia, urine immunoelectrophoresis demonstrating monoclonal light chains (Bence Jones protein), and cellulose acetate protein electrophoresis showing an M spike and a much larger peak of albumin. The patient is found to have myeloma with renal amyloid causing nephrotic syndrome.

Four months after institution of chemotherapy for the myeloma, Helen's arm and shoulder pain is almost completely relieved. The quantity of urinary light chains has diminished, but the albumin excretion remains unabated and her serum creatinine has risen from 1.0 to 1.6 mg/dl.

SUGGESTED READINGS

Birch DF, Fairley KF, Becker GJ, Kincaid-Smith P: A Color Atlas of Urine Microscopy. London, Chapman and Hall Medical, 1994.

Coggins CH: Membranous nephropathy. *In* Schrier RW, Gottschalk CW (eds): Diseases of the Kidney, 5th ed. Boston, Little, Brown, & Co, 1993.

Coggins CH: Glomerulonephritis and the nephrotic syndrome. *In* Dale DC, Rubenstein DD (eds): Scientific American Medicine. New York, Scientific American, 1995.

Kaysen GA: Nonrenal complications of the nephrotic syndrome. Annu Rev Med 45:201–210, 1994.

Kyle RA: Monoclonal proteins and renal disease. Annu Rev Med 45:71–77, 1994.

Rose BD: Approach to the patient with renal disease. *In* Dale DC, Federman DD (eds): Scientific American Medicine. New York, Scientific American, 1992.

Schapner HW, Robson AM: Nephrotic syndrome: Minimal change disease, focal glomerulosclerosis and related disorders. *In* Schrier RW, Gottschalk CW (eds): Diseases of the Kidney, 5th ed. Boston, Little Brown, & Co, 1993.

3 ▌ ACUTE NEPHRITIC SYNDROME

Daniel C. Cattran

The objective of this chapter is to enable the reader to

1. Recognize the features of the acute nephritic syndrome
2. Differentiate between primary and secondary forms
3. Assess the severity of the process
4. Be aware of initial management issues based on severity and etiology
5. Assess prognosis

Acute nephritic syndrome is the most serious and potentially devastating form of the various renal syndromes. Renal failure can develop over a period of days to weeks. The clinical and laboratory findings reflect the pathology. The expansion produced by the cellular proliferation of both intrinsic glomerular cells and extrinsic (invading) mononuclear and polymorphonuclear neutrophils (PMNs) within the glomerular tuft results in a reduction in the glomerular filtration surface area and subsequent filtration rate, a rising serum creatinine level associated with salt and water retention, peripheral edema, and frequently systemic hypertension. The inflammatory mediator release from the invading monocytes and PMNs damages the glomerular basement membrane and always results in some degree of proteinuria. This damage is also reflected in the urine sediment, where dysmorphic (abnormally shaped) RBCs and RBC and granular casts are commonly found.

Despite the generality of this definition of the acute nephritic syndrome, it is crucial to distinguish between primary and secondary forms and to estimate the pathologic severity of the process, because prognosis and therapy depend on both these factors.

PATIENT NUMBER 1

Mr. Hank C., a 63-year-old recently retired engineer, presented to his family doctor with a 4-day history of increasing shortness of breath on exertion and a 3-day history of difficulty in getting his slippers on at night and swollen eyes in the morning. He had initially attributed these problems to a new mattress and inadequate rest at night. On direct inquiry, he admitted to both a decrease in the amount of urine he was passing and that its color had been like Coca-Cola for the past couple of days. He thought this was because of something he ate. His only recent illness had been a severe sore throat 2 weeks ago; it had resolved spontaneously. On examining him, his family doctor found a blood pressure of 180/100 mm Hg, raised jugular venous pressure 4 cm above the sternal angle, fine crepitations in both lung bases, some minor costovertebral angle tenderness on percussion, and 1+ swelling of the ankles. Dipstick urinalysis showed 3+ blood, 2+ protein, trace glycosuria, and on microscopic examination of a fresh urine specimen 30 to 40 dysmorphic RBCs, 3 to 5 WBCs, and 2 RBC casts. The doctor asked for determinations of serum creatinine, urea, and electrolytes, as well as a complete blood count, to be done urgently through the laboratory located in his building. Hank's serum creatinine level was 180 μmol/L and urea was 13.5 mmol/L, but serum electrolyte values and complete blood count results were normal.

APPROACH TO PATIENT NUMBER 1

The first issue is **determining the severity of the process.** The history suggests the disorder is acute with no symptoms except the sore throat 2 weeks before presentation. Hank was known to be in previous good health. The rapid development of the symptoms suggests the process is severe. His clinical findings also reflect the extent of the disease—that is, a decrease in GFR in the absence of a reduction of fluid intake results in expansion of the intravascular volume first, often resulting in raised arterial blood pressure and increased venous pressure, as in this patient. The subsequent transudation into the extravascular space from the increased hydrostatic pressure produces edema in the lower limbs and around the eyes in the morning. Often, in older patients with some cardiac disease, the increased intravascular volume leads to pulmonary congestion and increasing shortness of breath. Hank's complaint of oliguria reflects the worsening GFR; the cola-colored urine and proteinuria suggest renal parenchymal damage.

> The quantity of proteinuria is often not an accurate reflection of the extent of the process. With the most severe glomerular injury, the filtration rate may be so low or renal function deteriorating at such a rate that even large molecules such as the major protein species cannot be filtered.

The variation in the size and shape of the RBCs in the urine is presumed to be a result of the trauma to RBC membranes during the passage through the damaged glomerular structure. This, taken together with the observed RBC casts (which are whole RBCs incorporated into a protein matrix), is consistent with active cellular proliferation and injury within the glomerular tuft. In rare circumstances, when the GFR is very low, even the urine sediment may be surprisingly inactive because of the minimal passage of any fluids or cells across this injured membrane. The glycosuria likely reflects an abnormal tubular handling of glucose secondary to the interstitial infiltrate and subsequent tubular damage that can occur in the most severe cases of the acute nephritic syndrome.

The second issue is the **cause of the process.** The only potential etiologic agent suggested by review of the history is the previous throat infection. The absence of any other system involvement on either history or physical examination supports a diagnosis of primary renal disease.

> Examination of the urine sediment is crucial. The finding of RBC casts and dysmorphic cells suggests that the glomeruli are the pri-

> mary target of injury. Remember that prolonged standing of the urine or imprecise preparation of the urine sediment for examination can lead to serious errors because both the casts and dysmorphic cells can degenerate.

PATIENT NUMBER 1 (continued)

Hank, accompanied by his anxious wife, was immediately referred to a nephrologist and was admitted to the hospital for further management of his acute renal failure. An 0.8 g/kg low-protein, low sodium (50 mmol), 80-mmol potassium, 1000 ml/day fluid restriction diet was ordered. He was also started on furosemide, 120 mg daily, and the antihypertensive medication extended-release nifedipine, 30 mg daily. His serum creatinine level increased daily and reached 500 μmol/L by day 3. A 24-hour urine collection showed 2 g of protein and a creatinine clearance of 0.4 ml/sec. Laboratory tests included a negative antinuclear factor (ANF) and negative antineutrophilic cytoplasmic antibody (ANCA) test but a low C3 value and an ASOT result of 1:400. Renal ultrasonography showed only bilateral large, engorged kidneys with no obstruction. A closed renal biopsy was carried out on day 3. This showed diffuse endocapillary proliferation on light microscopy (Fig. 3–1), and immunofluorescence showed large, irregularly shaped deposits along the capillary loops and in the mesangium of IgG and C3. Subsequent electron microscopy revealed subepithelial deposits of various sizes. Symptomatic management only was continued based on this information. The creatinine level rose to 700 μmol/L by day 8 and then slowly declined to normal by week 4. Fluid balance and blood pressure improved during the same time frame, and the diuretics and hypertensive agents were tapered and then stopped. Hank was reviewed at month 3 and was found to have normal blood pressure with no edema and a bland urine sediment with no proteinuria. His creatinine level was 105 μmol/L. He and his wife were very relieved at his recovery of renal function and were delighted to hear it was highly unlikely to happen again. He felt he could now plan his long-anticipated postretirement trip to Africa.

APPROACH TO PATIENT NUMBER 1 (continued)

The admitting physician, given Hank's history and initial assessment, concluded that the data were most compatible with acute disease and the cause being infectious in origin. Hank had no systemic disease features, and his only symptoms paralleled his acute decline in GFR. Laboratory test results that helped rule out secondary causes included the negative ANF (lupus), negative ANCA (vasculitis), negative hepatitis serology, and lack of cryoglobulins. Both the low C3 complement component and the positive ASOT result of 1:400 supported the diagnosis of an acute poststreptococcal infectious process.

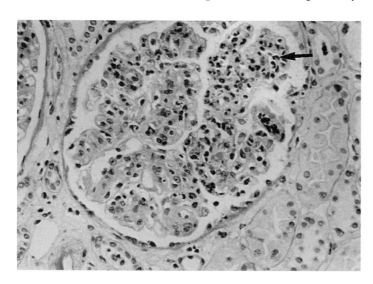

Figure 3–1. Proliferation of the intrinsic mesangial and endothelial cells of glomerular tuft plus increase in extrinsic cells, i.e., polymorphonclear leukocyte *(arrow)*, produces a reduced filtration surface and occluded capillary loops. Note no proliferation in Bowman's space and hence the name endocapillary proliferation.

A decrease in ASOT level at 8 to 12 weeks would be required to verify this, because a single positive titer indicates only previous exposure and not necessarily acute disease.

The laboratory tests of renal function confirmed progression of Hank's disease. The creatinine level rising at a rate exceeding 100 μmol/L/day, with a comparable increase in plasma urea, indicated ongoing severe damage to the kidneys. Ultrasonography was performed to help confirm the acuity and to ensure that obstruction was not present. The bilaterally equal-sized but slightly enlarged kidneys with no pelvicalyceal dilatation are typical of acute renal parenchymal disease. Ultrasonography also defines the depth and position of the kidneys in preparation for a closed renal biopsy. It is preferable to an intravenous pyelogram (IVP) or radioisotope scan. IVP is likely to be both noninformative, because no dye is likely to be taken up by severely impaired kidneys, and dangerous owing to the osmotic load given by the contrast material. Radioisotope scanning, although not dangerous, would show the decreased perfusion, but it cannot accurately estimate renal size or adequately assess obstruction under conditions of low renal blood flow.

The changes in serial serum creatinine level most clearly reflect the severity of the underlying disease. The one quantitative measurement of proteinuria of 2 g/day is really nondiagnostic, although it does support parenchymal injury.

> Both creatinine clearance and proteinuria underestimate the severity of the renal failure in patients with the acute nephritic syndrome presentation, because both poorly reflect renal function under conditions of rapid change.

The decision to perform a biopsy on Hank is based on the balance between risks versus benefits. The risk of bleeding after a closed biopsy is increased in the presence of renal failure; however, evaluation of the coagulation status and use of prophylactic DDAVP ensure a morbidity risk of significant bleeding of less than 5%. It was elected to proceed to a biopsy, given that benefits of knowing the exact histology would influence both therapy and prognosis.

Light microscopic examination of the tissue determines the major histologic groupings (Table 3–1). Pure endocapillary proliferation of the intrinsic glomerular mesangial and endothelial cells, with or without PMNs, carries the best prognosis. Extension of the process into Bowman's capsule, with subsequent crescent formation, or the presence of an interstitial nephritis significantly worsens the outlook. Immunofluorescence revealing a starry sky pattern of deposition of IgG and complement-containing complexes, combined with the subepithelial deposits on electron microscopy, supports a postinfectious etiology in Hank's case, although the specific bacterial or viral antigen cannot usually be determined.

Symptomatic management of fluid and electrolytes, maintenance of acid-base balance, and control of systemic hypertension, plus a tincture of time, are all that is required in this case once the pathology is determined. Ninety-five percent or more of these patients recover with minimal residual damage, and a recurrence of this disorder is extremely uncommon.

On the basis of the clinical history, physical examination, and laboratory testing, it would have been impossible, before a decline in creatinine clearance, to distinguish this presentation from idiopathic crescentic glomerulonephritis. In

TABLE 3–1. Primary Renal Diseases Associated with the Acute Nephritic Syndrome: Clinical and Laboratory Features, Prognosis, and Treatment

| Pathologic Classification | Mean Age (Range) | Gender (M/F) | BP | Urinalysis | 24-hr Protein | Creatinine Clearance | C3 | Renal Survival (%)° | | Acute Treatment |
								5 Years	10 Years	
Diffuse proliferative	20 (5–80+)	2/1	↑	Active	0.5–5 g	↓	↓	95	90	Symptomatic
Idiopathic crescentic glomerulo-nephritis	55 (10–80+)	2/1	↑	Active	<2 g	Markedly ↓	N/↓	50	30	Pulse steroid plus cytotoxic agent
IgA/IgG nephropathy	25 (10–70)	2–3/1	↑/N	Active	0.1–5 g	↓	N	75	40	Pulse steroid
MPGN										
Type I	18 (5–60)	1/1	↑/N	Active	0.1–5 g	↓	N/↓	75	50	Symptomatic
Type II	12 (3–35)	1/1	↑/N	Active	0.1–5 g	↓	↓↓	80	50	Symptomatic

°This prognosis and treatment refers *only* to patients in these histologic categories who present with the acute nephritic syndrome (see text). Key: N = normal; ↑ = increased; ↓ = decreased.

such a case, on biopsy, the endocapillary proliferation can be obscured by the proliferation of cells within Bowman's space (Fig. 3–2). The extracapillary proliferation is a consequence of rupture of the tuft's basement membrane, with leakage of both cells and plasma into Bowman's space. Mononuclear cells may also infiltrate the renal interstitium either as part of the primary process or related to subsequent rupture of the capsular membrane surrounding the glomerulus. Immunofluorescent microscopy, in addition to the previously described glomerular tuft deposits, may show fibrin deposition in the area of the crescent. Electron microscopy may show breaks in the basement membrane of both the tuft and capsule. When crescents are found, the prognosis is quite different from that of pure endocapillary proliferative type, despite the same cause. As the crescent enlarges, it compresses and often causes irreversible ischemia of the glomerular tuft. **Delays in diagnosis by only short periods (days to weeks) can result in irreversible scarring.** Crescents are initially cellular, but with time they become fibrocellular and finally acellular.

A patient's prognosis is closely tied to the percentage of glomeruli with crescents and their

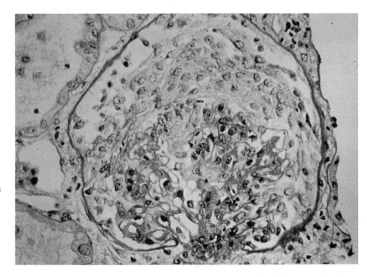

Figure 3–2. Crescentic glomerulo-nephritis. A large fibrocellular crescent occupies Bowman's space and compresses the glomerular tuft. This is also called extracapillary proliferative disease, and the cellular elements of the crescents are from both the lining parietal cells of the capsule and extrinsic mononuclear cells that have come from the blood through the breaks in the capillary basement membranes.

potential reversibility. This, in turn, is directly proportionate to their cellularity.

MANAGEMENT

Active cellular crescents associated with an interstitial nephritis warrant aggressive therapy despite an unknown cause. A number of studies have indicated that the natural history is altered by the use of Solu-Medrol, 5 to 10 mg/kg given on alternate days on three or four occasions, followed by high-dose daily prednisone starting at 1 to 1.5 mg/kg for 2 to 4 weeks and tapered to zero over 3 to 6 months. The addition of cytotoxic therapy such as azathioprine (Imuran), 1 to 2 mg/kg daily or monthly, plus cyclophosphamide, 500 mg/m^2 for 3 to 6 months, has also been advocated. Evidence supporting the addition of cytotoxic agents is less compelling, and these should not be added if the patient's life risk is heightened (i.e., age > 70) or if comorbid serious medical conditions or infection is present. The absence of any response within 2 to 4 weeks indicates a need for repeat renal biopsy to help determine if irreversible disease has occurred. Remember that **acceptance of end-stage renal disease, given the available treatment options, is preferable to death secondary to iatrogenic infection.** In the majority of cases of idiopathic crescentic glomerulonephritis, no therapy is warranted after 3 to 6 months.

PATIENT NUMBER 2

Mr. Yan C., a 36-year-old architect of Asian origin, presented to the emergency room with a history of gross painless hematuria on his last two voidings. On direct inquiry, he appeared very anxious and admitted to having a moderate sore throat and a slight cough for about 2 days but no fever or sputum. He had taken some over-the-counter cough syrup for the cough, with no relief, and thought this might have given him the blood in the urine. He admitted that a similar episode had occurred 3 years earlier and had lasted for 4 days. Results of investigations at that time had shown normal renal function and normal findings on renal ultrasonography and cystoscopy. Although no therapy had been given, Yan had been advised to obtain follow-up. He had become very busy, and because it didn't hurt and had not happened again, he had not returned to see his family doctor. On systems review, he denied all symptoms, and in particular he reported no history of joint discomfort, gastrointestinal upset, or skin rash. He had no

---

known family history of renal disease. The patient was a nonsmoker and denied any significant alcohol or street drug intake. On physical examination, he was a well-nourished man in no acute distress. His blood pressure was 130/90 mm Hg with no postural change, and his jugular venous pressure was normal. His chest was clear to auscultation. He had only trace peripheral edema. No arthritis or skin rash was found on examination. His urine was red on visual inspection and showed 4+ blood and 2+ protein on dipstick. Microscopic analysis of an unspun urine specimen showed RBCs too numerous to count, with some dysmorphic forms and an occasional RBC cast.

APPROACH TO PATIENT NUMBER 2

First, let us **consider the severity and target of the process.** There are more subtle signs of the acute nephritic syndrome suggesting a mild to moderate pathologic process in Yan's case, when compared to Hank's case (above). The jugular venous pressure is not elevated, and the lung fields are clear, but for his age and size, Yan has modest hypertension and there is trace peripheral edema. The findings in the urine sediment of dysmorphic RBCs, RBC casts, and protein strongly suggest a renal parenchymal disorder, focused at the glomerular level and associated with cellular proliferation on pathology.

Second, we need to **look for clues to the underlying etiology.** Gross hematuria can be seen in several types of primary renal disease such as IgA nephropathy, postinfectious glomerulonephritis, membranoproliferative glomerulonephritis (MPGN types I and II), and rarely focal segmental glomerulosclerosis. Macroscopic hematuria simultaneous with or very shortly after an upper respiratory tract infection is an important clue. Our patient Yan presents a classic case of IgA nephropathy, and although this was considered the most likely diagnosis, other information was necessary before drawing this conclusion.

PATIENT NUMBER 2 (continued)

Yan's serum creatinine value, measured in the emergency room, was elevated at 150 μmol/L, his urea level was 10 mmol/L, and his serum electrolyte values were normal. Given his renal insufficiency and his acute presentation, hospitalization was recommended. Yan had never been in the hospital before and claimed he was too busy (and perhaps a little frightened), but after discussion with the doctor about the need to have more information to help determine the diagnosis and prognosis, he agreed to the admission. Subsequent laboratory tests showed a normal complement profile, but serum immunoglobulin determinations revealed an elevated IgA level. Other test results included a negative ANCA and ANF, no cryoglobulins, and negative serology for hepatitis B and C. Renal function tests showed protein excretion of 0.75 g/day and a creatinine clearance of 1.1 ml/ sec. Renal ultrasonography revealed bilaterally normal-sized kidneys and normal Doppler results in renal arteries and veins. Yan's gross hematuria settled within 2 days, and his creatinine level started to fall at the same time. His creatinine was 100 μmol/L by day 3, and the dipstick reaction was only 1+ for protein, so Yan was discharged to be monitored as an outpatient. The creatinine clearance was estimated at 1.6 ml/sec, serum creatinine level was 95 μmol/L, and urine protein excretion was normal at 0.05 g/day at the 3-month follow-up visit. Urinalysis, however, still revealed microscopic hematuria, although no casts were seen.

The attending nephrologist believed that no renal biopsy was warranted; however, the patient now wanted to know exactly what disease type he had and what to expect long term. He was also having trouble getting any disability insurance because of the persistent hematuria. A biopsy was carried out. This revealed 2 out of 30 obsolescent glomeruli, but the rest had only mild mesangial cell proliferation and matrix expansion on light microscopy, as well as mesangial IgA immunoreactants and lesser amounts of IgG in the same location by immunofluorescence microscopy. One small segmental crescent was seen (Fig. 3–3). Electron microscopy confirmed mesangial deposits. No tubular, interstitial, or vascular changes were observed. Yan was reassured that the biopsy confirmed the diagnosis. He was told that he would, however, need regular follow-up at 6- to 12-month intervals because (1) the gross hematuria could recur,

(2) hypertension might develop in some cases, and (3) the disease process can progress to kidney failure over a 10- to 15-year period in some patients.

APPROACH TO PATIENT NUMBER 2 (continued)

First let us continue the assessment of the severity of the process and the related management issue. Yan's borderline hypertension and edema are abnormal but minor. A diastolic pressure of 90 mm Hg is marginal and can safely be observed, given the acuity of the event and the ability to monitor it closely in the hospital. Initial results of renal function tests parallel the clinical findings and suggest the severity is mild to moderate. Daily measurements of weight and fluid balance would suggest if diuretics are needed. Because Yan had no elevation of jugular venous pressure and only trace edema, the introduction of dietary sodium restriction and perhaps a modest amount of diuretics, such as furosemide, 40 mg/day, is all that is required at this point. Ongoing monitoring of renal functional parameters would be essential to assess the direction of the disease process. Investigation into etiology should occur *pari passu* with the severity issue, because it may independently influence therapy. The rapid resolution of the gross hematuria, the falling serum creatinine level, and the spontaneous correction of the hypertension would make the crescentic variant, either primary or secondary type, unlikely. The laboratory evaluation failed to identify a secondary cause. The elevated IgA level would support IgA nephropathy, and it is unlikely that the IgA deposits are secondary to

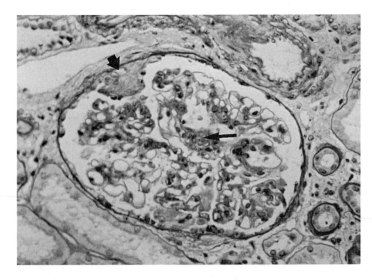

Figure 3–3. IgG/IgA nephropathy. The background mesangial proliferation and mesangial expansion give a prominence to the axial structure of the glomerulus (*long arrow*). The segmental (*short arrow*) crescents are more commonly present when the clinical presentation is with the acute nephritic syndrome.

either Henoch-Schönlein purpura or underlying liver disease because the patient had no arthritis, gastrointestinal symptoms, or purpura and described no history of alcohol intake.

The subsequent biopsy confirmed mild IgA nephropathy, although it is possible that during the acute phase of the gross hematuria, segmental or small crescents could have been present in a few glomeruli, thus explaining the occasional obsolescent one seen at the time of biopsy 3 months later.

Specific therapy in primary IgA nephropathy currently is poorly defined. A major problem is the wide variations in the natural history. Although initially described as a benign disorder, it is now the most common biopsy-proven primary glomerulonephritis in the world, with some series reporting progression to end-stage renal disease in as many as 40% of patients older than 10 to 15 years. Given the rapid return to normal of both Yan's clinical state and his renal function, no specific treatment is warranted. Poor prognostic features include persistent renal insufficiency, proteinuria $\geq$ 1 to 2 g/day, systemic hypertension, and, on biopsy, the degree of glomerular obsolescence and tubular/interstitial or vascular changes. When these features are present, several studies, although not randomized, report an improvement with aggressive antihypertensive treatment and perhaps an added benefit when angiotensin-converting enzyme (ACE) inhibitors are used for blood pressure control. Recent studies have suggested a benefit from fish oil high in omega 3 fatty acids, although other reports have failed to confirm these results. Treatment protocols using aggressive short-term, high-dose steroids with or without cytotoxic agents, similar to the protocol in idiopathic crescentic glomerulonephritis, are probably warranted when marked interstitial inflammation or extensive crescent formation is found in association with an acute nephritic presentation. The majority of patients, however, present with modest hypertension and mild renal insufficiency. In these cases, specific immune therapy has not been proved to be of benefit.

Careful attention to the management of systemic blood pressure, again with ACE inhibitors and perhaps a modest restriction in dietary protein to 0.8 to 0.9 g/kg, especially if the proteinuria is in the nephrotic range, is warranted. In rare instances, an explosive onset of the nephrotic syndrome occurs. This type of presentation is not usually associated with hypertension or impaired creatinine clearance, and biopsy tissue shows only the features of mild IgA nephropathy with mesangial cell and matrix increase and no tubular interstitial disease. Electron microscopy reveals diffuse effacement of the epithelial foot processes.

> **Many of these patients seem to have either a variant of minimal change disease (MCD) or a combination of IgA plus MCD. They tend to respond to a course of steroids in a manner similar to that in pure MCD.**

Both type I and type II MPGN may present with the acute nephritic syndrome in about 20% of cases, but asymptomatic proteinuria (30%) and the nephrotic syndrome (30%) presentations are more common. The typical histologic picture is illustrated (Fig. 3–4). The C3 component of complement is frequently depressed in both types but particularly in type II. Although spontaneous partial or complete remission occurs in approximately one third of these patients, the long-term prognosis must be guarded: 10-year kidney survival is still in the range of 50% to 60%.

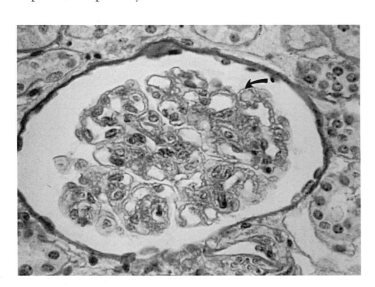

Figure 3–4. The classic histology of MPGN. The proliferation of the mesangial cells is segmental. The clue to the disease type is the apparent double contouring of the basement membrane *(arrow)*. The "space" between the layers is composed of the mesangial matrix material pushing up and around the capillary loops as it expands.

Treatment of the idiopathic type with cytotoxic agents combined with anticoagulants has not been shown to be of benefit. Long-term low-dose alternate-day steroids may modify the prognosis, especially in children, although their use has not been proved in randomized clinical trials. Conservative management with diet, diuretics, and strict antihypertension control is advocated. ACE inhibitors may confer a special benefit, especially if proteinuria is heavy. The absence of cryoglobulins, negative serology for hepatitis B or C, and normal C3 and C4 levels are evidence against a secondary MPGN. Until recently, the major cause of this histology was unknown, but the association of hepatitis C and cryoglobulins with the type I is increasing in frequency and should be excluded in every case. A postinfection etiology is possible, but the temporal relationship between infection and renal symptoms in these cases is usually in the range of 10 to 14 days not 1 or 2 days, as in our patient Yan. Lastly, focal segmental glomerulosclerosis can present with gross hematuria, but it is usually accompanied by proteinuria in the nephrotic range and often by a rising creatinine value.

ACUTE NEPHRITIS AS PART OF A SYSTEMIC DISORDER

PATIENT NUMBER 3

Mr. Al B., a 68-year-old garage manager, presented to his family physician with a 2-month history of feeling "lousy." Al complained of no appetite, a constant aching in his joints, a stuffy nose, and a recurrent ache in his left ear. Four days before this, the patient noticed that he was very short of breath when he was helping to change some tires at his garage. **He thought he was just getting too old for that type of work.** He did admit to coughing up some blood-tinged sputum on the morning of his visit. His wife added that he had also been complaining of stomach pains for the past 3 to 4 months and that she had noticed a 10-lb weight loss during that same period. She had found a low-grade fever up to 38°C in the past week, and after he coughed up the blood, she insisted that he visit his family doctor.

On clinical examination, Al appeared older than his stated age and was fatigued by simply undressing. His family doctor noted tenderness over the right maxillary sinus on percussion and an erosion on the medial aspect of the left naris. His conjunctivae were pale. Both fine and coarse crepitations were heard in both the left lung base

and the right midlung field. Al's blood pressure was 180/100 mm Hg, with no postural change, and his pulse was 78 and regular. Jugular venous pressure was not raised. Abdominal examination revealed some tenderness in the right upper quadrant but no organomegaly. The patient had 2+ peripheral edema. Peripheral pulses all were present, and no femoral or abdominal bruits were heard. There was no evidence of a neuropathy. Urinalysis showed 3+ blood and 2+ protein on dipstick testing, and microscopic examination showed 15 to 20 RBCs per high-power field (hpf) and both coarse heme granular and RBC casts.

From the family doctor's previous record, it was noted that on his annual physical 1 year before, Al was in good health and had normal levels of hemoglobin, BUN, and creatinine. He was taking no medication. The family doctor sent Al to his local hospital emergency room and arranged an urgent nephrology consultation.

Initial laboratory results revealed a normocytic normochromic anemia of 90 g/L, a creatinine level of 480 μmol/L, a urea value of 35 mmol/L, and a mild hyperchloremic metabolic acidosis.

Subsequent serologic laboratory tests showed a positive P-ANCA result, negative ANF, and negative anti-GBM antibody. Al was begun immediately on pulse Solu-Medrol, 7 mg/kg, and on day 3 cyclophosphamide, 1.0 g IV, was given. A closed biopsy showed extensive segmental necrotizing glomerulonephritis without crescents (see Fig. 3–4). Bolus Solu-Medrol was repeated on days 3, 5, and 7. Oral prednisone at 1 mg/kg was then begun. A single-strength tablet of Septra was started on day 5. The cyclophosphamide dose was repeated at monthly intervals for 6 months, then every 3 months for another four treatments.

Al's creatinine level rose to 700 μmol/L on day 5 but then fell slowly to 300 by day 12, and he was discharged feeling very well. The ANCA result became negative by day 8, and his electrolytes slowly corrected. Fluids and acid-base status were balanced by adjusting therapy daily. Al remained hypertensive but was controlled on an ACE inhibitor plus the diuretic furosemide, 160 mg daily. The patient remained well and had returned to part-time work by 6 weeks. He was advised to continue regular follow-ups with his nephrologist at 2- to 4-week intervals.

APPROACH TO PATIENT NUMBER 3

Our patient Al presents with features of a multisystem disorder affecting the kidneys and both the upper and lower respiratory systems. These features associated with an active urine sediment are consistent with a vasculitis (Table 3–2). Upper respiratory tract involvement com-

TABLE 3–2. Secondary (Systemic) Diseases Associated with the Adult Nephrotic Syndrome: Clinical and Laboratory Features, Prognosis, and Treatment

Disease	Mean Age (Range)	Gender (M/F)	Associated Features	Renal Survival°		Acute Treatment
				5 Years	10 Years	
Polyarteritis nodosa (microscopic variant)	55 (20–70+)	2/1	Petechiae/purpura, myalgia, arthralgia, weight loss, fever, neuropathies C-ANCA + dominant	85%	70%	Pulse steroid plus cytotoxic agent
Wegener's granulomatosis	50 (40–80+)	2/1	Sinusitis, otitis media, epistaxis, pulmonary infiltrates, P-ANCA + dominant	80%	65%	Pulse steroid plus cytotoxic agent
Anaphylactoid purpura (Henoch-Schönlein purpura)	15 (3–70)	1/1	Dependent purpura, arthralgia, abdominal pain, IgA level ↑	85%	—	Pulse steroid
Goodpasture's syndrome	30 (15–60)	5/1	Pulmonary hemorrhage Anti-GBM-antibodies present	70%	—	Plasma exchange, pulse steroid, cytotoxic
Lupus nephritis—class IV, diffuse proliferative ± crescents	30 (10–50)	1/5	Skin rash, arthritis, cerebritis pleuritis, C3 ↓, + anti-DNA antibodies	70%	50%	Pulse steroid plus cytotoxic agent
Mixed essential cryoglobulinemia	50 (30–75+)	1/1	Liver dysfunction, purpura, peripheral neuropathy, cryoglobulins present	60%	—	Pulse steroid plus cytotoxic agent ?α-interferon

°This prognosis and treatment refers *specifically* to patients in these categories who present with the acute nephritic syndrome (see text).

bined with lower tract involvement and renal disease makes Wegener's granulomatosis the most likely diagnosis. It is a necrotizing granulomatous vasculitis of uncertain cause. Upper respiratory tract involvement can be diverse and can include otitis media, sinusitis, conjunctivitis, and even gingivitis. Pulmonary involvement can present with cough, hemoptysis, and increasing shortness of breath. Characteristic pulmonary findings on radiographs include interstitial infiltrates and occasionally cavitation. Histologic examination of lung tissue usually reveals focal necrotizing lesions involving the small arteries and veins and, rarely, a dense inflammatory infiltrate with an actual granuloma. A nonspecific skin rash has been reported in 10% to 20% of patients with Wegener's, but it is usually mild and is rarely a presenting feature. Renal disease is found in the majority of patients with Wegener's. Early in its course, the disease tends to be mild, with modest proteinuria and minor elevations of serum creatinine level accompanying an active urine sediment. The renal involvement at this stage is usually a focal segmental necrotizing glomerulonephritis with or without an interstitial infiltrate (Fig. 3–5). Immunofluorescence tends to reveal negative findings or only trace C3 and IgG or IgM deposits in the glomerular tuft. Elec-

tron microscopy shows no deposits in this so-called *pauci-immune variant* of rapidly progressive glomerulonephritis. The disease tends to progress for periods of weeks or months, and in the most severe cases, the number of segmental lesions increases and can be associated with focal crescent formation occurring above the areas of tuft necrosis.

Polyarteritis nodosa (PAN) would also be included in the differential diagnosis. The macroscopic type is more common in the elderly, and vascular involvement tends to be of the large vessels, including those of the liver and gut. Aneurysms may form, and ischemic bowel symptoms may occur. Mononeuritis multiplex as well as peripheral neuropathies may also develop secondary to vascular involvement of the blood supply to the nerves. Microscopic polyarteritis variant is more common in young and middle-aged persons and affects men more often than women. Lesions are in smaller arterioles, capillaries, and venules. Churg-Strauss syndrome is the type associated with a major pulmonary component, often a history of asthma and findings of bilateral pulmonary infiltrates on radiographs, with or without a peripheral eosinophilia. Although the absence of skin petechiae in our patient Al argues against polyarteritis, the symptoms of ar-

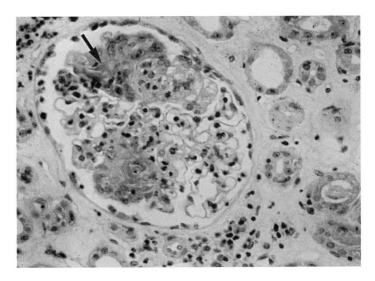

Figure 3–5. Segmental necrotizing glomerulonephritis. This glomerulus shows two areas of segmental proliferation surrounding two areas of necrosis *(arrow)*. This lesion is commonly associated with vasculitis.

thralgias, myalgias, abdominal pain, and weight loss with fever still make this diagnosis a strong possibility.

> **Antibodies to neutrophil cytoplasmic antigen by indirect immunofluorescence can be found in more than 90% of active cases of both of these types of vasculitis. The C-ANCA pattern with diffuse stippling in the cytoplasm is more commonly associated with PAN; the increased perinuclear cytoplasmic staining, or P-ANCA, is more common in Wegener's.**

Both tests can now be performed by an enzyme-linked immunoadsorbent method that allows a more accurate quantitation of the antibody. Nonspecific laboratory findings in both types include leukocytosis, thrombocytosis, and an elevated sedimentation rate.

Treatment for either Wegener's or microscopic polyarteritis with severe renal involvement is similar. A combination of high-dose prednisone and a cytotoxic agent for maintenance, most commonly cyclophosphamide, is now almost standard therapy. In acute fulminant disease, such as Al's case with acute renal failure and lung infiltrates, steroids are begun in the form of intravenous methylprednisolone (Solu-Medrol) in doses of 5 to 10 mg/kg on alternate days for three to five cycles, with subsequent initiation of oral prednisone at 1 to 1.5 mg/kg. Cyclophosphamide is often initiated 2 or 3 days later, when the diagnosis is confirmed, in the form of pulse intravenous therapy at 0.5 to 1 g/m^2.

Prednisone is usually tapered slowly to a low dose or discontinued, dependent on the clinical course, during a 4- to 6-month period. Cyclo-

phosphamide is given as a bolus every 4 to 6 weeks for 12 to 18 months. Optimum response requires prolonged therapy, and generally neither the prednisone nor the cytotoxic agent is completely discontinued until clinical disease activity has been quiescent for at least 6 to 12 months. This combined therapy has resulted in an 80% to 85% induced remission rate, although as many as 50% of patients eventually suffer a relapse.

> **These disease processes should be considered lifelong conditions, and monitoring should be continued even if no disease activity is apparent.**

A major risk in these patients is infection due to the intense immunosuppression required in the early phases of treatment. Prophylactic Septra therapy to prevent *Pneumocystis carinii* pneumonia (PCP) is an important adjunct. In the first 3 to 6 months, constant vigilance for infection must be maintained. Infection can include the common bacterial types, as well as the opportunistic ones including PCP, cytomegalovirus infection, atypical tuberculosis, and certain fungal diseases. The ANCA test results can remain positive despite disease quiescence, and in this situation it has little meaning.

> **The development of a positive ANCA test result, however, in a patient who had previously had a negative result, should alert the clinician to a possible impending clinical relapse, even if the other laboratory test results appear stable.**

PATIENT NUMBER 4

Mr. Jim S. was a previously healthy 22-year-old university physics student who presented with an 8-hour history of coughing up blood-tinged sputum and increasing shortness of breath. He had noticed some minor difficulty playing pick-up basketball 1 day before admission but had become acutely short of breath only on the day of admission. On arrival at the emergency room, he had an episode of massive hemoptysis. A brief review of symptoms revealed no other features. He did report a history of being a heavy smoker for several years but had no history of illicit drug use or exposure to hydrocarbons. The patient did note that he had passed little urine for the 24 hours preceding his admission but thought it was because of the hot weather and his previous day's exercise. On examination, he appeared acutely ill and had a respiratory rate of 34 breaths per minute. He was pale and diaphoretic, his blood pressure was 100/80 mm Hg, and his pulse rate was 108 and regular. His jugular venous pressure was below the sternal angle, although both fine and coarse crepitations were heard throughout both lung fields. Abdominal examination was unremarkable, and he had no peripheral edema. No skin or joint abnormalities were found. Urine was scanty but did show 1 + blood and 1 + protein, and the sediment had 30 to 50 RBCs/hpf and numerous RBC casts. Emergency laboratory tests revealed normal electrolyte values but a urea level of 15 mmol/L, a creatinine level of 250 μmol/L, and a modest respiratory acidosis with an oxygen saturation on blood gas analysis of only 60% on room air. Chest radiographs showed bilateral pulmonary infiltrates in an alveolar pattern compatible with pulmonary hemorrhage.

APPROACH TO PATIENT NUMBER 4

The severity of the process is evident with life-threatening pulmonary hemorrhage as well as acute renal failure. The explosive onset of the pulmonary hemorrhage indicates the urgency of management. The minor amount of proteinuria and hematuria can be deceptive and might not reflect the rapidly deteriorating renal function (discussed earlier).

Although the severity is not suggested by the laboratory values on admission, the history of the oliguria and the creatinine already being two to three times normal in a young man with no past history would support that the disease process is so severe that the glomerular filtration is already approaching zero.

Etiology

Although the differential diagnosis would include all of the pulmonary renal syndromes, the working diagnosis on admission would be Goodpasture's syndrome. Smoking increases the severity of the pulmonary hemorrhage in this disease and, if continued beyond the initial phase, is associated with a higher rate of relapse. The precise mechanism for this is unknown, although a "double hit" on the alveolar basement membrane from the antibodies to basement membrane that develop in this disease, combined with the injury from the inhaled pollutants of smoking, seems logical. Patient transfer to an intensive care setting with constant monitoring, including blood gases, should be undertaken immediately. Massive pulmonary hemorrhage can ensue in a small percentage of patients presenting in this fashion and can cause death. Blood should be immediately sent for an estimate of circulating antiglomerular basement membrane antibodies as well as for ANCA, anti-DNA antibodies, and C3 and C4 complement component, because both vasculitis and acute lupus can present in this fashion.

Specific therapy must often be started before confirmation of the diagnosis by specific laboratory tests or by histology. In Goodpasture's syndrome, antibodies directed against both alveolar basement membrane and glomerular basement membrane (and occasionally tubular basement membrane) are generated, and thus the clinical presentation can be predominantly lung or renal. **Institution of plasma exchange can be life saving under conditions when pulmonary hemorrhage dominates.** This is the most rapid method of reducing the antibody load. Each plasma exchange volume is generally 4 to 5 L and is given on alternate days, with a total course equal to 7 to 10 exchanges. Plasma exchange is often continued until the antibody titer is significantly lowered or has disappeared from the circulation. This therapy must be combined with high-dose steroid treatment in the form of pulse Solu-Medrol, 5 to 10 mg/kg on alternate days for two to three courses. This is generally changed to oral prednisone treatment after 8 to 10 days, usually beginning at 1 mg/kg and tapering over 4 to 6 months to zero. Cytotoxic agents such as pulse or oral cyclophosphamide are also introduced at this time in much the same manner as in vasculitis. Cyclophosphamide is generally continued for 4 to 6 months beyond the period when disease activity has abated. It is generally safe to discontinue both these medications after this period. It is important to strongly recommend to our patient Jim that he stop smoking. The incidence of relapse is relatively low in nonsmokers, i.e., between 10% and 20%.

Disseminated lupus erythematosus would also be in the differential diagnosis. Diffuse proliferative or crescentic glomerulonephritis can occur in this disease. It can present with the acute nephritic syndrome as well as with pulmonary features. A female-to-male predominance of 5:1 is noted in this disease, with a peak incidence between 15 and 45 years of age. Systemic manifestations can be protean and include skin rash, often in the malar areas, arthralgias or arthritis, serositis with pericarditis or pleuritis, and neurologic features including cerebritis. Other evidence of the systemic nature of the disease includes bone marrow involvement with anemia, leukopenia, and thrombocytopenia. Laboratory abnormalities that would support this diagnosis include a positive ANF result, suppression of C3 and C4 complement components, and elevation of anti–double-stranded DNA antibodies. Management of this, the most acute form of renal lupus, includes intravenous Solu-Medrol, followed by a course of oral corticosteroids in a dose similar to that used in vasculitis. Some evidence supports the addition of pulse cyclophosphamide, 0.5 to 1.0 g/m^2 every 4 to 6 weeks, in this disorder and when diffuse proliferative or crescentic glomerulonephritis is identified on biopsy, especially when accompanied by severe renal impairment. This has been shown in a limited number of patients to reduce future scarring and to lead to better long-term preservation of renal function. It must be recalled that therapy beyond 6 to 8 months with this drug, especially in patients older than 30 years, has a very high incidence of inducing permanent sterility. This is in addition to the commonly associated adverse effects of alopecia, leukopenia, and nausea. Involvement of the germinal tissue is directly proportional to age, and thus prolonged treatment eventually sterilizes all age groups. The use of birth control pills and other therapies directed at preventing this have been tried and, although not guaranteed, might be considered once a course of cytotoxic therapy has been begun, if the individual is in the susceptible age range. Late malignancy is also a possibility, although this may be an effect of the disease process not of just the treatment. **Plasma exchange has been shown to have no role in the treatment of lupus,** and although total lymphoid irradiation has been tried in resis-

tant cases, it must still be considered experimental. Cyclosporine has been used in some cases, as have immune globulin infusions, but the data in acute cases are still very preliminary. Therapy is often continued with both steroids and a cytotoxic agent for prolonged periods in this disease. Lupus should be considered a lifelong disorder, although the incidence of exacerbation of the process seems to decrease after the first 10 years, and all medication can be withdrawn if done carefully in a small percentage of patients beyond this time. Azathioprine is not as popular as cyclophosphamide as an immunosuppressive agent but has been used successfully in many cases. It should be considered as an alternative, especially if the patient's desire to have a family is strong, because it infrequently induces sterility.

Regardless of the rate and the degree of response, it is important to maintain careful and ongoing monitoring for infection and accelerated vascular disease. These remain the most common causes of both morbidity and mortality in the latter stages of lupus.

PATIENT NUMBER 4 (continued)

Goodpasture's syndrome was strongly suspected on clinical grounds. Pulse Solu-Medrol, 10 mg/kg, and plasma exchange were begun immediately. The diagnosis was confirmed within 24 hours with the finding of circulating antibodies to glomerular basement membrane in the patient's serum. Oral cyclophosphamide, 2 mg/kg, was begun on day 4. Jim's pulmonary hemorrhage had improved by that time, but his creatinine level continued to rise by 100 μmol/L/day. Renal biopsy confirmed crescentic glomerulonephritis with circumferential, cellular crescents seen in 50% of his glomeruli. Immunofluorescence microscopy showed intense linear staining of both IgG and C3 along the basement membrane, and some fibrin was seen in the crescents. Results of serologic tests for vasculitis and disseminated lupus erythematosus were negative. Plasma exchange was continued for a total of eight treatments during the first 3 weeks. Solu-Medrol was switched to oral prednisone (1 mg/kg/day) at day 7, and oral cyclophosphamide was maintained at 2 mg/kg. The creatinine peaked at 850 μmol/L by day 12 and fell to 175 μmol/L by day 30. Jim's chest radiograph remained clear. Urinalysis still showed a trace protein, occasional granular casts, and 10 to 15 RBCs/hpf. Both cyclophosphamide and prednisone were gradually tapered to zero by the end of month 6. At 2 years, the creatinine was still stable at 170 μmol/L, the urine sediment was benign, but the patient remained hypertensive but controlled on treatment. No relapses had occurred, and the patient continued to avoid smoking.

OTHER CAUSES OF THE ACUTE NEPHRITIC SYNDROME

Mixed cryoglobulinemia can also present with the acute nephritic syndrome. This disorder may be idiopathic (essential mixed cryoglobulinemia) or associated with infectious, autoimmune, or tumoral disorders (secondary mixed cryoglobulinemia). The cryoglobulin consists of two or more immunoglobulin classes, one of which is a monoclonal paraprotein, usually IgM, and the other a polyclonal of the IgG class. Systemic features may include purpura, arthritis or arthralgia, fevers, weight loss, and other manifestations suggestive of a vasculitis. Complement components are often depressed. As many as one third of these patients may present with either an acute nephritic or a nephrotic/nephritic picture.

> **Detection of cryoglobulins in the serum requires special attention to maintaining the sample at body temperature (37°C) until the laboratory is able to process the specimen.**

The histology on renal biopsy is usually a membranoproliferative pattern on light microscopy, typical double contouring of the basement membrane, and large irregular-sized deposits in the capillary loops, mostly in the subendothelial area of IgM, IgG, IgA, and complement-containing immune complexes. In cases of progressive disease, especially associated with a high cryocrit value, pulse steroid combined with cyclophosphamide treatment and plasma exchange similar to that in Goodpasture's syndrome has been used. The natural history is extremely vari-

able, and hence efficacy studies using such combined therapy are not available. Many researchers have found a high incidence of antibodies to hepatitis C virus in these patients, suggesting that a strong relationship exists between this virus and mixed cryoglobulinemia, especially in patients with renal involvement. Studies have advocated interferon-alpha therapy under these conditions, with or without plasma exchange. Although short-term benefits seem to accrue, the relapse rate approximates 100% once the interferon is stopped. Patients with this disorder are prone to serious life-threatening infections, which may well be heightened by too aggressive immunosuppressive treatment. A balance must be struck between the extent of the disease and the dangers (and cost) of treatment.

SUGGESTED READINGS

Balow JE: Renal vasculitis. Curr Opin Nephrol Hypertens 2:231–237, 1993.

Boumpas DT, Austin HA III, Fessler BJ, et al: Systemic lupus erythematosus: Emerging concepts. Part I: Renal, neuropsychiatric, cardiovascular, pulmonary, and haematologic disease. Ann Intern Med 122:940–950, 1995.

Cattran DC, Greenwood C, Ritchie S: Long-term benefits of angiotensin-converting enzyme inhibitor therapy in patients with severe immunoglobulin A nephropathy: A comparison in patients receiving treatment with other antihypertensive agents and to patients receiving no therapy. Am J Kidney Dis 23:247–254, 1994.

D'Amico G: Hepatitis C virus and essential mixed cryoglobulinaemia. Nephrol Dial Transplant 8:579–581, 1993.

Kallenber CGM, Brouwer E, Weening JJ, Tervaert JWC: Anti-neutrophil cytoplasmic antibodies: Current diagnostic and pathophysiological potential. Kidney Int 46:1–15, 1994.

Kelly PT, Haponik EF: Goodpasture syndrome: Molecular and clinical advances. Medicine 73:171–185, 1994.

Waldo FB, Wyatt RJ, Kelly DR, et al: Treatment of IgA nephropathy in children: Efficacy of alternate-day oral prednisone. Pediatr Nephrol 8:394–395, 1994.

Washio M, Oh Y, Okuda S, et al: Clinicopathological study of poststreptococcal glomerulonephritis in the elderly. Clin Nephrol 44:265–270, 1994.

Zent R, Van Zyl Smit R, Duffield M, Cassidy MJ: Crescentic nephritis at Groot Schuur Hospital, South Africa—not a benign disease. Clin Nephrol 42:22–29, 1994.

4 | SODIUM AND POTASSIUM DISTURBANCES

IN RENAL PATIENTS

Biff F. Palmer, Robert D. Toto, and Robert J. Alpern

Despite large variations in dietary salt and water, the tonicity of the body's fluid compartments is maintained within well-defined limits. Total body potassium and its distribution within the body are tightly regulated such that the serum concentration is similarly maintained within a narrow range. In disease states, those factors that govern the serum concentration of sodium and potassium are disrupted. In fact, disorders of serum sodium and potassium concentration are common problems in clinical medicine. In this chapter, a series of cases illustrating disorders of serum sodium and potassium concentration that are commonly encountered in clinical practice serve as the starting point for how one can approach and treat patients with these electrolyte disorders.

PATIENT NUMBER 1

Raymond, a 54-year-old man, presents with symptoms characteristic of new-onset congestive heart failure. He is currently the chief executive officer of a publishing house that he had an instrumental role in starting nearly 20 years ago. He has always been a tireless worker and takes great pride in the success of his business. His past medical history is significant for two prior myocardial infarctions. He used to smoke heavily but stopped 2 years ago, shortly after his second infarction. On admission, the physical examination is remarkable for bibasilar rales and 2+ pedal edema. Raymond's serum chemistry results are (mEq/L) Na 128, Cl 90, K 4.9, and HCO$_3$ 24. His BUN is 35 mg/dl, and his serum creatinine concentration is 1.8 mg/dl. His serum osmolality is 270 mOsm/L, and his urine osmolality is 625 mOsm/L.

APPROACH TO THE HYPONATREMIC PATIENT
(Fig. 4–1)

Step 1: Is the Hyponatremia Representative of a Hypo-Osmolar State?

Hyponatremia not associated with a hypo-osmolar state has two general causes. The first of these is pseudohyponatremia, which involves an abnormal measurement of the serum sodium level. This occurs in patients who have hyperglobulinemia or hypertriglyceridemia and in whom plasma water relative to plasma solids is decreased in blood, leading to less sodium in a given volume of blood. In general, hyperglobulinemia sufficient to cause pseudohyponatremia is rare and occurs only in Waldenstrom's macroglobulinemia. Triglycerides must be in the thousands to cause this condition, which most commonly occurs in diabetic persons. In general, this problem is becoming less prevalent because many laboratories are using sodium electrodes without diluting the blood, and thus the plasma sodium measurement becomes independent of plasma water and solid contents.

The other cause of hyponatremia in the absence of a hypo-osmolar state involves true hyponatremia but with elevations in the concentration of another osmole. Clinical examples include hyperglycemia as encountered in uncontrolled diabetes or rarely hypertonic infusion of mannitol used in the treatment of cerebral edema. The increases in plasma glucose level raise serum osmolality, thus pulling water out of cells and diluting the serum sodium. **For every 100 mg/dl rise in glucose or mannitol, the serum**

32

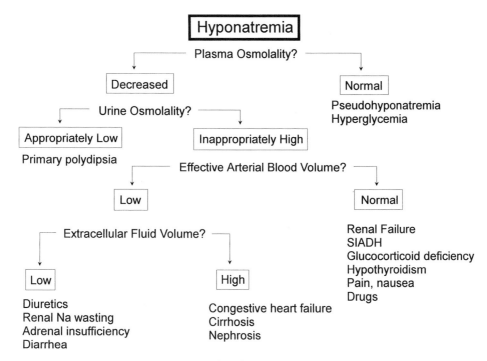

Figure 4–1. Approach to the patient with hyponatremia.

Na quickly falls by 1.6 mEq/L. The increased tonicity also stimulates thirst and arginine vasopressin (AVP) secretion, both of which contribute to further water retention. As the plasma osmolality returns toward normal, the decline in serum Na is 2.8 mEq/L for every 100 mg/dl rise in glucose. The net result is normal plasma osmolality but low serum sodium level. The serum osmolality in our patient Raymond is low, confirming the presence of hypotonic hyponatremia.

Step 2: Is the Kidneys' Ability to Dilute the Urine Intact?

The presence of hypotonic hyponatremia implies that water intake exceeds the ability of the kidneys to excrete water. In unusual circumstances, this can occur when the kidneys' ability to excrete free water is intact. However, because a normal kidney can excrete 20 to 30 L of water per day, the presence of hyponatremia with normal renal water excretion implies that the patient is drinking more than 20 to 30 L of water per day. This condition is referred to as primary polydipsia. These patients should have a urine osmolality less than 100 mOsm/L. **Although primary polydipsia is a common condition that leads to polyuria and polydipsia, it is uncommon as a sole cause of hyponatremia.**

In the absence of primary polydipsia, hyponatremia is associated with decreased renal water excretion and a urine that is inappropriately concentrated. **It is important to note that in the presence of hyponatremia, urine should be maximally dilute and a urine osmolality higher than 100 mOsm/L is inappropriate.** Inappropriately concentrated urine implies a defect in renal water excretion (Table 4–1).

Excretion of water by the kidneys is dependent on three factors. First, delivery of filtrate to the tip of the loop of Henle must be adequate. Second, solute absorption in the ascending limb and the distal nephron must be normal so that the tubular fluid is diluted. Finally, AVP levels must be low in the plasma. Of these three requirements for water excretion, the one that probably is most important in the genesis of hyponatremia is the failure to suppress AVP levels maximally. In many conditions, decreased delivery of filtrate to the tip of the loop of Henle also contributes.

TABLE 4–1. Factors That Lead to an Impairment in Renal Water Excretion

- Decreased glomerular filtration rate
- Decreased delivery of filtrate to the diluting segment
- Inhibition of NaCl reabsorption in the diluting segment
- Nonsuppressed antidiuretic hormone

Defective solute absorption in the ascending limb and distal nephron is probably relevant only to hyponatremia encountered with chloriuretic diuretics. In our patient Raymond, the urine osmolality is inappropriately concentrated, suggesting a defect in renal water excretion.

Step 3: Assess the Patient's Volume Status

In patients with hypotonic hyponatremia with inappropriately concentrated urine, one needs to define whether effective arterial volume is decreased. **Most of the causes of hyponatremia result from a decrease in effective arterial volume, which causes baroreceptor stimulation of AVP secretion and leads to decreased distal delivery of filtrate to the tip of the loop of Henle.** If effective arterial volume is low, ECF volume can be low in a volume-depleted patient (hypovolemic hyponatremia) or can be high in an edematous patient (hypervolemic hyponatremia). If effective arterial volume is normal, one is dealing with the euvolemic causes of hyponatremia (isovolemic hyponatremia).

Clinical determination of effective arterial volume is usually straightforward. On physical examination, the best index of effective arterial volume is a patient's pulse and blood pressure. Urinary electrolyte values are also useful in the assessment of effective arterial volume. Patients with a low effective arterial volume tend to have low levels of urinary sodium and chloride and low fractional excretions of sodium and chloride in the urine. Patients with euvolemic hyponatremia, however, are in balance and excrete sodium and chloride at rates that reflect dietary intake of sodium and chloride. Thus, they generally have urinary sodium and chloride values >20 mEq/L and fractional excretions of these electrolytes >1%.

Plasma composition can also be used to assess effective arterial volume. The BUN is particularly sensitive to effective arterial volume. In patients with normal serum creatinine levels, a high BUN suggests a low effective arterial volume and a low BUN suggests a high effective arterial volume. The plasma uric acid value can also be used as a sensitive index of effective arterial volume. In comparing patients with the syndrome of inappropriate ADH secretion (SIADH) and other causes of hyponatremia, patients with low effective arterial volume tend to have an elevated serum uric acid level. In patients with SIADH, serum urate value is not only not elevated but is *depressed*. This is because these patients are volume expanded, although it is clinically difficult to detect the degree of volume expansion.

CLINICAL DISORDERS ASSOCIATED WITH HYPONATREMIA AND AN INAPPROPRIATELY CONCENTRATED URINE

Hypovolemic Hyponatremia

Diuretics

Diuretics are a common cause of hypovolemic hyponatremia. The hyponatremia in this setting is often accompanied by a hypokalemic metabolic alkalosis. In addition to a decreased effective arterial blood volume, diuretics such as furosemide, ethacrynic acid, and thiazides decrease free-water excretion by directly inhibiting Na reabsorption in the thick ascending limb and early distal tubule. Urinary Na is high. Because loop diuretics inhibit generation of a hypertonic medullary interstitium leading to inhibition of ADH-mediated water reabsorption, hyponatremia is much less common than with thiazide diuretics (when urinary concentration is unaffected).

Salt-Losing Nephropathy

Certain interstitial renal diseases can result in a salt-losing nephropathy with resultant hypovolemic hyponatremia. In these diseases, Na loss in the urine is significantly increased despite a contracted effective arterial volume. Examples include medullary cystic disease, analgesic nephropathy, partial urinary tract obstruction, and chronic interstitial nephritis. These patients may need to ingest supplemental NaCl to avoid depletion of ECF volume and secondary hyponatremia.

Mineralocorticoid Deficiency

Patients with Addison's disease develop a decreased effective arterial blood volume as a result of renal salt wastage secondary to lack of mineralocorticoid activity. These patients are hyperkalemic.

Hypervolemic Hyponatremia

The edematous states of congestive heart failure, cirrhosis, and in some cases nephrotic syndrome all share in common a shrunken effective arterial blood volume, which sets into motion the same pathophysiologic effects as with a contracted ECF volume. Thus, delivery of filtrate to the diluting segment is decreased, ADH levels are inappropriately elevated, and thirst is increased. Urine Na concentration is low, reflective of the low effective arterial volume. These patients are recognized clinically by the presence of edema.

Isovolemic Hyponatremia

This condition is noted by the absence of edema and signs of a contracted ECF volume. Because effective arterial volume is not contracted, urine Na level is not low (i.e., >20 mEq/L).

Renal Failure

In the setting of total suppression of ADH and normal renal function, the kidneys can excrete large quantities of water. For example, assuming that 20% of the normal GFR rate of 120 ml/min can be excreted as free water, one can calculate that a normal individual has the capacity to excrete 30 L of water per day. In the setting of renal failure, this capacity to excrete free water is truncated by limited delivery of filtrate to the diluting segment. A patient who has a GFR of 5 ml/min and who excretes 20% of the filtered load of water excretes only 1.4 to 1.5 L/day. **Thus, patients with chronic renal failure can develop hyponatremia by drinking more water than they deliver filtrate distally.**

Syndrome of Inappropriate Secretion of Antidiuretic Hormone

In the setting of euvolemia, concentrated urine and high ADH levels are inappropriate. The most common cause of this condition is SIADH. SIADH is generally associated with diseases of the CNS, usually those that affect the base of the brain, pulmonary diseases, and neoplasms (Table 4–2). These conditions lead to ADH secretion that is inappropriate from the standpoint of both plasma osmolality and effective arterial volume. A number of other factors cause a condition of hypo-osmolality associated with euvolemia and can mimic SIADH.

Glucocorticoid Deficiency

With isolated glucocorticoid deficiency (normal mineralocorticoid activity), isovolemic hypona-

TABLE 4–2. Disorders Associated with the Syndrome of Inappropriate Secretion of Antidiuretic Hormone

- Tumors
  - Oat cell carcinoma
  - Adenocarcinoma of the pancreas
  - Hodgkin's disease
  - Thymoma
- Pulmonary diseases
  - Tuberculosis
  - Lung abscess
  - Viral and bacterial pneumonia
- Central nervous system disorders
  - Brain tumor
  - Encephalitis
  - Subarachnoid hemorrhage
  - Acute intermittent porphyria

tremia can occur. This situation is encountered in states of secondary hypoadrenalism resulting from decreased secretion of ACTH from the pituitary gland. These patients do not have salt wasting and possess an intact ECF volume. Persistent ADH secretion and decreased delivery to the diluting segment are responsible for the hyponatremia. Serum K level is normal.

Hypothyroidism

Lack of circulating thyroid hormone can result in hyponatremia. A decrease in GFR and increased circulating ADH account for the hyponatremia. Thyroid replacement corrects the abnormalities.

Emotional Stress, Pain, Nausea

Emotional stress, pain, and nausea can result in nonosmotic release of ADH. If water ingestion occurs at a time of nausea, pain, or acute psychosis, hyponatremia may ensue.

Drugs

Various drugs have been associated with either increased ADH release or augmented response of the kidneys to ambient ADH levels. These drugs are listed in Table 4–3.

In our patient Raymond's presentation, the low urine Na concentration and the disproportionate increase in BUN suggest a contracted effective arterial blood volume. The physical examination confirms an edematous state. Thus, this patient can best be categorized as having hypervolemic hyponatremia. Patients with congestive heart failure are prone to hyponatremia because of increased circulating levels of ADH stimulated by

TABLE 4–3. Drugs Associated with Hyponatremia According to Major Mechanism of Action

---

- Stimulate antidiuretic hormone (ADH) release
    - Chlorpropamide
    - Clofibrate
    - Cyclophosphamide
    - Vincristine
    - Carbamazepine
    - Amitriptyline
    - Thiothixene, haloperidol, thioridazine
- Potentiation of ADH effect on kidneys
    - Chlorpropamide
    - Carbamazepine
    - Nonsteroidal antiinflammatory drugs
    - Cyclophosphamide
- ADH-like action
    - Oxytocin
    - Deamino-D-arginine vasopressin (DDAVP)

---

a contracted effective arterial blood volume. A decrease in delivery of filtrate to the diluting segment further contributes to an impairment in free-water excretion.

TREATMENT OF HYPONATREMIA

The principal danger of hyponatremia or hypernatremia relates to effects on CNS function due to changes in brain size. Hyponatremia initially leads to cell swelling driven by the higher intracellular osmolality. The net result is equilibration of intracellular and extracellular osmolality at the expense of increased brain volume. Cells in general, and brain cells in particular, then respond by decreasing the number of intracellular osmoles, and as intracellular osmolality decreases, cell size returns toward normal despite the presence of hyponatremia. If the decrease in ECF osmolality is slow, no measurable cell swelling occurs. This pathophysiologic sequence correlates well with clinical observations. If hyponatremia is slow in onset, neurologic symptoms and permanent brain damage are unusual, even if the decreases in Na concentration and ECF osmolality are large. Conversely, if hyponatremia is rapid in onset, cerebral edema and significant CNS symptoms and signs can occur with lesser changes in serum Na concentration.

When a patient with hyponatremia is treated, the Na concentration should be raised at the rate at which it fell. **In a patient whose serum Na concentration has fallen slowly, neurologic symptoms are generally minimal, brain size is normal, and the number of intracellular**

osmoles **is decreased. Sudden return of ECF osmolality to normal values leads to cell shrinkage, neurologic symptoms, and possibly permanent brain damage. Rapid correction has been associated with central pontine myelinolysis. Thus, it is recommended that serum Na level be corrected slowly in these patients.** Patients whose serum Na concentration has decreased rapidly frequently have neurologic symptoms and cerebral edema. In this setting there has not been sufficient time to remove osmoles from the brain, and rapid return to normal ECF osmolality merely returns brain size to normal. In general, the development of hyponatremia in an outpatient setting is more commonly chronic and should be corrected slowly. By contrast, hyponatremia of short duration is more likely to be encountered in hospitalized patients receiving intravenous free water. In symptomatic patients, rapid correction may be necessary. The unusual patient with psychogenic polydipsia can also develop hyponatremia of short duration and, if symptomatic, may similarly require rapid correction.

Therapy of hyponatremia depends on several factors, including the underlying cause, the rapidity of development, and the severity of symptoms and signs. The initial approach in all cases is fluid restriction so that the degree of hyponatremia does not progress. The treatment of hypotonic hyponatremia is outlined in Table 4–4.

Rapid Correction of Hyponatremia

In patients who have acute hyponatremia and who are demonstrating CNS signs or symptoms, rapid correction is indicated. Rapid correction of hyponatremia involves intravenous administration of hypertonic saline (usually 3% NaCl). Generally, an infusion rate that raises serum Na concentration at a rate of 1 mEq/L/hr is used. Present evidence suggests that correction at a more rapid rate may be dangerous. To calculate the amount of Na required, one should use a volume of distribution of total body water (TBW). Although Na is confined to the ECF space, in disorders of osmolality one is replacing an osmolar deficit present throughout the TBW.

$$(\text{Desired Na} - \text{actual Na}) \times \text{TBW}$$
$$= \text{amount of Na required}$$

Assume a patient presents with a serum Na

TABLE 4–4. Treatment of Hyponatremia

Correction	Low ECF Volume	Edema	Euvolemic
Acute Onset			
Slow	Normal saline	Fluid restriction	Fluid restriction
Rapid	Hypertonic saline	Hypertonic saline + furosemide	Hypertonic saline + furosemide
Chronic	Remove cause	Remove cause	Remove cause
		? demeclocycline	Discontinue drug
			Hormone replacement
			Treat cause of SIADH
			Demeclocycline

level of 110 mEq/L, has symptoms of stupor, and demonstrates seizure activity. To raise his serum Na level to 130 mEq/L, one can calculate the amount of 3% saline needed:

$$\text{TBW} = 70 \text{ kg} \times 60\% = 42 \text{ L}$$
$$(130 \text{ mEq/L} - 110 \text{ mEq/L}) \times 42 \text{ L}$$
$$= 840 \text{ mEq Na}$$

Because each liter of 3% saline contains 513 mEq of Na, one would administer 1.6 L of 3% NaCl over 20 hours to raise the serum Na value by 1 mEq/L/hr.

Use of hypertonic saline alone may be associated with volume expansion that would be dangerous in the elderly or in patients with compromised cardiac function. Patients with impaired renal function are particularly prone to volume overload with such Na loads. In this instance, a furosemide diuresis can be used. Hypertonic saline is infused at a rate equal to the urinary loss of Na, chloride, and K that is induced by furosemide.

To calculate the total net negative fluid balance necessary to achieve the desired Na concentration, one can use the following formulas:

$$\text{Body weight} \times 60\% = \text{TBW}$$
$$\text{or } 70 \text{ kg} \times 60\% = 42 \text{ L}$$
$$\text{TBW} - (\text{actual [Na] / desired [Na]}) \times \text{TBW}$$
$$= \text{amount of excess water}$$
$$\text{or } 42 - (110 / 130) \times 42 = 6.5 \text{ L}$$

When a serum Na concentration of 130 mEq/L is obtained, one can simply place the patient on fluid restriction. In this manner, neurologic sequelae resulting from rapid correction of the serum Na can be avoided.

It should be emphasized that these formulas are to be used as guidelines only and that **frequent monitoring of the patient and serum [Na] is needed during these rapid changes in fluid balance.** With advanced renal failure, dialysis is required to correct the hyponatremic state rapidly. Interestingly, patients treated with dialysis for hyponatremia frequently correct their hyponatremia very rapidly; this is, however, generally well tolerated.

PATIENT NUMBER 1 (continued)

Raymond, our publishing house executive, was treated with diuretics and placed on an angiotensin-converting enzyme inhibitor for treatment of his congestive heart failure. As his forward cardiac output increased, his serum sodium concentration slowly returned to normal. Raymond decided that he would now consider retirement but only after he felt comfortable that his son was ready to take over the business.

PATIENT NUMBER 2

Arthur, a 70-year-old man with known chronic renal insufficiency, is brought to the emergency room in a stuporous state. He was a railway worker who had retired 5 years earlier after a successful 30-year career with the Pacific Northwest Railroad. He was recently widowed when his wife of 60 years died of breast cancer 2 years earlier. He lived at home alone. His past medical history was significant for long-standing poorly controlled hypertension and adult-onset diabetes mellitus. On admission, the physical examination shows evidence of a right-sided dense hemiparesis. Laboratory examination is significant for a serum sodium concentration of 170 mEq/L. The urine osmolality is 550 mOsm/L. Urine electrolyte values (mEq/L) are Na <10 and Cl <10. The approach to the hypernatremic patient is outlined in Figure 4–2.

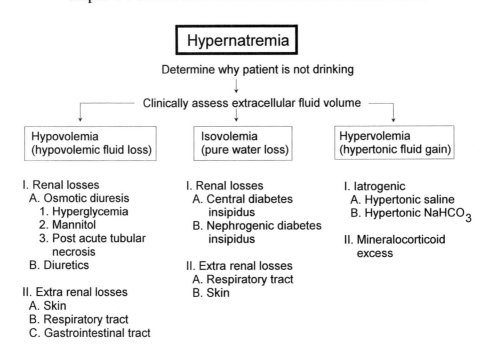

Figure 4–2. Approach to the patient with hypernatremia.

APPROACH TO THE HYPERNATREMIC PATIENT

Step 1: Why Is the Patient Not Drinking?

The initial approach to any patient with hypernatremia is to determine why his or her water intake has been inadequate. **Hypernatremia is rare in conscious patients who have free access to water because of the extreme sensitivity of the thirst mechanism.** Inadequate water intake may result from conditions associated with a specific lesion of the thirst center. More commonly, the level of consciousness is altered so that patients become unaware of thirst or cannot adequately communicate the need for water. In some instances, thirst is adequately sensed but water is unavailable or access to water is restricted because patients are restrained. Reduced sensation of thirst also occurs in otherwise normal individuals as a feature of increasing age, **rendering the elderly particularly susceptible to the development of hypernatremia.**

PATIENT NUMBER 2 (continued)

Arthur's altered mental status and physical disability were responsible for his failure to drink water. He was found at home by one of his two daughters, who immediately summoned help and transported him to the hospital. As a result of ongoing insensible water loss, hypernatremia ensued. Increased urine osmolality is an appropriate response to the free-water deficit. Normally, the kidneys can concentrate the urine to as high as 1200 mOsm/L in the setting of free-water deficits. Arthur's urine osmolality of only 550 mOsm/L is reflective of the known age-related decline in the ability to concentrate the urine maximally. The decreased urinary Na and Cl concentration allow one to conclude that Arthur has hypovolemic hypernatremia (discussed later).

Step 2: Has There Been Accelerated Water Loss or Increased Sodium Gain?

The next step in the evaluation of hypernatremia is to search for the presence of accelerated water loss or increased sodium gain, both of which increase the likelihood of a patient's developing hypernatremia. This can be accomplished best by clinically assessing the patient's ECF status (see Fig. 4–2).

Hypovolemic Hypernatremia

Hypernatremia in a volume-depleted patient results from fluid losses in which the urine sodium concentration is less than the plasma concentration. Extrarenal losses of salt and water from the gastrointestinal tract or from profuse sweating or renal losses due to osmotic diuresis are the major causes. Diuretics can also predispose to the development of hypernatremia because these agents are associated with renal salt and water loss but water loss to a greater extent. It should be emphasized, however, that **hypernatremia develops only if there is an associated impairment in water intake.** Urine sodium concentration should be low with extrarenal fluid losses, whereas the concentration is typically high with an osmotic diuresis or during the administration of a diuretic.

Hypervolemic Hypernatremia

Hypernatremia in the setting of hypervolemia can result from iatrogenic administration of hypertonic NaCl or hypertonic sodium bicarbonate or from mineralocorticoid excess. Administration of hypertonic fluids is usually evident from the clinical setting and is associated with a high urine sodium concentration. Mineralocorticoid excess is suggested by the presence of hypertension and hypokalemic metabolic alkalosis. Urine sodium concentration varies according to dietary intake.

Isovolemic Hypernatremia

Pure water loss, whether from mucocutaneous routes or from the kidneys, causes isovolemic hypernatremia. Because two thirds of pure water loss is sustained from within cells, patients do not become clinically volume depleted unless the water deficit becomes substantial. Insensible losses from the respiratory tract or skin result in concentrated urine. Inappropriate water loss by the kidneys, whether from central or nephrogenic diabetes insipidus, results in dilute urine. Although renal water loss can lead to hypernatremia in patients with impaired thirst or restricted access to water, most patients with diabetes insipidus have neither of these defects, and patients typically present with polyuria and polydipsia and a normal serum sodium concentration. As a result, the initial clue to the presence of diabetes insipidus usually comes not from the detection of hypernatremia but rather during the evaluation of the polyuric patient.

PATIENT NUMBER 3

Cara, a 35-year-old black woman who was employed as a track coach at a local high school, presented with dyspnea on exertion 2 years before admission. At that time, an extensive evaluation revealed that she had sarcoidosis. Her symptoms markedly improved with steroids, and she has been symptom free for the past 18 months. She is married and has two children. Cara now presents with polyuria and polydipsia, which began 2 to 3 weeks ago after returning from a successful track meet at a nearby town. Her urine volumes average 5 to 6 L/day. Her serum sodium concentration is 143 mEq/L. Her urine osmolality is 80 mOsm/L.

EVALUATION OF POLYURIA AND POLYDIPSIA

Polyuria can result from an osmotic diuresis or from a water diuresis. In turn, a water diuresis may result from inappropriate water loss, as in either central or nephrogenic diabetes insipidus, or may represent appropriate water loss, as in primary polydipsia (Table 4–5). As depicted in Figure 4–3, the initial steps in differentiating these processes are to consider the clinical setting and to examine the urine osmolality.

Step 1: Is the Polyuria a Result of a Water Diuresis or an Osmotic Diuresis?

The presence of an osmotic diuresis causing polyuria is often evident from the clinical setting. Poorly controlled glucose levels in a diabetic patient, administration of mannitol to a patient with increased intracranial pressure, and high-protein enteral feedings all are examples in which polyuria is a result of an osmotic diuresis. When not clinically obvious, the finding of isosmotic or hyperosmotic urine (>300 mOsm/L) in a poly-

TABLE 4–5. Etiology of Central and Nephrogenic Diabetes Insipidus

Central Diabetes Insipidus	Nephrogenic Diabetes Insipidus
Familial	Familial (X-linked recessive)
Trauma	Amyloid
Tumors	Sjögren's syndrome
Pituitary tumors	Sickle cell disease
Craniopharyngioma	Postobstructive
Metastatic (breast, lung)	Hypokalemia
Granulomatous disease	Hypercalcemia
Sarcoidosis	Drugs
Eosinophilic granuloma	Lithium
Encephalitis	Demeclocycline
Ischemic encephalopathy	Methoxyflurane

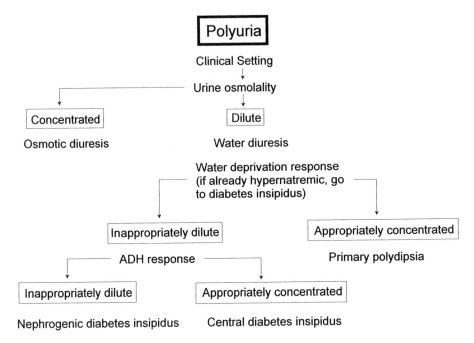

Figure 4–3. Approach to the patient with polyuria.

uric patient is suggestive of a solute or osmotic diuresis. The low urine osmolality in our patient Cara is consistent with a water diuresis.

After excluding the presence of an osmotic diuresis, one must then discriminate between the causes of a water diuresis. Some features of the clinical history may provide a clue to the correct diagnosis. In patients with central diabetes insipidus, the onset of symptoms is characteristically abrupt in nature, whereas patients with nephrogenic diabetes insipidus typically have a more gradual onset of symptoms. Patients with primary polydipsia are much more vague in dating the onset of their symptoms. Both nephrogenic and central diabetes insipidus are characterized by severe and frequent nocturia, a feature that is typically absent in patients with primary polydipsia. Patients with central diabetes insipidus seem to have a craving for ice water, which is not typical in the other two conditions. Finally, the finding of a serum sodium concentration <140 mEq/L is suggestive of primary polydipsia because these patients tend to be in mild positive water balance. By contrast, a serum sodium concentration >140 mEq/L is more suggestive of either central or nephrogenic diabetes insipidus because these patients tend to be in mild negative water balance.

Step 2: Water Deprivation Test

Primary polydipsia and central and nephrogenic diabetes insipidus can be distinguished by com-

paring the response of urinary osmolality to water deprivation and subsequent ADH administration. Typically, a patient is fluid restricted until urine osmolality changes by <30 mOsm/L on three consecutive measurements or until body weight falls by 3% to 5%. At this point, 5 units of AVP is administered subcutaneously and urine osmolality is measured 30 and 60 minutes afterward. In normal persons, the urine reaches a maximal concentration of approximately 1000 to 1200 mOsm/L over the course of 12 to 16 hours and demonstrates no further rise in urine osmolality on AVP administration. In patients with central diabetes insipidus, the urine concentrates to approximately 200 to 300 mOsm/L by AVP-independent mechanisms but fails to concentrate maximally owing to the lack of circulating AVP. When exogenous AVP is administered, a dramatic reduction in urine volume and a simultaneous increase in urine osmolality result. In nephrogenic diabetes insipidus, circulating AVP levels are high but urine osmolality remains low and unresponsive to parenteral administration of AVP. Patients with primary polydipsia demonstrate only a submaximal ability to concentrate the urine in response to fluid deprivation. Because circulating levels of AVP are normal, these patients demonstrate no further rise in urine osmolality in response to supplemental AVP. The inability to concentrate the urine maximally is a result of medullary washout induced by the preceding chronic polyuria. With sustained fluid restriction, the hypertonicity of the renal medulla becomes reestablished and the concentrating ability of the kidneys returns to normal.

PATIENT NUMBER 3 (continued)

*Water was restricted until Cara's serum sodium increased to 145 mEq/L. Despite the rise in serum sodium concentration, the urine osmolality increased to only 200 mOsm/L and urine flow rates remained high. The inability to concentrate the urine further excludes primary polydipsia as a cause of Cara's polyuria. After 5 units of aqueous AVP was administered, her urine osmolality increased to 640 mOsm/L during the next several hours. This response confirms the diagnosis of central diabetes insipidus. Sarcoidosis is a known cause of central diabetes insipidus as a result of granulomatous disease in the hypothalamus. Although not present in Cara's case, sarcoidosis-induced hypercalcemia can cause nephrogenic diabetes insipidus as well. **The patient was started on intranasal DDAVP, with complete resolution of her symptoms. She continues to be quite active and enjoys great success in her coaching career.***

TREATMENT OF HYPERNATREMIA

Increases in ECF osmolality initially cause cell shrinkage within the brain. Signs and symptoms include lethargy, weakness, fasciculations, seizures, and coma. **This reduction in brain size may also cause rupture of cerebral veins with intracerebral and subarachnoid hemorrhage.** The cells respond to this by the generation of intracellular osmoles, which pull water back into the cells, returning brain size to normal. These new intracellular osmoles include ions transported into cells, as well as other more poorly defined osmoles, referred to as *idiogenic osmoles.*

If extracellular osmolality is rapidly returned to normal during the therapy of hypernatremia, the extra intracellular osmoles pull water into the brain cells, resulting in cerebral edema. Thus, in general, hypernatremia should be corrected slowly by water administration at a rate that leads to half correction in 24 hours.

Calculation of Water Deficit

One can calculate the water deficit using a volume of distribution of TBW, assuming that total body cations remain constant.

$$TBW_{present} \cdot [Na]_{present} = TBW_{normal} \cdot [Na]_{normal}$$

The differences between the two TBWs is the amount of water required to correct the serum Na concentration. The water deficit in patient 2 would be as follows:

$$75 \text{ kg} \times 0.60 = 45 \text{ L (TBW)}$$
$$45 \text{ L} \times 170 \text{ mEq/L} = TBW_{normal}$$
$$\times 140 \text{ mEq/L}$$
$$TBW_{normal} = 54.6 \text{ L}$$
$$54.6 \text{ L} - 45 \text{ L} = 9.6 \text{ L water deficit}$$

Correction of the water deficit would require 9.6 L of positive water balance. In order to avoid the development of cerebral edema, chronic hypernatremia in particular should be corrected slowly. The water deficit should be replaced at a rate that leads to half correction in 24 hours. As with the treatment of hyponatremia, frequent monitoring of the patient and serum Na concentration is essential. The previous calculation should be considered only a rough estimate.

PATIENT NUMBER 4

Jean-Pierre is a 43-year-old man with a history of diarrhea that has lasted for several weeks. He is a 10-year employee of the United States State Department, where he specializes in agricultural development in developing countries. During the past 2 years, he has been stationed in Katmandu, Nepal. He returned to the United States 2 weeks ago with his wife and two children and is currently awaiting his next assignment. The diarrhea began while in Nepal and has continued up until the time of admission. During the past 3 days, Jean-Pierre has noted progressive weakness. Laboratory examination reveals the following (mEq/L) results: Na 140, Cl 110, HCO_3 16, and K 2.0. An arterial blood gas determination shows a pH of 7.28 and a PCO_2 of 30 mm Hg. The urine potassium concentration is 15 mEq/L.

APPROACH TO THE PATIENT WITH HYPOKALEMIA

Step 1: Is the Hypokalemia Due to a Cell Shift?

In the absence of physical and historical evidence of gastrointestinal or renal K losses, either a redistribution of K at the cellular level or laboratory error accounts for a low serum K value. The only spurious cause of hypokalemia is leukemia.

In patients with WBC counts of 100 to 250,000, the WBCs extract K from the serum.

The regulation of K distribution between the intracellular and extracellular space is referred to as *internal K balance*. Although the kidneys are ultimately responsible for maintenance of total body K, factors that modulate internal balance are important in the disposal of acute K loads. Cell shifts are critical, in that only 2% of total body K is located in the ECF. A high-potassium meal could potentially double extracellular potassium were it not for the rapid shift of the potassium load into cells. The kidneys cannot excrete K rapidly enough in this setting to prevent life-threatening hyperkalemia. Thus, it is important that this excess K be rapidly shifted and stored in cells until the kidneys have successfully excreted the K load. **The major regulators of K shift into cells are insulin and catecholamines, with a lesser effect mediated by metabolic and respiratory alkalosis.**

Insulin excess, whether given exogenously in a diabetic patient or as endogenous secretion in a normal person given a high-glucose load, lowers the serum K level. Beta agonists used in the treatment of bronchospasm or in treating premature labor effect similar K shifts. In the setting of an acute myocardial infarction, hypokalemia may result as a sequela of high circulating epinephrine levels and might predispose to arrhythmias in this clinical setting. Other clinical disorders resulting in intracellular sequestration of K are treatment of megaloblastic anemia with vitamin B_{12}, hypothermia, and barium poisoning. Hypokalemic periodic paralysis is inherited in an autosomal dominant pattern and is characterized by episodic hypokalemia resulting in muscle weakness. A similar but noninherited syndrome has been observed in thyrotoxic patients, often those of Japanese descent.

In Jean-Pierre's case, neither the clinical history nor laboratory findings suggest a cellular shift as the cause of his hypokalemia. Hypokalemia that results from cellular shifts is usually transient. Hypokalemia that is chronic always reflects a decrease in total body K content.

Step 2: What Is the Cause of Decreased Total Body Potassium?

In the absence of a cellular redistribution, low serum K level can result from inadequate dietary intake, extrarenal losses (e.g., gastrointestinal or skin), or renal losses. It should be emphasized that factors overlap among these groups. The urinary K concentration serves as a useful guide in discerning between these possibilities. A urine K concentration of <20 mEq/L is suggestive of extrarenal losses, whereas a urine concentration of >20 mEq/L suggests renal K losses.

Inadequate Dietary Intake

Inadequate dietary intake is an unusual cause of hypokalemia. However, extended lengths of time without K ingestion lead to hypokalemia. Clinical situations associated with extremely K-deficient diets include anorexia nervosa, crash diets, alcoholism, and intestinal malabsorption. Increased renal K excretion owing to magnesium deficiency (which is often present in these clinical situations) may contribute to the observed hypokalemia.

Extrarenal K Losses

Loss of K in sweat, with its low concentration of K, is an unusual cause of K depletion. However, during physical training, sweat losses can become substantial and K depletion may result. Gastrointestinal syndromes are the most common clinical disorders of extrarenal K losses. Diarrhea truly leads to fecal K wastage and is associated with a normal anion gap acidosis. Although usually associated with a low urinary K concentration, the acidosis per se can lead to some degree of renal K wasting through increased distal delivery of Na. As discussed later, the acidosis results in K redistribution out of cells, leading to a degree of hypokalemia that is not as severe as the degree of K depletion.

PATIENT NUMBER 4 (continued)

The low urinary K concentration in our patient Jean-Pierre suggests an extrarenal source of potassium loss. The patient has developed a decrease in total body potassium as a result of fecal K losses. The normal gap acidosis in this patient has the effect of shifting K into the extracellular space. As a result, the serum K concentration tends to be higher than it would be in the absence of acidosis and can mislead one into underestimating the magnitude of the total body K deficit. The administration of bicarbonate without first correcting the K deficit in such a patient can precipitate symptomatic hypokalemia, because alkalemia has the effect of shifting K into cells. Thus, in patients with hypokalemic acidosis, one should correct the serum potassium value before correcting the acidosis.

Renal Potassium Losses

Potassium is freely filtered by the glomeruli but is extensively reabsorbed by the proximal tubules and loops of Henle so that approximately 10% of the filtered load reaches the distal nephron. The distal nephron secretes K into the tubular fluid, which is excreted. Under most physiologic and pathologic conditions, K delivery to the distal nephron remains small and does not vary, but rather the rate of secretion by the distal nephron varies. Thus, the rate of K secretion in the distal nephrons determines the rate of K excretion. **Two of the most important physiologic determinants of renal K excretion are mineralocorticoid secretion and distal sodium and fluid delivery.**

Aldosterone is a major determinant of K secretion. Aldosterone-induced stimulation of Na reabsorption in the collecting tubules makes the luminal potential more negative, thus stimulating K secretion. In addition, mineralocorticoids directly stimulate K secretion in the distal nephron. Increased distal delivery of Na stimulates distal Na absorption, which makes the luminal potential more negative and thus increases K secretion. In addition, increased luminal flow rate lowers luminal K concentration, secondarily stimulating K secretion.

The dependence of K secretion on distal delivery and aldosterone levels helps to make K excretion independent of volume status. When patients are volume overloaded, distal delivery is increased but aldosterone is suppressed. When patients are volume depleted, aldosterone is increased (secondary hyperaldosteronism) but distal delivery is decreased. In both of the foregoing states, K homeostasis is maintained. Disruption of this balance explains many of the renal forms of hypokalemia. The causes of hypokalemia, grouped according to the physiologic determinants of renal K excretion, are listed in Table 4–6.

PRIMARY MINERALOCORTICOID EXCESS

In conditions classified as primary mineralocorticoid excess, increases in mineralocorticoid activity cannot be attributed to decreased ECF volume or hyperkalemia. An increase in mineralocorticoids in the absence of volume contraction leads to a high incidence of hypertension, but edema is unusual. A so-called escape occurs before sufficient salt is retained for edema formation. In these conditions, normal or increased ECF volume leads to normal or increased distal delivery in the presence of high mineralocorticoid levels and thus renal K wasting.

TABLE 4–6. Renal Causes of Hypokalemia

- Primary mineralocorticoid excess
  Adrenal adenoma
  Bilateral adrenal hyperplasia
- ↑ Renin → ↑ Aldosterone
  Renin secretion tumor
  Renovascular hypertension
  Accelerated hypertension
- ↑ Nonaldosterone mineralocorticoid
  Cushing's syndrome
  Licorice ingestion
- Decreased salt absorption proximal to the collecting tubule
  Diuretics
  Osmotic diuretics
  Bartter's syndrome
  Mg deficiency
  Distal delivery of nonreabsorbable anion
    Penicillins (carbenicillin, ticarcillin)
    Ketoacidosis
    Metabolic alkalosis
    Proximal renal tubular acidosis
    Acetazolamide

DECREASED SALT ABSORPTION PROXIMAL TO THE COLLECTING TUBULE

Inhibition of salt absorption proximal to the collecting tubule increases distal delivery and leads to small degrees of volume depletion that secondarily elevate aldosterone levels. The combination of increased aldosterone levels and increased distal delivery leads to increased renal K wasting and hypokalemia. This group of disorders is different from the previous group in that elevated aldosterone levels are appropriate for the mildly decreased ECF volume.

The most common cause of renal K wasting is diuretic ingestion. As is obvious from the foregoing discussion, any diuretic that acts proximal to the cortical collecting tubule increases renal K excretion. This includes diuretics that act in the proximal tubule, such as acetazolamide; diuretics that act in the loop of Henle, such as furosemide and ethacrynic acid; and diuretics that work in the early distal tubule, such as the thiazides. Osmotic diuresis also leads to K wasting by this mechanism. Osmotic diuresis occurs in poorly controlled diabetes mellitus when serum glucose rises to higher levels than the proximal tubule can absorb. In addition, osmotic diuretics are used therapeutically in some conditions.

Bartter's syndrome is a rare condition in which there appears to be a primary defect in loop of Henle salt absorption. This leads to chronic increases in distal delivery and a chronic state of mild volume contraction. Patients are hypokalemic and have very high renin and aldosterone levels.

In certain conditions, Na is delivered distally with a nonreabsorbable anion. This increases the lumen negative potential difference and leads to K wasting. All penicillins are nonreabsorbable anions, but only a few, such as carbenicillin, are given in sufficient quantities to lead to significant K wasting. Ketoacids act as nonreabsorbable anions in patients with ketoacidosis due to diabetes, alcoholism, or starvation. Bicarbonate can function as a nonreabsorbable anion if it is delivered to the distal nephron in greater amounts than can be reabsorbed proximally. This occurs in active vomiting, in proximal renal tubular acidosis, and with acetazolamide administration.

ACID-BASE CHANGES

All chronic acid-base disorders can lead to some degree of renal K wasting. However, metabolic alkalosis, both acute and chronic, clearly leads to the most marked degree of hypokalemia. This is because of increased collecting tubular cell K concentration, distal delivery of bicarbonate (behaving as a nonreabsorbable anion), and redistribution of K into cells. Metabolic acidosis may also lead to mild degrees of K depletion (due to decreased proximal salt absorption), but redistribution of K out of cells frequently prevents hypokalemia.

CLINICAL FEATURES OF HYPOKALEMIA

The most important clinical manifestations of hypokalemia occur in the neuromuscular system. Low serum K level leads to cell hyperpolarization, which impedes impulse conduction and muscle contraction. A flaccid paralysis typically develops in the hands and feet and moves proximally, eventually including the trunk and respiratory muscles. **Death may result from respiratory insufficiency.**

A myopathy may also occur and in its most severe form can lead to frank rhabdomyolysis (muscle cell lysis) and renal failure. K deficiency has also been thought to contribute to rhabdomyolysis occurring secondary to strenuous exercise. Hypokalemia can also lead to CNS changes with confusion and affective disorders and to smooth muscle dysfunction including paralytic ileus.

Cardiac complications of hypokalemia may also be important. The typical electrocardiogram (ECG) change is ST depression, T-wave flattening, and an increase in the amplitude of the U wave. This change, often misread as a widened QT, is nonspecific, often absent, and of little clinical use. It is well known that **patients on cardiac glycosides have an increased incidence of premature ventricular contractions and supraventricular and ventricular tachyarrhythmias when hypokalemic.** A concern is that hypokalemia may predispose to these arrhythmias in patients not on these drugs.

Hypokalemia also causes a renal concentrating defect due to both a decrease in the medullary gradient and resistance of the cortical collecting tubule to ADH. This leads to polyuria and polydipsia. Hypokalemia can cause Na retention and in some circumstances can contribute to metabolic alkalosis. Prolonged hypokalemia can also lead to tubulointerstitial nephritis and renal failure. Because insulin release is regulated partially by serum K, hypokalemia can lead to glucose intolerance.

TREATMENT OF HYPOKALEMIA

In treating patients with hypokalemia, it is useful but often difficult to ascertain the size of the K deficit. Serum K determinations can at times be misleading about the degree of deficit, because a normal or even increased K level can occur with significant total body K depletion. In the absence of significant K shifts, a decline in the serum K level from 4 to 3 mEq/L generally is associated with a deficit of 300 to 400 mEq intracellular K per 70 kg of body weight. A serum K concentration of 2 mEq/L reflects a deficit of approximately 600 mEq. Despite these guidelines, **one should monitor the serum K level frequently during replacement therapy.**

K can be given orally or intravenously as the KCl salt. K bicarbonate or citrate can be given if a patient has concomitant metabolic acidosis. The safest way to administer KCl is orally. KCl can be given in doses of 100 to 150 mEq/day. Liquid KCl is bitter tasting and, like the tablet, can be irritating to the gastric mucosa. The microencapsulated or wax-matrix forms of KCl are better tolerated.

Intravenous administration of K may be necessary if a patient cannot take oral medications or if the K deficit is large and is resulting in cardiac arrhythmias, respiratory paralysis, or rhabdomyolysis. Intravenous KCl should be given at a maximum rate of 20 mEq/hr and maximum concentration of 40 mEq/L. Higher concentrations result in phlebitis. Replacement of KCl in dextrose-containing solutions can actually lower the serum K further, secondary to insulin release. Thus, saline solutions are preferred. **On rare** occasions, higher concentrations of K may have to be given; frequent measurement of serum K and continuous ECG monitoring are essential in this case to prevent iatrogenic hyperkalemia, which may be fatal.

Additional therapy of chronic hypokalemia involves the use of K-sparing diuretics such as amiloride, spironolactone, or triamterene. These agents are useful in situations of primary or secondary hyperaldosteronism. One must be cautious in using these agents in patients with renal insufficiency or in patients with other disorders that impair renal K excretion.

TABLE 4–7. Causes of Hyperkalemia

- Pseudohyperkalemia
- Cellular redistribution
  - Acidosis
  - Cell shrinkage (hypertonicity)
  - Deficiency of insulin
  - Beta blockers
  - Hyperkalemic periodic paralysis
  - Cell injury
- Excess intake (very rare)
- Decreased renal excretion
  - Decreased distal delivery of Na (oliguric renal failure)
  - Mineralocorticoid deficiency
  - Defect of cortical collecting tubule

PATIENT NUMBER 5

Willy, a 30-year-old man with known insulin-dependent diabetes mellitus, is admitted with a diagnosis of diabetic ketoacidosis. The patient was first diagnosed with diabetes 10 years ago. Willy is unemployed and lives with his mother in a small apartment. He has had several prior admissions for ketoacidosis and on several occasions has admitted to poor compliance with taking his prescribed insulin regimen. Willy has had difficulty dealing with his illness ever since his father died of cardiovascular disease 3 years ago. His father was also diabetic and had undergone amputations of both legs secondary to marked peripheral vascular disease. On physical examination, evidence of cellulitis is noted on Willy's right lower extremity. His serum electrolyte values (mEq/L) are Na 135, K 6.2, Cl 95, and HCO_3 10. His serum glucose level is 850 mg/dl. His arterial blood gas shows a pH of 7.29 and a PCO_2 of 20 mm Hg.

APPROACH TO THE PATIENT WITH HYPERKALEMIA

Like the hypokalemic disorders, a high serum K level can occur in the setting of normal or altered body stores of K. The body has a marked ability to protect against hyperkalemia. This includes regulatory mechanisms that excrete excess K quickly and mechanisms that redistribute excess K into cells until it is excreted. All causes of hyperkalemia therefore involve abnormalities in these mechanisms. The causes of hyperkalemia are listed in Table 4–7.

Step 1: Does the Patient Have Pseudohyperkalemia?

In approaching a patient with a high measured serum K concentration, it is important to remember that not all of these patients have true hyperkalemia. Because cell K concentrations are large and plasma K concentrations are small, small leaks of K out of blood cells can have large effects on measured serum K. Normally, when blood is allowed to clot before centrifugation, enough K is released from platelets to raise serum K by approximately 0.5 mEq/L. This is accounted for in the limits of normal. However, excessive errors can occur in the presence of marked thrombocytosis, marked leukocytosis, or hemolysis on obtaining blood samples. These conditions are referred to as *pseudohyperkalemia*. None of the causes of pseudohyperkalemia were present in Willy, our diabetic patient.

Step 2: Is the Hyperkalemia a Result of a Cellular Shift?

Cellular redistribution is a more important cause of hyperkalemia than of hypokalemia. One should realize that as little as a 2% shift of intracellular K to the ECF results in a serum K of 8 mEq/L. Metabolic acidosis promotes K exit from cells dependent on the type of acid present. Mineral acidosis (NH_4Cl or HCl), by virtue of the relative impermeability of the chloride anion, results in the greatest efflux of K from cells, whereas organic acidosis (i.e., lactic, β-hydroxybutyric, or methylmalonic acid) results in no significant efflux of K. Acute respiratory acidosis also results in a small shift of K out of cells.

With regard to our patient Willy, sudden increases in osmolality cause K to move out of cells. This shift is most often noted in diabetic persons. In fact, it is the hypertonic state as well as insulin deficiency that accounts for the relative hyperkalemia encountered in patients who have diabetic ketoacidosis and are K depleted. Thus, K shifts out of cells are due to hyperosmolarity and insulin deficiency in ketoacidosis.

Beta-adrenergic-blocking agents can interfere with the disposal of acute K loads. Hyperkalemia can also be caused by the depolarizing muscle relaxant succinylcholine and by severe digitalis poisoning. Hyperkalemic periodic paralysis is a rare autosomal dominant disorder characterized by repeated bouts of paralysis associated with hyperkalemia.

Because 98% of body K is located within cells, cell death can result in substantial endogenous loads of K. Muscle breakdown due to crush injury or rhabdomyolysis can be associated with a substantial increase in serum K concentration. Cell death as occurs in tumor lysis syndromes can also be a source of substantial K loads. These syndromes are often associated with compromised renal function.

PATIENT NUMBER 5 (continued)

Willy was treated with intravenous fluids and insulin, and his serum K concentration decreased rapidly to 2.0 mg/dl. The increased K on admission that was a result of a cellular shift induced by insulin deficiency and hyperosmolality was in the setting of total body K depletion. Patients with diabetic ketoacidosis frequently have total body K depletion due to renal K losses that result from increased distal Na delivery in the setting of high aldosterone levels.

Before discharge, Willy was evaluated by the entire health care team. The social worker was successful in arranging for a job for the patient. Willy was quite appreciative and stated that he was going to pay much more attention to his health than he had in the past. Subsequent follow-up was significant for much improved glycemic control. On routine laboratory evaluation, however, persistent hyperkalemia was noted. The patient's only medications include split-dose insulin therapy and 600 mg ibuprofen, which he takes for occasional joint pain. Laboratory examination reveals the following results (mEq/L): Na 140, K 6.2, Cl 106, and CO_2 22. The serum creatinine level is 2.5 mg/100 ml. Blood pressure is 150/105 mm Hg. A 24-hour urine collection reveals a creatinine clearance of 35 ml/min. An ECG is obtained and is normal.

Although redistribution of K can result in hyperkalemia, the rise in K is generally mild and nonsustained. Prolonged and severe hyperkalemia implies the presence of concomitant decreases in renal K excretion. After precluding pseudohyperkalemia and a cell shift, one has to consider a disorder in renal potassium excretion.

Step 3: Why Does the Patient Have a Disturbance in Renal Potassium Excretion?

Decreased renal excretion of K can be due to one or more of three abnormalities: decreased

distal delivery of Na, mineralocorticoid deficiency, and abnormal cortical collecting tubule function.

Decreased Distal Delivery of Sodium

As discussed previously, most of filtered K is reabsorbed before the distal tubule. K excretion is then determined by the rate at which K is secreted in the distal nephron. Acute decreases in GFR, as occur in acute renal failure, would therefore not be expected to have a marked effect on K excretion. Acute decreases in GFR may, however, lead to marked decreases in distal delivery of salt and water, which may secondarily decrease distal K secretion. Thus, when acute renal failure is oliguric, hyperkalemia is a frequent problem; when acute renal failure is nonoliguric, distal delivery is usually sufficient and hyperkalemia is unusual.

Chronic renal failure is more complicated than acute renal failure. In addition to the decreased GFR and secondary decrease in distal delivery, nephron dropout occurs and less collecting tubule mass is available to secrete K. However, this is counterbalanced by a K adaptation, in which the remaining nephrons develop an increased ability to excrete K. In addition, these patients possess two other defenses against hyperkalemia. First, in response to a K load they redistribute the K into cells faster than do normal people. Second, they have a markedly increased rate of K excretion in their stool. Thus, although patients with chronic renal failure do not excrete a K load as fast as do normal persons, hyperkalemia is unusual until chronic renal failure has progressed to a GFR <5 ml/min. The occurrence of hyperkalemia with a GFR of >10 ml/min should raise the question of decreased mineralocorticoid activity or a specific lesion of the cortical collecting tubule.

DECREASED MINERALOCORTICOID ACTIVITY

Aldosterone deficiency can occur alone or in combination with decreased cortisol levels. Addison's disease is the deficiency of aldosterone and cortisol due to destruction of the adrenal glands. Certain enzyme defects can result in either isolated deficiency of aldosterone or adrenogenital syndromes associated with decreased mineralocorticoid activity. Heparin administration is associated with decreased adrenal secretion of aldosterone (Fig. 4–4).

Angiotensin-converting enzyme inhibitors lead

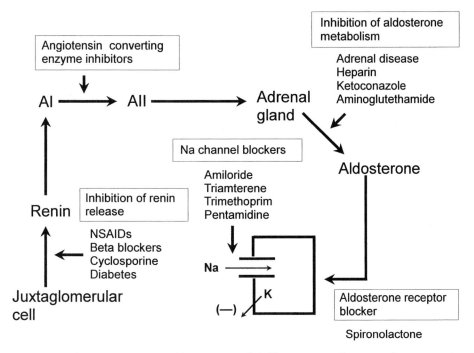

Figure 4–4. The renin–angiotensin–aldosterone cascade. Aldosterone stimulates Na reabsorption in the collecting duct, which in turn generates a lumen negative potential. The luminal electronegativity serves as a driving force for potassium excretion. Drugs that interfere in this process are depicted according to mechanism of action.

to hyperkalemia by decreasing angiotensin II levels, a critical mediator of aldosterone secretion. Renin levels are high and aldosterone levels are low in all of these conditions. The syndrome of hyporeninemic hypoaldosteronism accounts for the majority of unexplained hyperkalemia in patients in whom the GFR and K intake would not be expected to result in hyperkalemia. Diabetic nephropathy and interstitial renal disease are the most common clinical entities associated with this syndrome. Other causes of renal disease associated with hyporeninemic hypoaldosteronism include analgesic nephropathy, urinary tract obstruction, sickle cell disease, systemic lupus erythematosus, and amyloidosis. Nonsteroidal antiinflammatory drugs are associated with decreased renin secretion. Additionally, these agents can cause hyperkalemia by decreasing GFR and reducing distal delivery of Na. Cyclosporine administration is associated with the development of hyperkalemia in renal transplant recipients. Although cyclosporine has a direct effect on the renal tubules, many patients taking this drug have low renin and aldosterone levels. These patients additionally may have a primary tubular defect at the level of the tubule independent of cyclosporine. Beta$_1$ receptor blockade also results in a hyporeninemic state.

DISTAL TUBULAR DEFECT

Certain interstitial renal diseases can affect the distal nephron specifically and lead to hyperkalemia in the presence of mild decreases in GFR and normal aldosterone levels. Many of these diseases are the same ones that can cause hyporeninemic hypoaldosteronism, and the impaired renin release and defect in tubular secretion frequently coexist. Examples include renal transplantation, lupus erythematosus, amyloidosis, urinary obstruction, and sickle cell disease.

The K-sparing diuretics impair the ability of the cortical collecting tubule to secrete K (see Fig. 4–4). Amiloride and triamterene inhibit Na reabsorption, thus abolishing the lumen negative potential and therefore inhibiting K secretion. Other compounds that block the Na channel and that have been clinically associated with hyperkalemia include trimethoprim and pentamidine. Spironolactone competes with aldosterone and thus blocks the mineralocorticoid effect. Although the potassium-sparing diuretics are useful in patients with a hypokalemic tendency, they weaken an important defense mechanism against hyperkalemia. They should therefore be avoided in patients with other defects that predispose to hyperkalemia (i.e., diabetes mellitus, chronic renal insufficiency).

CLINICAL FEATURES OF HYPERKALEMIA

All of the clinically important manifestations of hyperkalemia occur in excitable tissue. Because the potential across cell membranes is in part determined by the ratio of intracellular to extracellular K, hyperkalemia leads to depolarization of the resting membrane. Conduction velocity is markedly slowed as a result of this resetting of the threshold potential.

The heart is certainly the most sensitive to this depolarizing effect, and changes are observable in the ECG. The progressive changes of hyperkalemia are:

1. Peaking of T waves
2. ST segment depression
3. Widening of the PR interval
4. Widening of the QRS interval
5. Loss of the P wave
6. Sine wave pattern

The appearance of a sine wave pattern is ominous and is a harbinger of impending ventricular fibrillation and asystole. The correlation of ECG changes with the serum K depends on the rapidity of onset of the hyperkalemia. Generally, with acute onset of hyperkalemia, ECG changes appear at a serum K of 6 to 7 mEq/L. With chronic hyperkalemia, however, the ECG may remain normal up to a concentration of 8 to 9 mEq/L. The treatment of hyperkalemia is based more on the ECG findings than the absolute serum value. All patients should have their serum K corrected, but patients with ECG changes should be treated emergently. The presence of hypocalcemia, hyponatremia, and acidemia worsens the cardiac manifestations of hyperkalemia.

Neuromuscular manifestations may also be observed with hyperkalemia. Paresthesias and fasciculations in the arms and legs are initially noted. As the serum K level continues to rise, an ascending paralysis with eventual flaccid quadriplegia supervenes. Trunk, head, and respiratory muscles are classically spared, but rarely respiratory failure can occur.

TREATMENT OF ACUTE HYPERKALEMIA

The goals of therapy of acute hyperkalemia fall into three categories: first, to counteract the depolarizing effect on the myocardium; second, to shift K into cells; and third, to effect a net loss of K from the body.

Treatment to Effect Stabilization of Cell Membranes

Calcium in the form of intravenous 10% calcium gluconate/chloride, 10 ml, is given. The immediate treatment of life-threatening hyperkalemia is administration of calcium, usually in the form of calcium gluconate or calcium chloride. Calcium reduces the threshold potential (makes it less negative) and reduces the propensity for cardiac arrhythmias. The presence of late ECG changes such as an increasing PR interval or a widening QRS complex warrants treatment with calcium.

Treatment with Resultant Potassium Movement into Cells

Glucose and Insulin Therapy. $D_{50}W$, 50 ml, can be given either as an intravenous bolus with 10 to 20 units of regular insulin or as a continuous infusion over 1 to 2 hours. Administration of glucose and insulin shifts K into cells. Acute administration of glucose without insulin can potentially worsen hyperkalemia in diabetic patients by raising extracellular osmolality and causing K to shift into the extracellular space. If patients have a normal capacity for insulin secretion, however, glucose infusion lowers serum K level by shifting K into cells. **The effect of insulin and glucose can last for several hours**.

Na Bicarbonate: 100 mmol (mEq) IV. Na bicarbonate administration through expansion of the ECF space results in dilution of the serum K. Additionally, however, K is shifted into cells. The effects of Na bicarbonate are short lived, usually lasting <1 hour. Complications of Na bicarbonate therapy include volume overload, hypernatremia, and the precipitation of hypocalcemic tetany.

Beta₂ Agonists. Although not yet widely used, inhalation of beta₂ agonists such as fenoterol and albuterol or parenteral use of salbutamol can effect significant K shifts into cells. One study demonstrated that albuterol administered in a nebulized saline solution produced significant decreases in serum K levels without adverse effects in dialysis patients.

Treatment with Decreases in Total Body Potassium

The effects of calcium, bicarbonate, glucose and insulin, and beta₂ agonist therapy only temporarily correct the problem if excessive K stores have resulted in hyperkalemia. Therefore, measures to reduce total body K must soon be initiated. Although a decrease in the serum K from 4 to 3 mEq/L is associated with a 300 to 400 mEq total body K deficit, only a 100 to 200 mEq excess of K is required to raise the plasma K concentration from 4 to 5 mEq/L.

- Na polystyrene sulfonate (Kayexalate), 30 to 50 g resin PO dissolved in 50 to 100 ml 20% sorbitol, repeated every 2 to 4 hours
- 50 to 60 g resin in 200 ml 20% sorbitol administered rectally and retained 45 to 60 minutes; repeat every 2 to 4 hours

This resin acts as an Na-K exchange resin and is usually given with sorbitol to promote rapid transfer through the gastrointestinal tract. One must monitor patients closely for evidence of volume overload because significant Na absorption can eventuate. When administered as an enema, K removal begins within 30 to 60 minutes and 0.5 mEq of K is bound for every gram of resin. When given orally, 1 mEq of K is bound for every gram of resin and onset begins in 3 to 4 hours.

Dialysis. Patients with serum K levels that are rapidly rising (rhabdomyolysis) or significant hyperkalemia associated with renal failure frequently require hemodialysis. As a patient is being readied for this procedure, the foregoing treatments should be initiated. Hemodialysis can remove approximately 25 to 30 mEq of K per hour. Peritoneal dialysis is less efficient in removing K.

TREATMENT OF CHRONIC HYPERKALEMIA

Measurement of serum aldosterone level is valuable in a patient with chronic hyperkalemia. If a low value is obtained, administration of 9 α-fludrocortisone at doses of 0.1 to 0.3 mg daily is given. If aldosterone levels are normal, treatment with a diuretic such as furosemide or a thiazide to increase distal delivery of Na is effective. However, aldosterone measurements are not rapidly obtainable, and a more practical approach can be used. One first assesses the volume status. Patients with a contracted ECF volume are best treated with fludrocortisone. If a patient is volume expanded or hypertensive, therapy with a diuretic is indicated. In the setting of metabolic acidosis, therapy with $NaHCO_3$ is indicated. Administration of $NaHCO_3$ increases renal K excretion by increasing distal Na delivery. In addition, correction of the acidosis shifts K into the intracellular space. Patients should be counseled about low-K diets. Finally, some patients may have to be maintained on long-term Kayexalate therapy, titrating the dose and frequency to the desired K level.

PATIENT NUMBER 5 (continued)

Normally, the kidneys' ability to excrete K is maintained until the GFR falls below 10 ml/min. Hyperkalemia in a setting of a GFR >20 ml/min implies a defect in mineralocorticoid activity or a lesion within the cortical collecting duct. Diabetic patients such as Willy have a high incidence of hyporeninemic hypoaldosteronism resulting from disease of the juxtaglomerular apparatus. Additionally, Willy's use of a nonsteroidal antiinflammatory drug would predispose him to a hyporeninemic state. Therapy in the setting of a normal ECG would include discontinuation of ibuprofen and Kayexalate and dietary restriction of K. Such patients are often hypertensive, and thus a diuretic such as furosemide or a thiazide might be helpful in treating both the hypertension and hyperkalemia.

SUGGESTED READINGS

Anderson RJ: Hospital-associated hyponatremia. Kidney Int 29:1237–1247, 1986.

DeFronzo RA, Bia M: Extrarenal potassium homeostasis. *In* Seldin DW, Giebisch G (eds): The Kidney Physiology and Pathophysiology. New York, Raven Press, 1985, pp 1179–1206.

Linas SL, Berl T: Clinical diagnosis of abnormal potassium balance. *In* Seldin DW, Giebisch G (eds): The Regulation of Potassium Balance. New York, Raven Press, 1989, pp 177–205.

Mitch WE, Wilcox CS: Disorders of body fluids, sodium, and potassium in chronic renal failure. Am J Med 1982; 72:536–550.

Narins RG, Jones ER, Storm MC, et al: Diagnostic strategies in disorders of fluid, electrolyte, and acid-base homeostasis. Am J Med 72:536–550, 1982.

Robertson GL: Abnormalities of thirst regulation. Kidney Int 25:460–469, 1984.

Saxton CR, Seldin DW: Clinical interpretation of laboratory values. *In* Kokko JP, Tannen RL (eds). Fluids and Electrolytes. Philadelphia, WB Saunders, 1986, pp 3–62.

5 | ACID-BASE DISORDERS IN AZOTEMIC

PATIENTS

David Z. Levine and Kevin D. Burns

OBJECTIVES

This chapter describes our approach to the diagnosis and management of common acid-base disturbances in people with kidney disease. It does not discuss infrequent presentations or detail mechanisms of transport. Six patients with interesting stories have been selected. Among these is a sad gentleman, living alone in a rural area, who develops symptoms mostly due to profound metabolic acidosis. Another is a truck driver, hauling loads from a quarry, who has had years of stone disease and frequent colic because of the gravel *he* passed. This problem is associated with an acidification defect. We also meet a patient who has undergone long-term dialysis and who comes to the emergency room because of severe hypotension and acidosis and seems to enjoy the efforts made to solve the mystery of his presentation: He knows the cause of his predicament.

DIFFERENT PRESENTATIONS OF METABOLIC ACIDOSIS IN RENAL DISEASE

PATIENT NUMBER 1

Connie, well known to the nephrology service, is a 55-year-old woman with lupus nephritis of 15 years' duration. A renal biopsy performed at initial presentation revealed membranoproliferative glomerulonephritis. Now, on a routine clinic visit, we find arterial blood pH 7.33, plasma [HCO_3^-] 21 mmol/L, and $PaCO_2$ 38 mm Hg. The serum [K^+] is normal. Creatinine clearance is 8% of the lower limit of normal. Ultrasonography of her abdomen reveals a reduction in renal size with increased echogenicity of the cortices. She feels quite well, adores her physician, and loves line dancing and playing with her grandchild.

Diagnosis of Acid-Base Disturbances in Renal Patients

Many disorders of acid-base balance are initially detected from an evaluation of the arterial blood gas or serum electrolyte data in asymptomatic renal patients. In fact, it is usual to encounter a well-managed patient in a clinic setting with little residual function—like Connie—with only a mild reduction of plasma bicarbonate concentration.

Let's first review the way we diagnose acid-base disorders and then turn to processes that may lower the plasma bicarbonate concentration.

What Is the Primary Acid-Base Disturbance in Patient Number 1?

If the reported values are consistent (see Appendix at the end of this chapter), the principal acid-base disturbances can be readily determined.

If the [H^+] is increased, the patient has an acidemia, for which two explanations are possible:

1. **Metabolic acidosis:** a primary reduction in [HCO_3^-] and increase in [H^+]
2. **Respiratory acidosis:** a primary increase in both $PaCO_2$ and [H^+]

If the [H^+] is decreased, the patient has an alkalemia, for which there are also two possible explanations:

1. **Metabolic alkalosis:** a primary increase in [HCO_3^-] and decrease in [H^+]
2. **Respiratory alkalosis:** a primary decrease in both $PaCO_2$ and [H^+]

Is There an Appropriate Compensatory Response?

In each of these disorders, a physiologic compensatory change minimizes the derangements in [H^+]. This compensation need not return the blood [H^+] to normal. In fact, only in chronic respiratory alkalosis does the $[H^+]$ return to the normal range with the compensatory response.

The data on expected degrees of compensation are derived from normal persons. Patients with renal disease may not compensate to the same extent, especially in respiratory disorders, in which the expected changes in renal $[H^+]$ secretion may not occur.

Compensatory Responses for Acid-Base Disorders

Metabolic Acidosis: For every 1 mEq/L reduction in $[HCO_3^-]$ from 25 mEq/L, expect a 1 mm Hg reduction in $Paco_2$.

Metabolic Alkalosis: For every 1 mEq/L increase in $[HCO_3^-]$ from 25 mEq/L, expect a 0.6 mm Hg increase in $Paco_2$.

Acute Respiratory Acidosis: For every 1 mm Hg reduction in $Paco_2$, expect a 0.77 nEq/L increase in $[H^+]$. Or, for every 10 mm Hg increase in $Paco_2$, expect a 1 mEq/L increase in $[HCO_3^-]$.

Chronic Respiratory Acidosis: For every 1 mm Hg increase in $Paco_2$, expect a 0.33 nEq/L increase in $[H^+]$. Or, for every 10 mm Hg increase in $Paco_2$, expect a 3 mEq/L increase in $[HCO_3^-]$.

Acute Respiratory Alkalosis: For every 1 mm Hg increase in $Paco_2$ from 40 mm Hg, expect a 0.74 nEq/L decrease in $[H^+]$. Or, for every 10 mm Hg reduction in $Paco_2$, expect a 2 mEq/L decrease in $[HCO_3^-]$.

Chronic Respiratory Alkalosis: For every 1 mm Hg reduction in $Paco_2$, expect a 0.17 nEq/L decrease in $[H^+]$. Or, for every 10 mm Hg reduction in $Paco_2$, expect a 5 mEq/L decrease in $[HCO_3^-]$.

PATIENT NUMBER 1 (continued)

In Connie's case, the pH is lower than normal (7.33), the plasma $[HCO_3]$ likely fell about 5 mEq/L from normal, and the $Paco_2$ is in the lower part of the normal range. Thus, Connie has an acidemia because of the low pH, and this is due to a low $[HCO_3]$ as opposed to a high $Paco_2$. The acid-base diagnosis is metabolic acidosis, albeit mild.

PATIENT NUMBER 2

Charley is a 63-year-old recluse who rarely saw his physician. He was known to have chronic renal failure for many years. He presented to the emergency room, hyperventilating and confused. On physical examination, no evidence of ECF volume contraction was found. Laboratory studies revealed a serum creatinine result of 950 μmol/L. Arterial blood gas analysis showed pH 7.02,

---

$[HCO_3^-]$ 4 mmol/L and $Paco_2$ 15 mm Hg. Electrolyte values were Na^+ 140 mmol/L, Cl^- 110 mmol/L, K^+ 6.0 mmol/L, and an anion gap of 26 mmol/L. An ultrasound examination of his abdomen revealed bilateral shrunken kidneys, with no evidence of obstruction. On further inquiry, no evidence of ingestion of nephrotoxic drugs was elicited, nor were any factors known to precipitate acute renal failure identified.

Mechanisms of Metabolic Acidosis in Renal Patients

In normal persons, about 40 to 80 mmol H^+ is produced daily by hepatic metabolism of the dietary protein load. To maintain plasma $[HCO_3^-]$ at a constant level, H^+ must be excreted. The kidneys excrete the daily acid load in the form of ammonium (NH_4^+) and titratable acid, mainly acid phosphate, with little HCO_3^- normally appearing in the urine. Free H^+, reflected by the urine pH, represents a trivial amount of acid.

The process of net acid excretion is impaired in renal failure, leading to metabolic acidosis. Renal net acid excretion, the sum of NH_4^+ plus titratable acid minus bicarbonate, is reduced as a result of an impairment in the ability either to generate NH_4^+ in proximal tubular cells and therefore an inability to generate new bicarbonate, or to deliver NH_4^+ to the final urine. Delivery of HCO_3^- out of the proximal nephron may also be increased in renal failure, leading to a relatively alkalotic distal tubular fluid, which further impairs NH_4^+ trapping. Despite this, the urine pH in chronic renal failure is often less than 5.5, indicating that NH_4^+ availability is more impaired than is H^+ secretion. The consequence of this impaired ability to excrete acid is that dietary and endogenous acid production progressively titrate the plasma $[HCO_3^-]$ downward until a new steady state is reached. The fact that a new steady state is reached, despite impaired renal HCO_3^- regeneration, indicates that either $[H^+]$ production is reduced or some other source of acid buffering is mobilized. Negative calcium balance has been reported in renal patients, suggesting that acid is buffered by bone apatite, with H^+ displacing calcium ions.

In contrast to Connie (patient number 1), Charley was in distress on presentation, with a profoundly lowered plasma bicarbonate concentration and an elevated anion gap $\{Na^+ - (Cl^- + HCO_3)\}$. Despite the very high anion gap (discussed later), no other cause of metabolic acidosis was discovered other than his end-stage renal failure. Indeed, **in severe metabolic acidosis, patients exhibit Kussmaul's respirations (tachypnea and increased tidal volume) and perhaps frank signs of congestive heart failure.** Bradycardia and hypotension may also be noted. Severe alkalemia, on the other hand, may induce neuromuscular irritability (positive Trousseau's and Chvostek's signs), mental confusion, and cardiac arrhythmias.

> **Suspect *severe* metabolic acidosis in renal patients with Kussmaul's breathing, bradycardia, or hypotension.**

Assuming that the two patients described earlier have no diarrhea, sepsis, circulatory failure, ketoacidosis, or exogenous poisons, the source of acid addition is presumed to be the metabolism of ≈ 1 mEq/kg/day of dietary acid. In both patients, to a greater or lesser degree, there is an inability of the damaged kidneys to excrete dietary-derived acid, so that the plasma [HCO_3^-] is progressively titrated downward. However, patient 2, Charley, has seemingly exceeded the limits of adaptation and, over a period of many days or weeks, has titrated his plasma [HCO_3^-] down to very low levels. **Therefore, it must be recognized that patients with chronic renal failure may present with either mild or severe depression of the plasma [HCO_3^-].**

What accounts for the difference in clinical presentations of these patients, both with severe reductions in renal function? Patient 1 has only a mild degree of metabolic acidosis despite a significant depression of the GFR. In fact, this patient, who appeared relatively well, with a mild metabolic acidosis, is entirely typical of a large number of patients who are approaching end-stage renal disease and who are carefully treated in outpatient renal clinics. Indeed, they may remain asymptomatic, with no symptoms due to acid-base imbalance, virtually up to the point of initiation of dialysis. In these patients, the surviving nephrons must have remarkably adapted to do the acid excretory work of normal kidneys. In contrast, Charley, patient 2, has small kidneys, severe metabolic acidosis, and no reversible component to his renal failure. His profound acidemia and breathlessness are marked because of near total nephron loss. On the other hand, certain renal diseases such as chronic pyelonephritis and analgesic nephropathy may be associated with severe metabolic acidosis, with only moderate decreases in GFR, because of a reduction in tubular H^+ secretion or decreased NH_3 availability as a result of a damaged renal medulla.

MIXED ACID-BASE DISTURBANCES IN CHRONIC RENAL FAILURE

Patients with chronic renal failure may develop a superimposed metabolic acidosis after use of certain medications, as illustrated in the following case and discussed in more detail in the later section on renal tubular acidosis (RTA).

PATIENT NUMBER 3

Jane, a 75-year-old woman, presented to the emergency room with a chief complaint of general malaise for several days. She had a history of diabetes mellitus and regularly visited her ophthalmologist for 20 years for treatment of diabetic eye disease. Physical examination in the emergency room was unremarkable. Laboratory results were as follows: Na^+ 140 mmol/L, K^+ 3.3 mmol/L, HCO_3^- 19 mmol/L, Cl^- 109 mmol/L, anion gap 12 mmol/L, serum creatinine level 350 μmol/L, pH 7.36, Pa_{CO_2} 33 mm Hg, and HCO_3^- 19 mmol/L. This level of renal function had been stable for the previous year and was thought to be secondary to diabetic renal disease. Jane's condition subsequently deteriorated, as described later.

It is certainly not unusual for patients with chronic renal failure to develop superimposed acid-base disturbances as renal function deteriorates. Perhaps the most common uremic symptoms are anorexia and nausea, which may progress to frank vomiting. Indeed, we see patients who present with virtually no renal function but have almost normal plasma [HCO_3^-] and [K^+]. Here, metabolic alkalosis is superimposed on uremic acidosis, which may "normalize" blood pH and plasma bicarbonate concentration. The underlying mechanism is loss of gastric HCl, which alkalizes the ECF, offsetting the acidifying effect of retained dietary acid. Similarly, patients with diabetic gastroparesis may have protracted vomiting and thus may present with frank metabolic alkalosis despite the presence of renal failure. The impaired glomerular filtration of HCO_3^- contributes to maintenance of the alkalosis in these patients.

Diagnosis of the Presence of More Than One Acid-Base Disturbance in a Renal Patient

A mixed acid-base disturbance is diagnosed when two or more acid-base disturbances coexist. This is often evident clinically only when the expected compensatory responses outlined earlier are not present for a given set of acid-base parameters.

Mixed acid-base disturbances can also be identified by calculating the anion gap:

$$\text{Anion gap} = [\text{Na}^+] - ([\text{HCO}_3^-] + [\text{Cl}^-])$$

The normal plasma anion gap is 12 ± 2 mEq/L and is due to the negatively charged proteins, phosphate, sulfate, and other organic anions. An increase in the anion gap by greater than 5 mEq/L usually represents metabolic acidosis. Examples are lactic acidosis, ketoacidosis, the acidosis of end-stage renal disease, and metabolic acidosis due to intoxications. In these instances, the increase in the anion gap is approximately equal to the decrease in $[\text{HCO}_3^-]$. Otherwise, the patient has a mixed disturbance. That is, if the plasma anion gap has risen less than the decrease in $[\text{HCO}_3^-]$, a second process is lowering the $[\text{HCO}_3^-]$, either a normal anion gap type of metabolic acidosis or respiratory alkalosis.

If the increase in plasma anion gap greatly *exceeds* the decline in $[\text{HCO}_3^-]$, a second process has raised the $[\text{HCO}_3^-]$. The patient has either coexistent metabolic alkalosis or chronic respiratory acidosis.

PATIENT NUMBER 3 (continued)

In Jane's presentation, the mild hypokalemia and metabolic acidosis with normal anion gap were thought to be consistent with ingestion of acetazolamide, prescribed by her ophthalmologist. She was advised to stop taking the drug and to return to her ophthalmologist for follow-up of the glaucoma. Unfortunately, there was some confusion about these instructions, and the patient continued to take the acetazolamide. One week later, she returned to the hospital with increasing malaise. Laboratory studies revealed Na^+ 140 mmol/L, K^+ 4.0 mmol/L, HCO_3^- 9 mmol/L, Cl^- 115 mmol/L, anion gap 16 mmol/L, and serum creatinine level 650 μmol/L. The patient had developed severe metabolic acidosis: Because the plasma $[HCO_3^-]$ fell more than the increase in the anion gap, she had both normal anion gap and high anion gap acidosis. The increase in anion gap is consistent with her degree of renal dysfunction.

This patient demonstrates that patients with reduced renal capacity to handle daily dietary acid load are at risk of developing severe metabolic acidosis. In our patient Jane, H^+ excretion is impaired further by the addition of an inhibitor of carbonic anhydrase, acetazolamide. Elderly patients with chronic renal failure are particularly prone to develop severe metabolic acidosis after use of this agent, and further deterioration of renal function may ensue. Thus, in a patient who has chronic renal failure and who presents with a metabolic acidosis in which the decrease in plasma $[\text{HCO}_3^-]$ exceeds the increase in the anion gap, the clinician should be alerted to the possibility of ingestion of drugs impairing renal HCO_3^- reabsorption or should consider other sources of HCO_3^- loss, such as diarrhea.

Four Clues to the Presence of Superimposed Acid-Base Disorders in the Renal Patient

1. **A rapid fall in plasma bicarbonate concentration**
2. **An anion gap greater than 30 mmol/L**
3. **A high plasma osmolal gap**
4. **Paco_2 inappropriate for the degree of reduction in plasma bicarbonate concentration**

ACUTE RENAL FAILURE AND MIXED ACID-BASE DISORDERS

PATIENT NUMBER 4

Edgar, a 54-year-old attorney who couldn't play golf because of leg pains, underwent right femoral popliteal bypass surgery. Preoperative renal function and acid-base status were normal. Twenty-four hours postoperatively, he was noted to be oliguric, cold and clammy, and poorly responsive. Physical examination revealed a blood pressure of 90/60 mm Hg, pulse of 126, and absent pulses in his right foot. Laboratory studies revealed these results: arterial pH 7.00, $[\text{HCO}_3^-]$ 8 mmol/L, Paco_2 32 mm Hg, serum creatinine 220 μmol/L, serum K^+ 6.4 mmol/L, and anion gap 31 mmol/L.

In uncomplicated renal failure, metabolic acidosis progresses slowly, and generally, the degree of increase in the anion gap does correlate, but only to a limited degree, with the fall in plasma $[\text{HCO}_3^-]$. The increase in the anion gap is thought to be the result of reduced GFR with accumulation of filtered anions (e.g., HPO_4^{-2}). However, clinicians should not be surprised to find only minor elevations in the anion gap in patients with chronic renal failure, despite very severe reductions in GFR. In contrast, when the anion gap is greatly elevated (> 30 mmol/L) in a patient with chronic renal failure, one should be alerted to the presence of another process causing high anion gap–type metabolic acidosis.

For example, a diabetic patient with renal disease may be prone to cardiovascular catastrophes leading to hypoperfusion (lactic acidosis), sepsis (lactic acidosis), or diabetic ketoacidosis. In each case, **the marked elevation in the anion gap, associated with a rapid fall in the plasma [HCO$_3^-$], provides a valuable clue to the presence of a serious nonrenal process contributing to life-threatening metabolic acidosis.**

Rate of Fall of Plasma [HCO$_3^-$]

The rate of fall of the plasma [HCO$_3^-$] also provides a clue to the cause of the metabolic acidosis. Consider Edgar, patient 4, who developed oliguric renal failure with a high anion gap type of metabolic acidosis within 24 hours of surgery. Could this be explained solely by a deterioration of renal perfusion? The answer is clearly no. Because the daily ingested acid load is approximately 70 mEq of H$^+$/day, in a 70-kg man, the plasma [HCO$_3^-$] can fall by only about 2 mEq/day: The apparent bicarbonate space is about half the body weight (i.e., about 35 L). Because the plasma [HCO$_3^-$] has fallen to 8 mmol/L in 24 hours, more rapidly than can be explained by failure of the kidneys to excrete net acid normally, another process must explain the fall in plasma HCO$_3^-$ from about 25 to 8 mmol/L. The anion gap of greater than 30 mmol/L is also inconsistent with uncomplicated renal failure; thus, the clinician must rule out sepsis or other causes of lactic acidosis, diabetic ketoacidosis, or exogenous poisons.

Severe Metabolic Acidosis in Acute Renal Failure	
Causes	*Clinical Context*
"Excess" H$^+$ production	Hypercatabolic states, burns, rhabdomyolysis
Lactic acidosis	Sepsis, hypovolemic shock
Diabetic ketoacidosis	Diabetic patients also experience renal failure
Ethylene glycol intoxication	Acute renal failure with anion gap >30 mEq/L, osmolal gap >15 mOsm, oxalate crystals in urine

Edgar developed a severe metabolic acidosis, complicated by a component of superimposed respiratory acidosis (the Paco$_2$, assuming normal compensation, should have been 24 to 26 mm Hg). In this postoperative patient, respiratory acidosis was likely secondary to oversedation. The cause of the metabolic acidosis was multifactorial and could not be attributed solely to development of renal failure. Elevation of the anion gap suggests increased organic acid production. Indeed, this patient had lactic acidosis from impaired perfusion of his right leg, and acute renal failure was due to rhabdomyolysis in combination with impaired renal perfusion.

Because acute renal failure is often accompanied by lactic acidosis (sepsis, hypovolemic shock, severe congestive heart failure), clinicians can expect profound high anion gap metabolic acidosis in some of these patients. In addition, acute renal failure may occur in hypercatabolic states (e.g., burns, rhabdomyolysis) in which increased production of sulfuric and phosphoric acids contributes to the high anion gap acidosis. Finally, the finding of an unusually high anion gap (> 30 mmol/L), elevation of the osmolal gap, and the presence of oxalate crystals in the urine should alert a clinician to ethylene glycol poisoning as a cause of acute renal failure.

ACID-BASE DISTURBANCES IN PATIENTS UNDERGOING DIALYSIS

PATIENT NUMBER 5

Gerald, 71 years old, a gaunt patient undergoing chronic hemodialysis, comes to the emergency room complaining of dizziness and anorexia. His blood pressure is 105/72 mm Hg. His plasma [HCO$_3^-$] is 14 mmol/L, and serum [K$^+$] is 3.9 mmol/L. He was last dialyzed 2 days earlier and states that he drinks a lot of fluids. His anion gap is 16 mmol/L.

Patients undergoing continuous ambulatory peritoneal dialysis (CAPD) and hemodialysis often have multiple disease processes and are therefore, perhaps, more susceptible to acid-base disturbances than other patient groups. Indeed, if it is recalled that patients with no residual renal function cannot excrete the daily acid load, it follows that maintenance of a normal plasma [HCO$_3^-$] depends on the addition of alkali to the ECF by the dialysis procedure. In patients on hemodialysis, acetate, but more commonly HCO$_3^-$, added to the blood during dialysis, raises predialysis plasma $[HCO_3^-]$ from approximately 19 to 23 mmol/L to 28 mmol/L during the typical 4-hour dialysis session. Patients undergoing CAPD, exposed during the day to lactate-containing dwell solutions, obtain their base from the metabolism of lactate to HCO_3^- (note that acetate is converted to HCO_3^- in hemodialysis patients). However, patients undergoing CAPD tend to have nearly normal plasma $[HCO_3^-]$, in contrast to the mild metabolic acidosis that characterizes hemodialysis patients just before dialysis.

Gerald actually knew his diagnosis, enjoying the confusion of the emergency room physician. Could simply too much fluid have been removed during the last dialysis? This is unlikely, because it would not explain the superimposed metabolic acidosis in a patient with good cardiac output. What about the normal serum $[K^+]$ 2 days after the last dialysis? When asked about his urinary output, Gerald said he had none.

What kind of metabolic acidosis is associated with a loss of HCO_3^-, fluid, and presumably K^+? This patient had long-standing Crohn's disease with ileal diarrhea and had neglected to take his $NaHCO_3$ supplements.

Metabolic Alkalosis in a Patient Undergoing Dialysis

Metabolic alkalosis can rapidly progress to frank alkalemia in patients with established renal disease. This is because any process that *initiates* metabolic alkalosis is perpetuated by the inability of the poorly functioning kidneys to excrete excess HCO_3^- in the urine. This is especially important when the GFR is severely reduced (<20 ml/min). As already noted, patients with end-stage renal disease often experience nausea and vomiting as the major symptoms heralding the need for dialysis. In this setting, loss of acid caused by vomiting first tends to correct the preexisting metabolic acidosis of renal failure and then progresses to alkalemia. An increase in blood pH exceeding 7.60 is potentially life threatening and must be corrected promptly.

We recently cared for a 27-year-old woman who was on chronic hemodialysis and was asymptomatic but for occasional hand cramps. Predialysis plasma $[HCO_3^-]$ was 38 mmol/L, with arterial pH 7.60 and $PaCO_2$ 37 mm Hg. This young woman was in no distress when assessed. She had undergone regular, uneventful, HCO_3^- hemodialysis, with a 38 mmol/L bath concentration. Review of her past laboratory results revealed variable elevation of her plasma $[HCO_3^-]$, al-

though metabolic alkalosis was never so severe. Metabolic alkalosis in patients undergoing dialysis is invariably due to HCl loss, either by nasogastric suction or vomiting. This patient was a surreptitious vomiter, leaving us with the lingering alkalemia as a diagnostic clue. Treatment involved counseling, as well as dialysis against a 28 mmol/L HCO_3^- bath.

Another common example of rapidly progressing metabolic alkalosis occurs in patients who undergo nasogastric suction without sodium chloride replacement. ECF volume depletion and decreased GFR reduce the body's ability to excrete HCO_3^-, causing sustained metabolic alkalosis.

Management. The treatment of renal patients with metabolic alkalosis depends on the severity of the alkalosis and the degree of depression of GFR. Severe alkalemia can cause cardiac arrhythmias, soft-tissue calcification, and neuromuscular irritability. Patients with severe alkalemia may require intravenous administration of a source of acid such as dilute HCl, arginine HCl, or ammonium chloride, over several hours. Alternatively, patients can be dialyzed with a high Cl^-/low HCO_3^- dialysate to correct the disturbance.

Patients who have mild renal insufficiency (whether due to prerenal azotemia or established renal disease) and who also have metabolic alkalosis respond to cautious administration of sodium chloride or indeed potassium chloride, bearing in mind the hazards of potassium supplements in renal patients. If gastric acid loss is the cause of the alkalosis, use of antiemetics and H_2 blockers and discontinuation of nasogastric suction (if permissible) also diminishes HCl loss.

RESPIRATORY ACID-BASE DISTURBANCES IN RENAL PATIENTS

Although the ventilatory response to metabolic acidosis appears to be normal in patients with varying degrees of renal insufficiency, it is not clear whether appropriate changes occur in plasma $[HCO_3^-]$ when renal patients have superimposed respiratory disturbances. For example, can a kidney with a GFR of 30 ml/min generate sufficient HCO_3^- to prevent severe acidemia in a patient with severe chronic hypercapnia? No data are available to answer this question, although one might expect to find coexistent metabolic acidosis in patients who have renal failure and respiratory acidosis. This combination is particularly hazardous, because it can lead to profound acidemia.

Respiratory alkalosis occurs commony in renal patients. This is especially true in patients on hemodialysis, because arterial carbon dioxide can diffuse across the dialyzer and cause alkalemia. Renal patients not uncommonly develop triple acid-base disturbances, in which metabolic acidosis and metabolic alkalosis accompany respiratory acidosis and alkalosis.

DISTAL RENAL TUBULAR ACIDOSIS

PATIENT NUMBER 6

Claude, a 52-year-old quarry driver, presented to our hospital with a long-standing history of bilateral flank pain and dysuria. The patient, a particularly stoic individual, had a 10-year history of nephrolithiasis, passing two to three small stones per day. On admission, an IVP revealed multiple discrete calcifications in both kidneys and abnormal renal papillae, consistent with medullary sponge kidney disease. His serum creatinine level was normal. Random past urinalyses were reviewed: Urinary pH values were 8.5, 7.5, 8.0, 6.5, and 7.0. However, his plasma $[HCO_3^-]$ was always within normal limits, as were serum $[K^+]$ and $[Ca^{2+}]$.

The syndromes of RTAs are a heterogeneous group of disorders characterized by the presence of hyperchloremic metabolic acidosis (normal anion gap) due to impaired renal net acid excretion, in association with minimal or absent reduction in GFR. Distal RTA represents a group of conditions characterized by defective distal nephron acidification mechanisms. The distal convoluted tubule and collecting duct reclaim 10% to 15% of the filtered HCO_3^- and are responsible for lowering the urine pH to its final value, and titrating nonbicarbonate urinary buffers. The distal nephron is able to maintain steep pH gradients of 10- to 100-fold, compared with the limited capacity of the proximal tubule. In the cortical collecting duct, acidification is partly dependent on Na^+ transport and is therefore influenced by the transepithelial voltage. Na^+ reabsorption in this segment generates a lumen negative electrical potential, which facilitates active secretion of H^+. Aldosterone increases H^+

secretion and Na^+ reabsorption and, hence, cortical collecting duct acidification.

Distal RTA is associated with impaired renal NH_4^+ excretion, which in the end remains the basis for the acidification defect. The two reasons for impaired NH_4^+ excretion are

1. Impaired distal nephron H^+ secretion (discussed earlier)
2. Impaired availability of NH_3 at the distal nephron site

The urine pH can give insights into which mechanism is operative. Impaired H^+ secretion is generally associated with urine pH >5.3, whereas NH_3 defects are associated with urine pH <5.0. Combined defects may be associated with an intermediate urine pH.

Further insights into the pathogenesis of distal RTA can be gained from the plasma $[K^+]$. In patients with hypokalemia, an H^+ secretory defect is more likely, whereas with hyperkalemia, some process interfering with the generation or maintenance of the lumen negative potential difference is thought to be the basis of the problem. These would include the following:

1. Impaired distal sodium delivery
2. Mineralocorticoid deficiency
3. Impaired response to mineralocorticoid
4. Chloride shunt disorder

The steps involved in distal nephron H^+ secretion are as follows:

1. H^+-ATPase secretes H^+ into the distal lumen. This H^+ secretion is promoted by mineralocorticoid and inhibited by a lumen positive potential difference.
2. The minimization of a lumen positive potential difference requires the following:
   A. Distal delivery of sodium
   B. Reabsorption of sodium, which requires mineralocorticoid secretion, normal receptor and postreceptor responses to mineralocorticoid
   C. Anion impermeability

Isolated H^+ pump disorders are associated with hypokalemia, as the lumen negative potential is normally generated and K^+ flows down its electrochemical gradient into the distal nephron lumen.

Any process reducing the biologic response to mineralocorticoid (see 2A and B, earlier) is associated with hyperkalemia, because the lumen negative potential difference favoring K^+ addition to the luminal fluid is absent.

Abnormal anion reabsorption in this nephron segment (chloride shunt disorders) is also associated with hyperkalemia due to dissipation of the lumen negative potential difference. These patients also have hypertension due to ECF volume expansion secondary to the sodium reabsorption with chloride rather than with potassium secretion (potassium excretion is equivalent to loss of sodium from the ECF; as potassium leaves the intracellular fluid for excretion, sodium enters the intracellular fluid).

In patients with hyperkalemia, ammoniagenesis may be inhibited, resulting in a lower urine pH (<5.0) if some H^+ secretion is preserved.

The clinical approach to patients with a normal anion gap metabolic acidosis should proceed as follows: Evaluate the urine $[NH_4^+]$ from the urine electrolytes and osmolal gap.

1. If the urine $[NH_4^+]$ is adequate (urine $[Na^+] + [K^+] << $ urine $[Cl^-]$), look for a non-renal cause of the acidemia (gastrointestinal HCO_3^- loss, acetazolamide, occult high anion gap acidosis [e.g., hypoalbuminemia masking the high anion gap], posthypocapnia, or acid ingestion).

2. If the urine $[NH_4^+]$ is low (urine $[Na^+] + [K^-] > $ urine $[Cl^-]$ and there is no osmolal gap, evaluate for RTA as detailed next.

Evaluation of Patients Suspected of Having Renal Tubular Acidosis

1. Obtain urine pH while patient is acidemic.
   - If it is alkaline (>7), the patient has a proximal RTA, characterized by failure of the proximal tubule to reclaim filtered HCO_3^-.
   - If <5, the patient probably has a defect in NH_3 availability. Confirm by proceeding with the steps listed next.
2. Administer $NaHCO_3$ and correct hypokalemia if present.
   - If urine pH was *not* initially alkaline, administer HCO_3^- until urine pH is >7.4. Assess plasma $[HCO_3^-]$; if it still is low, the patient has proximal RTA.
   - If plasma $[HCO_3^-]$ returns to normal before the urine becomes alkaline, proximal RTA is ruled out.
3. Once urine pH is >7.4, assess urine P_{CO_2}.
   - If the urine P_{CO_2} is <50 mm Hg, the patient has a H^+ pump defect (classic distal RTA).
   - If the urine P_{CO_2} is >70 mm Hg, the H^+ pump is normal.
   - If the initial urine pH was <5.0, the

patient's RTA is due to an ammoniagenesis disorder.
- If the initial urine pH was >5.3, the patient's RTA is due to back-diffusion of H^+ from the lumen (e.g., amphotericin B).
- If blood acid-base status is normal but RTA is suspected, an NH_4Cl challenge may be performed, as in patient 6, described next.

PATIENT NUMBER 6 (continued)

Further inquiry revealed no history of urine infection. The urine was sterile on admission, and the stones were analyzed and shown to contain calcium, magnesium, and phosphate. The patient was loaded with NH_4Cl to determine if distal acidification was impaired. IVP showed classic findings of medullary sponge kidney.

NH_4Cl Loading of Patient Number 6, with Medullary Sponge Kidneys and Recurrent Nephrolithiasis

	Time (hour)							
	0	1	2	3	4	5	6	7
p$[HCO_3^-]$°	26	22	19	23	24	22	22	22
Blood pH	7.34	7.25	7.22	7.23	7.22	7.25	7.27	7.26
Urine pH	6.98	6.93	6.52	6.52	6.30	6.33	6.35	6.54

mmol/L

Note carefully that despite the fall in plasma $[HCO_3^-]$ and blood pH, 19 mmol/L and 7.22, respectively, at hour 2, urine pH never approaches 6.0, confirming an inability to excrete acid. In this patient with renal stones, nephrocalcinosis might induce interstitial renal scarring, which could impair NH_3 diffusibility into the tubular lumen. Accordingly, Claude, patient 6, has a distal RTA, revealed only by acid loading.

Renal Tubular Acidosis in Renal Transplant Recipients

Normal anion gap metabolic acidosis is the most common acid-base disturbance in renal transplant recipients. These disorders can be classified into those occurring early after transplantation and those in long-standing renal allografts. In the first few weeks after transplantation, proximal RTA can occur, with urinary HCO_3^- wasting due to resolving secondary hyperparathyroidism. This defect is typically transient, resolving within a few months. In addition, development of Fanconi's syndrome soon after transplant surgery has been described and appears to be transient.

Acute tubular necrosis is not uncommon in the early posttransplant period. In these cases, the capacity of the distal nephron to acidify the urine may lag behind recovery of GFR, manifesting as a temporary hyperchloremic metabolic acidosis. In long-standing renal transplants, chronic allograft rejection may be accompanied by distal RTA. Indeed, distal RTA is also associated with acute allograft rejection in the early posttransplant period. In patients with chronic rejection and distal RTA, distal H^+ secretion is defective. Renal biopsies of these patients reveal interstitial mononuclear cell infiltrates, resembling specimens from patients with Sjögren's syndrome or hypergammaglobulinemia. Thus, it is interesting to speculate that as with Sjögren's syndrome, H^+-ATPase activity in chronic rejection may be deficient. In addition, however, aldosterone deficiency and hyperkalemia have been reported.

Cyclosporin A induces distal RTA in as many as 20% of renal transplant recipients. These patients typically have hyporeninemic hypoaldosteronism and thus present with hyperkalemic distal RTA. In addition, distal tubular response to aldosterone may be impaired, and human data exist to suggest augmented distal Cl^- reabsorption as a pathogenetic mechanism in some patients. Adjustment of the cyclosporine dose, plus thiazides or loop diuretics, is the mainstay of therapy.

In our own renal transplant population, development of RTA has been unusual. We retrospectively studied 38 renal transplant recipients, all treated with cyclosporin A. At the time of discharge from the hospital after transplantation, 8 of 38 patients (21%) had mild hyperchloremic metabolic acidosis, with plasma $[HCO_3^-]$ < 20 mmol/L, out of proportion to any degree of renal dysfunction. By 6 months after transplantation, no patient in this group had metabolic acidosis.

De novo normal anion gap metabolic acidosis developed in 5 of 38 patients (13%), from 1 to 6 months after transplantation. Two of these patients continued to have plasma $[HCO_3^-]$ < 20 mmol/L at 12 months, associated with mild hyperkalemia. Base supplements were not required in any other patients.

Thus, in our center, serious acid-base disturbances in renal transplant recipients are infrequent. We agree, however, that in patients with persistent proven distal RTA, one should suspect chronic rejection or cyclosporin A toxicity.

THERAPY OF METABOLIC ACIDOSIS IN ACUTE AND CHRONIC RENAL FAILURE

In acute renal failure, treatment of metabolic acidosis is indicated when the plasma $[HCO_3^-]$ is low (<10 mmol/L) or when a patient is fatigued or dyspneic from respiratory compensation. Initial therapy must remove patients from immediate danger by raising the plasma $[HCO_3^-]$ to 10 mmol/L (**see precautions below**). The amount of $NaHCO_3$ required is determined by assuming that the volume of distribution of HCO_3^- is at least 50% of the body weight. With increasing acidemia, the volume of distribution of HCO_3^- progressively increases and, accordingly, more $NaHCO_3$ is required for correction. Each ampule of $NaHCO_3$ contains 50 mEq of HCO_3. Therefore, an 80-kg patient with a plasma $[HCO_3^-]$ of 5 mmol/L requires at least 4 ampules of $NaHCO_3$ to raise the $[HCO_3^-]$ to 10 mmol/L, assuming no ongoing H^+ generation.

Of course, it is critical to arrest ongoing H^+ production in conditions with a rapid rate of H^+ addition to the ECF. For example, improving tissue oxygenation in lactic acidosis may be life saving, as can other measures to improve the cardiac output.

In patients with renal failure and diabetic ketoacidosis, the organic acids that are overproduced are not excreted in the urine as they are in patients with normally functioning kidneys. Thus, these patients can regenerate HCO_3^- consumed in buffering excess acid production, if production can be halted and metabolism of the organic anions to carbon dioxide and water proceeds in a normal way. If acidemia is not severe in these situations, insulin therapy alone is often sufficient to restore acid-base status.

How can $NaHCO_3$ be administered to patients with acute renal failure? Because the majority of these patients have limited ability to excrete Na^+, alkali therapy is usually accompanied by a procedure to remove fluid simultaneously—that is, dialysis. Dialysis against a HCO_3^- bath is extremely effective in increasing plasma $[HCO_3^-]$ and, indeed, is most effective when predialysis plasma $[HCO_3^-]$ is low. Hemodialysis is also particularly useful in those patients with acute renal failure and severe metabolic acidosis associated with toxic ingestions. Hemodialysis against an acetate bath should not be used in critically ill patients, because they may have impaired ability to metabolize acetate to HCO_3^-, and acetate may depress cardiac contractility.

In some hypercatabolic patients, acid generation may exceed the removal rate by daily hemodialysis. In these patients, institution of peritoneal dialysis or continuous arteriovenous hemofiltration elevates plasma $[HCO_3^-]$. In both instances, lactated Ringer's solution is used to replace the filtrate. In situations with diminished ability to metabolize lactate, the clinician can substitute HCO_3^--containing solutions.

Should a patient with chronic renal failure and a stable reduction in plasma $[HCO_3^-]$ receive alkali therapy? Studies suggest that the metabolic acidosis of uremia may contribute to development and maintenance of renal osteodystrophy. Bone is the largest reservoir of base in the body and, as noted earlier, appears to be a source of buffer in states of chronic metabolic acidosis. It has been suggested that significant losses of calcium and carbonate from the bones of uremic patients are proportional to the duration of disease and to the duration of acidosis.

In children with RTA, alkali therapy reduces urinary calcium and phosphate excretion and causes a sharp increase in bone growth. However, alkali therapy in chronic renal failure does not appear to have the same beneficial effects as it does in RTA. This may relate to the differences between uremic acidosis and other forms of chronic metabolic acidosis. Uremic acidosis is associated with major alterations in calcium, phosphate, parathyroid hormone, and vitamin D metabolism not found in other forms of metabolic acidosis. Thus, for example, negative calcium balance in chronic renal failure is due to decreased gastrointestinal reabsorption of calcium rather than increased urinary loss, as seen with chronic metabolic acidosis of other etiologies. Alkali therapy has only a modest effect on gut calcium reabsorption. Nevertheless, alkali therapy and correction of metabolic acidosis may be of significant benefit to renal patients (see also Chapter 13).

To return to the original question posed earlier, based on the existing body of evidence, it seems reasonable to try to maintain plasma $[HCO_3^-]$ above 20 mmol/L. This can be achieved with $NaHCO_3$ tablets at a dose of 600 mg q.i.d. (28.8 mEq of HCO_3^- per day), although as much as 1200 mg q.i.d. may be necessary to correct acidemia. The clinician must be alert to the complications of $NaHCO_3$ therapy: exacerbation of edema and hypertension from the Na^+ load, hypokalemia (especially in patients on CAPD), and tetany induced by a decrease in ionized calcium concentration.

SUGGESTED READINGS

Fagen TJ: Estimation of hydrogen ion concentration. N Engl J Med 288:915, 1973.

Halperin ML, Goldstein MB: Fluid, Electrolyte and Acid-Base Physiology: A Problem-Based Approach. Philadelphia, WB Saunders, 1994.

Kassirer JP, Bleich HL: Rapid estimation of plasma carbon dioxide from pH and total carbon dioxide content. N Engl J Med 272:1067, 1965.

Narins RG, Emmett M: Simple and mixed acid-based disorders: A practical approach. Medicine 59:161, 1980.

APPENDIX

AN APPROACH TO EVALUATION OF BLOOD GAS AND ELECTROLYTE VALUES: WHAT IS THE RELATIONSHIP BETWEEN pH AND $[H^+]$?

The $[H^+]$ of the ECF is usually reported as its negative log, the pH. Because the negative log transformation results in data that are difficult to manipulate mentally and obscures the magnitude of the change in $[H^+]$ in either direction, we encourage readers to think in terms of the $[H^+]$ rather than the pH. A number of bedside methods can be used to convert the pH to $[H^+]$.

Fagen has pointed out that an *increase* of pH of 0.1 is equal to 0.8 × $[H^+]$, knowing that pH 7.00 = $[H^+]$ of 100 nEq/L. This therefore yields the following relationship:

pH	$[H^+]$ (nEq/L)
7.00	100
7.10	80
7.20	64
7.30	51
7.40	41
7.50	32
7.60	24

The values in between can be obtained by interpolation—for example, pH 7.15 = $[H^+]$ of 64 + 0.5 (80 − 64) = 72 nEq/L. Similarly, the values of pH less than 7.00 ($[H^+]$ = 100 nEq/L) are obtained by multiplying the $[H^+]$ by 1.25—for example, pH 6.90 = $[H^+]$ of (100 × 1.25) = 125 nEq/L, pH 6.80 = $[H^+]$ of (125 × 1.25) = 156 nEq/L.

Another method of conversion (see Kassirer and Bleich) recognizes the fact that in the pH range often encountered clinically (7.28 to 7.45), a near linear relationship exists between pH and $[H^+]$, with a change of 0.01 pH unit leading to a 1 nEq/L change in $[H^+]$ in the opposite direction. Beginning with a normal pH of 7.40 equivalent to a $[H^+]$ of 40 nEq/L, other values become as follows:

pH	$[H^+]$ (nEq/L)
7.46	34
7.44	36
7.40	40
7.36	44
7.33	47

ARE THE REPORTED VALUES INTERNALLY CONSISTENT?

The Henderson equation gives the relationship between the $[H^+]$, $P_{CO_2}/[HCO_3^-]$ and can be used to verify the accuracy of the reported blood gas values.

$$[H^+] = K \times P_{CO_2}/[HCO_3^-]$$

The value of the constant, K, is 23.9. This simple equation allows one to check for laboratory errors and to calculate the $[HCO_3^-]$ when provided with the P_{CO_2} and pH.

Many laboratories report the total carbon dioxide concentration ($[tCO_2]$), to represent $[HCO_3^-]$. However, the $[tCO_2]$ is the sum of the $[HCO_3^-]$ plus dissolved carbon dioxide and carbonic acid (H_2CO_3). Because the latter two values are small in the absence of severe hypercapnia, $[tCO_2]$ usually is close to the value for $[HCO_3^-]$. However, the $[HCO_3^-]$ calculated from the pH and P_{CO_2} is in mEq/L plasma water, whereas the $[tCO_2]$ determined with other electrolytes is in mEq/L total plasma volume. Therefore, any process that reduces the water portion of the plasma (e.g., hyperlipidemia) results in a $[tCO_2]$ that is *lower* than the $[HCO_3^-]$ (compare factitious hyponatremia).

Another useful way to check for internal consistency is to rearrange the Henderson equation and to use the value 25 for K, as follows:

$$P_{CO_2} = \frac{[H^+][HCO_3^-]}{25}$$

Because the value of K is 25, the relation between the P_{CO_2} and HCO_3^- is the relation between the $[H^+]$ and 25. Note that for pH 7.00, $[H^+] = 100$ nEq/L.

Therefore, $P_{CO_2} = \dfrac{100 \times [HCO_3^-]}{25}$

$$(100{:}25 = 4)$$

or approximately 4 times the $[HCO_3^-]$ at this pH.

Similarly, other *approximate* relations are as follows:

When pH = 6.90 ($[H^+] = 125$ nEq/L), P_{CO_2} is 5 times the $[HCO_3^-]$.
When pH = 7.20 ($[H^+] = 64$ nEq/L), P_{CO_2} is 2½ times the $[HCO_3^-]$.
When pH = 7.30 ($[H^+] = 51$ nEq/L), P_{CO_2} is twice the $[HCO_3^-]$.
When pH = 7.60 ($[H^+] = 24$ nEq/L), P_{CO_2} equals $[HCO_3^-]$.

Using either this technique or the Henderson equation, it should be immediately apparent that one of the parameters is incorrect, when provided with the following laboratory results:

pH = 7.30	$[H^+] = 51$ nEq/L
$[HCO_3^-] = 6$ mEq/L	$P_{CO_2} = 32$ mm Hg

The P_{CO_2} should be twice the $[HCO_3^-]$ in this case. The test should be repeated.

Therapy can be initiated in patients with a life-threatening disorder while the results are being checked, using clinical judgment to decide which of the three parameters is the most likely discrepant value.

For example, if a patient has acute respiratory acidosis ($Pa_{CO_2} = 60$ mm Hg), we would expect the $[H^+]$ to be 55 nEq/L. The calculation follows: *In acute respiratory acidosis, we expect a 0.77 nEq/L rise in $[H^+]$ for each 1 mm Hg increase in Pa_{CO_2}. Normal Pa_{CO_2} is 40; therefore, the increase in $[H^+]$ is 0.77 × 20 = 15.4. Because the normal $[H^+]$ is 40 nEq/L, the expected $[H^+]$ is 40 + 15.4 = 55 nEq/L. We can calculate the patient's expected $[HCO_3^-]$ from the Henderson equation, and it is 25 × 60/55 = 27 mEq/L. If this patient's actual blood gas values were pH 7.10, $[H^+] = 80$ nEq/L, and $P_{CO_2} = 60$ mm Hg, the $[HCO_3^-]$ is 25 × 60/80 = 19 mEq/L.*

The patient's $[HCO_3^-]$ is much lower than expected, with an acute increase in Pa_{CO_2} to 60 mm Hg. Therefore, he has metabolic acidosis in addition to the acute respiratory acidosis.

6 ▮ OBSTRUCTIVE UROPATHY

Saulo Klahr

Obstructive uropathy is of great importance to clinicians because it is a common entity that is treatable and often reversible. Patients with obstructive uropathy may be asymptomatic or may exhibit a diversity of clinical syndromes (Table 6–1). Patients with obstructive uropathy very often present with symptoms and signs of acute or chronic renal failure. This chapter describes the approach to the diagnosis and management of urinary tract obstruction. Although the diagnosis of obstructive uropathy should be considered in various clinical settings, particular attention should be given to patients presenting with acute renal failure. **In most instances, the renal failure due to obstructive uropathy is reversible, and surgical procedures or instrumentation may completely resolve the clinical picture.**

TABLE 6–1. Clinical Presentations of Obstructive Uropathy

Presentation	Cause
Acute renal failure	Complete bilateral obstruction (or complete obstruction of a solitary kidney)
Chronic renal failure	Severe partial bilateral obstruction
Flank pain and/or enlarged, tender kidney	Unilateral obstruction, partial or complete
Polyuria, polydipsia, sodium wasting, and/or renal tubular acidosis	Chronic partial obstruction or postobstructive diuresis
Bladder symptoms: hesitancy, incontinence, decreased caliber of urine stream	Obstruction of lower urinary tract (bladder neck, bladder pathology)
Repeated or refractory urinary tract infections	Any obstructive lesion but most commonly lower urinary tract
Hypertension	Increased ECF volume (bilateral obstruction); increased renin-angiotensin (unilateral obstruction)
Polycythemia	Increased renal production of erythropoietin (presumably due to renal ischemia during obstruction)

PATIENT NUMBER 1

Alfred, an 81-year-old white man, presented to the emergency room with a chief complaint of no urine output for 36 hours. The patient had been in obvious discomfort for the past day and had been unable to pursue even the leisurely paced activities of his sedentary life, such as playing cards and reading the newspaper, because of the sensation of a bladder that was much too full. He had a history of recurrent urinary tract infections and a slightly elevated serum creatinine level. He had an indwelling Foley catheter, which had been irrigated and then replaced the previous evening at the nursing home where he resides. This was done because the nurses had noted no urine output from the patient during the afternoon shift. Unfortunately, the procedure brought no improvement. The patient also had oral hydration without improvement. In the emergency room, he had a blood pressure of 200/120 mm Hg.

APPROACH TO PATIENT NUMBER 1

This elderly patient presented with anuria—that is, no urine output, which is frequently encountered in the setting of complete bilateral obstruction or with unilateral ureteral obstruction in patients with a solitary kidney. In addition, anuria (defined as <100 ml urine per day) can result from complete obstruction at the level of the urethra. It can also occur in patients with extensive acute tubular necrosis or with cortical necrosis. The medical history from the nursing home where Alfred lived indicated quite clearly that he had not passed urine for approximately 36 hours. His blood pressure was adequate—as a matter of fact, somewhat elevated—and he had been hydrated fully, suggesting that prerenal causes of acute renal failure (dehydration, hypotension) would be unlikely.

PATIENT NUMBER 1 (continued)

In the emergency room, Alfred's BUN was 65 mg/dl and his serum creatinine level was 3.7 mg/dl; baseline values before this episode were creatinine

1.8 mg/dl and BUN 30 mg/dl. Percussion of the hypogastrium revealed dullness and suggested the presence of a distended, full bladder; the possibility of acute urinary retention was considered. Examination also revealed that the Foley catheter had been incorrectly placed. It extended no farther than the meatus. After proper placement of the catheter, approximately 1400 ml of cloudy urine was obtained. Blood pressure decreased to 152/100 mm Hg subsequently.

Hypertension may be coincidental in patients with acute urinary tract obstruction or can occur as a consequence of the obstruction. **Hypertension may be due to expansion of the ECF or to increased secretion of renin and angiotensin.** In Alfred, the oral hydration during the period of anuria resulted very likely in expansion of extracellular volume and an increase in blood pressure. The decrease in blood pressure that followed the diuresis supports this explanation. In patients with unilateral ureteral obstruction without acute renal failure, hypertension may be due to increased secretion of renin and generation of angiotensin II, a vasoconstrictor.

PATIENT NUMBER 1 (continued)

The urine obtained after adequate placement of the Foley was cloudy. Specific gravity was 1010, and the urine sediment revealed 20 RBCs, 10 to 20 WBCs, and many bacteria. A subsequent culture grew gram-negative organisms, and the patient was given the appropriate antibiotics.

Patients with obstruction may occasionally present with acute pyelonephritis, high fever, and costovertebral angle pain and tenderness. Bacteremia may occasionally be the presenting picture. In men, the presence of a urinary tract infection suggests possible obstruction and an IVP may be required. This may not be the case in women, in whom urinary tract infection is common in the absence of obstruction. In Alfred, the possibility of benign prostatic hyperplasia (BPH) or prostatic cancer was considered, and appropriate follow-up was carried out: prostate-specific antigen (PSA) levels were obtained; these were within the normal range. It was concluded that Alfred's difficulties were due to BPH, inadequate placement of the Foley catheter at the nursing home, and acute urinary retention. The nursing home was advised not to use anticholinergic agents and to try to discontinue phenobarbital and other sedatives that might result in urinary retention. In this case, adequate placement of the Foley catheter resulted in relief of the acute urinary retention and an improvement in renal function with a decrease in blood pressure as ECF volume

was normalized. A concomitant urinary tract infection was treated with appropriate antibiotics. Alfred exhibited three clinical findings commonly associated with urinary tract obstruction: (1) anuria, (2) an increase in blood pressure, and (3) a urinary tract infection. It should be emphasized that **emergency medical treatment may be required when gram-negative septicemia is present in patients with complete or partial obstruction.**

LOWER URINARY TRACT OBSTRUCTION

Our patient Alfred presented with lower urinary tract obstruction, most likely due to BPH. In men, BPH is the most common cause of obstruction of the lower urinary tract. In fact, about 80% of men older than 60 years may have BPH and some evidence of bladder dysfunction. Other causes of lower urinary tract obstruction include lesions of the urethra and the bladder. Urethral strictures are usually secondary to chronic instrumentation or gonococcal infection. Neurogenic vesical dysfunction (neurogenic bladder) can result from brain or upper spinal tract damage and can produce involuntary micturition (spastic bladder dysfunction) or lower spinal tract injury and give rise to a flaccid, atonic bladder. In both settings, significant residual urine may accumulate, resulting in ureteral vesical reflux, ureteral dilatation, and increased pressure in the upper urinary tract. Drugs such as tranquilizers (diazepam), anticholinergics, antihistamines, and alpha-adrenergic stimulators can cause bladder dysfunction and urinary retention. Lower urinary tract obstruction may be manifested by difficulties in micturition, including a decrease in the force and caliber of the urinary stream, intermittence, postvoid dribbling, hesitancy, and nocturia. Urgency, frequency, and urinary incontinence can be due to incomplete emptying of the bladder. Obstruction of the lower urinary tract can be evaluated by the use of cystoscopy, radiologic tests, and urodynamic tests. When obstruction is due to abnormal bladder function, dynamic studies are essential to determine therapy.

The main goals of therapy should be (1) to establish the bladder as a urine storage organ without causing renal parenchymal injury and (2) to provide a mechanism for bladder emptying that is acceptable to the patient. The best treatment for patients with significant residual urine and recurrent bouts of urosepsis is clean intermittent catheterization at regular intervals. The goal should be to catheterize four to five times per day, such that the amount of urine drained from the bladder does not exceed 400 ml. This technique is successful but requires that patients accept treatment and be carefully trained. Obstruction secondary to BPH does not always progress. Therefore, a patient with minimal symptoms, no infection, and a normal upper urinary tract may be safely monitored until he and his physician agree that surgery is desirable. Urethral and bladder neck obstruction in patients who have recurring infections and are ambulatory requires surgery, particularly when reflux, renal parenchymal damage, total urinary retention, repeated bleeding, or other severe symptoms are present. In the presence of lower urinary tract obstruction, surgical diversions are indicated if (1) deterioration of renal function occurs despite conservative measures, (2) the patient has intractable incontinence, (3) the bladder is small and contracted, and (4) multiple bladder fistulas are a factor. An ileal conduit is the operation of choice for permanent diversion.

PATIENT NUMBER 2

Jacob, a 72-year-old black man, presented to the emergency room with a tonic-clonic seizure. He was given diazepam, 5 mg IV, which stopped the seizure activity, and was admitted to the hospital. Although the patient progressed from incoherent to rational speech within an hour of the diazepam injection, he also became quite apprehensive, believing that he had suffered a stroke and complaining that his blood was "racing" through his body. His blood pressure was 150/110 mm Hg. He had these serum values: sodium 147 mEq/L, potassium 5.6 mEq/L, chloride 106 mEq/L, CO_2 19 mEq/L, BUN 102 mg/dl, creatinine 6.2 mg/dl, and uric acid 12.4 mg/dl. An ultrasound examination of his abdomen revealed bilateral hydronephrosis.

APPROACH TO PATIENT NUMBER 2

In our patient Jacob, obstructive uropathy occurred without symptoms directly referable to the genitourinary tract. Laboratory findings, however, were highly suggestive of pathology of the urinary tract. These included the presence of marked renal insufficiency, as reflected by the elevations in levels of serum creatinine and BUN and the presence of bilateral hydronephrosis. Jacob's medical history was also useful. He had been diagnosed with adenocarcinoma of the

prostate 2 years before and had refused surgery. He also had chronic renal insufficiency thought to be secondary to long-standing hypertension. BUN and creatinine values 2 years before were 47 and 1.9 mg/dl, respectively. Renal ultrasonography performed at that time showed no hydronephrosis. Because of the bilateral nature of the obstruction and the difficulty in identifying the site at which obstruction had occurred, a urologist was called in consultation and recommended cystoscopy and retrograde pyelography. These were performed 1½ days after admission. Retrograde pyelography identified an area approximately 5 cm long on either side, and the areas appeared to be aperistaltic and narrow. Above the narrowing, hydroureteronephrosis was observed on both sides. Bilateral stents were placed. The impression derived from the pyelogram was of bilateral, symmetrical, smooth narrowing of the distal ureters, most likely as a consequence of extension of the adenocarcinoma of the prostate to the ureters. The following day, the BUN and creatinine values had decreased to 88 mg/dl and 4.5 mg/dl, respectively. These changes indicated that bilateral ureteral obstruction contributed significantly to the decrease in GFR. Placement of bilateral stents led to a marked decrease in levels of serum creatinine and BUN during a 24-hour period, indicating an increase in GFR as a consequence of drainage of the obstructed areas. Importantly, urinary tract obstruction occurred in this patient in the setting of underlying chronic renal insufficiency. The availability of ultrasonography results from a previous examination that demonstrated the absence of obstruction was most helpful. Also, the previous levels of serum creatinine and BUN and their subsequent elevation suggested that either progression of the underlying chronic renal disease or a superimposed event had occurred.

Although in some instances the diagnosis of obstruction of the urinary tract is obvious, in other cases it is difficult to establish. When obstructive uropathy is strongly suspected, as in Jacob's case, appropriate tests should be performed. **Because obstruction may result in irreversible renal damage, the sooner the diagnosis is made and the sooner appropriate therapy is instituted, the better the prognosis.** Obtaining a detailed history with emphasis on some of the clinical manifestations previously described is of great importance, as in Jacob's case. Rectal examination is essential in elderly men to rule out the presence of a markedly enlarged prostate. Pelvic examination in women is necessary to preclude pelvic malignancy. It is clear that when urinary tract obstruction is suspected, certain laboratory determinations should be obtained, including BUN, creatinine, and electrolytes in serum. Serum electrolytes may reveal hypernatremia in patients with partial obstruction due to severe water losses, the presence of hyperchloremic hyperkalemic acidosis, as in our patient Jacob, or the presence of acidosis due to renal tubular defects in hydrogen secretion. A urine culture should be obtained to identify infection of the urinary tract.

RADIOLOGIC TESTS IN UPPER URINARY TRACT OBSTRUCTION

Several radiologic techniques can be used to diagnose suspected upper urinary tract obstruction as described in patient 2, Jacob. These techniques include plain abdominal radiographs, ultrasonography (Fig. 6–1A), computed tomography (Fig. 6–1B), excretory urography (Fig. 6–2), retrograde pyelography (Fig. 6–3), isotopic renography, pressure flow studies, and voiding cystography. In our patient Jacob, sonography, a noninvasive test, was used as the initial screening procedure in the diagnosis of obstruction. The main finding detected by sonography is dilatation of the urinary tract (see Fig. 6–1), which is encountered in 90% of instances even in the absence of excretory function. In a few instances, sonography may give false-positive results, suggesting obstruction because anatomic variations

of the pyelocalyceal system may be interpreted as dilatation of the urinary tract. In patients with acute obstruction (<24 hours), on the other hand, dilatation of the urinary tract may not occur and sonography may be unrevealing. Sonography may also provide false-negative results in patients with obstruction and severe dehydration or in those with a frozen pelvis due to malignancy. Retrograde pyelography (see Fig. 6–3) requires retrograde injection of radiocontrast and is used to visualize the ureters and collecting system when an IVP cannot be performed or is not justified because of a history of allergic reactions to contrast material or other contraindications. Retrograde pyelography may help to identify both the site and the cause of the obstruction. However, urinary tract infections may be a consequence of retrograde pyelography. If obstruction is present, the risk of producing infection that is difficult to control with conventional therapy is great. Hence, **if obstruction is diagnosed during retrograde pyelography, it is imperative to provide adequate drainage to avoid the development of infection in an obstructed urinary tract.**

CHRONIC RENAL FAILURE

Severe partial bilateral obstruction may cause chronic renal failure. Patients with chronic, slowly progressive urinary tract obstruction, such as those with retroperitoneal fibrosis, may not report any symptoms. Compulsive water drinking

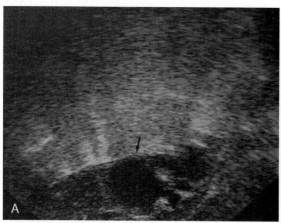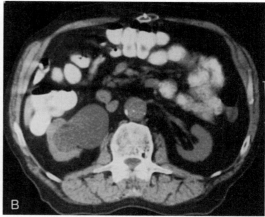

Figure 6–1. *A.* Ultrasonogram, longitudinal section, illustrating chronic urinary tract obstruction secondary to a large recurrent cancer of the bladder. The different echogenicity is indicated by the arrow. *B.* A computed tomogram obtained in the same patient revealed, in the absence of injection of contrast material, chronic hydronephrosis. The attenuation value of the widened pyelocalyceal system equals that of water. There is also thinning of the renal parenchyma, which is a characteristic of long-standing severe hydronephrosis. (Reproduced with permission from Klahr S, Bander SJ: Obstructive nephropathy. *In* Massry SG, Glassock RJ (eds): Textbook of Nephrology, 2nd ed., Vol. 1. Baltimore, Williams & Wilkins, 1989, pp. 889–909.)

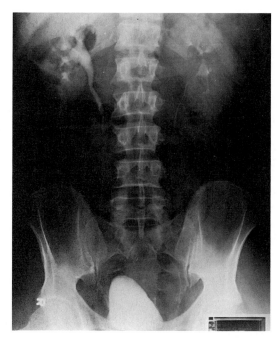

Figure 6–2. Intravenous pyelogram (IVP) of a patient admitted with the chief complaint of renal colic. A flat film of the abdomen (KUB) revealed the presence of a radiopaque density suggestive of a ureteral stone. The IVP reveals dilatation of the upper right ureter, the pelvis, and calyceal system of the right kidney (notice the difference between the renal pelvis and calyces of the right and left kidneys). There was an abrupt change in the diameter of the right ureter below the site where the stone had been impacted. At this site, the dye stopped and the stone is now seen as a radiolucent area. (Reproduced with permission from Klahr S, Bander SJ: Obstructive nephropathy. *In* Massry SG, Glassock RJ (eds): Textbook of Nephrology, 2nd ed., Vol. 1. Baltimore, Williams & Wilkins, 1989, pp. 889–909.)

(psychogenic polydipsia), a well-recognized clinical entity often noted in patients with psychiatric disorders, may result in urinary tract abnormalities including hydronephrosis and an enlarged bladder. Singh and Linas have reported four cases of psychogenic polydipsia presenting with chronic renal failure, presumably as a consequence of a combination of excessive water ingestion, enlarged bladder volume, and use of anticholinergic drugs.

PATIENT NUMBER 3

Juan, a 54-year-old Colombian physician visiting this country, developed left flank pain radiating to his left testicle 2 days before admission to the hospital. This was accompanied by frequency of urination and hematuria. The symptoms were not incapacitating, but when he found that he could not comfortably participate in the sightseeing or the social gatherings he had planned, he decided to seek medical attention. On admission, an ultrasound examination revealed a slight degree of hydronephrosis and suggested the presence of a renal stone in the left ureter. An IVP was performed; urinalysis showed few WBCs and RBCs in the urine and many oxalate crystals. A 24-hour urine collection yielded 180 mg of calcium. Blood analysis revealed a BUN of 16 mg/dl and a creatinine level of 1 mg/dl.

APPROACH TO PATIENT NUMBER 3

Pain is a frequent symptom in obstructive uropathy, particularly in patients with ureteral calculi. Acute ureteral obstruction may be manifested by a steady crescendo flank pain radiating to the labia, the testicles, or the groin. The acute attack

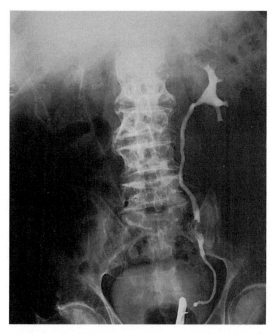

Figure 6–3. Retrograde pyelogram in a patient who was admitted with the chief complaints of hematuria and dull flank pain. A computed tomogram revealed mild dilatation of the pelvis and calyces of the left kidney. The same computed tomogram, at the level of the pelvis, revealed a soft-tissue density located on the left side. When a retrograde pyelogram of the left ureter and pelvis was performed, an irregular mass was detected in the ureter at the level of the pelvis. At surgery, this was found to represent a transitional cell carcinoma of the ureter. (Reproduced with permission from Klahr S, Bander SJ: Obstructive nephropathy. *In* Massry SG, Glassock RJ (eds): Textbook of Nephrology, 2nd ed., Vol. 1. Baltimore, Williams & Wilkins, 1989, pp. 889–909.)

may last less than half an hour or as long as a day. IVP is used to investigate suspected upper urinary tract obstruction. Visualization of dye may be delayed in patients with a low GFR because of a decrease in the filtered load of the contrast medium. In such cases, the examination should be extended until the collecting system and the site of obstruction are identified. This was not a problem in our patient Juan because the partial obstruction was unilateral and had not substantially affected overall renal function. Ultrasonography already had suggested the presence of a stone, but the IVP confirmed the presence of such a stone and located the exact site of it in the ureter. **Stones are the most frequent cause of ureteral obstruction.** Therapy includes relief of pain, elimination of obstruction, and treatment of infection. Pain can be relieved by intramuscular injection of a narcotic analgesic. Stones less than 5 mm in diameter, as was the case in our patient Juan, usually do not require surgical intervention or instrumentation because about 90% of these calculi pass spontaneously; in fact, this patient passed a stone, about 4 mm in diameter, 2 days later, after aggressive hydration. If the stones are 5 to 7 mm in diameter, however, only about half pass spontaneously. Stones larger than 7 mm in diameter usually are not passed spontaneously. Increased fluid intake to achieve urine volumes of at least 1.5 to 2 L/day may help to mobilize the stone. Surgery or instrumentation for calyceal ureteral stones is indicated in patients with persistent colic, urinary tract infection, complete obstruction, a calculus greater than 7 mm in diameter, or a smaller calculus that has not moved despite a prudent waiting period and increased fluid intake. Endourologic techniques and the application of extracorporeal shock wave lithotripsy have allowed for the management of ureteral stones without the need for open surgery. Calculi located distal to the pelvic brim can be approached from below. They can be removed from the ureter using various loops or baskets, and this procedure is successful in about 70% of patients. If it fails, dilatation of the ureter or ultrasonic disintegration of the stone can be accomplished using a ureteral renoscope. Thus, the need for open surgery for distal ureteral calculus is rare. Broad-spectrum antibiotics are useful when infections complicate the presence of renal calculi. Choice of antibiotics depends on appropriate urine cultures and sensitivities. It should be remembered, however, that relief of obstruction is indispensable for successful antimicrobial therapy. Before an IVP is performed, a serum creatinine level should be obtained. An IVP is not helpful in patients with severely compromised renal function (serum creatinine level >5 mg/dl) because visualization of the urinary tract is poor in these individuals.

What the Patients Taught Us

1. The clinical manifestations of obstructive uropathy are variable.

2. It is essential to obtain a detailed history and conduct a careful physical examination.

3. In many instances, the renal failure due to obstructive uropathy is reversible.

4. Complete bilateral ureteral obstruction presenting as acute renal failure requires rapid intervention.

5. Pain is a frequent symptom in "acute" obstructive uropathy, particularly in patients with ureteral calculi.

CAUSES OF OBSTRUCTIVE UROPATHY

The specific causes of obstructive uropathy are numerous. A simple classification is provided in Table 6–2. Obstruction of the urinary tract can occur in the upper tract (above the ureterovesical junction) or in the lower tract (below the ureterovesical junction). Upper urinary tract obstruction can be due to intrinsic causes (intraluminal or intramural) or to extrinsic causes. As exemplified by the cases described, the clinical manifestations of obstructive uropathy vary, depending on the location, duration, and degree (complete, partial) of the obstruction. **A pattern of changing urine output, particularly alternating periods of oliguria and polyuria, strongly suggests the presence of obstructive uropathy.**

DIFFERENTIAL DIAGNOSIS

The differential diagnosis varies, depending on the clinical presentation and clinical symptoms.

TABLE 6–2. Causes of Obstructive Uropathy

Bladder outlet
Prostatic hyperplasia
Bilateral ureteral obstruction
Tumor invasion
Retroperitoneal fibrosis
Calculi
Surgical accident
Renal pelvic and intrarenal obstruction
Staghorn or other calculi
Papillary necrosis
Acute uric acid nephropathy (tumor lysis syndrome)

Patients presenting with anuria and acute renal failure should be evaluated for other potential causes of acute renal failure such as ischemia, administration of nephrotoxins, and so on. Partial obstruction and polyuria may mimic the entity of nephrogenic diabetes insipidus. Patients with obstruction presenting with hyperchloremic hyperkalemic metabolic acidosis should be distinguished from patients who have the same syndrome on the basis of low levels of renin and aldosterone secretion. Renal colic due to stones may mimic flank pain due to gastrointestinal pathology. In children, the manifestations of obstructive uropathy can include gastrointestinal symptoms such as nausea, vomiting, and abdominal pain.

TREATMENT OF POSTOBSTRUCTIVE DIURESIS

Postobstructive diuresis is the marked natriuresis and diuresis that follow relief of obstructive uropathy. This diuresis is characterized by the excretion of large amounts of sodium, potassium, magnesium, and other solutes. Although of self-limited duration, the losses of salt and water may result in hypokalemia, hyponatremia or hypernatremia, hypomagnesemia, or marked contraction of the ECF volume with peripheral vascular collapse.

In many patients, however, a brief diuresis after relief of obstruction may represent a normal response to expansion of the ECF volume that occurred during the period of obstruction. This postobstructive diuresis is physiologic and does not compromise a patient's volume status. However, diuresis in this setting can be prolonged by overzealous administration of salt and water after relief of obstruction. Fluid replacement is justified only when excessive losses of sodium and water are inappropriate for the volume status of a patient and are presumably due to an intrinsic tubular defect for sodium and water reabsorp-

tion. Fluid replacement is guided in large part by the volume and composition of the urine. Intravenous fluid replacement should be provided when tachycardia and orthostatic hypotension are present. **To distinguish between inappropriate diuresis and appropriate excretion of fluid retained or excess fluid administered, it may sometimes be necessary to decrease fluid replacement to levels less than those of urine output and observe patients carefully for signs of volume depletion.**

Weighing patients daily and making laboratory determinations of the electrolyte composition of the plasma are necessary to adjust fluid replacement. Urine losses of salt and water are usually replaced with half normal saline to which sodium bicarbonate and potassium chloride are added. Magnesium can be replaced by adding magnesium sulfate (supplied as 2-ml ampules containing 8 mEq of magnesium) to the NaCl solution. In some instances, phosphate replacement may be necessary. Either 42% sodium phosphate (15-ml ampules containing 45 mmol of phosphate and 60 mEq of sodium) or 46% potassium phosphate (15-ml ampules containing 45 mmol of phosphate and 66 mEq of potassium) may be added to 5% dextrose or half normal saline.

SUGGESTED READINGS

Klahr S: Obstructive uropathy. *In* Greenberg A (ed): Primer on Kidney Diseases. San Diego, Academic Press, 1994, pp 184–189.

Milam OF: Causes of upper urinary tract obstruction. *In* Jacobson HR, Striker GE, Klahr S (eds): The Principles and Practice of Nephrology, 2nd ed. St Louis, Mosby-Year Book, 1995, pp 298–306.

Pollack HM, Banner MP: Diagnostic uroradiology. *In* Hanno PM, Wein AJ (eds): Clinical Manual of Urology, 2nd ed. New York, McGraw-Hill, 1994, pp 89–136.

Singh H, Linas SL: Compulsive water drinking in the setting of anticholinergic drug use: An unrecognized cause of chronic renal failure. Am J Kidney Dis 26:586–589, 1995.

Wein AJ: Benign prostatic hyperplasia and other anatomic causes of bladder outlet/urethral obstruction. *In* Hanno PM, Wein AJ (eds): Clinical Manual of Urology, 2nd ed. New York, McGraw-Hill, 1994, pp 379–401.

Wilson D, Klahr S: Urinary tract obstruction. *In* Schrier RW, Gottschalk CW (eds): Diseases of the Kidney, 5th ed. Boston, Little, Brown & Co, 1993, pp 657–687.

7 ▎ DIABETIC NEPHROPATHY

Sharon G. Adler, Stella Feld, and Richard J. Glassock

DEFINITIONS AND TERMINOLOGY

Diabetic nephropathy is an all-encompassing term used to identify disorders of kidney structure and function that arise secondary to diabetes mellitus, either of the insulin-dependent (type 1) or non–insulin-dependent (type 2) variety. As such, this definition includes disorders that affect the glomeruli, tubules, interstitium, and intrarenal vasculature. The term *kidney disease of diabetes mellitus* is often used interchangeably with diabetic nephropathy. *Diabetic glomerulopathy* is a more specific term that refers to the disorders of glomerular structure and function that arise as a consequence of long-standing diabetes mellitus.

Two principal morphologic variants of diabetic glomerulopathy are recognized: (1) diffuse diabetic intercapillary glomerulosclerosis and (2) nodular diabetic glomerulosclerosis (the Kimmelstiel-Wilson lesion) (Fig. 7–1). Although morphologically distinct, these two forms of diabetic glomerulopathy are viewed as part of a continuum of diabetes-induced abnormalities of the glomerular capillaries and associated supporting structures.

In addition to its associated disorders of renal structure and function, diabetes mellitus may also be implicated in extrarenal diseases involving the genitourinary tract. These disorders, which have important clinical consequences, include unilateral or bilateral extrarenal arterial vaso-occlusive disease (atherosclerosis), ascending urinary tract infection, ureteric obstruction secondary to sloughed papillae or localized mycelial fungal growths, bladder dysfunction secondary to autonomic neuropathy, and vulvovaginal infections. In addition, functional disorders, in part related to extrarenal abnormalities, may influence renal function in important ways. Examples might include congestive heart failure, renal tubular acidosis, abnormalities of adrenal steroidogenesis secondary to insulin deficiency, and diarrhea or nausea and vomiting secondary to visceral

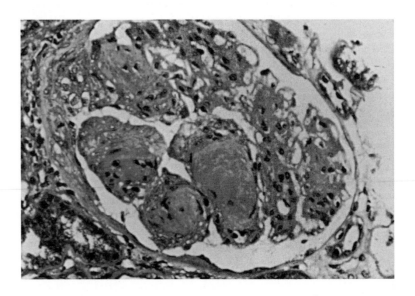

Figure 7–1. Nodular diabetic glomerulosclerosis—Kimmelstiel-Wilson lesion (PAS, × 500).

autonomic insufficiency (e.g., diabetic gastroparesis). Thus, it is important to recognize that diabetes mellitus may be attended by a wide variety of kidney and urinary tract disorders. The fluid and electrolyte abnormalities that accompany diabetes, such as diabetic ketoacidosis and hyperosmolar coma, are beyond the scope of this brief discussion. The principal focus of this chapter is on the progressive renal disease that is the direct consequence of the abnormal milieu engendered by diabetes mellitus *per se*. Because diffuse diabetic glomerulosclerosis and nodular diabetic glomerulosclerosis are found to be the underlying causes of progressive renal failure in most patients with long-standing diabetes mellitus (either type 1 or type 2), the clinical features, natural history, and management of diabetic glomerulopathy are discussed.

STAGES IN THE EVOLUTION OF DIABETIC NEPHROPATHY, WITH AN EMPHASIS ON TYPE 1 DIABETES

Incipient Nephropathy

PATIENT NUMBER 1

Rena is a 20-year-old woman who developed insulin-dependent diabetes mellitus at age 8. She has been noncompliant with her medical regimen and has been hospitalized repeatedly for episodes of ketoacidosis. She now presents with a severe episode of *Candida* vulvovaginitis. She takes 18 units of NPH insulin in the morning and 10 units of regular insulin in the evening.

Physical examination reveals a thin woman with a blood pressure of 136/90 mm Hg, pulse of 90, and temperature of 37°C. The optic fundi reveal only grade 1 background diabetic retinopathy. Other than vulvovaginitis, results of the examination are normal.

Laboratory studies reveal hemoglobin of 13.6 g/dl, hemoglobin A1c of 13.6%, and a WBC count of 6800 mm³. Serum creatinine level is 0.8 mg/dl, serum electrolyte values are normal, and nonfasting blood glucose level is 300 mg/dl. The urinalysis reveals 4+ glucose, many WBCs, no RBCs, and no protein.

Rena's vulvovaginitis was treated and resolved, and strategies to achieve better glycemic control implemented. After these interventions, several timed urine specimens revealed urinary albumin excretion consistently greater than 30 μg/min.

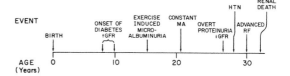

Figure 7–2. The natural history of diabetic nephropathy in insulin-dependent diabetes mellitus (type 1). MA, microalbuminuria, HTN, hypertension, RF, renal failure.

Diabetic glomerulopathy evolves over many years (often decades) (Fig. 7–2). The clinical manifestations of the disorder depend on the stage of evolution in which it is detected. It is believed that diabetic glomerulopathy evolves through these states in a similar fashion in both type 1 and type 2 diabetes mellitus, although longitudinal studies of the progress of diabetic glomerulopathy have largely been conducted in type 1 (insulin-dependent) diabetes mellitus. Diabetic glomerulopathy evolves gradually in four fundamental stages.

The initial stage begins with the onset of clinically recognized abnormalities in glucose homeostasis or sometimes before overt hyperglycemia. This initial stage is characterized by a substantial increase in GFR (sometimes as much as 40% to 50% greater than normal), increased renal plasma flow, and increased renal length and volume. A transient increase in albumin excretion, above the normal range (> 15 μg/min) but below what is readily detectable by standard qualitative tests, is also often present. This transient "microalbuminuria" quickly disappears on institution of insulin therapy and partial correction of hyperglycemia. This initial proteinuria may also be associated with a rise in β₂-microglobulin excretion, suggesting that it may at least in part be of tubular origin. However, with partial correction of hyperglycemia, the increase in GFR does not return to normal and renal size remains increased. Renal biopsies at this stage demonstrate some mild thickening of the capillary basement membranes and perhaps an increase in mesangial volume.

Among patients who have type 1 diabetes mellitus and who maintain excellent glycemic control (hemoglobin A1c values <8%), no further progression beyond this stage may be noted. In fact, approximately 30% to 40% of all patients with type 1 diabetes mellitus *never* develop any overt signs of diabetic glomerulopathy. In addition to having excellent glycemic control, these patients seem to lack a family history of hypertension and themselves remain normotensive. However, the majority of patients with type 1 diabetes mellitus and an unknown but probably similar fraction of patients with type 2 diabetes mellitus eventually progress to the second stage, designated as *incipient* or *early diabetic glomerulopathy*. The usual period between the onset of abnormal glucose homeostasis and the onset of incipient glomerulopathy is 7 to 10 years. If incipient glomerulopathy has not developed within 15 years of the onset of abnormal glucose homeostasis, it is increasingly unlikely that it will ensue thereafter.

The second stage of diabetic glomerulopathy, incipient glomerulopathy, is heralded by the onset of *persistently* abnormal urinary excretion rates of albumin, usually >30 μg/ min. This excretion rate is well below the limit of detection of the usual qualitative tests for albumin excretion. Detection of this microalbuminuria depends on more sensitive colorimetric, radioimmune, or immunoenzymatic assays. On occasion, persistent microalbuminuria may be preceded by intermittent episodes of microalbuminuria exacerbated by intercurrent illness or exercise. Microalbuminuria is not associated with an increase in the excretion rate of β_2-microglobulin, indicating its glomerular origin.

At the onset of this stage, the GFR remains elevated, the kidneys continue to be enlarged, and a slight increase in blood pressure (mean arterial pressure) is observed. This rise in arterial pressure is usually 5 to 10 mm Hg, and many patients may remain within the so-called normotensive range (e.g., <140/90 mm Hg). Background retinopathy may begin to demonstrate a transition to proliferative retinopathy during this stage. In the absence of dramatic improvement in glycemic control or antihypertensive therapy, urinary albumin excretion rates continue to increase slowly during the next several years, and at the end of 5 to 10 years most cases have progressed to overt proteinuria (albumin excretion rates >200 μg/min and urinary total protein excretion rates of >500 mg/day). As the urinary albumin excretion rate rises, blood pressure rises further and in most patients reaches frank hypertensive ranges. GFR simultaneously declines from supranormal levels into the range of normal values for nondiabetic persons of comparable size, age, and sex. During the stage of incipient glomerulopathy, the rate of increase of albumin excretion can be influenced by glycemic control and by reduction of arterial pressure by antihypertensive agents. The rate of rise of albumin excretion and the relationship between albumin excretion rate, blood pressure, and progressive renal disease are better defined for type 1 than for type 2 diabetes mellitus.

Excellent glycemic control combined with rigorous control of blood pressure may arrest the disease at the stage of incipient glomerulopathy; however, many cases continue to progress to the next stage of overt glomerulopathy. The time that elapses between the onset of incipient nephropathy and the onset of overt nephropathy averages 7 to 10 years. More rapid progression may occur in those patients who develop more severe hypertension, particularly when combined with very poorly regulated glycemia.

A detailed discussion of the management of hyperglycemia, ketoacidosis, nonketotic hyperosmolar coma, and other fluid and electrolyte problems that occur in patients with diabetes mellitus is beyond the scope of this chapter. Nevertheless, it is extremely important to emphasize that many of the renal complications of diabetes mellitus can be avoided or substantially decreased by rigorous attention to the management of the diabetic state *per se*. For example, strict control of blood glucose levels to maintain the hemoglobin A1c levels below 8% seems to diminish substantially the risk of subsequent development of diabetic glomerulopathy. It may also reduce the risk of the attendant extrarenal complications, particularly retinopathy, neuropathy, and large vessel atherosclerosis, the latter by returning lipid levels toward normal. For now, clinicians (and patients) need to recognize the importance of metabolic control in the prevention of later complications, particularly those affecting the kidneys and blood vessels. For patients with type 1 diabetes, this degree of **tight glycemic control is achievable by careful and frequent consultation with nutritionists along with three to four insulin injections daily with concomitant glucose monitoring, or insulin pump therapy.** Risks of tight glycemic control include the attendant complications of hypoglycemia and weight gain. Ultimately, successful whole or segmental pancreas or islet cell transplantation may avoid all of the late complications of diabetes mellitus, including renal disease. Additionally, early treatment of newly diagnosed type 1 diabetes mellitus with immunosuppressive agents (e.g., cyclosporine) may ultimately prevent irreversible damage to beta cells and lead to a cure for diabetes mellitus.

Because fewer than 60% of patients with diabetes mellitus ultimately develop diabetic glomerulopathy, it would be helpful to be able to identify those patients at risk at the onset of their disease. At present, such risk stratification at the onset of disease is not possible; however, patients with diabetes mellitus and a strong family history of hypertension seem to have a significantly increased risk of later developing glomerulopathy. Perhaps in the future, genetic analysis (e.g., HLA genotype) may uncover a genetic basis for susceptibility to diabetic glomerulopathy. For now, clinicians must rely on careful follow-up observation to detect the earliest manifestations of diabetic glomerulopathy.

Serial measurements of urinary albumin excretion appear to be the best method for early detection of incipient glomerulopathy. For such measurements to be interpreted reliably, they need to be carried out under carefully controlled conditions of activity, glycemic and blood pressure control, protein and water intake, and medications. Studies performed during urinary tract infection are of no value. Decisions should be based on measurements repeated on several occasions. Twenty-four-hour urine collections or timed overnight urine collections seem to be most reliable. Accurate and quantitative measurement of albumin in urine samples is essential. This can be accomplished by radioimmunoassay, enzyme-linked immunoadsorbent assays, or specialized colorimetric techniques. Screening may be accomplished by the use of special, highly sensitive dye-impregnated paper strips. Persistent albumin excretion of >20 to 30 $\mu g/$min can be regarded as evidence of early or incipient glomerulopathy and identifies patients with type 1 diabetes mellitus. These patients, in the absence of intervention, have an 80% or greater likelihood of evolving to overt glomerulopathy in the next 5 to 10 years.

The exact relationship between the development of microalbuminuria and overt glomerulopathy is best established in type 1 diabetes mellitus and is less well understood in type 2. Periodic screening for microalbuminuria should be initiated after 5 years of insulin dependence in type 1 diabetes mellitus. Exercise-induced microalbuminuria in diabetic patients seems not to have great prognostic value. Greatly elevated GFRs, especially in conjunction with high hemoglobin A1c values, may also be used to stratify patients into a high-risk category.

Patients with persistent microalbuminuria should be treated with an intensive regimen of insulin to secure optimal glycemic control without an unacceptable occurrence of hypoglycemic episodes. Careful attention to concomitant lipid disorders is also important.

Blood pressure should be monitored carefully and frequently. Although such treatment is controversial, **many researchers believe that antihypertensive agents, particularly angiotensin-converting enzyme (ACE) inhibitors,** **should be prescribed to diabetic patients (particularly those with type 1 diabetes mellitus) at the onset of persistent microalbuminuria irrespective of the actual blood pressure level.** Because most patients with microalbuminuria will have experienced a significant rise in blood pressure, compared with values obtained in the premicroalbuminuric stage, an argument could be made that hypertension actually exists even though the absolute values are less than the conventional definition of abnormal blood pressure (i.e., 140/90 mm Hg).

Further support for this argument comes from ambulatory blood pressure recordings in diabetic patients and in age-matched healthy controls, showing significantly higher blood pressure measures in diabetic individuals despite values in the traditionally normal range. It should be emphasized that the renal circulation in diabetes mellitus is in a vasodilated state (primarily at the afferent arteriole); therefore, systemic arterial pressure is being transmitted to a greater extent to the glomerular capillaries in diabetic individuals than in nondiabetic persons. Certain agents, particularly ACE inhibitors, may reduce this capillary hypertension (by relaxing efferent arterioles) even in the absence of an effect on the prevailing systemic arterial pressure.

Numerous studies seem to indicate that rigorous metabolic control, combined with lowering of the capillary or systemic mean arterial pressure, decreases microalbuminuria or retards its progression to overt proteinuria and thus may delay or prevent the evolution of overt glomerulopathy. Whether this scenario also applies to type 2 diabetes mellitus is unknown.

Dietary protein restriction may have effects similar to those of ACE inhibitors but seems to reduce capillary hypertension by increasing afferent arteriolar resistance. Thus, the effects of ACE inhibitors and protein restriction may be additive. Unfortunately, because many patients with type 2 diabetes mellitus present with overt glomerulopathy, the opportunity for intervention at an earlier stage may not be available.

Approach to Patients with Incipient Nephropathy

PATIENT NUMBER 1 (continued)

Given this background, it is evident that our patient Rena has incipient diabetic nephropathy manifested by persistent microalbuminuria. Her glycemic control should be managed vigorously to achieve optimal hemoglobin A1c levels, using continuous subcutaneous insulin pump therapy if necessary. Data from the

Diabetes Control and Complications Trial suggest that this value should be as close to 7% as possible, although data from the Joslin Clinic suggest that large increases in risk for diabetic renal complications begin to appear with HbA1c values >8%. Rena's blood pressure should be better controlled, with a goal of maintaining it at approximately 130/80 to 135/85 mm Hg. An ACE inhibitor may be the preferred agent to achieve this. Modest dietary protein restriction may be instituted at or near the recommended dietary allowance of 0.8 g/kg/day. Rena's albumin excretion rate should be monitored yearly, because she is at high risk for developing overt diabetic nephropathy. She should have careful ophthalmologic follow-up.

Management Guide for Type 1 Diabetes 5 to 20 Years After Onset

- **Strive for euglycemia**
- **Screen for microalbuminuria yearly—consider treatment with an ACE inhibitor if present**
- **Screen for hypertension—attempt to maintain blood pressure at <135/85 mm Hg, preferably with a regimen that includes an ACE inhibitor**
- **Consider modest dietary protein restriction, 0.6 to 0.8 g/kg/day**
- **Treat hyperlipidemia**
- **Monitor for proliferative retinopathy**

Overt Nephropathy

PATIENT NUMBER 2

Christine is a 35-year-old woman with insulin-dependent diabetes since age 11 years. She has had laser therapy of both eyes for proliferative diabetic retinopathy. She has occasional bouts of abdominal fullness followed by vomiting, as well as occasional episodes of diarrhea. Paresthesias in her feet are troublesome, and she has diminished perception of light touch. She presented because of the gradual onset of leg edema and was noted to have blood pressure of 170/100 mm Hg. Her serum creatinine level is elevated, suggesting a substantial reduction in her GFR.

The onset of the stage of overt glomerulopathy is heralded by the development of qualitatively detectable abnormal proteinuria, usually in excess of 500 mg/day (or >200 μg/min of albumin excretion). At the onset of this stage, most if not all patients have unequivocal hypertension, which at times may be severe. The GFR will have decreased to normal or slightly subnormal values. The rate of decline of the GFR is variable from patient to patient but overall averages about 0.8 to 1.1 ml/min/mo. In this regard, it is important to emphasize that **creatinine is a very poor marker for glomerular filtration in the presence of proteinuria and renal disease. Because of increasing tubular secretion of creatinine, the creatinine clearance *overestimates* the true GFR (sometimes by a factor of 2 or more), and a substantial decline in GFR can occur even with a normal serum creatinine concentration. The kidneys remain enlarged.**

Most patients progress to frank nephrotic syndrome with urinary protein excretion rates of >3.5 g/day and accompanying hypoalbuminemia, hypercholesterolemia, and edema. Proliferative retinopathy appears and progresses. Blood pressure continues to rise and may require multiple antihypertensive agents for management. The GFR continues to decrease, and by definition, when this decline is accompanied by a distinct rise in serum creatinine and blood urea nitrogen above normal levels, the patient has entered the final stage of azotemic glomerulopathy. The time elapsed from the onset of overt glomerulopathy to azotemic glomerulopathy averages 3 to 5 years. However, the rate of progression can be significantly influenced by vigorous antihypertensive therapy, and rates of progression as low as 2 ml/min/yr have been achieved in some clinical trials, albeit over relatively short follow-up periods.

Renal biopsies at this stage reveal further expansion of the mesangial zones by the accumulation of an acellular matrix and distinct thickening of the glomerular capillary walls. Some biopsy specimens reveal a distinct intercapillary nodular glomerulosclerosis at this stage. In addition, substantial degrees of vascular and tubulointerstitial disease are found.

The treatment of patients with overt glomerulopathy is focused primarily on rigorous control of blood pressure. All patients with overt glomerulopathy should have blood pressure monitored at frequent intervals. ACE inhibitors are the agents of choice for therapy because they have been shown in prospective randomized trials to slow the rate of loss of renal function and diminish mortality and morbidity. On rare occasions, the use of ACE inhibitors may be associated with an aggravation of type 4 hyperkalemic renal tubular acidosis. Quite commonly but not universally, urinary protein excretion rate falls significantly (by 50% or more) after treatment with ACE inhibitors. Nondihydropyridine calcium channel blockers may also decrease urinary protein losses. No decrease or only slight decline in urinary protein excretion rates is observed when most other antihypertensive agents are used. Other agents, including beta blockers, calcium channel antagonists (other than dihydropyridine class), vasodilators, and sympatholytic drugs may slow the progression of renal insufficiency if excellent blood pressure control is achieved. The goal of blood pressure lowering should be to maintain mean arterial pressure below 100 mm Hg. Somewhat higher values might be accepted in patients with serious underlying cerebral or coronary arterial occlusive disease, because of the theoretic concern that too great a reduction in mean arterial pressure in these patients might induce ischemia. The latter has not to date been clearly shown to be a risk in diabetic patients, although studies are currently under way to determine optimal mean arterial pressures in patients with type 1 diabetes.

Limited studies have shown that protein restriction to 0.6 g/kg/day reduces the magnitude of proteinuria and stabilizes the GFR in patients with type 1 overt diabetic nephropathy. Because blood pressure control was also improved, it is difficult to be sure whether the limitation of protein intake or the salutary effect on blood pressure was responsible for the observed retardation of the progression of renal disease. Although the Modification of Diet in Renal Disease Study, a large national collaborative trial assessing the efficacy of dietary protein restriction in slowing the progression of renal functional decline, failed to clearly demonstrate benefit of protein restriction in patients with various kidney diseases, the result of that study may not apply directly to patients with diabetes. In the latter study, of more than 900 patients, fewer than 50 were diabetic, and type 1 diabetic patients were specifically excluded. Thus, currently, **modest dietary protein restriction (0.6 to 0.8 g/kg ideal body weight) may still be the most prudent option for patients with overt nephropathy and type 1 diabetes.** A vegetarian diet may be preferred to one with animal sources as the principal protein component of the diet. Control of hyperlipidemia is also advised.

Although it has been generally taught that tight glycemic control may not affect the rate of progression of renal disease at this point, newer data suggest that even at this late stage, glycemic control may still be beneficial with regard to renal function. Unfortunately, even with normalization of blood pressure and reasonable glycemic control, patients slowly and predictably develop end-stage renal disease (ESRD).

Approach to Patients with Overt Nephropathy

PATIENT NUMBER 2 (continued)

Christine has progressed from incipient to overt diabetic nephropathy and, like most patients with type 1 diabetes in this condition, has concomitant complications including retinopathy, gastroparesis, neuropathy, and potentially coronary, cerebral, or peripheral vascular disease. It is in this group of patients—that is, patients with type 1 diabetes and overt nephropathy—that the strongest data favoring benefits from ACE inhibitors emerged. Thus, patients in this group should be treated with ACE inhibitors as first-line therapy for hypertension and probably also for reduction of proteinuria even if they are not hypertensive. Studies demonstrate statistically significant reductions in the rate of rise in serum creatinine level, rate of progression to ESRD, and morbidity and mortality in ACE inhibitor–treated patients. Tight glycemic control should be continued but with very careful surveillance for hypoglycemia. Christine would be at increased risk for hypoglycemia with tight control owing to alterations in insulin metabolism in the presence of decreased renal function. Currently, there are no controlled data to indicate that tight control is beneficial for renal function at this stage. Dietary protein restriction (0.6 g/kg ideal body weight) may slow the progression of renal insufficiency. Control of hyperlipidemia may be beneficial for both the macrovascular and microvascular disease.

Management Guide to Patients with Type 1 Diabetes and Overt Nephropathy

- **Screen for hypertension frequently and treat with a regimen that includes an ACE inhibitor if possible.**
- **Maintain blood pressure below a mean arterial pressure of 100 mm Hg.**
- **Continue tight glycemic control with HbA1c values in the 7% to 8% range with caution. The risk of hypoglycemia is probably increased at this stage.**
- **Consider dietary protein restriction to 0.6 g/kg ideal body weight.**
- **Control hyperlipidemia with dietary and pharmacologic measures.**
- **Continue ophthalmologic surveillance.**
- **Monitor cerebral, coronary, and peripheral arterial circulations.**

End-Stage Diabetic Nephropathy

PATIENT NUMBER 3

Fred is a 46-year-old bank robber with longstanding insulin-dependent diabetes mellitus.

Approximately 4 years ago he developed severe proteinuria, edema, and hypertension. He was placed on an antihypertensive regimen, and despite a modest decline in his blood pressure, heavy proteinuria persisted and renal insufficiency gradually developed. One month ago, he began to develop symptoms of nausea and vomiting, particularly in the morning. His serum creatinine level was found to be 6.0 mg/dl; his serum electrolytes demonstrated mild hyperkalemia and metabolic acidosis. His visual acuity has recently been decreasing, and proliferative retinopathy has been noted by his ophthalmologist. This visual impairment interfered with Fred's work. He had to refrain from his vocation as a bank robber because his ability to achieve clean getaways was compromised by his retinopathy. He also complains of occasional numbness and tingling in his lower extremities at night.

Fred is a pale, chronically ill man who appears somewhat older than his stated age. Physical examination reveals a blood pressure of 170/105 mm Hg, a pulse of 72, and a temperature of 37°C (98.6°F). His optic fundi reveal advanced proliferative diabetic retinopathy. His heart is enlarged, and he has an atrial gallop. His extremities reveal 2+ pitting pretibial edema. Ankle and knee jerks are absent bilaterally. Laboratory studies reveal a hemoglobin value of 8.6 g/dl, hematocrit value of 26%, and WBC count of 9000/mm³. Serum electrolyte levels reveal modest hyperkalemia, metabolic acidosis, and hyponatremia. Serum creatinine level is 7.1 mg/dl; random blood glucose level is 190 mg/dl. ECG reveals left ventricular hypertrophy.

The onset of the phase of azotemic glomerulopathy is heralded by a distinct and abnormal elevation in serum creatinine level and/or BUN. The GFR has decreased to less than 30% to 50% of normal nondiabetic values corrected for age, sex, and body size. Patients at this stage have heavy proteinuria, hypertension, edema, and often hypoalbuminemia. In addition, they may also be suffering from extrarenal manifestations such as ischemic heart disease, congestive heart failure, peripheral vascular insufficiency, neuropathy, severe proliferative retinopathy, cerebral vascular accidents, or occlusive renal vascular disease. The kidneys remain large, although late in the stage of azotemic glomerulopathy they may gradually become smaller.

The rate of progression, as measured by the rate of decline in GFR, may accelerate in the last few months before ESRD develops. Severe nephrotic syndrome with marked hypoalbuminemia and difficult-to-manage edema may accompany the early phases of azotemic glomerulopathy. Proliferative retinopathy may progress rapidly, leading to blindness. Peripheral and autonomic neuropathy and peripheral and coronary artery disease may further complicate the picture. The time elapsed from the onset of azotemic glomerulopathy to ESRD averages 2 to 5 years but, in patients with very poorly controlled blood pressure, may be even shorter.

Diabetic nephropathy evolves to ESRD in approximately 40% to 50% of insulin-dependent and 30% to 60% of non–insulin-dependent patients with diabetes mellitus. Representation of diabetic patients in ESRD programs not only reflects the prevalence of end-stage diabetic nephropathy in a given population but also reveals the commitment of resource allocation of given societies to the treatment of ESRD in general and to diabetic patients within that group in particular. In the United States, diabetic nephropathy has become the most common primary renal diagnosis cited for patients with ESRD (33%), followed closely by hypertensive nephrosclerosis (30%). In the diabetic group, 40% of the patients are insulin dependent, 57% non–insulin dependent, and 3% unspecified. In contrast, the percentage of diabetic patients receiving renal replacement therapy in the United Kingdom was 11.1% in 1984. The differences between the United States and United Kingdom dialysis populations reflect differences in social priorities as well as differences in patient population base.

It should be appreciated, however, that not every diabetic patient approaching ESRD should necessarily undergo renal replacement therapy. In a minority of individuals with severe, untreatable, unrelenting diabetic complications (e.g., peripheral vascular disease with multiple amputations, debilitating cerebrovascular accidents, confining and untreatable cardiovascular ischemia, refractory congestive heart failure, uncontrollable fecal incontinence, severe gastroparesis, or autonomic or peripheral neuropathy), prolongation of life with dialysis or transplantation may be an inappropriate choice. Ideally, frank and informative sessions with patients and their families well in advance of the need for a decision should help to provide the perspective necessary to make an appropriate decision. For the majority of patients, however, renal replacement therapy sustains life and provides an acceptable quality of life.

Although survival for diabetic patients treated for ESRD has been improving, these individuals do not fare as well as their ESRD counterparts without diabetes. Taken together, actuarial survival of diabetic patients with ESRD treated with dialysis may be as low as 50% at 2 years, irrespective of the type of renal replacement therapy offered. In general, the older a patient with diabetes is at the time of initiation of renal replacement therapy, the worse the prognosis. Two-year survival of diabetic patients who are older than 65 years and are undergoing renal replacement therapy (other than renal transplantation) may be as low as 25%.

Patients with diabetes tend to require renal replacement therapy when they have higher levels of residual renal function than nondiabetic persons with ESRD. This is because of the additive effects of diabetes superimposed on uremia. Diabetic patients are more likely to experience intractable hyperkalemia (and acidosis) due to insulin deficiency, hyporeninemia, and hypoaldosteronism. Nausea, vomiting, and resultant malnutrition due to gastroparesis may be difficult to distinguish from that of uremia alone, although diabetic vomiting is more likely to be nocturnal whereas uremic vomiting tends to occur closer to mealtimes. Poor glycemic control can induce myopathy and simulate the fatigue and general malaise of uremia. Peripheral and autonomic neuropathy is common to both. Finally, the prevalence of left ventricular dysfunction in diabetic patients may limit the patients' tolerance for volume overexpansion, especially with superimposed uremia. Visual loss due to proliferative retinopathy with retinal or vitreous hemorrhages may occur during the azotemic stage. Earlier institution of renal replacement therapy may be important for the preservation of vision.

Hemodialysis

In the United States, approximately 80% of diabetic patients receiving renal replacement therapy are treated by in-center hemodialysis, compared with only 47% of these patients in the United Kingdom. In-center hemodialysis is a viable option for patients with impaired vision, who may otherwise have difficulty with self-care (approximately 25% of diabetic patients with ESRD are blind). Initial concerns that heparinization and increased ocular pressure during dialysis might worsen diabetic retinopathy appear now to be unfounded. However, placement of vascular access sites in diabetic patients with marked peripheral vascular disease continues to be a challenge. Arteriovenous fistulas with adequate flow rates are more difficult to create with the narrowed atheromatous arteries frequently encountered in diabetic patients, and these access sites

are slow in maturing. Arteriovenous grafts, although shorter lived, may be the access site of choice. However, both fistulas and grafts may induce steal syndromes causing ischemia in hands, legs, and feet. Rarely, the presence of a fistula or graft may induce high-output congestive heart failure in a patient previously in tenuous balance. Permanent indwelling subclavian vein Silastic catheters may occasionally be required if hemodialysis is the option of choice and fistulas and grafts meet with failure.

Additional difficulties in performing hemodialysis in diabetic patients include the problems arising from impaired autonomic responses during periods of rapid ultrafiltration, resulting in hypotension. Bicarbonate rather than acetate hemodialysis baths may help minimize the frequency of hypotension. Addition of glucose (200 mg/dl) to the bath prevents hypoglycemia during dialysis. Although continued maintenance of euglycemia and treatment of hypertension in the ESRD period should minimize progressive extrarenal disease and prolong survival in diabetic patients, cerebral, coronary, and peripheral vascular disease continues to take their toll in these patients earlier than in their nondiabetic counterparts with ESRD.

Continuous Ambulatory Peritoneal Dialysis

For a number of reasons, continuous ambulatory peritoneal dialysis (CAPD) offers theoretic advantages over hemodialysis as a treatment modality for ESRD in diabetic patients. No vascular access site is required. Dialysis can proceed without heparin, and rapid changes in fluid balance that induce cardiovascular stress do not occur. Insulin can be added to the peritoneal fluid, where it enters the portal circulation, a more physiologic route of entry than the subcutaneous route. Simplified transfer systems have been developed, allowing for the training of patients without vision. Thus, **CAPD offers diabetic patients the same advantages of self-reliance and freedom from a hemodialysis center that it offers nondiabetic persons, with additional benefits of specific importance to diabetes sufferers.** However, despite its theoretic advantages, the CAPD technique failure rate is higher in diabetic than nondiabetic individuals. This is largely because of **higher peritonitis rates in diabetic patients,** especially in those with impaired vision, and because of difficulties these patients have in the self-maintenance of fluid balance, alternately inducing hypotension or complications of fluid overload. In patients with many episodes of peritonitis, loss of peritoneal vascular surface area limits the success of the technique. Glucose absorption from the CAPD solutions may exacerbate hyperlipidemia, especially hypertriglyceridemia, a concern in patients with prevalent atherosclerotic disease. It is possible that amino acid– or polyglucose-containing CAPD solutions may lessen this problem to some extent. Finally, as in nondiabetic persons, the burden of three to four daily exchanges often results in emotional burnout and loss of enthusiasm for the technique. In the United States, a minority of diabetic patients undergo CAPD, whereas in the United Kingdom, this is the treatment modality of 51% of diabetic patients treated for ESRD.

Renal Transplantation

There is general agreement that in selected diabetic patients, early renal transplantation offers the best hope for achieving a near normal lifestyle. In eligible patients, transplantation should ideally be performed when the endogenous creatinine clearance is approximately 10 to 15 ml/min (corresponding to a GFR of 5 to 7 ml/min) and before malnutrition, severe vascular disease, or irreversible autonomic or peripheral neuropathy ensues. Candidates should be assessed for the presence of significant coronary artery lesions with radionuclide imaging or stress echocardiography, and angioplasty or bypass should be performed before elective renal transplantation when indicated. In one study, left main or three-vessel disease or severe left ventricular failure was associated with a 62% mortality rate after renal transplantation. In contrast, carefully selected, pretreated diabetic patients undergoing renal transplantation can have an excellent prognosis. At the University of Minnesota, 2-year graft survival in 360 diabetic recipients was 83% between 1979 and 1984 and is now even higher with more frequent and experienced use of cyclosporine.

In the past, transplants from living related donors were the modality of choice, but with increased graft survival with the use of cyclosporine, the timing rather than the source of the graft seems most critical. Undeniably, even carefully selected diabetic patients present greater problems than nondiabetic persons in the operative and postoperative periods. Graft anastomosis may be more difficult because of the presence of recipient atherosclerotic plaque lesions. The use of high-dose steroids in the treatment of acute rejection may make glycemic control difficult. Long-term steroid use may accelerate cataract formation and atherogenesis, and some have argued that progressive severe peripheral vascular disease requiring amputation may be even more common in diabetic transplant recipients than in patients undergoing maintenance dialysis. The presence of a neurogenic bladder may predispose an immunosuppressed diabetic renal transplant recipient to frequent urinary tract infections or even pyelonephritis.

Finally, progression of the vascular, retinal, and neuropathic disorders of diabetes continues unabated after renal transplantation. For this reason, there has been some interest in transplantation of the pancreas in diabetic patients. Data from the International Pancreas Transplant Registry show that **as of 1994, more than 5000 pancreas transplants were performed. Of those patients receiving simultaneous pancreas and kidney transplants, 91% of patients were alive 1 year postoperatively, more than 80% had functioning renal allografts, and 72% were insulin independent.** Pancreatic allograft survival was 72% at 1 year, 67% at 2 years, and 62% at 3 years. Pancreatic graft survival was superior in patients who had kidney and pancreas allografting performed simultaneously, compared with patients who had pancreas transplants alone or pancreas transplants after kidney transplants. Theoretically, a successful pancreas transplant might slow or reverse diabetic retinopathy, nephropathy, vasculopathy, and neuropathy. In practice, even successful pancreas transplantation may not prevent the progression of nephropathy. In a small number of patients, decrements in total glomerular volume compared with measurements before pancreas transplant have been reported. However, the fractional mesangial volume is not diminished in patients as long as 5 years after pancreas transplantation. Thus, it remains to be seen whether the presence of diminishing glomerular size without decreasing the disproportionately large mesangial volume will ultimately translate into long-term preservation of renal function. Preliminary evidence suggests that a successful pancreas transplant may improve autonomic neuropathy and cardiorespiratory reflexes. Despite its potential, pancreatic transplantation currently remains a therapy whose widespread application is limited owing to problems related to patient selection, technical surgical complications, and graft failure. Improvements in the latter two will likely make this therapy more commonplace.

In summary, in selected patients, early re-

nal transplantation, possibly with simultaneous pancreas transplantation, is the therapy of choice for diabetic patients. Such procedures would be especially useful in type 1 diabetic patients, who are very "brittle" and difficult to treat.

Approach to Patients with End-Stage Diabetic Nephropathy

PATIENT NUMBER 3 (continued)

Fred now has end-stage diabetic nephropathy and, as is often the case in patients with advanced renal insufficiency, has evidence of retinopathy, neuropathy, gastroparesis, cardiomyopathy, and peripheral vascular disease. A detailed discussion of the management of each of these entities cannot be pursued here. Readers are referred to other sources (see the later list of selected readings) for this information. Our patient Fred should be counseled about the various dialytic and transplantation options available to him. These discussions should certainly begin before Fred's creatinine clearance declines to approximately 25% to 30% of normal. A living related renal transplant should be considered, although currently, with the use of cyclosporine, the allograft survival advantage conferred by a living related donor compared with a cadaver donor is lessening. In preparation for a kidney transplant, Fred's coronary, cerebral, and peripheral vascular beds should be evaluated, because disease in these circulations may limit transplantation options. Significant vascular disease should be surgically or medically corrected before renal transplantation. Similar surveillance of these systems would be required for Fred in any event, because the general treatment of diabetic patients should be geared to minimizing (1) cerebral ischemia, (2) irreversible loss of myocardium through infarct, and (3) risk of amputation. Sexual dysfunction due to vascular compromise and autonomic neuropathy may also be problematic for Fred and can be treated in men by implantation devices or by local injections of vasodilator agents. Ophthalmologic care of Fred's proliferative retinopathy remains critical. Blindness due to proliferative retinopathy is almost entirely preventable by careful follow-up and appropriate prophylactic interventional care. Fred should not be dialyzed with heparin on days when retinal laser therapy is planned by the ophthalmologist. Use of agents such as cisapride, metoclopramide, and erythromycin may improve Fred's overall nutritional state and his quality of life by decreasing nausea and vomiting due to gastroparesis. He may also experience situational depression. This is particularly common among patients with type 1 diabetes, who experience these multisystem problems in their early to mid-30's. Depression is only modestly improved by antidepressants, which are occasionally also used to diminish the symptoms of neuropathy.

Management Guide for End-Stage Diabetic Nephropathy

- **Begin to discuss renal replacement therapy options *early* (e.g., renal transplantation, CAPD, hemodialysis).**
- **Attempt to perform transplantation in medically suitable patients just before the development of uremic symptoms.**
- **Vigilantly maintain patency of major vascular beds including coronary, cerebral, and peripheral vessels and treat medically and surgically as needed.**
- **Monitor for and treat retinopathy.**
- **Treat hyperlipidemia.**
- **Maintain glycemic control.**
- **Consider pancreatic or islet cell transplantation in patients who have brittle diabetes and whose metabolic control is difficult using exogenous insulin.**

Type 2 Diabetic Nephropathy

PATIENT NUMBER 4

Muriel is a 48-year-old woman who presents with lower extremity edema. She was diagnosed with diabetes mellitus 4 years ago and has been treated with diet and oral hypoglycemic agents. During the past 2 months, she has developed lower extremity edema and shortness of breath whenever she climbs more than one flight of stairs. She has not been to a physician for more than 2 years. Physical examination reveals a moderately obese woman appearing chronically ill. Her blood pressure is 170/100 mm Hg, pulse 86, and temperature 37°C. The optic fundi reveal grade 4 hypertensive retinopathy but no hemorrhages, exudates, or papilledema. Her heart is enlarged, and an atrial gallop can be heard. Her lungs are clear. She has no abdominal bruits. Pitting pretibial edema is noted. Laboratory studies reveal a hemoglobin value of 10.1 g/dl and a WBC count of 7800. Her serum level of creatinine is 2.2 mg/dl, albumin 2.6 g/dl, potassium 4.4 mEq/L, cholesterol 350 mg/dl, and glucose 180 mg/dl. Urinalysis reveals 4+ protein, 2+ blood, 1+ glucose, no ketones, and occasional broad waxy casts. An ECG shows left atrial enlargement and left ventricular hypertrophy with strain.

The most common form of diabetes in the United States is the type 2 variety, and it represents the fastest-growing diagnosis in the population with ESRD. Despite this, the natural history of type 2 is not as well defined or studied as that of type 1 diabetic nephropathy. In general, the nephropathy in the two entities appears to be pathogenetically and morphologically similar. However, some differences may be noted in clinical presentation and course. Although >90% of patients with type 1 diabetic nephropathy have significant retinopathy, as few as 50% of patients with type 2 diabetic nephropathy have concomitant proliferative retinopathy. In type 1 diabetes, overt proteinuria due to diabetes occurs only in patients who have been diagnosed with diabetes for many years, usually for more than a decade. In type 2 diabetes, because of its occasionally indolent manifestations, proteinuria may be present at the time of or even before the diagnosis of diabetes. The risk for chronic renal failure associated with the presence of persistent proteinuria at the time of the diagnosis of non–insulin-dependent diabetes is increased 12-fold. When persistent proteinuria develops after the diagnosis of non–insulin-dependent diabetes mellitus, the cumulative risk for chronic renal failure 10 years after the diagnosis of persistent proteinuria is 11%. Finally, although the rate of progressive loss of renal function is highly variable and is not well studied in type 2 diabetes, in certain subsets of patients with type 2 diabetic nephropathy (e.g., Native Americans), progression may be very rapid. Microalbuminuria is not useful in predicting the subsequent development of overt nephropathy in patients with type 2 diabetes. However, the presence of microalbuminuria in patients with type 2 diabetes is associated with increased risk of morbidity and mortality from macrovascular disease. Screening for microalbuminuria should be initiated at the time of diagnosis of type 2 diabetes mellitus.

The role of glycemic control in the pathogenesis of microalbuminuria in type 2 diabetes is unclear, although one study demonstrated a significant association between glycemic control (measured by glycosylated hemoglobin levels) and microalbuminuria. A link between lipid levels and microalbuminuria has also been demonstrated.

As in type 1 diabetes, aggressive control of blood pressure in type 2 appears to be important in slowing the rate of loss of renal function. Unlike in type 1 diabetes, hypertension in type 2 frequently precedes the diagnosis of diabetes. As previously demonstrated in patients with type 1 diabetic nephropathy, ACE inhibitors decrease proteinuria in patients with type 2 diabetes and overt nephropathy.

Diabetic nephropathy progresses to ESRD in 20% to 60% of patients with non–insulin-dependent diabetes mellitus. The wide range in the latter group is largely due to differences in the populations studied, the higher percentage noted in certain groups such as Native Americans, Hispanics, and African-Americans. The prevalence of comorbid conditions, most notably hypertension, also influences the likelihood of the development of renal failure.

Approach to Patients with Type 2 Diabetic Nephropathy

PATIENT NUMBER 4 (continued)

Muriel has type 2 diabetes mellitus and nephrotic syndrome. Although diabetic glomerulopathy is probably the most likely cause, one must consider other causes of her nephrotic syndrome in light of her relatively short history of diabetes mellitus, her hematuria, and the absence of retinopathy. In some patients, atypical features such as these may result in the need for renal biopsy in order to be certain of the diagnosis. Rigorous control of blood pressure is very important in our patient Muriel, and a target mean arterial pressure of <100 mm Hg may be appropriate. A diuretic (usually a loop diuretic if the creatinine clearance is <50 to 60 ml/min) should be used to decrease her edema and improve her blood pressure control. She should be counseled to lose weight, consume a low-sodium diet (2 g of sodium per day) and restrict her protein intake to 0.6 to 0.8 g/ kg/day. ACE inhibitors should be initiated, but Muriel should be closely monitored to ensure that she does not develop hyperkalemia, leukopenia, or a precipitous rise in her serum creatinine level. Serum levels of low-density lipoprotein, high-density lipoprotein, and triglycerides should be checked, and her hyperlipidemia treated aggressively. She should be appropriately evaluated for the presence of cerebral, coronary, and peripheral arterial disease.

Management Guide for Patients with Type 2 Diabetic Nephropathy

- **Screen for microalbuminuria.**
- **Institute rigorous blood pressure control (mean arterial pressure <100 mm Hg).**
- **Avoid severe hyperglycemia.**
- **Provide dietary and pharmacologic control of hyperlipidemia.**
- **Monitor the patient for the presence of coronary, cerebral, and peripheral vascular disease.**
- **Counsel patients to modify other cardiovascular risk factors (sedentary lifestyle, lipids, smoking, obesity).**

OTHER RENAL DISEASES IN PATIENTS WITH DIABETES MELLITUS

Although diabetic glomerulopathy is the most common renal parenchymal disorder encountered among patients with diabetes mellitus, it is important for clinicians to recognize that several other renal disorders may occur in diabetic patients and may contribute significantly to renal morbidity and mortality. A detailed description of these disorders is beyond the scope of this discussion, but brief mention and description of several of these entities are appropriate.

Renal Arterial Occlusive Disease

Patients with diabetes mellitus are subject to a dramatically increased risk of large vessel atherosclerotic disease. Such atherosclerosis may affect one or both renal arteries. Unilateral renal arterial stenosis, secondary to atherosclerosis, may dramatically aggravate the underlying tendency to hypertension. Afflicted individuals may present with sudden worsening of hypertension, difficult-to-control hypertension, grade 3 or 4 hypertensive retinopathy, lateralizing abdominal bruits, disparity in renal size, and hyperreninemia. A high index of suspicion is required in order to make the diagnosis. Bilateral renal arterial occlusive disease should always be suspected when acute renal failure or a substantial decline in GFR follows the administration of ACE inhibitors or an acute lowering of systemic arterial pressure with any antihypertensive agent. Captopril scintigraphy or duplex Doppler ultrasonography may be a useful screening test, but these have very limited usefulness in bilateral disease. Percutaneous transfemoral renal arteriograms or intraarterial digital subtraction angiography is required to substantiate the diagnosis. However, in the setting of incipient, overt, or azotemic glomerulopathy, administration of radiocontrast agents may induce acute renal failure. The use of magnetic resonance imaging (with an overall accuracy of 81%) or carbon dioxide angiography is a useful alternative that obviates the risk of acute renal failure, and these are preferred methods of investigation.

Acute Renal Failure Secondary to Contrast Media or Nonsteroidal Antiinflammatory Agents

Patients with diabetes mellitus, particularly those with early, overt, or azotemic glomerulopathy, are at **increased risk of developing acute renal failure** (acute tubular necrosis) after contrast media injection, such as with an IVP or a renal arteriogram. The renal failure is often mild and reversible and is chiefly of a nonoliguric variety. The risk of acute renal failure may be decreased by volume expansion before contrast media injection, diminishing the total dose of contrast media, using nonionic contrast media, and pretreating with calcium channel blockers before angiography. When appropriate, consideration should be given to avoid contrast agents altogether by the performance of magnetic resonance or carbon dioxide angiography.

Nonsteroidal antiinflammatory agents may also induce a functional form of acute renal failure in patients with diabetes mellitus, particularly those with concomitant congestive heart failure due to coronary artery disease. In such patients, the GFR rapidly declines on administration of the drug and usually quickly returns to baseline when the drug is discontinued. On rare occasions, tubulointerstitial nephritis may complicate the use of these drugs.

Renal Medullary or Papillary Necrosis

Patients with diabetes mellitus are at increased risk of developing medullary or papillary necrosis in association with partial lower urinary tract obstruction or with acute ascending bacterial pyelonephritis. Necrotic papillae may be passed into the urine, and acute renal failure may develop.

Urinary Tract Infection

The incidence and prevalence of urinary tract infection may be slightly increased in patients with diabetes mellitus, particularly females. Relapses of infection after treatment are common, especially in the presence of abnormal bladder emptying or impaired renal function. On rare occasions, such urinary tract infections may be complicated by the development of granulomatous pyelonephritis. This disorder principally affects one or the other kidney and results in an enlarged, poorly functioning, or nonfunctioning kidney. It is often mistaken for a renal malignancy. Rarely, fungal infection of the urinary tract may lead to ureteric obstruction from the mycelial phase growth of the organism (fungus ball). Diabetic patients are also at increased risk for developing the uncommon entity known as *emphysematous pyelonephritis*, in which gram-negative gas-forming bacterial organisms rapidly induce necrosis of the kidney.

Renal Tubular Acidosis

Patients with diabetes mellitus, particularly those with incipient or early overt glomerulopathy, may develop a form of renal tubular acidosis known as type 4 (hyperkalemic) renal tubular acidosis. These patients also have low plasma renin levels. Aldosterone secretion rates are abnormally low in relationship to the concomitant hyperkalemia. The pathogenesis of this syndrome is diverse. In some patients, a primary defect in renin secretion may be at fault; in others, an abnormality of aldosterone production may be the underlying cause. This complication seldom requires any direct therapy, although the hyperkalemia and acidosis may sometimes result in morbidity. Hyperkalemia is particularly hazardous in patients with coronary artery disease and disorders of atrioventricular conduction.

Nondiabetic Glomerular Disease

Because diabetes mellitus is a relatively common disorder, it is not surprising that a significant proportion of patients with diabetes presenting with overt renal disease are found to have non–diabetes-related lesions on careful investigation. These are most common in patients with type 2 diabetes mellitus presenting with proteinuria or hematuria but are also found among patients with type 1 diabetes mellitus presenting with proteinuria or hematuria 5 years or less from the onset of insulin dependence. **Primary renal disease unrelated to diabetes has been described in more than 20% of diabetic patients who begin renal replacement therapy and in as many as two thirds of patients who undergo renal biopsy because the clinical diagnosis of diabetic nephropathy is doubted.** Clues to the presence of a nondiabetic lesion underlying a disorder of renal function in a diabetic patient include rapid onset, absence of proliferative retinopathy (especially for type 1 diabetes; less important for type 2 diabetes), "active" urinary sediment (dysmorphic hematuria and RBC casts), absence of hypertension, small

kidneys, tubular proteinuria, or normal hemoglobin A1c values. The presence of either hematuria or tubular proteinuria may not be a reliable or discriminatory observation. However, it should be emphasized that **some patients (<15%) with diabetic glomerulopathy may present with hematuria and RBC casts in addition to glomerular proteinuria.** The origin of the RBCs in the urine of patients with diabetic glomerulopathy is unknown but could relate to concomitant hemorrhagic cystitis, papillary necrosis, or a ruptured glomerular microaneurysm. Dysmorphic hematuria is noted only when RBCs derive from a glomerular origin.

Clinicians should retain a high index of suspicion for nondiabetic glomerular disease in patients who have type 2 diabetes mellitus presenting initially with renal failure and proteinuria. Similarly, patients who have type 1 diabetes mellitus and who present with proteinuria or renal failure 5 years or less from the onset of insulin dependence may have a cause of renal failure that is separate from diabetes. The nondiabetic renal lesions that occur in patients with diabetes mellitus are heterogeneous, but the prevalence of idiopathic membranous glomerulopathy, minimal change disease, IgA nephropathy and poststreptococcal glomerulonephritis appears to be increased. Amyloidosis, for unknown reasons, is quite uncommon. Renal biopsies sometimes may be required for definitive distinction of diabetic glomerulopathy from nondiabetic glomerular disease. In otherwise typical cases of diabetic glomerulopathy, a clinical diagnosis is sufficient and renal biopsies are ordinarily not performed.

SUGGESTED READINGS

Adler SG, Nast CC, Artishevsky A: Diabetic nephropathy: Pathogenesis and treatment. Annu Rev Med 44:303–315, 1993.

Humphrey LL, Ballard DJ, Frohnert PP, et al: Chronic renal failure in non-insulin dependent diabetes mellitus. A population based study in Rochester, Minnesota. Ann Intern Med 111:788–796, 1989.

Lewis EJ, Hunsicker LG, Bain RP, et al: The effect of angiotensin converting-enzyme inhibition on diabetic nephropathy. N Engl J Med 329:1456–1462, 1993.

Mathiesen ER, Hommel E, Giese J, Parving H-H: Efficacy of captopril in postponing nephropathy in normotensive insulin dependent diabetic patients with microalbuminuria. Br Med J 303:81–87, 1991.

Nathan DM: Long-term complications of diabetes mellitus. N Engl J Med 328:1677–1685, 1993.

Slataper R, Vicknair N, Sadler R, Bakris GL: Comparative effects of different antihypertensive treatments on progression of diabetic renal disease. Arch Intern Med 153:973–980, 1993.

Sutherland D, Gruessner A: International Pancreas Transplant Registry Report. Transplant Proc 26:407–411, 1994.

8 | RENAL DISEASE AND HYPERTENSION IN PREGNANCY

Marshall D. Lindheimer and Jason G. Umans

This chapter discusses renal disorders and high blood pressure in pregnant women. After reviewing anatomic and physiologic changes that occur in gestation and that are pertinent to clinical circumstances, it focuses on acute renal failure (ARF) and chronic parenchymal diseases (including transplantation) and on features of urinary tract infection unique to pregnancy. Because most of the hypertensive complications of gestation are due to preeclampsia and essential hypertension, the final section is primarily devoted to these two disorders.

STRUCTURAL AND FUNCTIONAL CHANGES IN NORMAL PREGNANCY

Table 8–1 summarizes the renal changes in normal gestation and comments on their clinical relevance. During pregnancy, the kidneys increase in size and the intrarenal collecting system and ureters dilate. The latter change, present at the end of the initial trimester, may persist through the third postpartum month. However, despite the occasional presence of substantially marked ureteral dilation, it is unclear whether vesicoureteral reflux is increased during pregnancy. It also remains unresolved whether these changes are secondary to humoral (i.e., estrogen, progesterone, or prostaglandins) or to mechanical (i.e., the enlarged uterus) factors. Radiographic studies that demonstrate that ureteral dilatation terminates at the pelvic brim suggest an obstructive origin due to the compression of the ureters as they cross the iliac arteries. Pyelography may reveal a smooth cutoff or filling defect at this region, termed the *iliac sign*. Figure 8–1 is an example of the physiologic dilation of the ureters as it is often seen on ultrasound examination.

These physiologic alterations have several consequences: First, frank urinary obstruction may be difficult to diagnose. Urinary stasis in the dilated tracts may lead to errors in the collection of timed urine samples (minimized by hydrating patients and placing them in lateral recumbency before beginning and completing the collection) and may increase the frequency with which asymptomatic urinary tract infections progress to pyelonephritis. Finally, a rare distention syndrome is characterized by abdominal pain, marked hydronephrosis, a variable increase in serum creatinine levels, and mild hypertension. Some of these cases have been managed successfully through delivery by the placement of ureteral stents.

RENAL HEMODYNAMICS AND SOLUTE HANDLING

The most striking changes in normal pregnancy are increases in GFR and renal plasma flow (RPF), which occur during the initial trimester and rapidly reach values ~50% greater than those before conception. Near term GFR may fall by approximately 20% (measured as the clearance of creatinine), though on occasion the decrement reaches nonpregnant levels. The relevance of these changes are as follows: Norms for values of creatinine and urea nitrogen decrease from means of 0.7 and 12 mg/dl (62 μmol/L and 4.3 mmol/L) in a nonpregnant woman to 0.5 mg/dl and 9 mg/dl (44 μmol/L and 3.3 mmol/L), respectively. Levels of creatinine that would appear normal (i.e., a serum creatinine level of 0.9 mg/dl [81 μmol/L]) may reflect renal disease in a pregnant patient. Filtered loads of many solutes are increased. For example, both glycosuria and aminoaciduria are normal in gestation. Although the renal handling of urate is complex, its clearance, too, rises in pregnancy, and values ex-

TABLE 8–1. Gestational Alterations in Renal Structure and Function

Alteration	Manifestation	Clinical Relevance
Increased renal size	Renal length approximately 1 cm greater on roentgenograms.	Postpartum decreases in renal size should not be mistaken for parenchymal loss.
Dilatation of renal pelves, calyces, and ureters	Resembles hydronephrosis on intravenous pyelography or renal ultrasonography (usually more marked on right).	Do not mistake for obstruction; defer elective pyelography to at least 3 months postpartum; retained urine may lead to errors in timed collections; may be responsible for "distention syndrome"; upper tract infections are more virulent.
Increased renal hemodynamics	Both GFR and effective renal plasma flow increase 30%–50%.	Serum creatinine and urea nitrogen values decrease, with normal Cr ≤0.8 mg/dl; urinary protein, glucose, and amino acid excretion all increase; serum urate falls to <5 mg/dl.
Changes in acid-base regulation	Compensated primary respiratory alkalosis with decreased renal bicarbonate threshold.	$PaCO_2$ decreases 10 mm Hg, and serum bicarbonate falls by 4–5 mEq/L. An asthmatic patient with a $PaCO_2$ of 40 mm Hg already manifests CO_2 retention.
Water metabolism	Osmoregulation of vasopressin release is altered, and metabolic clearance rate of vasopressin is increased.	Plasma osmolality decreases 10 mOsm/L (serum sodium by 5 mEq/L). Increased vasopressin clearance may cause certain transient diabetes insipidus–like syndromes.
Volume homeostasis	Intravascular volume increases 40% early in pregnancy. Interstitial volume increases >2 L after midgestation.	Volume changes must be considered in the rare gravidas maintained on dialysis.
Blood pressure regulation	Arterial pressure normally decreases 10 mm Hg by second trimester.	Antecedent mild essential hypertension may be undiagnosed in early pregnancy and misdiagnosed as preeclampsia when pressure rises near term.

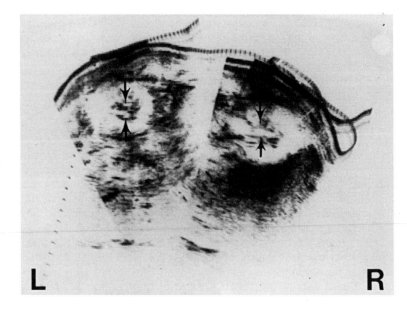

Figure 8–1. Renal ultrasonography demonstrating a dilated intrarenal collecting system in a normal gravida *without* obstructive uropathy.

ceeding 5 mg/dl (297 μmol/L) are abnormal. Protein excretion (but apparently not that of albumin) also increases in gestation, and the former may be partially due to the rise in GFR. In any event, during pregnancy, upper limits for normal proteinuria should be doubled to 300 to 500 mg/24 hr.

ACID-BASE REGULATION

Pregnant women normally hyperventilate to a P_{CO_2} of ~30 mm Hg and compensate for this respiratory alkalosis by decreasing their plasma bicarbonate levels to 20 to 22 mEq/L, resulting in a mean pH of 7.44. The renal bicarbonate threshold is decreased, and urine thus may be more alkaline during pregnancy; however, the kidneys' ability to augment excretion of titratable acid and ammonium after an acid load is unimpaired. Thus, measurement of a P_{CO_2} of 30 mm Hg during a severe asthmatic attack represents significant carbon dioxide retention, and a blood pH of 7.40 already suggests acidemia.

VOLUME HOMEOSTASIS AND OSMOREGULATION

Weight gain throughout pregnancy averages 12.5 kg, but there is a large standard deviation about this mean. Half of the gain is attributable to increments in total body water of 6 to 8 L, 4 to 6 L of which is in the extracellular compartment, including a 50% rise in plasma volume. The gestational volume expansion is accompanied by a cumulative retention of ~900 mEq of sodium. There is some controversy about how a pregnant woman senses her new volume status (i.e., under-, over-, or normal filled). Our view is that the physiologic hypervolemia is perceived as normal by the woman, who responds to salt depletion or volume loads in a manner that defends circulating volume and blood pressure around her new set-point. For reasons not completely understood, though, all elements of the renin-angiotensin-aldosterone system are increased in pregnancy. These systems, too, seem to respond to volume challenges around a new set-point. A pregnant woman's pressor responsiveness to angiotensin II (and perhaps to other vasoconstrictors) is quite blunted, however, and the elevated mineralocorticoid levels do not lead to hypertension, hypokalemia, or excess salt retention.

Osmoregulation is profoundly altered in gestation, plasma osmolality decreasing by ~10 mOsm/kg below nonpregnant values, the changes occurring very early in pregnancy. This hypotonic state, associated with a predictable fall in plasma sodium level of ~5 mEq/L, is maintained to term, normalizing during the first 2 weeks of the puerperium. These changes are due to decrements in the osmotic thresholds of both thirst and vasopressin (AVP) release, and as was the case in volume regulation, the gravida senses her new (hypotonic) set-point as normal, concentrating and diluting appropriately around a P_{osm} ~10 mOsm/kg lower than in the nonpregnant state. A fourfold increase occurs in the metabolic clearance rate (MCR) of AVP, in part a result of large quantities of vasopressinase produced by the placenta and secreted into the circulation.

The relevance of these osmoregulatory changes include the following: A P_{osm} in the nonpregnant range or even at its lower limit of normal in a polyuric gravida suggests diabetes insipidus (DI) but may mistakenly be diagnosed as primary polydipsia. There are several syndromes of transient DI of pregnancy, one due to the combined effects of subclinical central DI and the increased MCR of endogenously produced hormone and a second caused by excessive quantities of circulating vasopressinase. The latter disorder resists treatment with synthetic AVP, and both forms should be treated with DDAVP, a vasopressin analogue resistant to enzymatic degradation.

PATIENT NUMBER 1

You are requested to consult about a 23-year-old nullipara hospitalized at 33 weeks' gestation because of hypertension (140/95 mm Hg) and proteinuria (qualitative 1 to 2+). The immediate history taking and physical examination are nonrevealing except for confirmation of the hypertension (now 130/90 mm Hg), and the laboratory values in the chart reveal a creatinine of 0.9 mg/dl (81 μmol/L), a uric acid of 4.9 mg/dl (291 mmol/L), and serum electrolyte levels of sodium 143 mEq/L, potassium 4.2 mEq/L, bicarbonate 23 mEq/L, and chloride 110 mEq/L. Her hematocrit is 41%, and a platelet count is 133 × 10³/mm³. What have you forgotten to ask, and what further information do you want?

A plasma sodium level of 143 mEq/L may be uneventful in a nonpregnant patient but is high during gestation, suggesting hyperosmolality. Further questioning of patient 1 revealed the sudden onset of polyuria 2 weeks previously, associated with severe thirst. The volume in a 24-hour urine collection was 6.3 L with an osmolality of 155 mOsm/kg. Also, the creatinine level is abnormal for gestation, the uric acid level borderline, and as discussed later, this patient's hematocrit is actually high for pregnancy (hemoconcentration). In addition, her platelet numbers are decreased for pregnancy. Review of her blood smear revealed schistocytes, liver enzyme levels were discovered to be elevated, and her albumin level was 2.1 g/L. Thus, this woman with seemingly mild hypertension and proteinuria has a dangerous variant of preeclampsia that includes liver involvement and early signs of a microangiopathic hemolytic anemia (in which case the hematocrit of 41% might represent an even greater degree of hemoconcentration). Furthermore, the liver involvement and not the modest proteinuria may be the reason her serum albumin is low and may also explain the sudden occurrence of DI (decreased hepatic inactivation of vasopressinase).

This patient's pregnancy was terminated shortly thereafter by cesarean section under general anesthesia. Failure to diagnose DI might have resulted in life-threatening hypernatremia. How should her DI be treated? Obviously with DDAVP, because the polyuria in these women is resistant to vasopressin.

PRESSURE REGULATION

Mean arterial pressure decreases early in gestation, and by midpregnancy, diastolic levels are often 10 to 15 mm Hg below postpartum values. Blood pressure normally increases in the last trimester, approaching nonpregnant values near term. Thus, values that would appear normal in a nonpregnant patient may be abnormally elevated in a gravida, and likewise, the early gestational decrement in diastolic pressure may mask antecedent hypertension.

Cardiac output increases 30% to 50% in gestation, and thus the decrease in blood pressure denotes an even larger decrement in peripheral vascular resistance. The cause of this early, marked, and persistent systemic vasodilation is poorly understood, but attention has recently turned to the role of endothelium-derived relaxing factors, whose basal or induced concentrations may be considerably augmented throughout pregnancy.

RENAL DISORDERS
Urinary Tract Infection

The prevalence of asymptomatic bacteriuria during gestation is similar to that in nonpregnant

TABLE 8–2. Treatment of Asymptomatic Bacteriuria and Cystitis in Pregnancy

Agent°	Dose
Standard Courses of Treatment (Duration 7–10 Days)	
Ampicillin	500 mg q.i.d.
Amoxicillin	250 mg t.i.d.
Nitrofurantoin†	50 mg q.i.d.
Cephalexin	250 mg b.i.d.
Amoxicillin/clavulanic acid	250/125 mg t.i.d.
Long-Term Prophylaxis	
Nitrofurantoin†	50 mg at night
Cephalexin	250 mg at night
Amoxicillin	250 mg at night

°All antibiotics listed in this table are in FDA risk category B.
†Nitrofurantoin macrocrystals may reduce the incidence of gastrointestinal side effects.
Modified from Pedler SJ, Orr KE: Bacterial, fungal, and parasitic infections. *In* Barron WM, Lindheimer MD (eds): Medical Disorders During Pregnancy, 2nd ed. St Louis, Mosby-Year Book, 1995, pp 356–388.

women of reproductive age, ranging from 2% to 10%. However, the natural history of these two groups differs substantially, being benign in the nongravid population but progressing to acute pyelonephritis in 20% to 30% of pregnant women. Thus, in pregnancy, we recommend universal screening, preferably between gestational weeks 12 and 16, as well as treatment of significant bacteriuria with the appropriate antibiotic as determined by culture (Table 8–2).

Cystitis or pyelonephritis complicates 3% of all pregnancies. Interestingly, the incidence of acute cystitis (1% to 2%) does not appear to be influenced by universal screening, but the incidence of the more ominous infectious pyelonephritis has declined from 3% to ≤1%; it is this decrease that is ascribed to aggressive screening for covert bacteriuria and treatment of it. Pyelonephritis during gestation is associated with prematurity, growth retardation, fetal demise, and an increased incidence of maternal sepsis (often associated with hypotension or shock and, in a surprising number of cases, acute respiratory distress syndrome). Thus, treatment should be rapid and aggressive, using parenteral antibiotics in an inpatient setting. Because of an increase in the number of community-acquired pathogens resistant to ampicillin, many consultants recommend addition of an aminoglycoside (usually gentamicin) and clindamycin initially, adjusting therapy when culture results become available. The extended-spectrum penicillins have also been used in these women. (One should continually check the U.S. Food and Drug Administration [FDA] guidelines for up-to-date pregnancy risk classifications, which are usually listed in the *Physicians' Desk Reference* [PDR].)

Pregnant patients with pyelonephritis usually respond rapidly to treatment but often suffer a relapse or become reinfected later in gestation. Avoiding such an outcome requires appropriate oral antibiotic therapy for a minimum of 2 or 3 weeks, followed by either frequent surveillance urine cultures or suppressive antibiotic therapy (see Table 8–2).

Acute Renal Failure

ARF severe enough to require dialysis, which once had an incidence of 1 in 2000, now occurs rarely (i.e., <1 in 20,000). This decline has been attributed to the virtual disappearance of septic abortion in countries where women have easy access to sterile terminations. The pathology in almost all cases of ARF is acute tubular necrosis, although a minority present with patchy or sometimes bilateral renal cortical necrosis. Cortical necrosis, however, is a rare lesion (incidence 1 in 40,000), but when it occurs it is most likely to be associated with concealed uterine bleeding at 32 to 34 weeks. The causes of ARF in pregnancy are similar to those in nonpregnant populations, including bleeding, infection, volume depletion, obstruction, toxins, and various nephritides. ARF occasionally complicates preeclampsia, especially those cases manifesting the HELLP variant (discussed later). Two other forms of ARF are peculiar to gestation, acute fatty liver of pregnancy and idiopathic postpartum renal failure. The cause of renal dysfunction in the former disorder is obscure, recognition of the syndrome demanding prompt evacuation of the uterus. The cause of kidney failure in the idiopathic postpartum disease is also unknown, but the peripheral blood picture and renal pathology often resemble those in the thrombotic microangiopathies, especially adult hemolytic-uremic syndrome. Fortunately, both acute fatty liver of pregnancy and idiopathic postpartum renal failure are quite rare.

Dialysis During Pregnancy

Management of acute and chronic renal failure is similar to that in nonpregnant populations and may include either peritoneal dialysis or hemodialysis. A gravid uterus is not a contraindication to placement of a peritoneal catheter, which should be made under direct vision and high in the abdomen. Some believe ambulatory perito-

neal dialysis is better tolerated ("gentler") than hemodialysis. They also believe that because urea and presumed uremic "toxins" readily cross the placenta, early aggressive prophylactic or intense (daily) dialysis should be empirically instituted to attempt to maintain urea N levels less than 50 mg/dl (18 mmol/L). Very few data are available, but we, too, practice this aggressive approach.

Suggested alterations in the hemodialysis prescription during pregnancy are outlined in Table 8–3. A registry for women currently undergoing dialysis during pregnancy is being directed by Dr. Susan Hou, at Rush Presbyterian-St. Luke's Medical Center, in Chicago. Initial data suggest that at most 50% of the pregnancies in women undergoing chronic dialysis succeed and that maternal morbidity (and even mortality) is considerable. Therefore, we continue to counsel women with end-stage renal disease against conception (discussed later).

PATIENT NUMBER 2

A 27-year-old woman with end-stage renal disease secondary to focal and segmental glomerulosclerosis has been receiving dialytic therapy for 3 years. Her menstrual cycles have been irregular for 5 years, and during the past 18 months she has had no menstrual periods at all. She produced 1 L of urine a day, which contained 500 mg of protein. Her peritoneal dialysis regimen included four 2-L exchanges. Can this woman conceive, and if so, what are her contraceptive options?

It is important to know that women with end-stage renal disease are only relatively infertile. They can have both ovulatory and anovulatory cycles in the presence or absence of menstruation. Thus, they must receive contraceptive counseling. As for contraceptive options, intrauterine devices should be avoided. They often fail and are more likely to cause bleeding and infection in these patients. Otherwise, very few data are available, and we prefer the use of oral contraceptives with low-dose estrogen in these patients, believing any risks are outweighed by those associated with conception.

PATIENT NUMBER 2 (continued)

Shortly thereafter, the patient uncharacteristically complained of nausea and vomiting and had one episode of blood-tinged dialysate. Results of a pregnancy test were positive, and an ultrasound scan revealed a normal singleton 12-week gestation and a

TABLE 8–3. Modifications of Hemodialysis Prescription During Pregnancy

Modification	Rationale
Intensified or daily dialysis to keep BUN <50 mg/dl with increased dialysis may be required.	A fetus is exposed to uremic toxins of maternal origin, and fetal outcome is poor when dialysis merely avoids maternal uremic symptoms. A fetus produces >0.5 g of urea daily at term, and maternal BUN rises during the last trimester.
Monitor predialysis potassium level and increase dialysate potassium concentration to 3–3.5 mEq/L as needed.	Daily dialysis may lead to hypokalemia.
Lower dialysate sodium concentration to 134 mEq/L.	Attempt to mimic the normal hypo-osmolality of pregnancy.
Avoid large fluid shifts by daily dialysis and use of isolated ultrafiltration for excessive intradialytic weight gains. Treat intradialytic hypotension by liberal use of saline infusions.	Episodic hypotension or rapid fluid shifts may lead to fetal distress and premature labor.
Dose of calcitriol may have to be decreased and that of erythropoietin increased.	The placenta produces $1,25(OH)_2-D_3$, and more erythropoietin is required to sustain the normal gestational increase in RBC mass.
Increase estimated dry weight by 0.5–1 kg/mo during the first 6 months and by 0.25–0.5 kg/wk during the last trimester, while closely monitoring blood pressure and physical findings.	Attempt to mimic physiologic volume expansion of pregnancy.

small ovarian cyst. Termination was recommended but declined.

Her physicians decreased her exchanges to four 1.5-L exchanges daily, concerned that with the enlarging uterus greater quantities of fluid would be poorly tolerated. Table 8–4 summarizes blood pressure as well as several chemical values measured serially throughout gestation. When her creatinine and urea N levels were noted to rise, her dialysis prescription was increased to five 1.5-L exchanges daily. It was further noted that her urine protein excretion had increased to 1 g/day. Throughout gestation she manifested mild hypertension, which increased somewhat at 30 weeks' gestation. She also received 3 units of packed RBCs at 29 weeks. At 30 weeks, premature contractions were noted. They were resistant to tocolysis and were followed by ruptured membranes and the delivery of a growth-retarded 1.3-kg male. During labor, she also developed abdominal pain, and a retroplacental clot consistent with abruption was noted after delivery of the placenta.

This case demonstrates many of the problems when patients receiving dialytic therapy conceive. First, because of irregular or absent menses, these potentially high-risk pregnant patients fail to seek early prenatal care, the gestation remaining unnoticed sometimes until after mid-pregnancy. The woman described here was fortunate in that nausea and vomiting resulted in a diagnosis during the 12th week. Her physicians were not aware of the need to increase dialysis and initially let her azotemia worsen. Her anemia increased because erythropoietin demands rise during gestation. Her physicians were reluctant to use such therapy, and data on erythropoietin therapy during gestation currently are still scarce. Experience is increasing, however, and we believe its use might have spared this patient the need for transfusion. Hypertension often worsens in these patients, usually in the early third trimester. In this case, the rise was mild, but in many such women the increments are severe and life threatening. Her doctors did not prescribe antihypertensive drugs. This is because mild hypertension is usually not treated during gestation. We, however, believe that high-risk situations such as this one are exceptions and would have

TABLE 8–4. Blood Pressure and Chemical Values Throughout Gestation

	NP	Gestation (Weeks)								PP
		4	8	12	16	20	24	28	30	
Creatinine, mg/dl	5.1	4.5	4.3	4.3	5.1	5.6	5.7	6.8	6.7	5.6
Urea N, mg/dl	39	36	36	42	45	45	54	60	60	45
Hb, g/dl	8.5	8.5	8.0	7.5	7.0	7.0	7.5	7.0	9.0	6.5
Weight, kg	55	54	53	53	55	56	58	58	58	52
BP, mm Hg	130/80	130/80	130/90	140/90	140/90	140/90	140/90	140/95	150/100	130/90

treated her. Also note that despite end-stage renal disease, her proteinuria increased. This may be due to changes in the filtration barrier of the few surviving nephrons, but of importance here, it makes diagnosis of superimposed preeclampsia difficult in these women. Finally, note the premature labor, fetal growth retardation, and abruption, each a complication more likely to occur in these patients than in normal gravidas. In conclusion, this was one of the 50% "successes" in women receiving dialysis, underscoring why we still counsel against conception and recommend termination of pregnancies.

PREGNANCY WITH PREEXISTING RENAL DISEASE

Renal parenchymal disease was formerly considered a contraindication to pregnancy, whatever its severity. Publications dating from the 1980s, however, although largely retrospective and uncontrolled, revealed better prognoses than previously thought, suggesting guidelines for management of gravidas with underlying chronic renal disorders.

When GFR is well preserved and hypertension absent, pregnancy is successful more than 95% of the time, maternal complications are minimal, and gestation does not appear to affect the natural history of the kidney disorder adversely (or if it does, the effect is minimal). Such patients often manifest increases in GFR during gestation, a favorable prognostic sign. Patients with glomerular diseases frequently demonstrate nephrotic-range proteinuria, but this is rarely a sign of progressive disease. Although the foregoing generalizations are true for the majority of renal disorders, there are exceptions. Prognosis is poorer in women with collagen-vascular disease, and several entities provoke controversy (discussed later).

In patients with moderately decreased GFR (serum creatinine level ≥1.5 mg/dl, 132 µmol/L) or those with difficult-to-control moderate or severe hypertension, the prognosis is more guarded. Approximately one third suffer accelerated renal functional deterioration, of which at least 10% do not reverse after delivery. In addition, the incidence of late pregnancy hypertension (often superimposed preeclampsia) is high, and the increment in pressure may be severe and difficult to control. Nevertheless ~90% of the gestations succeed, although both prematurity and growth retardation are increased.

Severe renal dysfunction (serum creatinine level ≥3 mg/dl, 265 µmol/L), as noted, is often associated with infertility, and when such patients do conceive, their pregnancy success rate barely approaches 50% but maternal and fetal morbidity are substantial. We usually counsel against pregnancy in the presence of both moderate and severe renal insufficiency.

GENERAL GUIDELINES FOR EVALUATION AND MANAGEMENT

Pregnant women with renal disease are best treated by a team that includes both a maternal-fetal medicine subspecialist and a nephrologist. In addition to the usual prenatal tests, initial laboratory evaluation should include the following: an assessment of GFR by creatinine clearance, a careful urinalysis, screening urine culture, and a 24-hour collection to measure urinary protein excretion. Other tests include measurement of serum electrolytes, urea nitrogen, uric acid, albumin, glutamic oxaloacetic transaminase, lactic acid dehydrogenase, and platelet count. These data serve as a baseline to help evaluate the renal disorder and for later detection of superimposed preeclampsia as well (discussed later). Follow-up care includes biweekly visits until gestational week 32 and weekly visits thereafter. Renal parameters are reassessed every 4 to 6 weeks, and fetal assessment by electronic monitoring is usually commenced between weeks 30 and 32.

GLOMERULAR DISEASES

The course of most glomerular disorders in pregnancy is determined by the level of renal function and blood pressure before conception. There is disagreement, however, about the natural history of IgA nephropathy, most investigators observing little or no adverse effect on the course of the disease but some reporting deteriorating renal function, the *de novo* appearance or aggravation of hypertension, and progression of the lesions in renal biopsy specimens. Likewise, controversy surrounds the courses of focal glomerulosclerosis and mesangioproliferative glomerulonephritis, reflecting, in part, a paucity of data on these disorders. We believe, here too, that prognosis is favorable in normotensive women with preserved function.

Connective Tissue Disorders

The influence of gestation on activity and progression of both renal and extrarenal manifestations of systemic lupus erythematosus (SLE) is not uniformly predictable, not surprising in view of the lack of prognostic accuracy in nonpregnant patients with the disease. Although outcome is poorer than with many other glomerular disorders, most patients with preserved renal function fare well. Prognosis is most favorable when a patient is normotensive and the disease has been quiescent for at least 6 months. The course is less favorable if circulating lupus anticoagulants or antiphospholipid antibodies are present, this group of patients probably accounting for the increased incidence of spontaneous abortion with SLE.

Patients are treated as discussed earlier in the section on general guidelines, and both laboratory and clinical markers of disease activity are watched closely. Hypertension with increasing proteinuria and thrombocytopenia, especially when it occurs in late pregnancy, may be difficult to differentiate between an exacerbation of SLE and superimposed preeclampsia.

Pharmacologic management includes steroids, nonsteroidal antiinflammatory drugs, and azathioprine (even though the latter is in FDA class D). Nonsteroidal agents should be avoided near term because of their effects on the fetal ductus arteriosus. We also try to avoid chloroquine (FDA class C) and do not prescribe cyclophosphamide (FDA class D). Aspirin and heparin are usually prescribed for patients who have high titers of antiphospholipid antibodies; however, their efficacy is unclear. Because fetal exposure to specific maternal autoantibodies, especially anti-Ro (SS-A), is associated with congenital heart block, fetuses should have echocardiographic evaluation at midgestation and careful monitoring of their heart rates thereafter.

In contrast to the generally favorable outcome in patients with SLE, prognosis is markedly poorer in women with scleroderma or polyarteritis nodosa. Anecdotal reports of severe maternal morbidity and mortality during gestation suggest that pregnancy not be undertaken and that early unanticipated gestations be terminated.

DIABETIC NEPHROPATHY

Insulin-dependent diabetic patients often already have occult nephropathy when they conceive, are at greater risk for urinary tract infections, and are more susceptible to superimposed preeclampsia. Still, most of their gestations succeed without any other evidence of renal complications. Some state that screening for microalbuminuria helps predict late pregnancy hypertension as well as other complications (although data are scarce).

Pregnancy in patients with overt nephropathy and well-preserved function is usually successful, but these women often develop hypertension and heavy proteinuria and occasional decrements in renal function early in the last trimester, the latter usually reversible postpartum. The presence of hypertension with the nephropathy before conception denotes a poorer prognosis.

NEPHROTIC SYNDROME

Whether symptomatic nephrotic syndrome before or in early gestation is associated with progression of the underlying disease in pregnancy is controversial. It may be associated with a poorer fetal outcome. Although serum albumin level decreases and edema usually worsens during pregnancy, diuretic therapy should be minimized, if possible, because diuretic use may result in severe intravascular volume depletion and impaired uteroplacental perfusion. An exception is made for diabetic nephropathy, in which judicious use of saluretic therapy may counteract the tendency toward salt-sensitive hypertension and may help obviate early termination of the pregnancy.

Pregnancy is a hypercoagulable state that may be exacerbated in nephrotic syndrome owing to urinary loss of fibrinolytic proteins. Thus, some clinicians administer prophylactic heparin, although it may cause severe maternal osteoporosis. We prefer to treat such high-risk patients by serially assessing the patency of their lower extremity venous system using Doppler techniques. In the future, low-molecular-weight dextran may prove useful. The hyperlipidemia associated with nephrotic syndrome is rarely treated during gestation, and the hydroxymethylglutaryl-coenzyme A reductase inhibitors are contraindicated during gestation (FDA class X). Affected individuals are at greater risk for infection, and repeat screening for covert bacteriuria is recommended.

In the past, high-protein diets were recommended in an attempt to maintain serum albumin levels in gravid patients and theoretically counter their tendency to growth-retarded or low-birth-weight infants. It has been suggested that low dietary protein intake paradoxically lessens proteinuria, improves albumin kinetics, and minimizes glomerular hyperfiltration and intraglomerular pressure. **However, dietary protein restriction during pregnancy has been shown to have adverse developmental ef-**

fects in animal models. Therefore, dietary protein restriction should not be attempted in pregnant women.

Most of the glomerular lesions known to cause nephrotic syndrome in nonpregnant populations have been described in pregnant patients. However, preeclampsia remains the major cause of nephrotic proteinuria presenting during gestation. The importance of a specific diagnosis before institution of therapy in these patients is therefore emphasized.

PATIENT NUMBER 3

A 25-year-old gravida 2 para 1 presented at 11 weeks' gestation with intractable nausea and vomiting. History was at first nonrevealing, blood pressure was 130/80 mm Hg, and the remainder of the physical findings were unremarkable. Laboratory values were serum creatinine of 1.9 mg/dl (168 μmol/L) and urea nitrogen of 19 mg/dl (6.8 mmol/L), which decreased to 1.5 mg/dl (133 μmol/L) and 8 mg/dl (2.9 mmol/L), respectively, after intravenous hydration. Urinalysis was unremarkable except for 1+ proteinuria by dipstick test, and a 24-hour urine collection contained 750 mg of protein, with a calculated creatinine clearance of 43 ml/min (0.72 ml/sec). Serum albumin level was 2.6 g/dl (26 g/L), cholesterol level was 98 mg/dl (2.53 mmol/L), an antinuclear antibody titered at 1:50, and anti-DNA antibodies and serum complement levels were within normal limits for pregnancy. On further questioning, the patient revealed she had been told of proteinuria at a school physical examination 1 year ago but had not sought further evaluation.

What effect do you anticipate that the continuing pregnancy will have on her disease, and what is the expected gestational outcome? Would you recommend termination or a renal biopsy? Would you recommend low-dose aspirin therapy for preventing superimposed preeclampsia?

First, patient 3 has an underlying glomerular disorder, probably chronic, and her renal function is already moderately decreased. Thus, although fetal success will be near 90%, the risk of preterm birth and growth retardation is increased. More important, the chance that gestation will aggravate the maternal disease and result in accelerated loss of renal function is 30% to 40%. The diastolic level of 80 mm Hg, high for early pregnancy, is an additional adverse sign. We would actually suggest termination, especially with the knowledge that the first pregnancy had

been successful. However, this patient decided to proceed.

We do not recommend biopsy in such cases, because at present the results have little influence on management. However, although previous data highlighted bleeding complications, renal biopsy may be performed during gestation, and the risks are no different from those in nonpregnant populations. Although some recommend liberal use of renal biopsy in pregnancy, we limit its use to certain indications—first, in cases of sudden deterioration of function for no apparent reason (because certain forms of rapidly progressive glomerulonephritis when diagnosed early may respond to aggressive treatment such as steroid pulses and/or plasma exchange). Biopsy may also be useful in symptomatic nephrotic syndrome (or when chemical abnormalities are marked), if present before the 32nd gestational week. Although some consider therapeutic trials with steroids in such cases, we prefer to determine first if the lesion is likely to respond to the regimen, thus avoiding the potential complications of corticosteroids, such as fetal abnormalities, hyperglycemia, propensity to infection, and poor wound healing. Nephrotic range proteinuria alone would lead us to examine the patient frequently, deferring biopsy to the postpartum period, given that fetal and maternal prognosis are determined primarily by the level of renal function and the presence or absence of hypertension. We also defer biopsy to the postpartum period for pregnancies complicated by asymptomatic hematuria when a tumor seems to have been ruled out.

Finally, several large multicenter trials have failed to confirm the ability of low-dose aspirin to prevent preeclampsia in low-risk populations, but secondary analysis suggests the drug may be efficacious in women at higher risk (i.e., those with a history of severe preeclampsia in a previous gestation, diabetic patients, women with chronic hypertension or renal disease, and patients with multiple fetuses). Some therefore prescribe low-dose aspirin for these women. However, a number of large, multicenter, blinded, and placebo-controlled trials will end during 1995–1996, and we suggest awaiting the publication of their outcomes.

PATIENT NUMBER 3 (continued)

At 31 weeks' gestation, the patient was admitted in premature labor. Her blood pressure was now 150/100 mm Hg, serum creatinine level was 1.5 mg/dl (133 μmol/L), and protein excretion was 2.5 g/24 hr. Her creatinine levels rose to 2.5 mg/dl (221 μmol/L) during the next 4 weeks, at which time labor was *induced and a healthy 2190-g infant delivered. Three months postpartum, her creatinine level was stable at values between 1.8 and 2.1 mg/dl (158 to 184 μmol/L). A postpartum renal biopsy revealed focal glomerulosclerosis. What caused the increased blood pressure and proteinuria at 31 weeks, and would you have treated it?*

At gestational week 30, clinical criteria alone do not permit us to differentiate between superimposed preeclampsia or exacerbation of the primary disorder. Evidence of hemoconcentration, a disproportionate rise in uric acid, a decrease in platelet number, and liver enzyme abnormalities would point to the former complication (one reason for the baseline tests suggested earlier in the general guidelines section). Also, although this patient's physicians did not treat her hypertension, we would have. In general, mild hypertension during pregnancy is usually not treated. A Working Group Consensus Report on Hypertension in Pregnancy issued by the U.S. National High Blood Pressure Education Program (NHBPEP), for instance, stated that chronic hypertension need not be treated during gestation until diastolic levels reach 100 mm Hg. Exceptions exist, however, including end-organ damage and renal disease, the case here.

TUBULOINTERSTITIAL DISEASES AND NEPHROLITHIASIS

Polycystic kidney disease often remains undetected during pregnancy, because hypertension or functional deterioration in most cases is not manifested until after the childbearing years. Patients with the disease have an increased risk of preeclampsia, and many reports describe women whose liver cysts enlarged during gestation. Chronic pyelonephritis, especially the infectious variety, is more prone to exacerbation during gestation. Both frequent surveillance urine cultures and high fluid intake are prudent interventions.

Reflux nephropathy is one of the most common renal disorders occurring in young women. Although some investigators suggest that pregnancy has a negative impact on the course of this disease, it is more likely that the poor outcome is manifested in the subset of patients with hypertension and moderate renal insufficiency before conception. These patients, too, require frequent surveillance urine cultures and aggressive treatment of urinary tract infections throughout gestation.

The incidence of stone disease in pregnant women varies by geographic location and is estimated to occur in 1 of every 1500 gestations. The actual incidence may be higher, because patients are often not identified until their disease is symptomatic and may even be overlooked when the symptoms are subtle (i.e., repeated urinary tract infections). Of interest, though, is that the incidence or recurrence rate of nephrolithiasis does not appear to be increased in pregnant women. This fact is surprising because gravidas are usually hypercalciuric and their urinary supersaturation for calcium oxalate and brushite is increased. The lack of an expected gestational increase in stone formation, however, may be due to several factors, including enhanced urinary excretion of citrate, magnesium, and crystal growth inhibitory glycoproteins.

Clinical presentation of stone passage is similar to that in nongravid patients (pain, nausea and emesis, and hematuria). Complications may include urinary tract infection and premature labor. Ultrasonography may aid in the diagnosis, but its sensitivity may be impaired because most symptomatic stones in pregnancy are located in the ureters, which are already "physiologically" dilated. One should be aware that pregnancy does not preclude radiologic evaluation, because abdominal films or intravenous pyelography involves less than 0.4 rads, an acceptable risk, being less than that of a missed diagnosis.

Conservative therapy with bed rest, hydration, and analgesics results in passage of more than 75% of symptomatic stones. If possible, it is prudent to delay urologic intervention until after delivery. Pregnancy should not be a deterrent to necessary surgery, however, which requires a team approach including intraoperative fetal monitoring. Nephrostomy, rigid ureteroscopy, and ureteral stent placement all have been performed successfully in gravid women. The limited experience with lithotripsy currently precludes using this modality during gestation. Except for analysis of recovered stones, metabolic evaluation of patients should be delayed until at least 3 months after delivery and the cessation of lactation. Treatment of hypercalciuria with thiazide diuretics or of hyperuricosuria with xanthine oxidase inhibitors (allopurinol is in FDA class C) is best avoided during pregnancy. Reasonable therapy in a gravida includes adequate hydration to maintain a daily urine volume of 2.5 L and, in the rare case of uric acid stone disease, oral alkali intake to maintain a urine pH of 6.0. Finally, there is very little experience with cystinuria in pregnancy. No fetal effects have thus far been ascribed to penicillamine (FDA class D), but the drug is best withheld in the initial trimester.

RENAL TRANSPLANT RECIPIENTS

Much experience has been gained with successful pregnancies in renal transplant recipients, including European and American registries. However, the majority of the patients surveyed were those treated with prednisone and Imuran, and data on women receiving cyclosporine or several newer agents are limited. A substantial risk is posed for both fetal and maternal complications, including rejection, renal deterioration (~10% of the patients), or hypertension (~30% of the women) in pregnancies that continue beyond the first trimester. Preterm delivery and growth retardation are likewise increased. Nevertheless, more than 90% of these pregnancies have a successful outcome. These patients are at increased risk for infectious complications as a result of their chronic immunosuppression. The presence of a renal allograft poses no unique contraindications to spontaneous vaginal delivery. Guidelines for transplant recipients who desire pregnancy include good general health and stable renal function for at least 2 years after transplantation; a serum creatinine level ≤2 mg/dl (176 μmol/L), preferably ≤1.4 mg/dl (123 μmol/L); normal blood pressure or easily managed hypertension; and stable antirejection therapy at maintenance doses of prednisone (15 mg/day or less) and azathioprine (2 mg/kg/day or less). In the case of cyclosporin A, safe doses have not been clearly established, but we recommend doses less than 5 mg/kg day, which aim to maintain circulating levels between 100 and 200 ng/ml. In addition, patients should have no evidence of rejection or collecting system obstruction.

The common occurrence of third-trimester proteinuria (>2 g/day in 40% of these patients), hypertension (in ~30%), and drug-induced laboratory abnormalities all make the diagnosis of superimposed preeclampsia even more problematic in these patients. Likewise, considering the risks that aggressive antirejection therapy poses to a fetus, clinical suspicion of acute rejection is more likely to require renal biopsy for definitive diagnosis.

Whether pregnancy adversely affects the long-term health of the allograft is controversial. One case-control study suggested a small but definitive negative effect on graft survival, but two more recent studies contest this. Treatment of these patients is similar to that outlined in the general guidelines sections.

HYPERTENSION IN PREGNANCY

Hypertension complicates ~7% of all pregnancies and remains a major cause of morbidity and mortality of both the woman and fetus. Multiple schemas have been proposed to classify the hypertensive disorders of pregnancy, leading to considerable confusion in the literature. Also, by clinical criteria alone, it is extremely difficult to diagnose the cause of the high blood pressure complicating pregnancy. We use the schema endorsed by the 1990 NHBPEP Working Group on Hypertension in Pregnancy, which, because of its simplicity, is quite useful. It classifies hypertension occurring during gestation into only four categories: (1) **preeclampsia-eclampsia**, (2) **chronic hypertension** (essential and secondary), (3) **chronic hypertension with superimposed preeclampsia**, and (4) **transient hypertension of late pregnancy.**

Preeclampsia

Diagnosis and Clinical Spectrum. Preeclampsia is a disorder unique to pregnancy. It is most frequent in nulliparas and usually presents after gestational week 20, most frequently near term, and is characterized by hypertension and proteinuria, often accompanied by edema and sometimes by coagulation or liver functional abnormalities. High blood pressure in late pregnancy is defined as either a sustained blood pressure of 140/90 mm Hg (diastolic level measured as Korotkoff sound 5) or an increase of 30 mm Hg systolic and 15 mm Hg diastolic over measurements made earlier in pregnancy. Signs favoring a diagnosis of preeclampsia may include the sudden appearance of proteinuria, the rapid accumulation of edema, and the appearance and progression of one or more of the following: hemoconcentration, hypoalbuminemia, and liver function or coagulation abnormalities. The diagnostic accuracy of hypocalciuria, low antithrombin III levels, and increased serum iron concentration and high cytokine levels remains to be established.

Pathophysiology and Pathology. The cause of the hypertension in preeclampsia remains obscure, although alterations in the systemic vasculature (primarily in the endothelium) appear to

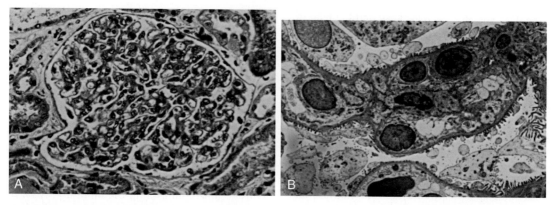

Figure 8–2. *A.* Light micrograph of a renal biopsy from a patient with preeclampsia. An enlarged and relatively bloodless glomerulus herniates into the proximal tubule ("pouting"). Its capillary lumen is obstructed by swollen endothelial cells. *B.* Electron micrograph from the patient's glomerulus in which the capillary lumen is filled with the hypertrophied endothelial cell and, despite proteinuria, the endothelial foot processes are quite well preserved.

favor vasospasm and contribute to blood pressure lability by rendering the arteries more sensitive to the effects of endogenous vasopressors. For instance, normal gravidas are relatively refractory to the vasopressor effect of infused angiotensin II, but preeclamptic patients have lost this refractoriness, and their vasculature may be more sensitive than that of nonpregnant women (perhaps because of a higher density of vascular AII receptors compared with those of nongravid populations). Both invasive and noninvasive hemodynamic studies limited to nulliparas have shown that untreated preeclamptic patients have decreased cardiac outputs, lower ventricular filling pressures, and markedly elevated systemic resistance compared with normotensive gravidas. Uteroplacental perfusion is often compromised, possibly explaining the increased incidence of fetal growth retardation associated with this disorder. Renal hemodynamics decrease 25% to 30% in patients with preeclampsia.

Alterations in prostaglandin metabolism may occur in preeclampsia, thus favoring vasoconstrictor over vasodilatory metabolism, events that may also relate to deficient antioxidant activity resulting in endothelial damage. The "prostaglandin imbalance" theory underlies the recent and ongoing clinical trials designed to evaluate the ability of low-dose aspirin to prevent preeclampsia. However, as noted in the description of patient 3, data to date are disappointing.

The pathology of preeclampsia involves multiple organs (primarily the liver, brain, kidneys, and placenta), but the focus here is on renal lesions. We recommend the classic monograph by Sheehan and Lynch (see the later list of selected readings) for those interested in further details.

Renal biopsy discloses a characteristic lesion: The glomeruli are typically enlarged and relatively bloodless as a result of endothelial (and occasionally mesangial) hypertrophy rather than proliferation. Figure 8–2 demonstrates the light and electron microscopic lesion termed *glomerular endotheliosis*. The relationship of immunohistochemical abnormalities or lesions of focal and segmental glomerular sclerosis to preeclampsia is unclear and subject to some debate. The renal lesions typical of preeclampsia appear to be reversible with time.

Renal biopsy studies have revealed how often the clinical diagnosis in women with hypertension complicating gestation is incorrect (in 25% of nulliparas and >50% of multiparas). However, it is rare for results of antepartum renal biopsy to modify management, and the procedure is not indicated in the hypertensive complications of gestation.

Complications. Preeclampsia is a potentially dangerous disease, one reason why clinicians should overdiagnose the disorder even when unsure of the cause of *de novo* hypertension in late pregnancy. Two life-threatening complications of the disorder must be recognized and treated promptly. The first is characterized by fulminant microangiopathic hemolytic anemia, hepatic dysfunction, and coagulopathy. **This syndrome, termed HELLP (for Hemolysis, Elevated Liver enzymes, Low Platelet count), is an emergency requiring prompt termination of the pregnancy.** The second complication is the progression of preeclampsia to a convulsive phase termed *eclampsia*. **Incipient or manifest eclampsia likewise requires immediate termination of pregnancy.**

Treatment. All patients in whom preeclampsia is suspected should preferably be hospitalized. Fetal maturity is assessed, and if the gravida is near term and the fetus is mature, induction is the therapy of choice. Temporizing measures appropriate earlier in gestation include bed rest (supervised and not restrictively "complete") and antihypertensive medication to decrease diastolic levels to ≤100 mm Hg. **Early termination is indicated in the setting of uncontrollable blood pressure, renal functional deterioration, hepatic dysfunction, coagulopathy, or fetal compromise.** (Table 8–5 summarizes some of the more ominous signs and symptoms of the disease, ones that lead clinicians to a decision to terminate the gestation.) Hyperreflexia and impending eclamptic convulsions should be treated with parenteral magnesium sulfate therapy monitored by serum determinations or assessment of deep tendon reflexes. Magnesium sulfate administration, the domain of fetal-maternal medicine specialists, usually commences with a slow intravenous loading dose of 4 g of $MgSO_4$ heptahydrate followed by a maintenance infusion of 2 to 3 g/hr as needed to maintain serum levels between 4.8 and 8.4 mg/dl. Decreased renal function may result in magnesium accumulation to toxic levels (i.e., >10 mEq/L), requiring dose adjustment. Such high levels may cause respiratory arrest, and the antidote, calcium gluconate, should be kept nearby.

Severe peripartum hypertension can usually be controlled with intravenous hydralazine, using low doses because patients' blood pressure is often quite sensitive to antihypertensive medications and precipitous declines may compromise the fetus. The initial parenteral dose should be but 5 mg, followed by 5 to 10 mg every 10 minutes. The few patients resistant to hydralazine are given labetalol (20 mg IV, then 20 to 80 mg every 20 to 30 minutes, up to 300 mg; or a constant infusion 1 to 2 mg, reduced to 0.5 mg/min when control achieved). Some recommend oral nifedipine, but this drug may interact with magnesium, resulting in precipitous decrements in pressure or enhancement of Mg toxicity, and we avoid its use prepartum.

Chronic Hypertension. Most pregnant women with chronic hypertension have essential hypertension, which may first appear during gestation. Although but a very small subset of these women have secondary hypertension, the extremely morbid course of pheochromocytoma in pregnancy makes screening of urinary catecholamines or metabolites prudent if any suspicion is aroused. Patients with chronic hypertension are more likely to develop superimposed preeclampsia, and the latter is responsible for most of the morbidity of the pregnant woman and her fetus.

Most women with essential hypertension have uncomplicated pregnancies, but there are exceptions. As noted, these women have an increased incidence of superimposed preeclampsia (and a greater propensity for its life-threatening complications, including cerebral hemorrhage), as well as abruption, growth retardation, and midtrimester fetal demise. The appearance of these complications seems to co-vary with maternal age and the duration of the hypertension. Thus, women at greatest risk are those who are older than 30 years or who have evidence of end-organ damage.

Antihypertensive Therapy. Treatment of mild hypertension in pregnancy remains the subject of ongoing debate. As noted in patient 3, the NHBPEP Working Group report suggested that chronic hypertension need not be treated until diastolic levels (Korotkoff 5) reached 100 mm Hg or higher, a policy many clinicians adhere to (though we often start therapy at 95 mm Hg at midpregnancy, especially if the gravida

TABLE 8–5. Ominous Signs and Symptoms in Women with Preeclampsia

---

Preeclampsia is always potentially dangerous, but particularly ominous findings may include:
- Blood pressure ≥160 mm Hg systolic or ≥110 mm Hg diastolic.
- Rapid increases in proteinuria, especially ≥3 g/24 hr.
- Increasing serum creatinine levels (especially >177 μmol/L [2 mg/dl], unless known to be elevated previously).
- Platelet count <10 × 10^9/L or evidence of microangiopathic hemolytic anemia (e.g., schistocytes and/or increased lactic acid dehydrogenase and direct bilirubin levels).
- Upper abdominal pain, especially epigastric and right upper quadrant pain.
- Headache, visual disturbances, or other cerebral signs.
- Cardiac decompensation (e.g., pulmonary edema). Usually associated with underlying heart pathology or chronic hypertension.
- Retinal hemorrhages, exudates, or papilledema. (These are extremely rare in the absence of other indicators of severity and when present almost always indicate underlying chronic hypertension.)
Signs of intrauterine growth retardation and decreasing urine volumes also require added vigilance.

Modified from Cunningham FGC, Lindheimer MD: Hypertension in pregnancy. N Engl J Med 326:927–932, 1992.

TABLE 8–6. Antihypertensive Drugs Used to Treat Chronic Hypertension in Pregnancy

Alpha-adrenergic receptor agonists	Methyldopa is the most extensively used drug in this group. Its safety and efficacy are supported in randomized trials and in a 7.5-year follow-up study of children born to treated mothers. *Methyldopa is the drug of choice recommended by the NHBPEP Working Group.*
Beta-adrenergic receptor antagonists	These drugs, especially atenolol and metoprolol, appear safe and efficacious in late pregnancy, but fetal growth retardation has been noted when treatment was started in early or midgestation. Fetal bradycardia can occur, and animal studies suggest that a fetus's ability to tolerate hypoxic stress may be compromised.
Alpha- and beta-adrenergic receptor antagonists	Labetalol appears as effective as methyldopa, but there is little or no follow-up information on children born to mothers treated with labetalol, and there is concern for maternal hepatotoxicity.
Arteriolar vasodilators	Hydralazine is used frequently as adjunctive therapy with methyldopa and beta-adrenergic receptor antagonists. Rarely, neonatal thrombocytopenia has been reported. Experience with minoxidil is limited; this drug is not recommended.
Calcium channel blockers	Studies with these agents, especially nifedipine, look promising. There is concern, however, that synergism between these drugs and $MgSO_4$ may lead to precipitous declines in blood pressure in labor.
Converting enzyme inhibitors	Captopril causes fetal death in various animal species, and several converting enzyme inhibitors have been associated with renal failure in neonates when administered to humans. *Do not use in pregnancy.*
Diuretics	Many authorities discourage their use, but others continue these medications if they were prescribed before gestation or if a chronically hypertensive woman appears to be quite salt sensitive. *The latter views have been endorsed by the Working Group.*

Modified from Lindheimer MD, Katz AI: Hypertension in pregnancy. N Engl J Med 313:675–680, 1985; and Cunningham FCG, Lindheimer MD: Hypertension in pregnancy. N Engl J Med 326:927–932, 1992. Copyright 1985 and 1992, Massachusetts Medical Society. All rights reserved.

has not demonstrated the anticipated physiologic decline in blood pressure associated with gestation). However, mild hypertension should be treated if there is evidence of end-organ damage or the presence of underlying renal disease. Individual drugs are discussed in Table 8–6. Note that the recommendations of the Working Group are based on the following considerations. Few well-designed trials assess the safety and efficacy of antihypertensive medications in pregnancy. Also, such trials require very large numbers of patients to ascertain that they do not provoke fetal anomalies or jeopardize their normal development. This is why methyldopa (considered antiquated by some) remains the drug of choice, based on its long use with few reported complications and one study reporting a 7.5 year follow-up of infants born to mothers receiving the drug.

Transient Hypertension of Late Pregnancy. This final category includes women with diverse underlying diagnoses. Patients typically present in the last trimester with nonproteinuric hypertension that normalizes during the first 10 days of the puerperium. At presentation, transient hypertension of late gestation cannot be reliably distinguished from early preeclampsia, and thus it is prudent to treat nulliparas as if they were preeclamptic. Some of the affected women may have previously undiagnosed chronic hyperten-

sion, unappreciated owing to the physiologic fall in blood pressure during early gestation, but with levels now returned to frankly hypertensive values. However, the greatest majority of the patients categorized as having hypertension of late pregnancy, especially the multiparous ones, are likely those women currently normotensive but destined to have essential hypertension later in life.

PATIENT NUMBER 4

A 33-year-old multigravida was found to be hypertensive 4 years before her current pregnancy when she presented with a blood pressure of 160/100 mm Hg. Evaluation failed to disclose secondary causes of hypertension or any evidence of end-organ disease. Her blood pressure was well controlled (~124/78 mm Hg) with propranolol, 160 mg/day, and hydrochlorothiazide, 25 mg/day, respectively. She is now 5 weeks pregnant. Would you modify her hypertensive drug regimen?

We would change patient 4's drug therapy. Beta-adrenergic inhibitor drugs are associated with fetal growth retardation. Diuretics started before pregnancy are acceptable to the

NHBPEP Working Group, but we are concerned that they may hamper the physiologic volume expansion of pregnancy. At any rate, this patient is in the phase of pregnancy when anomalies are most likely to develop. This is also the period when many women with essential hypertension experience spontaneous decreases in blood pressure. Thus, we would discontinue both drugs, measure the patient's blood pressure on a weekly basis (it is even better if she has a cuff at home and can notify us of the pressures several times during the week), and are prepared to commence therapy with methyldopa if necessary.

PATIENT NUMBER 4 (continued)

All medications were discontinued. Her blood pressure remained between 120/70 and 140/90 mm Hg until gestational week 26, at which time values increased, ranging from 140/100 to 150/105 mm Hg. Would you initiate therapy at this time, and what additional history and laboratory tests become important?

Treatment is definitively indicated, and methyldopa, 250 mg b.i.d., was started and increased to 1 g daily shortly thereafter. It is also necessary to ascertain that this is the third-trimester rise in pressure typical of both normotensive gravidas and chronically hypertensive women and not an early indication of superimposed preeclampsia. Thus, chronically hypertensive women should have baseline urine and blood tests performed in early gestation similar to those for women with underlying renal disorders (see the general guidelines section), and these had been performed on patient 4. The tests were repeated to establish whether proteinuria had developed and to seek evidence of hemoconcentration, a substantial decrease in platelet numbers, increments in serum creatinine concentration and a disproportionate rise in uric acid levels, or the appearance of liver function or coagulation test abnormalities with a decrease in serum albumin concentration (even in the absence of proteinuria). Patient 4 was also questioned about symptoms of preeclampsia including headaches, blurred vision, and epigastric pain. The evaluation was nonrevealing.

PATIENT NUMBER 4 (continued)

At 29 weeks of gestation, the patient complained of epigastric distress and nausea and was admitted to the hospital. She was afebrile, and her blood pressure, which had averaged 130/80 mm Hg with antihypertensive treatment, rose again and was now 150/95 mm Hg. Laboratory evaluation revealed a hematocrit of 40% and a platelet count of 120,000/mm³. Her urinalysis demonstrated 1+ proteinuria by dipstick; her serum creatinine level was 0.8 mg/dl (71

μmol/L) and uric acid value was 5.5 mg/dl (327 mmol/L). Her liver function values were a total bilirubin of 1.6 mg/dl (32 μmol/L), an oxaloacetic transaminase of 40 U/L (2.63 ukat/L; upper limit of normal 35 U/L or 0.58 ukat/L), and a lactic acid dehydrogenase of 276 U/L (5.4 ukat/L; upper limit of normal 225 U/L or 3.75 ukat/L). What is your differential diagnosis now, as well as a plan of management?

Patient 4 now has evidence of superimposed preeclampsia and signs and symptoms that suggest she may be developing the HELLP variant. Epigastric pain and nausea are serious symptoms in third-trimester pregnancy, most often associated with preeclampsia and rarely with the more ominous acute fatty liver of pregnancy. The patient is also hemoconcentrated, and her platelet count is low for pregnancy (a value of 230,000/mm³ had been measured during the initial trimester). She also shows early evidence of liver involvement. One of the first things her physicians did was to evaluate her peripheral blood smear, but no schistocytes were seen. Still, with her present manifestations, many physicians would worry about continuing the pregnancy. Preeclampsia, especially the HELLP variant, is explosive; platelet counts may plunge 50 to 100,000/mm³ in only 24 hours, and liver enzymes can rise to more than 1000 U/L during the same period.

PATIENT NUMBER 4 (continued)

Because she was only at gestational week 29, her physicians decided to temporize but set rigid limits. Platelet counts less than 100,000/mm³ or a rise in the transaminase or lactic acid dehydrogenase level above 100 and 400 U/L, respectively, would not be tolerated. She was also observed closely for signs and symptoms of cerebral irritability. Two days later, her epigastric pain worsened, she complained of severe frontal headache, and a blood pressure of 200/120 mm Hg was recorded. She was treated with parenteral hydralazine, and labor was induced. However, a cesarean section had to be performed when it was noted that her platelet count had decreased to 90,000/mm³ and liver enzyme values had virtually tripled. This resulted in the delivery of an 1800-g boy, who subsequently fared well. After delivery, her blood pressure had decreased to 140/80 to 140/90 mm Hg, but her platelet number continued to fall, reaching 22,000/mm³ on day 3 of the puerperium. Her liver enzyme levels had reached a nadir and plateaued 1 day previously, and levels now appeared to be decreasing. The epigastric pain had subsided, and the patient was relatively symptom free. Would you plasma-exchange this patient?

The answer is no. HELLP syndrome often

continues into the puerperium, the nadir for the platelet count occurring most often during the third postpartum day. Even at a count of 22,000/mm³, such patients rarely demonstrate petechiae or other signs of bleeding (despite the recent operation), and now that her blood pressure is under control, there is little concern about cerebral bleeding. The disappearance of epigastric pain and the stability of liver function are other favorable prognostic signs, and this optimism was rewarded because her platelet counts and liver enzyme levels rapidly normalized during the next 3 days.

This case demonstrates the explosiveness of preeclampsia. Chronic hypertension in this woman was well tolerated, and her need for antihypertensive medications actually declined until the third trimester. She was older than 30 years but had had her hypertension for only ~5 years, demonstrating no evidence of end-organ damage. However, once the first signs of superimposed preeclampsia occurred, she rapidly developed a life-threatening syndrome requiring immediate termination of the gestation. In essence, most of the morbidity associated with hypertension in pregnancy is related to pure or superimposed preeclampsia.

SUGGESTED READINGS

August P, Lindheimer MD: Pathophysiology of preeclampsia. In Laragh JH, Brenner BM (eds): Hypertension, Pathophysiology and Management, 2nd ed. New York, Raven Press, 1995, pp 2427–2450.

Brown MA, Gallery EDM: Volume homeostasis in normal pregnancy and pre-eclampsia: Physiological and clinical implications. Clin Obstet Gynaecol (Baillière) 8:287–310, 1994.

Cunningham FG, Lucas MJ: Urinary tract infections complicating pregnancy. Clin Obstet Gynaecol (Baillière) 8:353–373, 1994.

Cunningham FGC, Lindheimer MD: Hypertension in pregnancy. N Engl J Med 326:927–932, 1992.

Davison JM: Pregnancies in renal allograft recipients: Problems, prognosis, and practicalities. Clin Obstet Gynaecol (Baillière) 8:501–525, 1994.

Hou SH: Pregnancy in woman on haemodialysis and peritoneal dialysis. Clin Obstet Gynaecol (Baillière) 8:481–500, 1994.

Lindheimer MD: Hypertension in pregnancy (clinical conference). Hypertension 22:127–137, 1993.

Lindheimer MD, Grünfeld J-P, Davison JM: Renal disorders. In Barron WM, Lindheimer MD (eds): Medical Disorders During Pregnancy, 2nd ed. St Louis, Mosby-Year Book, 1995, pp 37–62.

Lindheimer MD, Katz AI: The normal and diseased kidney in pregnancy. In Schrier RW, Gottschalk CW (eds): Diseases of the Kidney, 6th ed. Philadelphia, WB Saunders (in press).

National High Blood Pressure Program Working Group report high blood pressure in pregnancy (consensus document). Am J Obstet Gynecol 163:1689–1712, 1990.

Sheehan HL, Lynch JP: Pathology of Toxaemia of Pregnancy. Baltimore, Williams & Wilkins, 1973.

9 ∎ PEDIATRIC NEPHROLOGY

Norman M. Wolfish

Although students learn in large academic centers, they often practice in smaller centers some distance from these institutions without the support of specialized personnel to assist with unusual cases. The purpose of this chapter is to highlight those aspects of pediatric nephrology commonly encountered in a primary care practice. We hope to show physicians some practical approaches to both diagnosis and management of either common or unusual presentations of renal problems in children. We outline some of the reasoning, including the pathophysiologic basis for these actions, rather than expect physicians to rely on a memorized, uncompromising approach to clinical problems. In this way, we hope to support practitioners in the problem-solving approach to common clinical nephrologic problems and provide assistance when the unusual occurs. Case scenarios are used to demonstrate the approach and management of some of these concerns.

We initially look at neonates and the common renal problems encountered in this age group. Next follows a discussion of some common clinical problems and the pitfalls experienced in management and assessment. A detailed discussion of pathophysiology is not included. The differences in management of both acute and chronic renal failure in children as opposed to that in adults are discussed, including dialysis and transplantation. Finally, no discussion of children would be complete without a comment on the fluid and electrolyte requirements of this age group.

MATURATION OF RENAL FUNCTION

At birth, renal function is related to gestational age rather than to birth weight, length, or surface area. Thus, the GFR of a prematurely born infant is much lower than that of a small-for-date neonate of equivalent weight. The secretory aspects of the placenta must be replaced postnatally by increasing renal function. Birth thus induces a functional maturation regardless of the gestational age. Fetal nephron development is complete by 32 weeks of gestation, and nephron maturation proceeds thereafter, induced by the excretory load.

At birth, GFR is quite low and slowly increases thereafter (Table 9–1). If the child's GFR is corrected to a surface area of 1.73 m², adult values are reached by 12 to 18 months of life. Uncorrected values may not reach adult levels until age 10 to 14 years. Neonatal GFR is depressed because of a combination of various physiologic circumstances, such as low renal fraction of cardiac output, low blood and renal perfusion pressure, high renal vascular resistance, and a decreased intraglomerular filtration pressure due to anatomic immaturity, low hydraulic permeability, and afferent arteriolar constriction. This is due to tubuloglomerular feedback mediated by the renin-angiotensin system. In concert with other parameters such as ADH, prostaglandins, catecholamines, and the sympathetic nervous system, GFR rises slowly during the first year of life.

TABLE 9–1. Normal Renal Values

Age	BUN		Creatinine		GFR
	mg/ml	mmol/L	mg/ml	μmol/L	ml/min/1.73 m²
Neonates	3–10	1.1–3.6	0.6–1.0	53.0–85.0	35–50
Infants 4 weeks to 2 years	5–10	2.0–4.0	0.25–0.5	25–50	45–90
Children 2–10 years	5–15	2.0–6.0	0.3–0.7	25–85	110–125
Adolescents	5–15	3.5–6.5	0.5–1.20	50–105	110–125

The placenta keeps the fetal and maternal serum chemistries similar *in utero*. Thus, the umbilical chord serum urea and creatinine levels reflect those of the mother at birth. During the first several neonatal days, the serum urea and creatinine levels slowly fall to reach expected neonatal values (see Table 9–1). Because the infant's metabolism is primarily anabolic, urea production is low and the infant's serum urea levels are less than in the adult. Because serum creatinine level reflects muscle mass, these values rise slowly throughout infancy and childhood to reach adult values only in adolescence. Concomitantly, the neonatal GFR is low and slowly rises throughout infancy and childhood to reach adult values only when growth and muscle mass are stable. To allow easy comparison, GFR is corrected to a standard 1.73 m² surface area. GFR (in ml/min/1.73m²) may be estimated by the formula

$$\frac{0.55 \times \text{length (cm)}}{\text{Serum creatinine (mg/dl)}} \text{ or } \frac{0.33 \times \text{length (cm)}}{\text{serum creatinine } (\mu\text{mol/L})}$$

Proximal tubular function is immature in neonates and infants and this is the controlling factor in actively keeping the GFR low through tubuloglomerular feedback, mediated by the renin-angiotensin system. Absolute and maximum rates (T_{max}) of reabsorption of glucose, phosphate, bicarbonate, and amino acids are lower in infants than in adults and in part account for the lower serum values in infants. For example, serum bicarbonate level is lower in an infant (20 to 22 mmol/L) than in an adult owing to the lower renal threshold for bicarbonate. Distal tubular acidification appears to be intact, however, because an infant is capable of excreting an acid load and reducing urinary pH to 4.8. However, although maximal urinary excretion of ammonia is less than adult values, an infant's higher serum and urinary phosphate level acts as a systemic buffer, minimizes the need for large increases in urinary ammonia excretion, and contributes to the infant's capabilities to maintain acceptable acid-base status.

An infant has a reduced ability both to dilute and concentrate the urine maximally (Table 9–2). This is partly because of the immature renal handling of sodium, the reduced content of osmotically active substances such as urea in an infant's urine, and the relatively short loops of Henle coupled with high rates of medullary blood flow. An infant's distal tubule is also relatively insensitive to ADH.

The serum phosphate level is also higher in infants and young children than in adults (4.5 to 6.0 mg/dl, or 1.1 to 1.6 mmol/L). Shortly after birth, a state of relative and transient hypoparathyroidism exists owing to a limited secretory capacity of the infant's parathyroid gland. When coupled with a low GFR, a reduced renal tubular responsiveness to PTH, and high dietary phosphate intake, an elevated serum level results. Serum calcium levels conversely tend to be slightly depressed by the elevated phosphate level, the relative hypoparathyroidism, the low serum bicarbonate level favoring the ionized form of calcium, the hypoactivity of the infant's renal 1α-hydroxylase activity, and reduced availability of 1,25-dihydroxycholecalciferol.

NEPHROLOGIC PROBLEMS IN THE NEONATE

Acute Renal Failure

Voiding occurs in the first 24 hours in 93% of full-term neonates and 90% of premature infants. Failure to pass urine thereafter is associated with an increasing risk of oliguria-anuria, most commonly as a result of abnormalities of perfusion-filtration (the failure to produce urine) or obstruction (Table 9–3).

PATIENT NUMBER 1

You have been called to see baby boy Jones, who was born after a 34-week gestation. His mom is concerned because it is 24 hours after birth and he has not yet passed urine. Although transient respiratory distress was initially encountered, he is now breathing normally. You have requested a serum creatinine determination, and it is 110 µmol/L at this time. The urinalysis shows a moderate amount of blood on dipstick, but the urine is not obviously bloody.

TABLE 9–2. Maximum Urine Concentration

Age	mOsm/kg	Specific Gravity
Neonate	600–800	1.018–1.021
2 months–2 years	700–1200	1.021–1.024
2–12 years	800–1200	1.024–1.030

A presumptive diagnosis of acute renal failure (ARF) can be made if the neonate's urine output is less than 1 ml/kg/hr and the serum creatinine and urea levels rise above the maternal values. ARF is most commonly secondary to perinatal

TABLE 9–3. Causes of Acute Renal Failure in the Newborn Period

---

Prerenal

Hypotension-hypovolemia
  Septic shock
  Maternal antepartum hemorrhage
  Twin-to-twin transfusion
  Surgery
Congestive heart failure
Hypoxia-asphyxia
Dehydration

Renal

Congenital anomalies
  Autosomal recessive polycystic kidney disease
  Multicystic dysplasia
  Hypoplasia
  Bilateral agenesis of aplasia
Acute tubular necrosis
  Asphyxia
  Dehydration
  Shock
  Nephrotoxins
Vascular
  Renal vein or artery thrombosis
  Cortical necrosis
  Disseminated intravascular coagulopathy
Inflammatory
  Pyelonephritis
  Toxoplasmosis
  Syphilis

Postrenal (Obstruction)

Posterior urethral valves
Urethral diverticulum
Ureterocele
Neurogenic bladder
Ureterovesical junction obstruction (adynamic segments)
Ureteropelvic junction obstruction
Tumors
  Nephroblastoma
  Mesoblastic nephroma

---

asphyxia or vascular hypoperfusion/shock syndromes, reducing both renal blood flow (RBF) and GFR. The reduction in GFR may be complete (anuria) but is usually reversible, provided renal parenchymal damage has not been extensive. The prognosis then is favorable. Normal renal function is usually quickly reestablished and should remain normal at the end of the first year of life.

ARF due to congenital structural abnormalities in the renal-urinary drainage system is almost always associated with obstruction of the urinary flow or with deficient functional renal parenchyma or dysplasia. Resumption of normal urine flow is more problematic, and attainment of normal renal function is dependent on the severity of the renal anomaly, the amount of functioning renal tissue, and the extent of associated renal dysplasia.

Clinical clues to the presence of structural anomalies in a neonate include a single umbilical artery; vertebral, sacral, or rectal anomalies; and low-set ears or other auricular anomalies. These may coexist in neonates with shock, dehydration, and respiratory or cardiac failure in which vascular volume is compromised. A palpable bladder suggests posterior urethral valves or other bladder obstruction, whereas enlarged kidneys, either palpable or demonstrated sonographically, may be associated with hydronephrosis, multiple cysts, renal vein thrombosis, or rarely tumor. Hematuria often accompanies ARF as a result of reduced renal perfusion due to hypoxic anoxia and is often associated with proteinuria or RBC casts. Seizures and ARF may be associated with disseminated intravascular coagulopathies or hypertension or may imply electrolyte disturbances such as hyponatremia, hypocalcemia, or hypokalemia.

> **A presumptive diagnosis of ARF in a neonate is made when serum urea and creatinine values exceed maternal values or remain at maternal values for more than 72 hours.**

Because the most common cause of oligoanuria is hypovolemia, a fluid challenge of 10 to 20 ml/kg of saline or 0.22% NS in 5% dextrose in water over 1 to 2 hours may be diagnostic in this circumstance. Continued failure to pass urine would necessitate a trial of furosemide, 1 to 2 mg/kg IV over 30 minutes. Further continued oliguria or anuria may require imaging studies such as ultrasonography, differential radionuclide scanning, or cystography for diagnosis. IVP should be only attempted cautiously in neonates because of the attendant risk of inducing ATN.

Reliance on the fractional excretion of sodium (FE_{Na}) to differentiate prerenal from postrenal failure should be with the understanding that neonatal handling of sodium differs from that in adults. In neonatal prerenal failure, FE_{Na} is 2% to 3% and is slightly higher in premature infants. Principles of fluid replacement in neonatal ARF are similar to those in adults—that is, balancing insensible, renal, and nonrenal losses with intake. For neonates, fluid requirements are insensible: (neutral environment) 60 ml/kg, fecal 20 mg/kg, plus urinary losses. Insensible losses are increased under radiant heat or phototherapy or with fever and are decreased with humidified ventilator therapy.

Urinary Tract Infection—Pyelonephritis

Urinary tract infections (UTIs) in neonates are commonly associated with renal parenchymal infection (i.e., pyelonephritis). Structural abnormalities are frequently but not invariably associated and occur with equal or greater frequency in boys than girls. Sepsis is a frequent accompaniment. The most common causative organism is *Escherichia coli*, and treatment should be initiated immediately with intravenous ampicillin and gentamicin or an appropriate cephalosporin until results of bacterial sensitivity tests are available. Sequelae include permanent parenchymal scarring in many cases, but differentiation from preexisting renal dysplasia is critical. Dysplasia is associated with major structural anomalies such as grade 4 to 5 reflux and can be bilateral, impairing overall renal function. Renal scarring, often encountered in older children with structural anomalies but with no previous history suggestive of renal infection, probably represents dysplasia rather than pyelonephritic scars.

PATIENT NUMBER 1 (continued)

This prematurely born infant has anuria due to renal failure because his serum creatinine level is elevated beyond maternal values. Foremost causes are hypotension and hypoxia as a result of respiratory distress or cardiac failure. However, structural anomalies such as posterior urethral valves, bilateral obstructive lesions, nonfunctioning renal cysts, or dysplasias must be precluded. The most helpful distinguishing investigation at this point would be a renal ultrasound examination.

HEMATURIA IN CHILDREN

Hematuria in children is not uncommon, the prevalence varying from 0.7% to 2.5% of school-aged children. The hematuria most often is microscopic and in many instances may be no more than a variant of normal. Gross hematuria in children, although more alarming to practitioner and parent alike, may have less serious consequences than in adults. An important clue to the site and cause of the hematuria is RBC morphology. Dysmorphic RBCs usually originate from the upper nephron, whereas isomorphic RBCs often come from the calyces and lower urinary tract. Although helpful, RBC morphology is not always reliable, because dysmorphic changes may develop even in freshly voided urine. The most helpful clue to the significance and thus the prognosis of hematuria is its association with protein-

uria. Isolated hematuria (or proteinuria) is of less concern than their coexistence.

PATIENT NUMBER 2

Penelope is a healthy 12-year-old girl who has come to your office for a precamp physical examination. Christine, the office nurse, reports trace to moderate amounts of blood on the urine dipstick. When asked, Penelope says she has never seen blood in her urine.

Dysmorphic RBCs usually imply glomerular bleeding and thus glomerular injury from inflammation. In these circumstances, diagnostic evaluation with imaging studies including renal ultrasound examination would thus not be informative and should be avoided unless alterations in renal size, density, or architecture are anticipated. Isomorphic RBCs have a nonglomerular origin such as stone, cysts, or tumor and are more easily identified by renal imaging.

The epidemiology of hematuria varies in the different age groups in children as it does in adults. In neonates, hematuria is most frequently associated with ATN induced by anoxic damage of the renal parenchyma. Respiratory distress, cardiac failure, and shock are the most likely causes of hypoxia. Renal vein thrombosis, polycystic disease, Wilms' and other tumors, and drug-induced nephropathies are less commonly encountered. Table 9–4 lists the more usual disorders associated with hematuria in the older infants and children. It is important to ensure that concentrated or colored urine is not mistaken by caregivers as hematuria. A common problem is the frequent misdiagnosis of precipitated urates in an infant's diaper as hematuria. Precipitated urates appear salmon-pink, especially in the first morning change.

> RBC morphology is often helpful in identifying the site of bleeding and thus the value of imaging. Dysmorphic RBCs have a glomerular origin, whereas isomorphic RBCs have a nonglomerular origin.

Isolated (i.e., in the absence of proteinuria) microhematuria in children is more likely to be benign, whereas gross hematuria is more likely to have a definable cause. IgA nephropathy is one of the most common causes of both microscopic and gross hematuria in an ambulatory setting. Because serum IgA levels are not always

TABLE 9–4. Common Causes of Hematuria in Children

Glomerular

Benign persistent or recurrent
  Sporadic, physiologic (fever, exercise)
  Familial
Glomerulopathies
  Postinfectious
  IgA nephropathy (Berger's)
  Membranoproliferative
  Rapidly progressive (crescentic)
  Lupus nephritis
  Hemolytic-uremic syndrome
  Anaphylactoid purpura (Henoch-Schönlein) nephritis
  Hereditary (Alport's) nephritis
  Nephrotoxins

Nonglomerular

Trauma
Cystic disease—polycystic, multicystic, microcystic
Neoplasm—Wilms' tumor (bilateral)
Sickle cell disease or trait
Idiopathic hypercalciuria
Nephrolithiasis
Pyelonephritis
Hydronephrosis
Interstitial nephritis

Nonrenal

Cystitis
Extra renal calculi
Foreign body
Meatal ulceration
Left renal vein compression

---

elevated, a definitive diagnosis can be made only by observing IgA mesangial immunofluorescence on renal biopsy. Progression to renal failure is unusual in children, in contradistinction to adults, unless the presentation is associated with significant proteinuria, azotemia, or hypertension. Idiopathic hypercalciuria without nephrolithiasis is emerging as a common associated finding in microhematuria. Whether these children are at greater risk for developing stones later in life has not been adequately resolved. Hypercalciuria is diagnosed when the urinary calcium-to-creatinine ratio exceeds 0.2 (0.6 in SI units) or the urinary excretion of calcium exceeds 4 mg/kg/day (0.1 mmol/kg/day). The finding of isolated hematuria without supporting evidence of WBCs or significant bacterial growth on culture ***does not*** imply UTI and should not be treated with antibiotics.

Investigation of a child who tests positive for blood on three occasions without a recent history of streptococcal infection should include study of cellular morphology to assist in the localization of the bleeding, a search for RBC casts, urine

culture, calcium-to-creatinine ratio, 24-hour urinary protein excretion, creatinine clearance, and serum immunoglobulin determinations. Further testing for serum complement, antistreptococcal antibodies, antinuclear antibodies, and anti-DNA antibodies should depend on the clinical situation. Imaging should be selective in the presence of dysmorphic RBCs but is indicated in isomorphic hematuria. Renal ultrasonography in experienced hands may point the way to further radiologic evaluation. The role of renal biopsy should be reserved for those situations in which management decisions will be altered by biopsy results.

> **Microscopic or gross hematuria associated with proteinuria has a worse prognosis than isolated hematuria.**

PATIENT NUMBER 2 (continued)

A previously healthy young girl with microscopic hematuria and absent proteinuria documented on three separate occasions most probably has idiopathic microscopic hematuria. The next likely diagnosis may be physiologic (i.e., menses). The next likely concern would be an IgA nephropathy. RBC morphology would be helpful in decision making in such circumstances. In this age group, systemic lupus erythematosus should be considered, but patients rarely present with only isolated hematuria.

PROTEINURIA IN CHILDREN

Isolated proteinuria, in the absence of hematuria, is one of the more common urinary findings in children and adolescents. Its prevalence in school-aged children varies from 0.1% to 1.5%, and it is more frequently encountered as age advances to adolescence. Thereafter, the prevalence diminishes. The value at which protein excretion becomes significant varies with advancing age, because premature infants and neonates excrete more protein per kilogram of body weight than do children and adults. The figure commonly cited for children older than 1 year is <0.1 mg/kg/hr. If protein excretion per square meter is calculated, then weight and age differences are minimized. Normal excretion is <4 mg/m²/hr; significant, 4 to 40 mg/m²/hr; and nephrotic, >40 mg/m²/hr. Because of the difficulties in collecting 24-hour samples in young children, the protein-to-creatinine (UPr/Cr) ratio has been used to estimate significant proteinuric states. A UPr/Cr ratio of <0.2 expressed in milligrams per milligram is normal for children older than 2 years. For children 6 months to 2 years, values up to 0.5 are acceptable. Because this ratio is dependent on creatinine excretion, it is affected by muscle mass and renal function.

PATIENT NUMBER 3

Mario is a 10-year-old boy whom you have been monitoring since birth. Other than a few respiratory infections each year, he has been in excellent health. He is again in your office for a mild upper respiratory tract infection when the nurse reports that his urine dipstick shows 100 mg/L of protein. You wonder what conditions could cause this and their significance.

Premature and newborn infants may have transient proteinuria for the first 2 weeks of life. Common causes of proteinuria in children are listed in Table 9–5. *Transient* or *physiologic* proteinuria may also occur in febrile illnesses, with infectious and inflammatory processes, or after exercise but rapidly resolves. Proteinuria may also occur with changes in posture or position, so-called *orthostatic* or *postural* proteinuria. This is noted more frequently in growing children

TABLE 9–5. Common Causes of Proteinuria in Children and Adolescents

Functional/Transient

Fever
Exercise
Stress
Infections/inflammations

Isolated

Orthostatic/postural proteinuria
Persistent asymptomatic proteinuria

Glomerular Disease

Minimal change nephrotic syndrome
Glomerulonephritides
  Postinfectious
  Membranoproliferative
  Membranous
  IgA nephropathy
  Henoch-Schönlein nephritis
  Systemic lupus erythematosus
  Hereditary nephritides

Tubulointerstitial Disease

Reflux nephropathy
Interstitial nephritis
Fanconi's syndrome
Ischemic or nephrotoxic tubular injury

and adolescents, and protein excretion is rarely greater than 1.0 g/day. *Persistent* or *fixed* proteinuria is detectable at all times and has a more ominous prognosis because it may increase and may be associated with a significant underlying renal process.

PATIENT NUMBER 3 (continued)

The workup of a child with proteinuria includes documentation of significant protein in at least three recumbent specimens. The importance of the investigative process is to differentiate acceptable physiologic causes from common pathologic disorders. A 24-hour collection to measure the amount of excreted protein, test for postural proteinuria, and determine creatinine clearance, serum urea, creatinine, and immunoglobulins is a first step. Other tests such as antistreptococcal antibodies, complement, lupus studies, total proteins, albumin, cholesterol urine culture, and imaging studies depend on the coexistence of such factors as family history and the presence of hematuria, hypertension, or edema. Positive results may warrant a full nephrologic assessment.

ENURESIS

Few problems in pediatrics are more disturbing to children and parents alike than enuresis. The reported incidence in 5-year-olds varies from 14% to 18%, less than 5% at age 10 years, and less than 1% by age 15, with boys outnumbering girls, increasing at each age group. It has a strong familial link. The cause is a delay of maturation of nocturnal bladder control induced by three mechanisms: a failure of the pons to inhibit spontaneous bladder contractions, a lack of augmentation of nocturnal ADH secretion, and an unusually elevated sleep arousal threshold resulting in an unarousable child. The bladder fills normally, exacerbated by low ADH levels inducing a spontaneous and uninhibitable bladder contraction in an unarousable child and resulting in bladder emptying. This process may be repeated throughout the night, depending on the rate of bladder filling. If bladder contractions are induced during the day, incontinence occurs, often without the child's awareness. Associated symptoms of urgency and frequency can also be present. No investigation is required other than a urine culture, and a careful history. Treatment is primarily to reassure both parent and child alike that there is no organic problem and that in time the problem will spontaneously resolve (the incidence in adults is unknown). The use of behavior modification programs in association with wet alarms is most effective. DDAVP is a useful

TABLE 9–6. Immune-Mediated Glomerulonephritis

Condition	Etiology/Chronicity	Serum C3	Immunopathologic Changes	Pathogenesis
Postinfectious	Streptococcal and other agents/acute	Low	Diffuse small subendothelial and subepithelial deposits	Immune complex
Systemic lupus erythematosus	Antinuclear (anti-DNA) low antibodies/acute and chronic	Low	Subendothelial, mesangial, subepithelial deposits	Immune complex/autoimmune
Membranoproliferative	Unknown/chronic	Low	Mesangial interposition and immune deposits	Immune complex
IgA nephropathy	Unknown/acute and chronic	Normal	IgA mesangial deposits	Immune complex
Goodpasture's autoimmune	Anti-GBM antibodies to NC_1 domain type IV collagen	Normal	Linear IgG deposits along GBM	Anti-GBM nephritis

GBM, glomerular basement membrane.

adjunct but often is effective only while the child remains on the medication.

GLOMERULONEPHRITIS

Most glomerulonephritides in children are immune related and can be classified on the basis of the glomerular immunopathologic findings and the presence of hypocomplementemia.

> **Glomerulonephritis is an inflammatory process characterized by the presence of hematuria and proteinuria. The nephritic syndrome is characterized by hematuria, proteinuria, and various degrees of azotemia, hypertension, and oliguria.**

The common glomerulonephritides encountered in the pediatric age groups are listed in Table 9–6.

Acute Postinfectious Glomerulonephritis

PATIENT NUMBER 4

Annabelle is a 12-year-old girl who is taken by her concerned parents to the emergency department of your hospital because she has had painless hematuria for the past day. She had the onset of an upper respiratory tract infection the day before. Your evaluation of her history and physical examination reveals a mild nasopharyngitis, and other findings are normal, including her optic fundi. Her blood pressure is normal in both arms. You order serum chemistry determinations and see her the next day in the ambulatory clinic. All results are normal,

including serum urea nitrogen, creatinine, complement (C3), and hemoglobin. Urinalysis shows 50 to 75 dysmorphic RBCs per high-power field and occasional RBC casts. What are you going to tell her parents?

These patients characteristically present some 5 to 14 days after a streptococcal infection with hematuria, usually gross, described as tea colored, cloudy urine. They may have various degrees of hypertension, oliguria, and edema, secondary to fluid overload. Confirmation of a streptococcal infection, usually a pharyngitis or pyoderma, with elevated antistreptococcal antibodies (ASOT anti-DNAase B antibody) and hypocomplementemia, establishes the diagnosis. Infection with certain other bacterial and viral pathogens can induce a similar clinical picture. During the course of the disease, careful fluid and electrolyte control is essential to forestall hypertensive complications. Once the antigenic stimulus has resolved, the prognosis is usually excellent, with no long-term sequelae. However, microhematuria may persist for 6 months to 2 years.

Systemic Lupus Erythematosus

When glomerulonephritis is present with evidence of persisting hypocomplementemia, systemic lupus erythematosus (SLE) must be suspected. The usual presentation is in a preadolescent or adolescent girl with prolonged fevers, arthralgias, skin rash, and glomerulonephritis. The diagnosis of SLE nephropathy is established by supportive serum antibodies, and renal biopsy is strongly recommended. The prognosis in children has improved with the aggressive use of steroids and immunosuppressive agents. Several accepted protocols are in common use.

Membranoproliferative Glomerulonephritis

Membranoproliferative glomerulonephritis (MPGN) has been classified into three forms, types 1, 2, and 3. All three conditions are associated with persisting hypocomplementemia and clinically may present with features of glomerulonephritis and the nephritic syndrome (hematuria, proteinuria, reduced renal function, and hypertension). Type 1 MPGN is a variably progressive form and on renal biopsy is characterized by mesangial cell interposition in peripheral glomerular loops and subendothelial immune deposits. There is evidence of activation of the alternate complement pathway (i.e., C_4 is depressed and C_3 is normal). Renal biopsy in type 2 MPGN, or dense deposit disease, is associated on light microscopy with a double contour or train track appearance of the glomerular basement membrane. This is due to double linear deposits of C3 as well as deposits in the lamina densa. Also seen is diffuse deposition of densely staining material throughout the basement membrane and mesangium. Type 3 MPGN is characterized by deposits mixed throughout the glomerular basement membrane. Treatment is with long-term steroids, and the prognosis in all three diseases is guarded, with type 2 having the worst overall.

IgA Nephropathy

IgA nephropathy, or Berger's disease, is characterized by various clinical presentations, including intermittent microhematuria, persistent microhematuria, or episodic gross hematuria with or without continuous microhematuria. It is probably the most common cause of hematuria in the pediatric age group and the most common form of glomerulonephritis. Classic presentation is with an episode of gross hematuria coincident with an upper respiratory tract infection (in contradistinction to postinfectious glomerulonephritis, which characteristically presents some 5 to 10 days later), normal renal function, and minimal proteinuria. Serum complement levels are normal. Because fewer than 50% of patients have an elevated serum IgA level, the diagnosis is often made by ruling out other causes of hematuria. Renal biopsy is indicated if renal function or protein excretion is abnormal and reveals focal segmental mesangial proliferation. The characteristic finding is IgA immunofluorescent staining of the mesangium and corresponding electron

dense deposits by electron microscopy. The course is often characterized by recurrent episodes of hematuria associated with upper respiratory tract infections. The disorder is usually benign in children, approximately 5% to 15% progressing to end-stage renal disease in adults. Poor prognostic signs at onset include black race, significant proteinuria, hypertension, male sex, older age at time of biopsy, and the finding of sclerosis or crescents on biopsy.

Rapidly Progressive Glomerulonephritis

The clinical term *rapidly progressive glomerulonephritis* is used to characterize those disorders that demonstrate a severe nephritic syndrome at onset and that rapidly progress to renal failure in a matter of weeks or months. Various clinical entities are associated, although the most common is Goodpasture's syndrome, renal failure associated with pulmonary hemorrhage and often CNS involvement. Glomerular crescents are typically seen on renal biopsy and are associated with diffuse cellular proliferation. Prognosis is often determined by the prevalence of crescents in the biopsy specimen. The most common finding in children is linear immunofluorescent deposition of IgG and C3 along the basement membrane. The autoimmune reaction is initiated by antibodies to the Goodpasture antigen, a noncollagen (NC-1) domain in type IV collagen, in the basement membrane. Patients may require dialysis to prevent uremic complications. Therapy is also aimed at reduction and elimination of circulating autoantibodies to the glomerular basement membrane by plasmapheresis plus immunosuppression with steroids and cytotoxic medication. Prognosis for renal recovery is guarded.

Hemolytic-Uremic Syndrome

Hemolytic-uremic syndrome (HUS) is a clinical syndrome characterized by progressing renal failure, hemolytic anemia, and thrombocytopenia. Age of onset is in late infancy and early childhood years. Two forms exist, one associated with diarrhea (D+) and one not associated with diarrhea (D−). The D+ is most often due to *E. coli* 0157:H7, found in contaminated meats, milk, and derived products. Other pathogens, such as *Salmonella, Shigella, Yersinia, Clostridium*, and *Campylobacter*, are found less commonly. Patients experience a prodrome of bloody diarrhea for several days before the onset of renal failure. The pathogenesis of the syndrome consists of localized intravascular coagulation and microthrombus formation due to endothelial damage caused by toxins (verutoxin) released from the *E. coli*. This may occur in any part of the vascular system but occurs with greater density in the glomerular capillary network, causing reduced glomerular filtration and ensuing renal failure. The progressive hemolytic anemia and thrombocytopenia also result from intravascular coagulation. This condition is difficult to distinguish from thrombotic thrombocytopenic purpura of adults, which is associated with CNS involvement, seizures, and frequently hemiparesis. The diagnosis of HUS is clinical once other causes of ARF have been excluded. Treatment is supportive, consisting of correcting any fluid or electrolyte abnormalities (i.e., hypokalemia and acidosis) and correction of any hematologic abnormalities by transfusion of blood or platelets. Progressive renal failure may require peritoneal dialysis or hemodialysis. No evidence shows that early dialysis shortens the course of the disease or lessens subsequent sequelae. High-dose furosemide therapy (3 to 4 mg/kg every 3 to 4 hours to maintain a urine volume greater than 2 to 3 ml/kg/hr) has been beneficial in circumventing the need for dialysis. Females often have a more severe clinical picture. The overall prognosis is favorable; most patients recover completely and eventually attain normal renal function. Poor prognostic indicators at disease onset include a severe clinical presentation (toxic enterocolitis), high WBC count, and a high hemoglobin value. The D − (nondiarrheal) form also has a poorer prognosis than D +. Long-term sequelae afflict 15% to 20% of children, who may develop either hypertension or proteinuria 3 to 5 years after the onset of the disease. Residual renal functional disturbance is due to patchy cortical necrosis present at the onset of the disease and may lead to eventual renal insufficiency and chronic renal failure.

PATIENT NUMBER 4 (continued)

Gross hematuria presenting after an upper respiratory tract infection is most likely caused by either an acute nephritic syndrome or IgA nephropathy. Laboratory evaluation should include complement and immunoglobulin assessment to help in differentiation. Most nephritic syndromes resolve after 5 to 10 days. Progressive creatinemia and oliguria should alert the practitioner to a rapidly progressing disorder or other grave renal disorders. Isolated gross hematuria may be familial, idiopathic, IgA nephropathy, or even

stones. Annabelle probably has an IgA nephropathy, based on the timing of the onset of hematuria and the normal C3 value.

NEPHROTIC SYNDROME IN CHILDREN

Nephrotic syndrome is defined as the association of proteinuria, hypoproteinemia, edema, and hypercholesterolemia. Alterations of the permeability of the basement membrane to serum proteins cause excess losses into the urine, with resultant decrease in serum oncotic pressure and thus transudation of water into the interstitial tissues.

PATIENT NUMBER 5

Bartholomew is a 2-year-old boy who is brought to your office because his mom has noticed swelling of his eyes each morning for the past week. He was seen in a community clinic and given medications for allergy, but to no avail. Today he presents with obvious swelling of his eyes and feet. His pants are too tight for him, and his weight is 4 kg heavier than usual.

Onset in children is usually between 18 months and 7 years, with minimal lesion prevailing as the most likely cause (Table 9–7). Patients have normal blood pressure, slightly elevated creatinine clearance, normal C3 and C4 levels, and, other than proteinuria, an acellular urinalysis. Only 3% to 5% of children have evidence of microhematuria, mild azotemia, or hypertension. Investigation should preclude causes such as hepatitis B and human immunodeficiency virus. As soon as the diagnosis is established, a clinical trial of steroids should be initiated. Studies suggest a benefit of longer treatment over short courses. Consequently, we recommend prednisone, 2 mg/kg in three divided doses daily for 4 weeks, followed by alternate-day therapy at the same dose for a further 8 weeks. Diuretics may be of value in assisting in the control of edema or ascites. Relapses are treated with daily therapy until the urine is protein free for 1 week or up to a maximum of 4 weeks, followed by a further 8 weeks of alternate-day therapy. Whether tapering steroids at this time has any benefit over abruptly stopping is still not well substantiated. Response to steroids within 4 to 6 weeks is observed in more than 85% of patients, but relapses are common. The number of relapses in the first 6

TABLE 9–7. Nephrotic Syndrome of Childhood

Clinical	Steroid Responsive	Steroid Resistant
Renal function	Normal	Normal or reduced
Blood pressure	Normal	Normal or reduced
Urinalysis	Occasional microhematuria, hyaline casts, proteinuria	Frequent hematuria, cellular or granular casts, proteinuria
Serology		
C3, C4	Normal	Normal or low
Biopsy		
Light microscopy	Minimal change	Focal sclerosis or proliferative glomerulonephritis
Immunofluorescence	Negative	Positive, often IgM
Electron microscopy	Foot process fusion	Immune deposits

months is highly predictive of future relapses. Steroid toxicity is common and may result in hypertension, fluid retention, susceptibility to infection, and growth arrest during the duration of steroid therapy, although the final height of children with minimal lesion nephrotic syndrome appears to be what would be predicted from their prenephrotic growth velocity and midparental heights. Resistance to prednisone therapy (i.e., failure to reduce protein excretion below significant levels) and persistence of proteinuria beyond 8 weeks are indications for renal biopsy. Most of these prednisone-resistant children are candidates for therapy with either cyclophosphamide or chlorambucil. Long-term prognosis is favorable for most children, however, with complete resolution of the disease before adolescence.

Pathologic findings reveal minimal lesion in 65% of cases; focal segmental glomerulosclerosis in 15%; proliferative glomerulonephritis, including pure mesangial proliferation in 15%; and membranous nephropathy in 4% to 5%. These latter disorders are most frequently found in the resistant group and may progress to renal failure. Focal glomerular sclerosis has been known to recur in transplants.

PATIENT NUMBER 5 (continued)

Significant isolated proteinuria in young children such as Bartholomew is unusual and must be considered to be due to nephrotic syndrome unless proven otherwise. In children older than 5 years, a multitude of conditions can result in proteinuria, most commonly postural or orthostatic proteinuria. A child with nephrotic syndrome should be considered to have a chronic relapsing disease because only 10% or less have one episode only. Although the majority respond to steroids, failure to respond often signifies a more ominous prognosis and may dictate the need for renal biopsy and cytotoxic medication.

CONGENITAL MALFORMATIONS OF THE URINARY TRACT

With the advent of prenatal ultrasonography, various congenital renal anomalies are being uncovered with a frequency approaching 0.45% to 0.9% of live births. Only some of these may have grave consequences to the fetus or neonate. As treatment programs improve, many children with severe congenital abnormalities of the renal urinary system are surviving for longer periods only to enter into renal dialysis programs as older infants and children. Congenital malformations of the kidneys can be grouped as abnormalities of morphogenesis (renal parenchyma), abnormalities of structure (the collecting system), or renal cysts (Table 9–8). The most significant prenatal renal lesions are obstructive: hydronephrosis, secondary to either ureteropelvic junction obstruction; or hydroureter, with ureterovesical junction obstruction or severe ureterovesical reflux. Bilateral hydronephrosis suggests either severe bilateral reflux or a central cause such as posterior urethral valves. Other prenatal structural anomalies not infrequently encountered are polycystic kidney disease, either the autosomal dominant or recessive form, and unilateral or bilateral multicystic dysplasia, associated with hypoplasia, aplasia, or agenesis (Potter's syndrome). Important gestational clues to renal anomalies include maternal polyhydramnios, suggesting poor fetal concentrating mechanisms. Oligohydramnios is a poor prognostic indicator because it implies a depressed fetal GFR. It is frequently associated with pulmonary hypoplasia. Potter's syndrome is an association of bilateral renal agenesis, pulmonary hypoplasia, and a characteristic flattened facies due to oligohydramnios. Most often it is incompatible with postnatal survival owing to the pulmonary hypoplasia.

Functional disturbances often accompany fetal renal malformations. Concentrating and acidification defects may occur with alterations of medullary architecture (hydronephrosis or cysts), whereas diminished GFR can accompany dysplasia and hypoplasia. Severe structural anomalies, especially if bilateral (i.e., hydronephrosis or multicystic disease) have associated dysplastic elements that result in combined glomerular (reduced GFR) and medullary functional defects (concentration, dilution, acidification). Kidneys with congenital hydroureter and hydronephrosis, if antenatal ultrasonography has not been performed, may escape detection and may present many months or years later, often with a patient in renal failure. These kidneys may be mistaken

TABLE 9–8. Congenital Renal Malformations

Abnormalities of Parenchymal Morphogenesis

Amount
  Agenesis
  Aplasia
  Hypoplasia
Differentiation
  Dysplasia
Location
  Ectopy
  Horseshoe kidney

Abnormalities of the Collecting System

Hydronephrosis
Hydroureter
Reflux

Renal Cysts

Nonhereditary
  Simple
  Multilocular
  Multicystic
Hereditary
  Cortical
  Medullary
    Autosomal recessive
    Autosomal dominant
  Polycystic
    Autosomal recessive
    Autosomal dominant

for chronic pyelonephritis because they have a similar imaging appearance, yet no history of infection can be obtained. The renal failure is due to unrecognized renal dysplasia.

Aplasia, Hypoplasia, Dysplasia

Prenatal sonographic screening has detected a large number of renal structural anomalies, but whether this has had a major impact on the prevention of eventual renal failure is moot. Renal hypoplasia is usually unilateral and inconsequential but may be bilateral and associated with reduced renal function or may be segmental, either unilateral or bilateral. Segmental hypoplasia is associated with a small arterial supply and is accompanied by hypertension. If present bilaterally, it is usually associated with dysplasia and reduced renal function. Renal dysplasia may also be unilateral or bilateral and can be associated with hypoplasia or multicystic disease. Observed clinically may be polydipsia, polyuria, reduced GFR, and hypertension. A unilateral multicystic dysplastic kidney, if present at birth, is either poorly functional or nonfunctional. These kidneys need not be removed, because more than 25% spontaneously involute over several years. There is no evidence that they are more prone to malignancy than normal kidneys.

Hydronephrosis

Routine antenatal ultrasonography has uncovered a wide range of renal structural abnormalities, the most frequent being a dilated renal pelvis. Postnatal ultrasonographic follow-up has shown spontaneous resolution in some of the milder cases; thus, a conservative initial approach is warranted. However, all such neonates require early evaluation and follow-up. Hydronephrosis is secondary to either structural or functional obstruction. Obstructive structural anomalies are most common at the posterior urethra (valves) or the ureterovesical or ureteropelvic junction. Functional obstruction is associated with gross reflux or the megacystis-megaureter syndrome. Bilateral hydronephrosis with hydroureter occurs with posterior urethral valves, megacystis syndromes, or bilateral ureteropelvic junction obstruction. The degree of renal functional disruption is often a factor of the severity of accompanying renal dysplasia and the amount of functional renal parenchyma remaining. To test for the likelihood of progressive obstruction and further degradation of GFR, sequential ultrasound examinations are recommended in association with a DPTA renal scan followed by furosemide (Lasix) infusion. If the radionuclide washout is acceptable, only conservative observation is required.

Reflux

Vesicoureteral reflux is a congenital anomaly associated with lateral displacement of the ureteral orifices and a short intravesicular canal. Moderate to severe grades of reflux are often associated with increasing degrees of dysplasia, and it is this feature (i.e., the dysplasia) that is responsible for the radiographic appearance of chronically shrunken kidneys that is mistaken for chronic pyelonephritis occasionally noted in very young infants. Clinically observed may also be concentrating defects, reduced GFR, and mild to moderate hypertension.

Reflux is the most common structural abnormality associated with UTI (30%) and is demonstrable by voiding cystography either during bladder filling (low pressure) or on micturition (high pressure reflux). Grade 1 reflux shows dye ascending to the renal pelvis, grade II reflux fills the pelvis and shows well-cupped calyces, grade III shows calyceal clubbing and some degree of pelvic dilatation, grade IV is accompanied by pyelonephritic scarring (loss of renal parenchyma), and grade V combines elements of extensive scarring, loss of renal parenchyma, and hydronephrosis. Prognosis of resolution is directly proportional to the degree of reflux; grades I and II are associated with an 85% spontaneous resolution, grade III with 60% to 75%, and grades IV to V with 5% to 10%. Urine must be maintained sterile during the intervening years, however, and this necessitates long-term antibiotic prophylaxis for a minimum of 6 months to many years. Surgical ureteral reimplantation thus is not indicated until after many years of antibiotic therapy and firm evidence of nonresolution. The frequency of repeated cystography should be kept to an absolute minimum, once every 3 to 4 years in children with persistent infections, and preferably using radioisotopes.

Posterior Urethral Valves

Persistence of redundant embryonic tissue in the posterior urethra of a male fetus forms valves that open during fetal micturition and thus cause intrauterine bladder outlet obstruction, increased intravesical pressure, bilateral hydroureters, and hydronephrosis. Almost always associated are bilateral renal dysplasia, reduced GFR, and various degrees of functional impairment. This condition is a common cause of renal failure in early infancy. Important clues to postnatal diagnosis are a readily palpable bladder and a history of straining on urination, with an interrupted urinary stream. Many affected infants present with acute pyelonephritis and bacteremia in infancy, and this diagnosis should be considered in the workup of all such patients.

Renal Cysts

Renal cysts (see Table 9–8) may occur singly, such as simple cysts or multilocular cysts; diffusely, as in polycystic or multicystic disease; in the cortex, associated with systemic syndromes; or in the medulla, such as juvenile nephronophthisis (or medullary cystic disease) and medullary sponge kidney.

Polycystic Kidney Disease

The pediatric polycystic kidney diseases occur most frequently as autosomal dominant (ADPKD) or less commonly as the autosomal recessive (ARPKD) form. They account for at least 10% of all end-stage renal disease in children. Although thought to be mostly confined to adults, ADPKD has been detected in utero. The earlier the cysts develop, the earlier the onset of renal insufficiency. The most sensitive method for their detection is ultrasonography, because IVP may not detect the presence of small cysts. Most children remain asymptomatic throughout childhood. The onset of renal insufficiency and hypertension is delayed until late adolescence to middle age. Screening family members for chromosomal markers on chromosome 16 is highly reliable and advisable for genetic counseling and for other at-risk family members. ADPKD presenting in utero or in early infancy must be differentiated from ARPKD. Because the cysts in the recessive form are usually smaller and frequently involve other organs, the in utero appearance may reveal only the presence of diffusely enlarged kidneys. Postnatally, the kidneys in ARPKD are enlarged and filled with multiple small cysts that are best seen at the edge of the renal shadows. The kidneys are palpable, and the liver may show multiple cysts as well. Hypertension and renal insufficiency are invariable accompaniments, but progression to end-stage renal disease is variable, some patients not requiring dialysis until adolescence.

Multicystic Kidney Disease

Multicystic kidney disease (discussed earlier) usually is unilateral. The cysts are multiple and diverse in size and are associated with dysplasia. These kidneys function poorly or not at all. The disease is usually accompanied by abnormalities of the ipsilateral ureter, such as severe reflux, stenosis, or aplasia, and contralateral ureteral abnormalities are also found in more than 35% of cases. Overall renal function may be acceptable unless involvement is bilateral. A child who has an obvious multicystic kidney and in whom the GFR does not reach the expected range should be suspected of having bilateral involvement.

PATIENT NUMBER 6 (continued)

When faced with enlarged kidneys on antenatal ultrasound examination, the practitioner should consider those entities that may diffusely cause renal enlargement in utero. ARPKD, because of the small size of the cysts, mimics diffuse enlargement. ADPKD should have a positive family history and usually is associated with observable cysts. Cysts are difficult to distinguish from dilatations on antenatal ultrasound examination; thus, multicystic (dysplastic) kidneys as well as obstructive hydronephrosis (ureteropelvic junction, ureterovesicular junction, posturethral valves) or hydronephrisis associated with reflux should be considered. Because some dilated renal pelves may resolve postnatally, they have been termed physiologic hydronephrosis, an unfortunate term. The association of a dilated renal pelvis with an enlarged bladder indicates outlet obstruction (i.e., posterior urethral valves). Considered together with oligohydramnios, this indicates poor renal function due to bilateral renal dysplasia. The prognosis for such fetuses is grave because of associated pulmonary hypoplasia.

URINARY TRACT INFECTION

UTI is the second most common infectious disease in children. The risk for females to develop symptomatic UTI during childhood is 2% to 3% and in boys is less than 0.1%. Recurrent UTI when complicated with major structural abnormalities and dysplasia can, if not properly treated, lead to chronic renal failure, whereas recurrent uncomplicated UTI (i.e., not associated with structural anomalies) probably does not. Structural abnormalities probably occur with equal frequency in both males and females, but because females have a shorter urethra, they tend to become infected more frequently. Thus, if males are infected, especially in infancy, they are highly likely to have major underlying structural problems.

PATIENT NUMBER 7

You are seeing Marlene, a 2-year-old girl, for a fever of 40°C, which she has had for the past 24 hours. Her dad says that she has complained of abdominal pain and has been voiding small amounts frequently. She appears ill, but little else is found on physical examination except diffuse abdominal discomfort. Her urine dipstick result is positive for leukocyte esterase and nitrites. What would be your treatment for Marlene?

UTIs tend to be recurrent. After the first infection, the chance of recurrence is 35%, but this climbs to more than 65% after the second infection. Investigation of these patients with multiple recurrences has demonstrated structural abnormalities in only 25% to 30%, usually reflux. New scars may develop in 5% to 10% of children with pyelonephritis but rarely develop after age 5 years. Children with frequent recurrences and normal urinary drainage systems are unusually susceptible to bacterial infection related to bacterial virulence and adherence sites to *E. coli* on the uroepithelium.

Clinical Presentation

Newborns with UTI present with signs of sepsis: fever (or hypothermia), poor feeding, vomiting, weight loss, and persistent jaundice. Older infants and young children present with a more classic picture of high spiking fevers, chills, diffuse abdominal or loin pain, and frequently lower tract symptoms consisting of dysuria, frequency, urgency incontinence, enuresis, and occasionally gross hematuria. Hematuria that accompanies UTI is evidence of a major inflammatory response and thus is invariably attended by dysuria or pyelonephritis. Asymptomatic hematuria is rarely a sign of UTI.

Pyelonephritis implies infection of the renal parenchyma. It is invariably accompanied by a spiking fever and, depending on the age, chills, rigors, flank or abdominal pain, and lower urinary tract symptoms (frequency, urgency, dysuria). Although structural abnormalities frequently are associated, most commonly ureteral reflux, as many as 40% to 60% of cases may have no demonstrable defect. In young children, pyelonephritis may be occasionally accompanied by nephronia, a round, well-circumscribed echodense area observed on ultrasound examination. Once thought to be a solid abscess, a precursor to liquefaction, it is now considered a localized area of pyelonephritic involvement, and therapy need not be prolonged.

Physical examination of young children with recurrent UTI or pyelonephritis should search for clues to an underlying congenital anomaly such as a history of a single umbilical artery in the neonate, ear tags or deformities, or abnormalities in the anorectum, spine, or genitalia (i.e., ectopic meatus or labial fusion). A history of a forced or interrupted urinary stream in boys suggests posterior urethral valves.

> Only 25% to 35% of children with recurrent UTI have an underlying structural defect.

Indications for Imaging Studies

Children with UTI should first be screened with ultrasonography before proceeding with voiding cystourethrogram. The indications for the combined study include the following:

A. First infections
1. First infection, especially if febrile, in all infants and toddlers up to age 3 years
2. Documented infections in boys up to age 10 years
3. A renal mass suggesting hydronephrosis or tumor
4. Hypertension or azotemia in a child with UTI
B. Recurrent infections
1. Children up to age 8 to 10 years of both sexes, realizing that the likelihood of an underlying anomaly decreases in relation to increasing age at first infections
C. Recurrent asymptomatic bacteriuria
1. If results of imaging studies are normal, no further evaluation is necessary (i.e., cystoscopy)

Treatment

Therapy for an acute afebrile UTI (i.e., cystitis) should last for 10 to 14 days. Single high-dose antibiotic therapy has not been a recommended protocol for children because relapses are frequent and doses may far exceed tolerance levels for this age group. Therapy for pyelonephritis in children other than infants, when sepsis may be an associated problem, need not always necessitate admission and intravenous antibiotics. When

TABLE 9–9. Antibiotics Commonly Used to Treat Urinary Tract Infections in Children

Antibiotic	Dose (mg/kg)	Interval
Amoxicillin	35–50	Every 8 hr
Nitrofurantoin	3–5	Every 6 hr
Trimethoprim-sulfamethoxazole	6	Every 8–12 hr
Cephalexin	30	Every 6 hr

structural anomalies coexist, therapy is continued for a minimum of 6 months as long-term low-dose prophylaxis (one dose per day) and in some cases for several years. Appropriate antibiotics should be chosen. Use of antibiotics with relative insensitivity or resistance is associated with a high rate of relapse or recurrence. Antibiotics in common use for prophylaxis are listed in Table 9–9.

PATIENT NUMBER 7 (continued)

Fever in a young child should alert the physician to a possible UTI. Typical symptoms in children are absent or sparse, and suspicion is often the best guide to diagnosis. Clean-catch urine samples are often difficult to obtain, and cultures should always be accompanied by a microscopic urinalysis. Bacterial contamination is common, but urine is not likely to contain WBCs. Ultrasonography should be carried out in all first infections, and voiding cystourethrography (VCUG) should be conducted according to the outlined protocol. Because reflux can be familial, a family history would be helpful in deciding whether a VCUG is appropriate for older children.

HYPERTENSION

Hypertension is not common in children but when detected requires confirmation and evaluation. Acute elevations are noted in the immediate postoperative period, probably secondary to the metabolic effects of anesthesia and fluid administration during surgery.

> Because acute hypertensive crises may be associated with seizures, congestive heart failure, and papilledema, blood pressure must be lowered quickly yet safely.

Other common causes include acute nephritic syndromes, fluid overload, unrecognized chronic renal failure, systemic vasculitis, aortic coarctation, renal dysplasia, and renal artery stenosis. Hypertension in neonates is frequently associated with renovascular disease (stenosis or thrombosis), structural defects associated with dysplasia, multicystic or polycystic disease, medications used for chronic lung disease, or in older infants, acute nephritic syndromes. Adrenal, thyroid, CNS, carcinoid, renal, and renovascular causes should be excluded in all children presenting with elevated blood pressure.

PATIENT NUMBER 8

Rock is a 10-year-old boy whom you are seeing in your office for headaches. His blood pressure is 150/100 mm Hg in both arms. Both his father and paternal uncle have been hypertensive for many years, and both are on medication.

Hypertension is unusual in infants but increases in frequency directly proportional to age, affecting a maximum of 3% to 5% of teenagers. Essential hypertension is more common than has previously been recognized, increasing in frequency after age 10 years to be the most likely cause in this and older age groups. A familial history is common, as are other epidemiologic factors such as smoking and obesity.

The first line of treatment of an acute hypertensive crisis is aqueous oral nifedipine (0.25 to 0.5 mg/kg/dose) given sublingually. In the event that blood pressure is not lowered successfully by the oral route, intravenous medication should be administered, often in the context of an intensive care environment to monitor the decline in pressures. Other effective intravenous medications for acute blood pressure control include labetalol (1 to 3 mg/kg/hr), diazoxide (2 to 5 mg/kg/dose) given rapidly over 15 to 20 seconds, and nitroprusside (0.5 to 0.8 μg/kg/min). Thiocyanate and cyanide intoxication and lactic acidosis are rarely encountered unless renal or hepatic function is impaired.

Because essential hypertension is unusual in young children, persistently elevated BP should be completely evaluated.

Treatment of persistent or chronic hypertension is related to the etiology of the problem. Drugs commonly used are outlined in Table 9–10. Medications in current use include the angiotensin-converting enzyme (ACE) inhibitors captopril and enalapril, as well as the calcium

TABLE 9–10. Antihypertensive Medications

Drug	Dosage (mg/kg/day)	Maximum mg/kg/day
Diuretics		
Hydrochlorthiazide	1	2–3
Furosemide	1	10
Metolazone	0.1	3
Bumetanide	0.02–0.05	0.3
Spironolactone	1	3
Triamterene	2	6
Converting Enzyme Inhibitors		
Captopril		
Neonates	0.03–0.15	2
Children	1.5	6
Enalapril	0.15	0.6
Calcium Channel Blockers		
Nifedipine	0.25	3
Nicardipine	0.25	2
Alpha-Adrenergic Blockers		
Prazosin	0.05–0.1	0.5
Alpha/Beta-Adrenergic Blockers		
Labetalol	1–3	1–3
Beta-Adrenergic Blockers		
Propranolol	1	8
Atenolol	1	8
Central Vasomotor Center (Alpha Agonist)		
Clonidine	0.05–0.1	
Vasodilators		
Hydralazine	0.75	7.5
Minoxidil	0.1–0.2	1

channel blockers verapamil, nifedipine, and long-acting amlodipine as first-line agents. The beta-adrenergic-blocking agents propranolol, atenolol, and metoprolol, which enjoyed extensive use in the past, have given way to the ACE inhibitors and calcium channel blockers but still remain useful additives. Other adrenergic agents such as the alpha$_1$-adrenergic blocker prazosin and the central alpha$_2$-adrenergic blocker clonidine have limited but important roles in patients with excessive sympathetic stimulation induced by vasodilating drugs. Diuretic agents are best used in children in combination with other antihypertensives such as the beta blockers. The thiazides are used in patients with relatively intact renal function, and the loop diuretics furosemide, metolazone, and bumetanide are best used when renal function is reduced. The potassium-sparing diuretics spironolactone and triamterene are useful when serum potassium levels are compromised. Particularly resistant hypertension may respond to the vasodilator minoxidil, which acts directly on the arterioles. Unfortunately, hypertrichosis is a common problem that negates long-term use, especially in females.

PATIENT NUMBER 8 (continued)

Blood pressure should be measured with a correctly sized cuff, especially important in obese individuals, in both arms and legs. If elevated, it should be repeated on three separate occasions, preferably in a relaxed environment. In the absence of adrenal, thyroid, CNS, and renovascular signs or symptoms, essential hypertension is the most likely cause even in this age group. Although smoking and alcohol are not major factors, obesity and family history are important predisposing causes.

ACUTE RENAL FAILURE

ARF is recognized clinically by an abrupt reduction in urine output. Oliguria has been defined as a urine output of less than 0.5 mg/kg/hr in neonates and young infants and less than 2.0 mg/kg/hr or 400 to 500 ml/m²/day in older infants and children. Common causes of ARF in children are listed in Table 9–11.

FE_{Na} is helpful in determining whether the ARF is prerenal or renal in origin. However, the values for children differ from those in adults, less than 2% to 3% acceptable for neonates and infants and less than 1% for older infants and children, similar to adults.

The importance of recognizing the presence and cause of prerenal ARF in children is related to the relative ease of producing hypovolemic prerenal failure in children secondary to diarrheal illnesses or heart failure. Renal causes of ARF are, as in adults, due to acute tubular necrosis, frequently associated with surgical, hypoxic-traumatic, or nephrotoxic events. Seen on pathologic study is necrosis of the renal tubular epithelium. In neonatal intensive care units, ARF is a relatively common event in infants with respiratory distress, sepsis, or shock due to any cause. Recovery in infants and children is usually complete, unless associated with severe tubular destruction and subsequent scarring.

> **Successful resolution or ARF in children is dependent on the correction and elimination of the causative factors and management of the fluid, electrolyte, and acid-base disturbances.**

Management of ARF in children follows simi-

TABLE 9–11. Causes of Acute Renal Failure in Children

Prerenal

Hypovolemia
Dehydration
Sepsis
Heart failure

Renal

Vascular
  Renal vein thrombosis
  Vasculitis
  Hemolytic-uremic syndrome
Glomerular
  Acute glomerulonephritis
  Rapidly progressive glomerulonephritis
Tubular
  Acute tubular necrosis
  Ischemic necrosis (shock, cardiac surgery, toxic nephropathies)
  Urate nephropathy
  Sepsis
Interstitial
  Acute interstitial nephritis
  Acute pyelonephritis

Postrenal

Obstruction
  Congenital—posterior urethral valves
    Ureterovesicular junction
    Ureteropelvic junction
    Megacystis-megaureter syndrome
  Acquired
    Wilms' tumor
    Lymphoma

lar principles as in adults, with special attention given to fluid, electrolyte, and acid-base imbalance. Volume replacement is calculated at insensible losses (400 ml/m²/day) plus urinary and other water losses. Forcing a diuresis is best accomplished with furosemide in large doses (1 to 4 mg/kg/dose every 3 hours). Metolazone and bumetanide are also useful and less likely to induce ototoxicity. Hyperkalemia is a common accompaniment of ARF and becomes an emergency if associated with ECG changes. All children with ARF and a serum potassium level elevated above 6.5 mmol/L should have cardiac monitoring. Treatment should include removal of all sources of potassium intake. An infusion of sodium bicarbonate at 3.3 ml/kg raises the plasma pH by causing an exchange of intracellular H^+ for extracellular K^+. An infusion of 25% to 50% glucose with 1 unit of insulin per 3 g glucose causes an intracellular shift of potassium as glucose is transported into the cell. A calcium chloride infusion of 10 mg/kg (0.1 mg/kg of a 10% solution) is cardioprotective and should be given along with the previous solutions. Kayexalate, an ion exchange resin, can be given either orally or by retention enema but should not be used in emergency situations because it takes many hours to lower serum potassium levels. The dose is 1 g/kg repeated every 4 hours as required. Oral doses should be accompanied by 70% sorbitol to maximize gastrointestinal excretion.

If renal failure is profound and persistent and is associated with intractable hyperkalemia, acidosis, hypertension, or fluid retention, then peritoneal or hemodialysis is indicated.

Peritoneal dialysis is not a difficult procedure in children and may be instituted in life-threatening circumstances if the child is to be transferred to another facility. Insertion of a peritoneal catheter can be performed percutaneously in the midline (linea alba) just below the umbilicus and directed toward the pelvis. Peritoneal fluid administration should start at 10 ml/kg/cycle and increased slowly, as tolerated, to 50 ml/kg/cycle. The glucose content of the fluids varies from 1.5% to 4.25%, and if hypervolemia, cardiac failure, or hyperkalemia is present, the initial fluid should be hypertonic (4.5% glucose). Potassium is added only after the serum levels have become normal, as solutions of 10 to 40 mmol/L. Systemic fluid, electrolytes, and acid-base status must be frequently monitored, and all sources of fluids adjusted accordingly. When circumstances dictate that intravenous fluids must be given rapidly, the concentration of the peritoneal dialysate can be increased to compensate for these excesses. Overall fluid balance is calculated by the difference of the total 24-hour fluid administered minus the urine and other fluid losses and the negative peritoneal fluid balance.

CHRONIC RENAL FAILURE

The prevalence of the causes of chronic renal failure in children differs from that in adults (Table 9–12). Renal structural malformations including the obstructive uropathies are the leading cause of ESRD in both children and adolescents, whereas chronic glomerulonephritis is more prevalent in adults. The overall incidence of ESRD in children varies from 4 to 8 per million child population per year, whereas in adults it varies from 60 to 120 per million population per year. This accounts for the major differences in dialysis and transplant populations in the two age groups.

Chronic renal failure causes unique complications specific to children. Failure to thrive in infants, reduced growth rates and short stature,

TABLE 9–12. Causes of End-Stage Renal Disease in Children Under 15 Years

Cause	Number	Percent
Renal malformations (including multicystic dysplasia, hypoplasia)	34	24
Chronic glomerulonephritis (including focal segmental glomerulonephritis, hemolytic-uremic syndrome, anaphylactoid purpura nephritis)	33	23
Obstructive uropathies (including hydronephrosis, pyelonephritis)	39	26
Hereditary disorders (including Alport's syndrome, cystinosis)	12	8
Miscellaneous disorders (polycystic, tubular necrosis, unspecified)	28	19
Total	146	100

From the Canadian Organ Replacement Registry, 1993–1994.

delayed puberty, infertility, and metabolic bone disease cause major disruptions for children and often induce profound adjustment problems for such individuals, as well as major health care concerns. Long-term management protocols must address these and many other health care concerns common to all patients with ESRD. High-calorie diets with protein intake restricted to only RDA levels are imperative in infants and young children to allow for growth. Calcium supplements, nonaluminum phosphate binders, and calcitriol are characteristically administered when the GFR falls below 25%. The early use of erythropoietin and iron supplements improves anemia and prevents clinical symptoms. The inclusion of ACE inhibitors early in the course of chronic renal failure slows the rate of decline of the GFR by causing efferent arteriolar vasodilatation and reducing elevated intraglomerular filtration pressures and hyperperfusion.

Long-term dialysis procedures, either peritoneal dialysis or hemodialysis, can be initiated at any age. The choice between peritoneal dialysis and hemodialysis should be both a patient and parental decision but is often tempered by pragmatic factors such as the age of the child (a younger child is more easily adapted to peritoneal dialysis), distance to the dialysis center, and so on. All children should be considered as candidates for transplantation before entry into a dialysis program, because growth on dialysis is marginal and pubertal development often is severely retarded. Growth is dependent on the age at which the chronic process began, the rapidity of its development, and the stage of growth and nutrition at entry into the dialysis program. These complications may persist or even worsen

TABLE 9–13. Water Balance in Children, Based on Surface Area

In			Out		
Source	*ml/m²/day*	*Tonicity (mOsm/kg)*	*Source*	*ml/m²/day*	*Tonicity (mOsm/kg)*
Water of metabolism	300	0	Skin	500–600	30–50
			Lungs	900	0
Usual dietary intake°	1500	Variable	Gastrointestinal	10–100	100
			Renal	300–800	300
Total	1800	0	Total	1800	100

°Represents usual maintenance requirements, i.e., 1500 ml/m²/day of fluids with a tonicity of 100 mOsm/kg one-third isotonic.

throughout the dialysis program. Thus, the expectation of minimizing or reversing these devastating problems is best attained through early transplantation. Results of pediatric transplantation are good but age dependent. The older the child at transplant, the closer the successes are to adult survival statistics. Living related donors offer a child the best chances of a long-lasting graft. Despite steroids and immunosuppressives, a well-functioning graft is usually associated with improved growth velocity and some pubertal development. Adjunctive use of human growth hormone improves stature, and selective use of hormonal therapy assists in pubertal development.

FLUID AND ELECTROLYTE THERAPY IN CHILDREN

Because infants have a higher metabolic rate, a higher ratio of surface area to weight, increased evaporative losses per unit of weight, a greater proportion of extracellular to intracellular water, and decreased ability to concentrate the urine, they are more prone to dehydration than adults. Fluid therapy in children must be based on the weight or surface area of the child to avoid overestimating or underestimating fluid and electrolyte requirements.

PATIENT NUMBER 9

Trevor is a 1-year-old infant whom you are seeing in the emergency room of your hospital for a 3-day history of vomiting and watery diarrhea. He has been unable to keep down any fluids for the past 24 hours. He appears severely dehydrated. His serum electrolyte values are Na^+ 133 mmol/L, K^+ 4.5 mmol/L, and Cl^- 115 mmol/L. Can you explain his serum electrolyte results?

The concept of *balance* is used in calculating fluid requirements of all age groups. Maintenance fluid requirements should equal the total amount of all body fluid losses (lungs, skin, gastrointestinal tract, and renal losses) minus the water gained through metabolism (Table 9–13). The usual volume and compositional losses are 1800 ml/m²/day of a fluid containing 100 mOsm/kg, and there is a net gain of 300 ml/m²/day of a fluid containing 0 mOsm/kg, resulting in an overall net loss of 1500 ml/m²/day of a fluid containing 100 mOsm/kg, equivalent to one-third isotonic. This fluid volume represents intravenous maintenance fluid requirements for infants and children older than 1 year and more than 10 kg in weight. Thus, usual body losses are hypotonic in nature. Large volume losses of a similar tonicity (one-third isotonic) induce compensatory mechanisms, primarily shifts of body water to either the intracellular or extracellular compartments, such that an isotonic dehydration is the end result. This is the most common dehydrational state. If net *osmolal* losses exceed the usual one-third isotonic losses, then a hyponatremic state ensues. Conversely, if net *osmolal* losses are less than the usual daily losses, then hypernatremia results.

> **Maintenance fluid requirements = 1500 ml/m²/day for all infants and children over 1 year of age and 10 kg in weight.**

Intravenous requirements for dehydrational states must include

1. Existing losses, as assessed by the degree of dehydration (Table 9–14)
2. Maintenance fluid requirements (1500 ml/m²/day)
3. Ongoing losses of equivalent volume and composition

TABLE 9–14. Degree of Dehydration as Percent of Weight Loss

	Mild	Moderate	Severe	Shock
Infants	<5%	5–10%	10–15%	>15
Children	<3%	3–8%	8–12%	>12%

In general, mild dehydration should be corrected by the oral route with appropriate hypotonic rehydration solutions containing 50 to 75 mOsm Na^+. Moderate and severe dehydrational states require intravenous fluid administration; the more severe the volume depletion, the more rapid is the replacement (Table 9–15).

Isotonic dehydration is generated by large hypotonic (one-third) fluid losses and is repaired with 0.25% (in neonates and very young infants) to 0.33% saline in 5% dextrose in water. Severe volume depletion causing shock is repaired with isotonic fluids (i.e., isotonic saline).

A general guide to the repair of hypotonic dehydration is as follows:

Serum Sodium (mmol/L)	NaCl in 5.0% DW
130–135	0.25%–0.33%
125–130	0.5%
120–125	0.9%
<120	3%–5%

Correction can also be calculated by the following formula:

$$\text{Amount of sodium required} = [\text{sodium deficit}] \times [\text{volume of distribution}]$$
$$= [135 - \text{serum } Na^+ \text{ observed}] \times [0.6 \times \text{body weight kg}]$$

Half is added to the initial replacement fluid and the remainder added during the next 24 hours, taking care not to raise the serum Na^+ level more than 10 mmol/24 hr to prevent the neurologic syndrome of central pontine myelinolysis.

Repair of hypertonic dehydration must be slow, over a period of 2 to 3 days. The tonicity of the fluid administered depends on the state of volume contraction. A hypotonic fluid (one

fourth to one sixth) is used if dehydration is mild to moderate and vascular volume is not compromised, because one can ignore the degree of dehydration and proceed with a slow repair at maintenance rates. However, if the degree of dehydration is more severe and the vascular volume is compromised, then larger volumes of fluid are required. The likelihood of inducing shifts of extracellular water to the intracellular compartment results if large volumes of hypotonic fluids are used, with resultant cerebral edema. When vascular volume is a concern, vascular compromise (degree of dehydration) should be repaired the first day with normal (0.9%) saline and at maintenance rates over the subsequent 2 to 3 days, with fluids of gradually decreasing tonicity to one-third isotonic, to lower the serum sodium level slowly.

Metabolic acidosis is the most common acid-base disturbance associated with dehydrational states in children. Correction is required when the serum bicarbonate level falls below 15 mmol/L according to the following formula:

$$\text{Bicarbonate required} = [\text{base deficit}] \times [\text{volume of distribution (i.e., bicarbonate space)}]$$
$$= [\text{desired bicarbonate}^\circ - \text{measured bicarbonate}] \times [\text{body weight kg} \times 0.5]$$

One half is administered over the next 2 to 4 hours, depending on the severity of the acidosis; the remainder over the next 18 to 24 hours. Persistent or profound acidosis such as salicylate intoxication may require repeated boluses or even continuous high-dose intravenous bicarbonate infusions. Caution must be exercised, because repeated bicarbonate infusions may induce hypertonicity and ensuing intracerebral hemorrhage and convulsions. Chronic acidosis must be corrected over several days because of the risk of inducing hypocalcemic tetany.

The addition of potassium to any infusion must await proof of adequate renal function. Potassium is added as KCl from 10 to 50 mmol/L.

°Desired bicarbonate level should not be greater than 10 mmol above the measured bicarbonate.

TABLE 9–15. Rate of Intravenous Replacement Therapy

Amount of Fluid Replacement	Moderate Dehydration	Severe Dehydration	Shock
½ of 24-hour replacement	6–8 hours	4–6 hours	20 ml/kg; ½ in ½ hour; remainder in 1–2 hours

PATIENT NUMBER 9 *(continued)*

Trevor weighs approximately 10 kg (body surface area, 0.45 m²). Because the most common form of dehydration is isotonic, generated from one-third isotonic losses, the concept of balance is maintained by replacing equivalent volume and compositional losses. Thus, one-third isotonic fluids should be given as maintenance if vascular volume is not compromised. Some prefer to expand the vascular volume with isotonic saline before administration of maintenance fluids. Acid-base status often self-corrects as dehydration is repaired.

SELECTED READINGS

Ettinger R: The evaluation of the child with proteinuria. Pediatr Ann 23:486–494, 1994.

Hogg FJ: Usual and unusual presentations of IgA nephropathy in children. Contrib Nephrol 104:14–23, 1993.

Holliday MA, Barratt TM, Avner ED: Pediatric Nephrology, 3rd ed. Baltimore, Williams & Wilkins, 1994.

Jose PA, Fildes RD, Gomez RA, et al: Neonatal renal function and physiology. Curr Opin Pediatr 6:172–177, 1994.

Leung AK, Robson WL: Urinary tract infections in infants and children. Adv Pediatr 38:257–285, 1991.

Sinaiko AR: Treatment of hypertension in children. Pediatr Nephrol 8:603–609, 1994.

Warshaw B: Nephrotic syndrome in children. Pediatr Ann 23:496–504, 1994.

Yadin O: Hematuria in children. Pediatr Ann 23:474–485, 1994.

10 ▮ STONE DISEASE

R. A. L. Sutton

Renal stone disease may require the attention of both an internist and a urologist. The treatment of patients presenting with a symptomatic stone, usually one causing renal colic, hematuria, or obstruction, or of patients in whom an asymptomatic stone is discovered on ultrasonography, radiography, or CT scan is generally undertaken by a urologist. The introduction of less invasive methods for treating stones, including percutaneous lithotripsy and extracorporeal shock wave lithotripsy (ESWL), has revolutionized the surgical management of stones. It may sometimes be appropriate to treat (e.g., by ESWL) a small, asymptomatic renal stone to avoid a future attack of renal colic or ureteric obstruction.

This chapter discusses the contribution of the internist (or nephrologist) to the treatment of patients with stones.

> **Stones are very common. About 10% of men and 5% of women will have had at least one stone by the time they reach 70 years of age.**

The majority of stones are calcium containing (mostly calcium oxalate, with or without calcium phosphate); as many as 20% consist of other compounds, including uric acid, pure calcium phosphate, triple phosphate (struvite or magnesium ammonium phosphate plus calcium phosphate), cystine, or other rarer constituents.

> **Stones commonly recur. A patient who has formed a single (first) calcium stone has a 35% to 40% chance of recurrence at 5 years and a 50% chance at 10 years.**

The primary role of the internist is to identify underlying causes of stones and to recommend appropriate measures to minimize the risk of recurrence. This involves a search for risk factors for stones in each patient, followed by advice on long-term prophylactic treatment, which might include dietary changes and/or medications.

In the case of uric acid or cystine stones, medical management can lead to dissolution of stones within the urinary tract. Unfortunately, this is very rarely possible with the common calcium-containing stone.

The intensity of investigation and treatment has traditionally depended on whether the patient was deemed to be an active (or multiple) stone former or whether the patient has had only a single stone. One study[1] has, however, questioned the validity of this approach, because it showed that the chance of relapse on medical therapy was in direct proportion to the number of pretreatment stones. If this is confirmed, the case will be stronger for more aggressive investigation, with a view to beginning therapy after the first stone rather than waiting for recurrences.

The objective of this chapter is to provide the background knowledge needed to undertake appropriate investigation of patients with stones, to identify risk factors, and to recommend and monitor prophylactic therapy.

PATIENT NUMBER 1

Ella, a 35-year-old married secretary on a visit from another city and with no significant past medical history and no previous pregnancies, came to the emergency room with typical right renal colic. A urine dipstick test showed microscopic hematuria but only a trace of protein. An IVP (excretory urogram) showed, on the plain film, a probable radiopaque stone, 4 mm in diameter, in the line of the right ureter; after dye injection, mild dilatation was observed in the right pelvicalyceal system and right ureter above the stone. The diagnosis of a right ureteric calculus was therefore confirmed; no other stones were visualized. She was given analgesics, the pain settled, and she was sent home with advice to see her family doctor on returning to her home city in 3 days. By the time she saw her family doctor, she thought she had passed the stone (though she had not retrieved it). The renal colic had not recurred. The patient was most anxious to know why she had formed a stone and wanted all possible measures to be undertaken to prevent a recurrence. As the family physician, how will you proceed to investigate and advise this patient?

APPROACH TO THE PATIENT WITH A SINGLE STONE EPISODE

As mentioned earlier, it has been traditional to defer elaborate metabolic investigations until patients prove to be recurrent stone formers. However, in any patient with a first stone, a relevant history taking and physical examination should be performed, as well as limited laboratory investigations.

> Rational preventive therapy requires knowledge of the chemical composition of the stone.

Stone Composition

The opportunity to obtain chemical analysis of a stone should never be missed. Our patient Ella should have been advised to strain her urine for a few days so that the stone could be retrieved when passed and subjected to analysis. This was not done, but some indirect information is available, in that the stone was radiopaque. Radiopacity precludes uric acid or other rare purine stones (which are radiolucent) but is consistent with calcium oxalate (the most common stone type), infection stones (triple phosphate), pure calcium phosphate, or cystine. Other indirect information pointing to the stone composition may include the observation on urine microscopy of typical hexagonal cystine crystals (specific to cystinuria) or "coffin-lid" struvite crystals (specific to urinary tract infection with urease-producing bacteria).

History

The history should focus on identifying remediable underlying causes of stone formation; the major causes of upper urinary tract stones are listed in Table 10–1.

The past medical history should include inquiry about features suggestive of primary hyperparathyroidism (e.g., bone disease, peptic ulcer, pancreatitis, symptoms of hypercalcaemia) or of sarcoidosis, and about chronic diarrhea or extensive small bowel disease or resection.

A family history of stones may point to inherited conditions, such as idiopathic hypercalciuria, cystinuria, hyperoxaluria, and occasionally primary hyperparathyroidism.

The history should identify a low fluid intake or an occupation that increases insensible fluid losses (e.g., working in a hot environment) or an excessive intake of calcium or vitamin D, oxalate (mainly present in green leafy vegetables, fruits, and nuts), or purine (meat, fish, and poultry). An unusually high intake of salt (which may exacerbate hypercalciuria or hypocitruria) or of protein (which can exacerbate most of the known risk factors for calcium stones) may also be important. Inappropriate calcium restriction may increase the risk for calcium stones, perhaps by enhancing the intestinal absorption of oxalate.[2]

> Dietary calcium restriction is therefore no longer recommended for long-term prevention of calcium stones, unless there is a specific indication.

With respect to drug history, acetazolamide (usually for glaucoma) or excessive ascorbic acid intake may be important.

PATIENT NUMBER 1 (continued)

Ella's history (including family history) was entirely negative, her diet was unremarkable, and (as is usually the case in patients with renal stone disease) results of physical examination were entirely normal. Her blood pressure was 120/70 mm Hg. With respect to further investigations, Ella was advised to have a renal ultrasound examination (to confirm that the mild hydronephrosis had resolved and that no stones were now detectable in her urinary tract), as well as a limited laboratory workup.

Laboratory Workup

A limited laboratory workup appropriate for a patient with a single stone (Table 10–2) should include determination of the serum creatinine to preclude renal impairment and accurate determination of the serum calcium, mainly to rule out underlying primary hyperparathyroidism. Most laboratories still determine the total serum calcium. This should be accompanied by determination of serum protein values, because an abnormality of the serum proteins, particularly hypoalbuminemia, can mask hypercalcemia. It is usually recommended that the serum calcium level be determined twice, on different occasions, particularly if the first value is borderline. Some laboratories now routinely determine the serum ionized calcium, which avoids the need for protein determinations but has not been shown to be superior to the accurate measurement of total serum calcium and proteins. A rule-of-thumb correction of the total serum calcium according to the serum albumin level is to add

TABLE 10–1. Causes of Renal Stones

Calcium Stones

Major known risk factors are hypercalciuria, hyperoxaluria, hyperuricosuria, hypocitruria, and low urine volume.

Hypercalciuria

 Specific causes
- Primary hyperparathyroidism (rarely familial)
- Sarcoidosis
- Dietary—excess calcium, vitamin D, salt, and protein
- Renal tubular acidosis (inherited or acquired)

Idiopathic hypercalciuria—may be hereditary

Hyperoxaluria

 Specific causes
- Hereditary hyperoxaluria
- Enteric hyperoxaluria (extensive small bowel disease, resection, or bypass)
- Dietary, including high oxalate, low calcium, and possibly high ascorbic acid

Idiopathic (mild) hyperoxaluria

Hyperuricosuria

 Usually dietary—excess purine ingestion

Hypocitruria

 Specific causes
- Renal tubular acidosis (inherited or acquired)
- Chronic diarrhea, ileostomy
- Dietary—high protein, high salt, and low fiber
- Acetazolamide ingestion

Idiopathic hypocitruria

Uric Acid Stones

Major risk factors are persistent low urine pH, hyperuricosuria, and low urine volume.

Persistent low urine pH
- Usually idiopathic
- Can also result from chronic diarrhea (stool bicarbonate loss)

Hyperuricosuria
- Endogenous uric acid overproduction in gout, inborn errors of metabolism
- Hematologic and other malignancies

Infection Stones

Result from the unique combination in the urine of a high pH (alkalinity) with a high ammonium content.
 Caused *only* by infection with urease-producing organisms, which split urea.

Cystine Stones

Caused only by hereditary cystinuria, generally inherited as an autosomal recessive trait.

---

or subtract 0.1 mg/dl (0.025 mmol/L) to the measured serum calcium value for each 0.1 g/dl (1.0 g/L) by which the serum albumin respectively falls below or exceeds a value of 4.0 g/dl (40 g/L). The limited laboratory workup should also include a qualitative urine test for cystine to preclude cystinuria (unless stone analysis has ruled out cystine stones) and urine microscopy and culture to preclude infection with a urea-splitting organism.

TABLE 10–2. Limited Workup of Single Stone Former

History and physical examination
Stone analysis
Determination of serum creatinine, total calcium, and
  serum proteins (or ionized calcium)
Qualitative urine test for cystine
Urine microscopy and culture

PATIENT NUMBER 1 (continued)

Ella's urine culture was sterile. Results of her cystine test were negative, and her serum creatinine level was normal. However, her serum calcium value was 10.5 mg/dl (2.62 mmol/L) (normal 8.9 to 10.3 mg/dl, 2.22 to 2.57 mmol/L) and her serum protein levels were normal (albumin 4.0 g/dl, 40 g/L). A repeat serum calcium determination was 10.8 mg/dl (2.70 mmol/L), again with normal serum protein levels, and her serum ionized calcium value was above the normal range.

The diagnosis in a patient with a renal stone and hypercalcemia is most likely to be primary hyperparathyroidism. Very rarely, this combination may result from sarcoidosis or vitamin D intoxication. Fewer than 10% of calcium stone formers have underlying primary hyperparathyroidism. It is a very important diagnosis to make, however, because the stone disease can usually be cured by parathyroidectomy.

If hypercalcemia is detected in a patient with a stone, the patient is usually referred to a specialist with an interest in calcium metabolism. Further investigation would include determination of the 24-hour urinary calcium excretion (usually high in primary hyperparathyroidism) and determination of the serum phosphate level (often low in primary hyperparathyroidism), as well as the parathyroid hormone (PTH) level. Modern (intact) PTH assays, which measure biologically active PTH, very reliably distinguish primary hyperparathyroidism (in which the PTH level is above normal) from other causes of hypercalcemia (in which the PTH level is usually suppressed).

In a patient who has primary hyperparathyroidism confirmed by laboratory tests, and who is actively forming renal stones, surgical parathyroidectomy is usually recommended.

Parathyroidectomy must be undertaken by a surgeon experienced in parathyroid surgery. At present, preoperative localizing techniques (including ultrasonography and radionuclide imaging) are not usually recommended before a first parathyroid exploration by an experienced surgeon.

PATIENT NUMBER 1 (continued)

Ella's investigations confirmed the diagnosis of primary hyperparathyroidism. She was referred for parathyroid surgery, which was successfully undertaken, with the removal of a left lower parathyroid adenoma. One month after surgery, her serum and urinary calcium levels were normal. Stone disease has not recurred.

Ella's case illustrates an approach to a patient who has formed a single renal stone. The recommended investigations identify a reduction of renal function, as well as several underlying causes of stones for which effective preventive treatment is available, including urinary tract infection, gross dietary indiscretions, relevant drugs, primary hyperparathyroidism, and cystinuria. In our patient Ella, the limited investigation led to the discovery and subsequent cure of underlying primary hyperparathyroidism, the cause of about 5% of renal stones in Western countries.

PATIENT NUMBER 2

Sandy is a 40-year-old businessman who is also an amateur pilot with his own small plane. He has a history of having passed renal stones, analyzed as calcium oxalate, on two occasions 6 and 3 years ago. One month before he sees you, he had a mild attack of what he is sure was renal colic, but findings on a subsequent excretory urogram were entirely normal. Because of his desire to determine the cause of his stones, as well as concern about whether he should be flying a plane solo while at risk of renal colic, he is referred for full investigation to try to institute effective preventive therapy.

He had been previously evaluated 6 and 3 years ago and was told that his urinary calcium excretion was a little above normal but that he had no other metabolic abnormalities. He was advised to maintain adequate urine output by drinking at least eight 8-oz glasses of water per day, but he found this difficult and did not comply. He had also been treated for a few months with a thiazide diuretic to reduce his urinary calcium excretion, but he thought that this made him feel weak and he discontinued it.

He is now referred by his family physician to you, a physician interested in the prevention of stone disease, for further investigation and treatment. A carefully taken history (including family history) is nonrevealing, except that he has difficulty maintaining high fluid intake. He eats a lot of salty food and restricts his intake of dairy products, because he has been told that this helps to prevent calcium stones. He does not take acetazolamide or extra vitamins D or C. He has no history of bowel disease. Findings on physical examination are entirely normal. Sandy's blood pressure is 130/80 mm Hg.

APPROACH TO THE RECURRENT CALCIUM STONE FORMER

Our patient Sandy presents the problem of identifying risk factors and introducing preventive measures in a patient with apparently idiopathic recurrent calcium oxalate stones. The laboratory investigation of such a patient is reasonably standardized and usually includes the studies listed in Table 10–3.

The purpose of these investigations is to iden-

TABLE 10–3. Investigation of a Recurrent Calcium Oxalate Stone Former

Blood:	Creatinine
	Calcium, serum proteins (or ionized calcium), phosphate
	Electrolytes (Na, K, Cl, CO_2)
	Uric acid
Urine:	Microscopy, culture, and sensitivity.
	24-hour urine chemistry—at least two 24-hour urine specimens collected with appropriate preservatives (as advised by the laboratory) while the patient is normally ambulatory and consuming his or her normal intake of food and fluids. Determination of

Constituent	*Normal 24-Hour Value*[7]
• Volume	Preferably >2 L
• Creatinine	Men >20 mg or 0.18 mmol/kg body weight; women >15 mg or 0.13 mmol/kg body weight
• Calcium	<300 mg (<7.5 mmol) in men; <250 mg (<6.25 mmol) in women
• Oxalate	<41 mg (<0.46 mmol)
• Uric acid	<800 mg (4.8 mmol) in men; <750 mg (4.5 mmol) in women
• Citrate	>210 mg (1 mmol) in men; >400 mg (2 mmol) in women
• Sodium	Up to 350 mmol—depends on diet
• Urea	Depends on dietary protein

tify the underlying disorders and risk factors listed in Table 10–1. The serum creatinine level gives an indication of the patient's GFR, which should be normal in the absence of renal obstruction. The serum calcium determination is primarily measured to preclude primary hyperparathyroidism. Serum determinations of electrolytes and uric acid identify rare underlying disorders such as complete distal RTA. (The incomplete form, which can cause renal stones, usually calcium phosphate, is not accompanied by serum electrolyte abnormalities. However, hypocitruria is usually present—discussed later.)

A 24-hour urinanalysis identifies the known risk factors for recurrent idiopathic calcium oxalate stones. Urine volume should be at least 2 L/day. Creatinine values should always be determined on a 24-hour urine collection, as a measure of completeness. The values for the two 24-hour urine specimens should not differ by more than 10%. Their normal values are indicated in Table 10–2. Additional useful information can be obtained by determining the sodium and urea contents of the 24-hour urine, as an index of the dietary salt and protein intake.

> The major risk factors for calcium oxalate stones normally determined in the 24-hour urine are calcium, oxalate, uric acid, and citrate.

Hypercalciuria is found in as many as 50% of recurrent calcium stone formers. In addition to specific causes, including primary hyperparathyroidism (see Table 10–1), several dietary factors

can contribute to hypercalciuria, including excessive intake of calcium or vitamin D, a high salt intake, and a high protein intake. A reasonable approach to the correction of hypercalciuria is to identify these dietary contributing factors from the diet history or from urinary determinations including sodium and urea. If any of these dietary contributing factors are present, they should be corrected before introducing drug therapy for the hypercalciuria, such as a thiazide diuretic.

With respect to dietary calcium intake, it is currently recommended that patients have a normal calcium intake of approximately 800 mg/day. Excessive intake should be moderated. However, the dietary calcium intake should not be severely restricted because this can enhance intestinal oxalate absorption, and it has been shown that the risk of stone formation is actually higher in patients who are self-selecting a low calcium intake than in patients with higher calcium intake.[2]

Urinary oxalate has, in the past, presented analytic problems. However, current enzyme kit methods are readily available and reliable.

> A small increase in urinary oxalate excretion is believed to be a more serious risk factor for calcium oxalate stones than is a proportional increase in calcium.

Even small elevations of urinary oxalate above the normal range require correction. Some causes of hyperoxaluria are listed in Table 10–1. Primary hyperoxaluria usually causes severe stone disease in early life, but mild, late-presenting adult forms have been described. Enteric hyperoxaluria occurs in association with extensive bowel disease or resection. It results from binding of calcium in the intestinal lumen to nonabsorbed fatty acids, leaving less calcium available to precipitate oxalate as insoluble calcium oxalate and thus rendering it nonabsorbable. Dietary factors that may contribute to mild hyperoxaluria include a high dietary oxalate intake, possibly a high ascorbic acid intake, and dietary calcium restriction (which enhances intestinal oxalate absorption). High protein intake may also contribute to increased oxalate excretion. Measurement of urinary glycolate, a metabolic precursor of oxalate, may be useful in differentiating these causes of hyperoxaluria, but testing is not widely available.

Glycolate is increased in the common form of hereditary hyperoxaluria and as a result of high protein intakes. Management of mild hyperoxaluria, after precluding underlying causes, includes avoidance of high-oxalate foods and a high protein intake, liberalization of dietary calcium intake, and occasionally other measures such as administration of pyridoxine.[3]

Hyperuricosuria is generally accepted as a risk factor for calcium oxalate stones, although the mechanism of this effect is unclear. Hyperuricosuria in these patients is usually related to a high intake of purine in the form of meat, fish, or poultry. An attempt can be made to correct the hyperuricosuria by restricting dietary purine, and if this fails, treatment should be with allopurinol.[4]

Citrate in the urine helps to prevent stone formation by complexing calcium and by inhibiting the agglomeration (clumping together) of calcium oxalate crystals. **The finding of a low urinary citrate level should lead to consideration of underlying causes such as chronic diarrhea, a high protein or high salt or low fiber intake, or distal RTA, complete or incomplete.** In RTA, the stones usually consist of pure calcium phosphate. In complete RTA, patients have a metabolic acidosis, whereas in incomplete RTA the serum electrolyte values are normal and the diagnosis is made by demonstrating a failure to acidify the urine normally, for example in response to an ammonium chloride test.

Urinary sodium excretion may be as high as 350 mmol/day in health. Sodium restriction may help to correct hypercalciuria or hypocitruria and can be monitored by checking the urinary sodium excretion, which should not exceed 100 mmol/day. The urinary urea excretion reflects the dietary protein intake.

> An attempt should be made to restrict dietary protein intake to less than 1 g/kg body weight per day in patients with hypercalciuria, hyperoxaluria, hyperuricosuria, or hypocitruria.

The conversion factor for urinary urea to dietary protein is

$$\text{Protein (g/day)} = 0.18 \times \text{mmol urea per day} + 14$$

The urine of normal persons contains inhibitors of stone formation, in addition to citrate, including several macromolecular inhibitors. It is suspected that abnormalities of these inhibitors may contribute to stone formation, particularly in patients in whom other risk factors are negative. However, these inhibitors are difficult to measure, and their assessment does not yet form part of the routine workup of patients with stones.

PATIENT NUMBER 2 (continued)

The results of these routine investigations in Sandy were as follows: normal levels of serum creatinine, electrolytes, calcium, and uric acid; urine microscopy and culture negative. His 24-hour urine results were as follows:

	24-Hour Urine # 1	24-Hour Urine # 2
Volume, ml	1550	1820
Creatinine, mg (mmol)	1450 (13.1)	1390 (12.5)
Calcium, mg (mmol)	408 (10.2)	350 (8.75)
Oxalate, mg (mmol)	40 (0.44)	42 (0.47)
Uric acid, mg (mmol)	715 (4.28)	650 (3.89)
Citrate, mg (mmol)	410 (1.9)	460 (2.2)
Sodium, mmol	305	254
Urea as urea N, grams (mmol urea)	13.8 (493)	17.2 (614)
Corresponding daily protein intake, grams	103	125

With regard to risk factors for calcium oxalate stones, Sandy's urine volumes are suboptimal, and he should benefit from increasing his fluid intake to ensure a urine output greater than 2 L/day. Sandy has hypercalciuria. His urinary oxalate level is at the upper limit of normal or just above it. His urinary uric acid and citrate values are normal. His urinary sodium level is high, confirming his preference for salty food. Urinary urea shows that protein intake is not excessive.

With respect to his hypercalciuria, our patient Sandy is already restricting his calcium (dairy product) intake, despite which he has hypercalciuria. Furthermore, his urinary oxalate level is borderline high, despite his avoidance of oxalate-rich foods. Some relaxation of the dietary calcium intake to around 800 mg/day may reduce urinary oxalate values by binding oxalate in the gut but may exacerbate the hypercalciuria. Because severe chronic calcium restriction is probably not advisable, Sandy was advised to relax his calcium intake to about 800 mg/day. At the same time, he was advised to restrict his salt intake by avoiding salty foods and added salt, aiming for a sodium intake of not more than 100 mmol/day.

PATIENT NUMBER 2 (continued)

One month after the introduction of these measures, two further 24-hour urine samples were collected and yielded the following results:

	24-Hour Urine # 3	24-Hour Urine # 4
Volume, ml	2520	3035
Creatinine, mg (mmol)	1365 (12.3)	1410 (12.7)
Calcium, mg (mmol)	305 (7.6)	315 (7.9)
Oxalate, mg (mmol)	28 (0.31)	31 (0.34)
Uric acid, mg (mmol)	630 (3.77)	680 (4.07)
Citrate, mg (mmol)	450 (2.11)	480 (2.3)
Sodium, mmol	110	96
Urea as urea N, grams (mmol urea)	16.9 (603)	14.5 (517)

These values show that Sandy's urine volume is now satisfactory. His hypercalciuria is much improved but is still present to a mild degree. His urinary oxalate level is now normal, and the urinary sodium determination shows that he is successfully restricting his salt intake. This measure is presumably responsible for the improvement in the hypercalciuria, and liberalization of his calcium intake is probably responsible for the reduction in urinary oxalate value.

Having taken all available dietary measures to correct the risk factors, consideration may now be given to additional drug therapy. At the same time, Sandy needs to be encouraged to sustain these dietary changes indefinitely.

Use of Medication for the Prevention of Recurrent Calcium Oxalate Stones

Medications of proven or suspected benefit are shown in Table 10–4, along with their specific indications. In hypercalciuria, some authorities have advocated the use of special tests to try to differentiate hypercalciuria of primarily absorptive origin from that of renal origin. It has been suggested that agents that bind calcium to render it nonabsorbable from the gut, such as cellulose phosphate, might be the preferred treatment for absorptive hypercalciuria, whereas thiazide diuretics might be preferable for so-called renal hypercalciuria. This differentiation is probably of limited practical value, however, and cellulose phosphate is not widely available. **If hypercalciuria persists despite the correction of dietary causes and active stone disease persists, the use of a thiazide diuretic is indicated.** This should be combined with sodium restriction, because a high salt intake reduces the efficacy of the thiazide to lower the urinary excretion of calcium. A dose of 25 mg of chlorthalidone per day is effective[5] and is unlikely to cause problems such as hypokalemia. If stone formation persists despite the addition of a thiazide diuretic, the urinary excretion of sodium should be checked, as well as that of citrate, because rarely a thiazide diuretic can induce hypocitruria secondary to potassium depletion. In this event, treatment with potassium citrate can be added in a dose of 20 mEq two or three times daily. It is also advisable to check the serum calcium level after 1 month of thiazide treatment, because the drug can make patients with mild or borderline primary hyperparathyroidism overtly hypercalcemic. The use of cellulose phosphate has largely been abandoned, and the drug is not generally available.

Neutral sodium phosphate has been widely recommended in a dose of phosphorus, 0.5 g two or three times daily, but it tends to cause diarrhea, and its efficacy has not been proved with a proper prospective trial. Of current interest is potassium phosphate for hypercalciuria.[6] Administration of phosphate should suppress the production of 1,25-dihydroxyvitamin D, which is believed to mediate most idiopathic hypercalciuria. It may be particularly indicated in patients with

TABLE 10–4. Medications for the Prevention of Calcium Oxalate Stones

Drug	Indication	Efficacy
Thiazide diuretic (e.g., chlorthalidone)	Hypercalciuria	Proven*
Cellulose phosphate	"Absorptive" hypercalciuria	Unproven
Neutral sodium phosphate	Hypercalciuria	Unproven
Potassium phosphate	Hypercalciuria	Unproven
Potassium citrate	Hypocitruria	Proven*
Potassium magnesium citrate	Hypocitruria	Unproven
Allopurinol	Hyperuricosuria	Proven*

*Significant efficacy has been proved in a prospective randomized double-blind trial.

a low serum phosphate level. It is undergoing current trials.

As already indicated, allopurinol in a dose of 200 to 300 mg/day should be given to patients with hyperuricosuria and calcium oxalate stones if dietary purine restriction has not corrected their hyperuricosuria.[4]

Hypocitruria not corrected by dietary means, including restriction of salt and protein, should be treated with potassium citrate, 20 mEq t.i.d., for example given as Urocit-K tablets. Potassium citrate may have advantages over sodium citrate because it does not increase the urinary calcium excretion. A new agent, potassium magnesium citrate, which may be more effective than potassium citrate, is currently under investigation.

PATIENT NUMBER 2 (continued)

Because of the importance of preventing further stones and the failure of the dietary interventions to correct the hypercalciuria completely, Sandy was placed on chlorthalidone, 25 mg/day. This resulted in correction of his urinary calcium level to less than 200 mg/day. No side effects occurred, and after 1 month his serum electrolyte values, including potassium and calcium, remained normal.

Our patient Sandy illustrates an approach to common recurrent calcium oxalate stone formers. Specific diseases that can cause calcium stones are first ruled out. Recognized risk factors are then sought in the urine, and dietary factors that may be exacerbating these risk factors are corrected.

> **Failure of dietary measures to correct risk factors is an indication to consider the use of medications for stone prophylaxis.**

PATIENT NUMBER 3

Harold is 48 years old. He has a previous history of a renal calculus, passed spontaneously 5 years previously and found to consist of uric acid. He now presents with a single episode of macroscopic hematuria, associated with mild right renal pain. He had been referred to a urologist, who requested an excretory urogram. This showed a 1-cm-diameter filling defect in the right renal pelvis. The radiologist could not distinguish clearly between a radiolucent calculus and a soft tissue mass, such as a tumor. An ultrasound examination was ordered and clearly showed that the lesion in the right renal pelvis was calculus. No other abnormality was observed on the excretory urogram or the ultrasound

examination. The urologist consults you for advice on medical management of the presumed uric acid stone.

> **The accepted risk factors for uric acid stones are a low urine volume, a persistently low urine pH, and hyperuricosuria.**

In any patient with uric acid stones, investigations should include a serum uric acid level, serum creatinine level (to preclude significant renal impairment), urine culture, 24-hour urine collection for volume and uric acid content, and assessment of urine pH. The latter can conveniently be done by providing the patient with urine pH test papers (e.g., nitrazine paper) and having the patient determine the urine pH at each voiding for a 24- or 48-hour period.

The effect of pH on the solubility of uric acid is such that at a urine pH above 6, even with very severe hyperuricosuria, it is unlikely that the urine will be supersaturated.

> **At a urine pH of 5.5 or below, uric acid supersaturation is likely, even at normal uric acid excretion rates.**

If any of these risk factors are identified, treatment can be introduced. Unlike calcium stones, uric acid stones can often be dissolved *in situ.* Cystine stones can also be dissolved, but with greater difficulty.

Treatment should include an increase in the urine volume to more than 2 L/day. If the urine pH is persistently 5.5 or below, sufficient alkali needs to be given to raise the pH above 6 for most of the day. An intelligent patient can be provided with alkali in the form of sodium bicarbonate or potassium citrate and advised to determine how much is required to achieve this result.

If the patient is severely hyperuricosuric or if increasing the urine volume and pH fails to prevent stones, allopurinol can be added to reduce the uric acid excretion.

PATIENT NUMBER 3 (continued)

Harold's urine volume was 1.5 L/day. His serial urine pH throughout 2 days showed persistently low values of 5.5 or less. The 24-hour urinary uric acid excretion was within the normal range, at 700 mg. Harold was advised to increase his fluid intake and was prescribed potassium citrate, 20 mEq t.i.d., after which his urine pH increased to 6.0 or above at virtually every voiding. One month later, a repeat ultrasound examination of the kidneys showed no evidence of a stone, indicating that the therapy had caused stone dissolution.

An alternative treatment for Harold could have been sodium bicarbonate tablets (375 or 500 mg), and he could have begun with 1 tablet t.i.d. and increased the dose to achieve the desired increase in urine pH.

REFERENCES

1. Parks JH, Coe FL: An increasing number of calcium stone events worsens treatment outcome. Kidney Int 45:1722–1730, 1994.
2. Curhan GC, Willett WC, Rimm EB, Stampfer MJ: A prospective study of dietary calcium and other nutrients and the risk of symptomatic kidney stones. N Engl J Med 328:833–838, 1993.
3. Sutton RAL, Walker VR: Enteric and mild hyperoxaluria. Miner Electrolyte Metab 20:352–360, 1994.
4. Ettinger B, Tang A, Citron JT, et al: Randomized trial of allopurinol in the prevention of calcium oxalate calculi. N Engl J Med 315:1386–1389, 1986.
5. Ettinger B, Citron JT, Livermore B, Dolman LI: Chlorthalidone reduces calcium oxalate calculous recurrence but magnesium hydroxide does not. J Urol 139:679–684, 1988.
6. Breslau NA, Padalino P, Kok DJ, et al: Physicochemical effects of a new slow-release potassium phosphate preparation (UroPhos-K) in absorptive hypercalciuria. J Bone Miner Res 10:394–400, 1995.
7. Lemann J Jr: Collection, Preservation and Analysis of Urine in the Evaluation of Mineral Metabolism, Bone Disease and Nephrolithiasis. Primer on the Metabolic Bone Diseases and Disorders of Mineral Metabolism, 2nd ed. New York, Raven Press, 1993.

SUGGESTED READINGS

Coe FL, Parks JH, Asplin JR: The pathogenesis and treatment of kidney stones. N Engl J Med 327:1141–1152, 1992.
Nephrolithiasis. Pathophysiology and prevention of renal calculi. Miner Electrolyte Metab 20:315–436, 1994.
Sutton RAL: Medical Management of Renal Stones. *In* Oxford Textbook of Nephrology, 2nd ed. Oxford, Oxford University Press (in press).

APPENDIX

CYSTINE STONES

Cystinuria, the cause of cystine stones, results from a mutation of the gene for the cystine transporter in the brush border of the proximal tubule epithelium. Cystine stones are uncommon but are important to recognize. They constitute 3% to 6% of childhood stones. The diagnosis should be suggested by a positive family history or by the commencement of stone disease at a fairly early age. The stones are radiopaque owing to their sulfur content. If not effectively treated, they may grow to form staghorn calculi and may ultimately damage renal function.

Determination of the 24-hour urine cystine excretion can be helpful in designing treatment. Milder cases of cystinuria can be managed by increasing urine volume, together with alkalization of the urine. More severe cystinuria requires the addition of a chelating agent such as penicillamine or alpha-mercaptopropionyl glycine (Thiola). Reports have suggested that captopril may be an effective alternative therapy.

STRUVITE STONES

Struvite (infection) stones in humans form only in the presence of urinary tract infection with urease-producing organisms. These stones consist of magnesium ammonium phosphate with calcium phosphate. They are radiopaque and often grow to staghorn configuration. They most commonly form in chronically infected, anatomically abnormal urinary tracts, for example in patients with bladder paralysis resulting from paraplegia. This type of stone disease has been described as malignant, meaning that the stones grow rapidly and often impair renal function. Optimal treatment consists of removal of stone material, often with a combination of percutaneous and extracorporeal shock wave lithotripsy, followed by long-term antibacterial treatment to suppress infection. The stones form because urease, produced by the bacteria, splits urea to form ammonium in a highly alkaline urine. Under this circumstance, the urine is supersaturated with magnesium ammonium phosphate. Drugs have been devised to inhibit urease and can be given by mouth, but none are sufficiently free of toxic side effects to have been introduced into routine use for the prevention of these stones.

11 | EDEMATOUS STATES AND HEPATORENAL SYNDROME

Mortimer Levy

EDEMA

ECF is normally partitioned so that about 25% of the total circulates within the vascular compartment as plasma and the remainder (75%) is found within the extravascular space as interstitial fluid and lymph. This volume, particularly the plasma component, is carefully regulated by the kidneys so that the ratio of the circulating plasma volume to the holding capacity of the arterial blood compartment is kept within a narrowly defined physiologic range, thus resulting in a normal arterial blood pressure. As physiologic requirements change, plasma volume is adapted by either altering the rate of urinary excretion of salt and water (compared with dietary intake) or by adjusting the transcapillary partitioning of the ECF.

The physiologic factors normally regulating this transvascular partitioning are collectively called the *Starling forces*. These factors include capillary hydrostatic pressure, plasma colloid oncotic pressure, free interstitial fluid hydrostatic pressure, and the integrity or hydraulic conductivity of the capillary membranes. Other important contributing factors are oncotic pressure within the interstitial fluid, the surface area of capillaries available for ultrafiltration, and the efficiency of regional lymphatic flow. When plasma ultrafiltrate accumulates to excess within the interstitial space, edema may occur.

Edema is defined as an excess of fluid within the interstitial or nonvascular extracellular space of an organ that is detectable by visual or other clinical means. When most physicians think of edema, they usually think of subcutaneous edema within the lower extremities, but of course edema may appear in numerous areas (e.g., periorbital, fingers, or within a serous cavity, as in pleural effusions or ascites). Edema appears when the volume of fluid leaving the capillaries overwhelms the ability of protec-

tive mechanisms within the interstitial space to retard such fluid accumulation. These protective mechanisms include binding of fluid to some of the proteins present in the interstitial compartment, reduction of the interstitial fluid oncotic pressure by a washout effect, and an increase in the regional lymphatic flow, returning fluid to the venous compartment. These mechanisms, in particular the effects of protein washout and lymph flow augmentation, together may add as much as 10 to 15 mm Hg to the effective transcapillary gradients for fluid ultrafiltration from the capillary bed. Therefore, in order for fluid to accumulate to any significant degree within the interstitial compartment, three conditions must be satisfied:

1. A significant disturbance must occur in the total sum of Starling forces.
2. The local protective mechanisms that normally afford a safety margin of 10 to 15 mm Hg must be overwhelmed (i.e., the extravascular space must be able to accept the edema fluid).
3. Urinary sodium retention must replenish the vascular compartment and allow progressive accumulation of edema.

Localized Edema

Edema may be localized to virtually any organ if that organ is caught up in an inflammatory response. Under these conditions, however, the edema may be a minor component of what is a more complicated and extensive disease complex. Although edema may be localized at some early phase, when there is a tendency to form generalized edema—for example, ankle edema, or pulmonary edema in early congestive heart failure (CHF)—edema is localized by and large to a given vascular territory when one of the following prevails:

1. An excess arterial inflow (e.g., immersing the hands in warm water)
2. Venous and/or lymphatic obstruction (e.g., thrombophlebitis)
3. A localized change in capillary permeability (e.g., angioedema)

In clinical practice, the most common cause of true localized edema is generally venous hypertension. **It is important to emphasize, however, that localized edema may appear as the first manifestation of generalized edema, largely because of normal postural considerations and the effects of gravity.** A good example of this is the periorbital edema that occurs in nephrotic syndrome when patients arise in the morning but that disappears during the day as they assume the orthostatic position. Ankle edema at the end of the day in patients with mild to moderate CHF is another example.

Collections of true localized edema (e.g., associated with a thrombophlebitis) rarely if ever are associated with significant perturbations in circulating plasma volume or with neuroendocrine disturbances such as increased plasma levels of renin, aldosterone, or catecholamines. This is probably because the fluid losses in localized edema from the vascular compartment are usually modest and because interstitial fluid from uninvolved areas may be mobilized to replenish the vascular compartment and so correct any tendency toward hypovolemia.

PATIENT NUMBER 1

Ezra is a 56-year-old obese gentleman gainfully employed as a pickle pusher in a local kosher foods company. It is his job to wedge the final pickle tightly into the jar before vacuum closure of the lid. This maneuver makes it virtually impossible to extract the pickle on opening the jar without squirting brine all over your clothes. A jovial individual, Ezra has been an insulin-dependent diabetic for 20 years and now presents to the hospital emergency room with severe dyspnea and extensive anasarca. On examination, he is found to have ascites, right pleural effusion, and 4+ edema of the lower extremities extending at least up to the level of his knees. Examination reveals blood pressure of 210/118 mm Hg, a pulse rate of 96, marked jugular venous distention, and rales in both lung bases. Urinary protein was 4+ on dipstick testing, and the sediment was considered active. His blood urea is 24 mmol/L, serum creatinine level is 205 μmol/L, and serum albumin level is 30 g/L. His recent shortness of breath has made it very difficult for him to continue his occupation

as a pickle pusher. What is the cause of his edema? Please note that Ezra detests sour pickles and all other deli foods and has not been surreptitiously ingesting large amounts of salt during his employment hours.

Approach to the Patient

Although Ezra's anasarca and the proteinuria as well as his underlying history of long-term diabetes initially suggested to the physicians that the patient had nephrotic syndrome, some discrepancies were apparent. The elevated venous pressure and the pulmonary edema in the presence of hypertension suggested an element of CHF. Moreover, considering the anasarca, Ezra's serum albumin level was remarkably well preserved at 30 g/L. Because the hypoalbuminemia seemed insufficient as a cause of anasarca, CHF with marked elevation of venous pressures was the next best choice. Indeed, subsequent therapy with antihypertensive agents, diuretics, bed rest, and control of dietary salt intake was associated with a rapid clearing of edema. When coupled with a restricted protein diet, in a situation such as this, angiotensin-converting enzyme (ACE) inhibitors would be the ideal drug to use because they could be expected to treat blood pressure, decrease afterload, and decrease intraglomerular pressures to effect a decrease in proteinuria.

PATIENT NUMBER 1 (continued)

After the treatment described, Ezra returned to his gainful employment as a pickle pusher, but a cautious company physician has installed a fan at Ezra's work station, thus ensuring that he does not inhale the salty fumes of the pickle brine. Though feeling quite well, Ezra is considering early retirement.

PATIENT NUMBER 2

Olga is an attractive 21-year-old brunette who models lingerie for a well-known firm. Olga is somewhat distressed because she has had significant ankle swelling for the past 2 days. This edema appeared to come on abruptly. She now presents to her physician with this 2-day history and complains of edema of the fingers and pronounced periorbital edema on arising in the morning. Swelling in the latter area appears to improve somewhat as the day wears on. Olga otherwise feels quite well but is somewhat distressed at the change in her body contour. What is the most likely cause of edema? Will Olga be able to return to her modeling position?

Approach to the Patient

Although any cause of generalized edema formation can present with ankle edema due to the effects of gravity, it is not common to encounter periorbital edema on awakening except under very special circumstances. The most prominent of these is hypoalbuminemia due to nephrotic syndrome. Hypoalbuminemia due to cirrhosis of the liver is rarely accompanied by periorbital edema because of the preferential accumulation of fluid within the peritoneal space. The other common cause of edema at this site is angi-oedema or localized cutaneous allergy. Even in the presence of severe CHF, it is unusual to detect any facial edema. The rapidity of the onset of Olga's edema, particularly in the absence of systemic symptoms, as well as the periorbital edema suggests that this is nephrotic syndrome, most likely due to minimal change disease. Uri-nalysis had indicated 4 + proteinuria with a normal microscopic examination, and the serum albumin level was reduced to 19 g/L.

PATIENT NUMBER 2 (continued)

Olga was given a short course of prednisone (40 mg/day), and within 10 days was edema free. She was able to return to her modeling job and can now frequently be seen on the pages of numerous popular fashion magazines in both North America and Europe. The initial prednisone regimen was maintained for only 3 months, and 2 years after the initial encounter, Olga remains free of edema.

PATIENT NUMBER 3

Sergio is a nervous auto mechanic who always seemed to be assigned to me whenever I took my 1985 Cavalier into the dealership for repairs. Sergio is 64 years old and has been smoking heavily for most of his adult life. Because of some hemoptysis and shortness of breath, Sergio was admitted to the hospital. After suitable investigation, he was subjected to thoracic surgery for partial pneumonectomy because of a bronchogenic carcinoma. During the course of this surgery, it was necessary to strip some of the pericardium from the right atrium. After this procedure, Sergio was somewhat oliguric, and although his serum creatinine level was within normal limits, his blood urea value was slightly elevated. In an attempt to improve Sergio's urine flow, his surgeon infused several liters of isotonic saline over a fairly short time. This procedure did not significantly affect urine flow, but it was noted that the patient's upper extremities and face had become more edematous. Sergio had no ankle edema. What is your interpretation of this pattern of edema formation?

Approach to the Patient

One would normally expect a saline infusion to accumulate in the legs and possibly in the presa-cral region of a patient who is lying supine in bed. Accumulation of edema in the upper extremities and the face represents a unique circumstance and suggests a probable venous obstruction in the vascular territory serving these areas. Given the nature of Sergio's surgery, it was assumed that Sergio had some obstruction of the venous return of the large veins or perhaps a partial herniation of the right atrium through the hole in the pericardium occasioned by the surgery.

PATIENT NUMBER 3 (continued)

Venous angiography confirmed the latter suggestion, and after corrective surgery the edema disappeared, urine flow increased dramatically, and Sergio's renal function remained normal, with disappearance of the urea-to-creatinine disproportion. Although making an uneventful recovery after the second procedure, Sergio has thankfully retired from being an auto mechanic. My Cavalier is now being repaired by a younger man who does not appear very nervous and seems quite stable when taking his lithium medication for a manic-depressive psychosis. Six months after his discharge from hospital, Sergio dropped into my clinic. He is still nervous, does not smoke, and, although the long-term prognosis appears poor, he should remain in good health for at least the next year.

Causes of Edema

Generalized edema most commonly occurs in association with acute or chronic renal failure, nephrotic syndrome, cirrhosis of the liver, or CHF. A more complete list is given in Table 11–1.

Therapy for Edema

Although therapy for the specific edema states is discussed in detail later in this chapter, several general principles may be applied to the treatment protocols of all edema states. Such therapeutic options are discussed in the paragraphs that follow.

TABLE 11–1. Some Common Causes of Generalized Edema

Diseases of the Kidney

Acute or chronic renal failure
Acute glomerulonephritis (GFR relatively well preserved)
Nephrotic syndrome

Diseases of the Heart

Low-output congestive heart failure
High-output congestive heart failure

Diseases of Hepatoportal Circulation

Cirrhosis of the liver
Budd-Chiari syndrome

Diseases of Women

Cyclic edema
Premenstrual syndrome
Ovarian hyperstimulation syndrome

Others

Capillary leak syndromes
Drugs: minoxidil, calcium channel blockers, valproate,
    estrogens, and others.

Dietary Manipulation

Because urinary retention of salt and water is characteristic of patients who are actively forming edema, attention must be closely paid to dietary intake. If the kidneys are capable of excreting only 40 to 50 mEq of sodium per day because of flagrant nephrotic syndrome or CHF, dietary intake in excess of this amount is simply retained, adding to the edema. In patients who have entered a phase of active edema formation, particularly those who are proving refractory to therapy, it is not inappropriate to document daily urinary excretion of sodium and to adjust the diet accordingly. **In practical terms, for ambulatory patients, it is very difficult to reduce sodium intake below 30 to 40 mEq/day. Less stringent curtailment, to approximately 50 to 60 mEq/day, is often sufficient** to ameliorate the situation. Reduction of salt intake often permits patients to achieve sodium balance. Restriction of salt intake is particularly effective in dialysis-independent uremic patients. Because in stable chronic renal failure urinary excretion of salt and water often remains fixed and at high values, dietary curtailment of salt and water intake often leads to rapid clearing of the edema, even without diuretics and particularly if a patient is given bed rest to help mobilize the edema.

In planning dietary restriction of sodium, it is helpful to recall that 1 g of NaCl contains 17 mEq sodium whereas 1 g of sodium contains 43 mEq Na$^+$. By avoiding the salt shaker at mealtime and by omitting salt from the preparation of foods and cooking water, as well as avoiding prepared and preserved foodstuffs that are notoriously high in salt, dietary sodium intake can easily be reduced to approximately 50 to 70 mEq/day.

For those patients who cannot tolerate a reduction in dietary salt but who feel they must have it, salt substitutes are available. These usually contain potassium salts, however, and great care must be taken before they are used in the presence of oliguric states or uremia and with concomitant use of potassium-sparing diuretics or ACE inhibitors. Fortunately, newer seasoning mixtures that contain neither Na$^+$ or K$^+$ are available in most grocery stores.

Postural Considerations

When patients assume the supine position from the standing, some 700 to 800 ml of blood that has been below the diaphragm is mobilized and returns to the central thorax. Bed rest, particularly with leg elevation, is an effective way of initiating diuresis and natriuresis (central activation of volume receptors) and thereby mobilizing edema. Indeed, some evidence suggests that slight head-down posture is even more effective in refractory cases.

Ultrafiltration

The widespread availability of various procedures for rapid removal of edema means that ultrafiltration from the vascular compartment can be achieved either rapidly for life-threatening pulmonary edema or more slowly for anasarca, which is not particularly life threatening. Acute peritoneal dialysis with 2.5% or 4.25% glucose solutions using 30- to 40-minute dwell times is one technique available; another is continuous arteriovenous hemofiltration using ultrapermeable cartridges. These techniques, particularly the latter, can easily remove 400 to 1500 ml/hr. Ultrafiltration using dialysis equipment is another option for rapid fluid removal. Modern machines with volumetric controls permit ultrafiltration rapidly and efficiently; 1.0 L/hr can easily be removed unless blood pressure falls too rapidly. Newer equipment allowing for effective and continuous venovenous hemofiltration is now becoming available.

Diuretics

Diuretics inhibit sodium reabsorption within the nephrons and increase the percentage of glomer-

TABLE 11–2. Complications of Excessive Diuresis

Azotemia
Hypotension with orthostatic exaggeration
Dizziness if hypotension with orthostatic exaggeration
  is sufficiently severe
Hypercalcemia
Hyperuricemia
Hyponatremia
Magnesium depletion
Hypokalemia and metabolic alkalosis (hyperkalemia and
  acidosis with potassium-sparing agents)
Weakness and easy fatigability

---

ular filtrate that is excreted as urine. The subsequent decrement in plasma volume and rise in colloid oncotic pressure then permit the mobilization of edema from the interstitial space into the vascular compartment, where it becomes available for renal excretion. The diuretic response has thus been translated into a mobilization response. Because any edema state imposes physiologic restrictions on the ease with which fluid may be returned to the vascular compartment, as a result of either the elevated venous pressures or reduced colloid oncotic pressures (or both in combination), overzealous diuresis poses the danger of producing hypovolemia. If this occurs, renal perfusion may then decline and the diuresis may come to an end. In addition to prerenal failure, relative hypotension (with further orthostatic decline) and biochemical features peculiar to hypovolemia may ensue (e.g., hyponatremia, hyperuricemia, hypokalemia, or hyperkalemia if sufficient azotemia and oliguria supervene). The complications of overzealous diuresis are summarized in Table 11–2. The nonhemodynamic complications of diuretics are summarized in Table 11–3.

Features of the diuretics most commonly used today are summarized in Table 11–4.

Another diuretic sometimes used is acetazolamide (Diamox). This agent, acting on the proximal tubule and producing a bicarbonate diuresis,

TABLE 11–3. Complications of Diuretics Unrelated to Fluid Losses

---

Hyperglycemia
Hyperlipidemia
Acute pancreatitis (thiazide group)
Skin rashes
Acute interstitial nephritis (thiazide, furosemide,
  triamterene)
Intratubular crystallization (stones)—triamterene
Gastrointestinal upset
Ototoxicity (furosemide, bumetanide)

---

is sometimes used in intoxications to alkalize the urine, as well as to treat hyperuricosuric states or even alkalemia. It has no place in the routine therapy of edema.

The potassium-sparing diuretics must be used cautiously in the elderly, particularly if they are obese or diabetic, because of the potential for provoking type 4 RTA and for aggravating hyperkalemia. **They should be used cautiously (or not at all) with ACE inhibitors because of the property of these antihypertensive drugs to increase serum potassium levels (inhibition of aldosterone effect).** Because they act at the most distal nephron sites, where perhaps only 1% to 2% of the available filtered sodium load is available for tubular reabsorption, they are, of necessity, weak diuretics. Their major uses are in the conservation of potassium and for causing mild sodium loss when a gentle diuresis is necessary to preserve the physiologic status of a patient (e.g., with cirrhosis of the liver).

PRINCIPLES OF DIURETIC MANAGEMENT

Except for life-threatening situations (e.g., acute pulmonary edema), diuresis should be judicious and fluid loss should probably not exceed 1 kg/day lest the problems of hypovolemia (described earlier) become predominant. **Diuresis should proceed at a pace that allows adequate mobilization from the extravascular compartment to keep pace with diuretic-induced losses from the circulation.**

When patients are proving refractory to these agents, they should preferably maintain bed rest and continue dietary salt curtailment to maximize the beneficial effects of the diuretics.

Edema of the gastrointestinal (GI) mucosa is often present and may reduce absorption of oral medication from the GI tract. If a patient is proving refractory to oral medication in the presence of extensive edema that could be affecting the GI mucosa, it may be worthwhile to switch to intravenous administration for a short time.

When a patient is proving refractory to a single diuretic (usually loop active), it may be wise to add a diuretic thought to be active at other sites. Useful additions include metolazone and other thiazides. Metolazone is thought to act at the level of the proximal convoluted tubule as well as the cortical diluting site. Moreover, unlike other thiazides, metolazone continues to be active even when the GFR is quite depressed (<35 ml/min). In this way, extra sodium is delivered to the loops of Henle, which may then be acted on by the loop-active diuretic. A thiazide added to

TABLE 11–4. Some Features of Commonly Used Diuretics

Common Brand Name	Generic Name	Usual Dosages	Remarks
HydroDIURIL	Hydrochlorothiazide	25–100 mg/day	Not recommended if GFR < 35 ml/min. Oral dose active within 2 hr; beware of hypokalemia and hyponatremia.
Lozide	Indapamide	2.5 mg/day	Acts on cortical distal tubule; rapidly absorbed—peak blood level within 1–2 hr; half-life = 14 hr. Do not exceed stated dose; useful in diabetics because of supposed lack of effect on blood sugar and lipids. May cause hyponatremia and hypothalemia. May increase serum urate; skin rashes.
Lasix	Furosemide	20–80 mg/day	Rapid onset, < 0.5 hr; potent; effective when GFR < 35 ml/min. Effects last 6 hr.
Edecrin	Ethacrynic acid	50–150 mg/day	Similar to furosemide, longer acting (~ 8 hr). May be used when patient allergic to thiazides or furosemide.
Zaroxolyn	Metolazone	1–10 mg/day	Effective with GFR < 35 ml/min. Potentiates action of loop-active diuretics. May cause profound diuresis and hypokalemia in susceptible patients.
Burinex	Bumetanide	0.5–2.0 mg/day	Loop active. May have additional proximal tubular effect. Half-life = 1.5 hr; 0.5–2 hr to peak blood levels. Diuresis complete within 3–4 hr (1 mg bumetanide = 40 mg furosemide). Complications as for other loop-active diuretics (volume depletion; electrolyte disturbances, potentiation of ototoxic antibiotics).
Potassium-Sparing Agents			
Aldactone	Spironolactone	25–100 mg q.i.d.	Gradual onset (2–3 days). Not recommended when GFR < 25 ml/min. Danger of hyperkalemia and acidosis.
Midamor	Amiloride	5–20 mg/day	Contraindicated when GFR < 25 ml/min. May cause hyperkalemia. Effects may last 2–24 hr.
Dyrenium	Triamterene	100–300 mg/day	Contraindicated when GFR < 25 ml/min. Long lasting, up to 16 hr. May cause hyperkalemia. Blood dyscrasias, triamterene stones, and interstitial nephritis may be a problem.
Dyazide	Triamterene/hydrochlorothiazide mixture	50 mg, 1 tab b.i.d. 25 mg	Commonly used in family practice when potassium sparing desired. Should not be used with K+ supplements or other potassium-sparing agents. Avoid use when GFR < 35 ml/min. Incidence of hyperkalemia rises with increasing age.

a loop-active diuretic such as furosemide often augments the natriuresis.

Specific maneuvers in specific disease states often potentiate the use of diuretics. These include

• Placing a pregnant woman in the third trimester in the left lateral position to improve renal hemodynamics

• Reduction of afterload in patients suffering from CHF with ACE inhibitors or other vasodilators, which often improves renal perfusion and suboptimal diuresis

• Infusion of albumin solutions to cirrhotic patients before initiating diuresis
• Keeping a woman with idiopathic cyclic edema at bed rest while initiating diuresis

Once "dry weight" has been reached, one should consider stopping the diuretic, reducing the dose, or even administering the drug on alternate days to minimize diuretic side effects.

As noted earlier, great care should be used when giving potassium-sparing diuretics so that concomitant clinical circumstances do not produce life-threatening hyperkalemia.

Treatment of Underlying Disorder

In addition to manipulating dietary salt, diuretic regimens, and activity, it is worthwhile to direct specific therapy to treatment of each of the underlying disorders responsible for generalized edema. Thus, in CHF, depending on clinical circumstances, the use of digoxin, antihypertensives, and ACE inhibitors for afterload reduction, together with antiarrhythmic agents, might be indicated, as well as agents to augment coronary artery perfusion.

In nephrotic syndrome, adjustment of protein intake and the use of specific agents such as prednisone and cyclophosphamide may be indicated to treat the underlying glomerulopathy.

In cirrhosis of the liver, refractory ascites may respond to LeVeen valve shunting or the placement of a hepatic-portal venous shunt (TIPS). Many centers have begun to perform large-volume (about 4.0 L) paracentesis every second or third day, supplemented by intravenous albumin infusion to compensate for the protein loss. This has proved to be an effective and safe way to control tense ascites.

Converting tense ascites to soft ascites has great advantages. By relieving excessive pressure on the abdominal vena cava, venous return and therefore cardiac output may be increased, and a previous refractory response may then prove amenable to the same diuretics.

It must be remembered in treating severe edema that major physiologic constraints (e.g., venous hypertension) or a reduction in the serum albumin level limits mobilization of interstitial fluid into the vascular compartment. Therefore, any maneuver that tends to empty the vascular space (e.g., diuretics or ultrafiltration) must be done cautiously to prevent significant hypovolemia with subsequent hypotension and reduced renal perfusion.

HEPATORENAL SYNDROME

Physicians have long recognized an intimate relationship between severe hepatobiliary disease and acute renal failure (ARF). Unfortunately, these relationships have often been poorly defined, and the term *hepatorenal syndrome* (HRS) thus has been inappropriately applied. We now recognize, for example, that the ARF frequently accompanying acute obstructive jaundice (particularly if a patient is subjected to surgery) most often takes the form of ATN and is less commonly functional in nature. The cause of ATN in this setting is not clear but probably includes a combination of factors, such as volume contraction, sepsis, endotoxemia, and jaundice.

HRS does not develop in acute biliary disorders and usually occurs in a clinical setting of advanced alcoholic cirrhosis with ascites. It may also be present in other causes of cirrhosis, in severe acute viral hepatitis, in fulminating alcoholic hepatitis, in Budd-Chiari syndrome, and in some patients with hepatic cancer, as well as in other conditions with acute and severe primary liver damage.

In a setting of severe liver disease, usually alcoholic cirrhosis of the liver, HRS may be defined as the onset of acute, progressive renal failure that shows two major features: (1) No clinical cause of the renal failure is apparent, and (2) the biochemical features of the urine indicate the presence of functional prerenal failure. This latter aspect implies severe underperfusion of the nephron mass.

This definition excludes clinical events such as polyarteritis, leptospirosis, shock, or drug intoxication, in which both the liver and kidneys may be the target of some common insult, but implies that the ARF is due to marked renal underperfusion brought about by some singular cause of renal vasoconstriction that is presumably related to the advanced liver failure.

Pathophysiology

The term HRS is widely abused and is often applied incorrectly to cases of ARF occurring in the presence of liver disease. The basis for such imprecision lies in the clinical setting in which HRS most commonly occurs, alcoholic cirrhosis of the liver with ascites. Consider the major pathophysiologic features involved. As alcoholic cirrhosis progresses, partial obstruction to hepatic venous outflow develops, eventually causing portal venous hypertension. As liver function continues to deteriorate, hypoalbuminemia supervenes. Because of these and other factors, large amounts of hepatic and splanchnic lymph form and cannot be drained away to the venous system by the regional lymphatics and thoracic duct. The overflow collects in the peritoneal space as ascites. We thus have a situation in which large volumes of blood may be sequestered within the mesenteric venous circulation and large volumes of fluid may be sequestered as a third space within the peritoneal compartment. These events lead to progressive arterial hypovolemia, which is invariably compounded by poor dietary intake of salt.

Once a patient is hypovolemic, the only reasonable source for vascular replenishment is the large ascitic depot. The disturbed Starling forces in the portal circulation (venous hypertension and low colloid osmotic pressure), however, do not favor reabsorption of ascites into the vascular compartment; indeed, continuing filtration of fluid is more likely to occur. Thus, by the very nature of the underlying disease, cirrhotic patients are prone to develop significant arterial hypovolemia. If, in this clinical setting, a prerenal type of ARF develops, it is grossly misleading to label this HRS, because causes of the renal ischemia are clearly identifiable. In other words, conferring a diagnosis of HRS on a cirrhotic patient suffering from arterial volume depletion is no more helpful than using the term *cardiorenal syndrome* to describe a patient who has severe CHF and progresses to ARF on a prerenal basis. **Strictly speaking, therefore, the diagnosis of HRS should be reserved for those circumstances in which renal underperfusion is not due to arterial hypovolemia but rather due to some unique cause of selective intrarenal vasoconstriction.**

Selective Renal Vasoconstriction: Possible Causes

Several lines of evidence suggest that a primary increase in intrarenal vascular resistance is the major cause of HRS.

Tristani and Cohn infused large volumes of iso-oncotic dextran into cirrhotic patients with oliguric renal failure. One group, clearly hypovolemic, responded to the infusion with an increase in cardiac output, a decrease in systemic vascular resistance, and a rise in renal blood flow. A second group, with higher plasma volumes, failed to respond with a change in cardiac output (already

normal), systemic vascular resistance, or renal blood flow. Therefore, there clearly is a group of cirrhotic patients with oliguric ARF in whom the cause of renal ischemia is not volume contraction but rather is selective renal vasoconstriction. Even in a group of patients who did respond to acute volume expansion with a marked increment in cardiac output and renal perfusion, renal vasoconstriction often persisted, requiring local intraarterial infusion of vasodilators to restore renal blood flow toward normal.

Epstein and colleagues have demonstrated that the renal blood flow in patients with HRS does not correlate with the level of cardiac output. Using radioactive xenon washout techniques, these investigators were able to demonstrate that comparable reductions of renal cortical blood flow are found in patients with either high or low cardiac output. This situation (i.e., in HRS) is unlike that in patients with another basic cause of arterial hypovolemia, CHF, in which cortical flow does correlate directly with cardiac output.

If cirrhotic patients with HRS are subjected to portal venous decompression by surgical means, renal perfusion often remains fixed despite large increments in cardiac output.

On removal of the diseased liver and transplantation of a healthy liver, the kidney commences forming urine. Alternatively, a kidney that is removed from a cirrhotic patient and transplanted into a new host attains normal function.

Selective angiography of the kidneys in patients with HRS reveals intense diffuse vasoconstriction. If this procedure is repeated postmortem, the vasculature is seen to be quite normal.

If local vasoconstrictor influences are the primary determinant of renal ischemia in HRS, what factors might mediate the vasoconstrictor response?

Table 11–5 summarizes the suggested possible causes of selective renal vasoconstriction in HRS. A discussion of the merits of each of these possibilities is beyond the scope of this chapter, and interested readers should consult recent reviews on the topic. At present, the view held by most investigators is that renal perfusion in health (and disease) is maintained by modulating vasoconstrictor influences of catecholamines and angiotensin II with the vasodilating influence of intrarenal prostaglandins and other autacoids such as kinins or nitric oxide. It has been suggested that if the intrarenal generation of vasodilator prostaglandins declines, unopposed vasoconstriction may cause HRS in a clinical setting of cirrhosis. Although there is some support for this view, this hypothesis is somewhat controversial and at the

TABLE 11–5. Possible Causes of Selective Renal Vasoconstriction in Hepatorenal Syndrome

Endotoxemia
Increased sympathetic activity and circulating catecholamines
Increased activity of the renin-angiotensin system
Hepatic encephalopathy
False neurotransmitters
Decreased intrarenal vasodilator prostaglandins or kinins
Increased intrarenal vasoconstrictor prostaglandins
Raised levels of endothelin
Disturbed nitric oxide synthesis/degradation
Release of unidentified humoral agents from diseased liver

moment must be considered speculative. Newer evidence supports a role for endothelin or nitric oxide involvement. No matter what the exact cause(s) of renal vasoconstriction, it is important to emphasize that **HRS cannot be diagnosed unless it is reasonably clear that arterial hypovolemia has been ruled out as a likely cause of the renal ischemia.**

Clinical Features

Table 11–6 summarizes the major clinical features usually observed in HRS. In North America, HRS occurs in an overwhelming number of patients with alcoholic cirrhosis of the liver. It is rarely observed in ambulatory patients (except those with alcoholic hepatitis) and usually occurs once a cirrhotic patient has been admitted to the hospital. It must be emphasized, however, that **because of profound and extensive muscle atrophy usually observed in these patients, the serum creatinine level does not accurately reflect GFR.** It has been determined as well that creatinine clearance in these patients probably overestimates true GFR by ap-

TABLE 11–6. Hepatorenal Syndrome: Major Clinical Features

Usually occurs only in hospitalized patients
No apparent clinical cause
Ascites usually present
No consistent relationship to jaundice
May have a temporal relationship to advent of hepatic encephalopathy
Marked oliguria is present
Relative hypotension may be present

proximately 20%. Thus, ambulatory out-of-hospital patients with severe cirrhosis but without overt oliguria may already have a profound reduction in GFR despite apparently normal levels of serum creatinine. The worsening of kidney function once admitted to hospital suggests that a reduction in salt intake or excessive diuresis by a managing physician may in reality be inducing relative arterial hypovolemia in a patient already partially volume contracted and with some degree of renal failure already present. Sequential observations of cirrhotic patients for many months and even years reveal that blood volume tends to decrease (from expanded levels), and this decrement is accompanied by the appearance of azotemia.

Oliguria as an isolated finding, without a progressive rise in serum levels of creatinine or BUN, does not imply ARF. There are many causes of oliguria in cirrhotic patients (poor dietary intake of salt, protein, and calories; inability of the liver to form urea; some degree of arterial hypovolemia; increased plasma levels of vasopressin and aldosterone), and low urinary output may be physiologic, considering the patient's condition. Only if the oliguria is accompanied by progressive azotemia or if creatinine clearance is depressed can a diagnosis of ARF be made.

It is difficult to know the true incidence of HRS in cirrhotic patients because the syndrome has been defined so many different ways and there may be so many different causes of renal failure. Probably 40% to 80% of all hospitalized cirrhotic patients have some degree of renal failure. True HRS is probably found in only 10% to 20% of those patients who present with ARF; the remainder probably have prerenal failure. A large teaching hospital (600 to 900 beds) probably encounters no more than six to eight cases of true HRS per year, depending on the type of community the hospital serves.

Laboratory Features and Diagnosis

Table 11–7 summarizes the major laboratory features of HRS.

Because HRS is due to intense renal underperfusion, it is no surprise that the composition of the urine is similar to that in prerenal failure. Moreover, if a patient is very jaundiced, the sediment may be quite active, because this latter condition often causes the appearance of an active sediment with RBCs, tubular cells, and granular casts in the absence of morphologic renal disease.

> **The diagnosis of HRS in a cirrhotic patient depends on the presence of at least two features: The ARF is prerenal in type, and significant arterial hypovolemia is not present.**

It may often not be possible to reach this conclusion until adequate intravenous fluid replacement has been administered. The biochemical features of the urine occasionally may be ambiguous, and it may not be possible to decide whether HRS or ATN is actually present.

The urine volume is usually quite depressed, and the urinary sodium concentration very low (usually <10 to 15 mEq/L) and sometimes may be 0 mEq/L. Despite the intense oliguria (100 to 600 ml/day), the serum creatinine may not reach very high levels and may stabilize at 600 to 700 μmol/L. Once renal failure is present and progressing, arterial blood pressure may decrease, and the serum sodium concentration may decline to very low levels (<125 mEq/L).

Several investigators have remarked on the relationship between spontaneously developing ARF in cirrhotic patients and the appearance of hepatic encephalopathy. Resolution of the renal failure has sometimes accompanied resolution of the hepatic coma or precoma. In some series, encephalopathy has been present in at least half the cases of HRS. Finally, **a diagnosis of HRS implies that other causes of ARF (obstruction, severe urinary sepsis, nephrotoxic drugs, or an acute glomerulopathy) have been ruled out.** Of course, HRS may, after some time (days or weeks), progress to ATN.

PATIENT NUMBER 4

Joe, a 62-year-old man with a chronic history of alcoholic cirrhosis, was admitted to the hospital for increasing ascites, increasing edema of the feet, and deterioration of renal function. He was hypotensive (88/60 mm Hg) and hyponatremic (plasma [Na$^+$] = 131 mEq/L), and his serum creatinine level was 299 μm/L. With bed rest, judicious diuretic therapy, and adjustment of diet, Joe's edema and ascites declined markedly over 10 days and his blood pressure rose to 96/72 mm Hg. His serum creatinine level declined to 98 μm/L, but his 24-hour creatinine clearance was only 47 ml/min. Joe was discharged but returned to the hospital 2 months later with similar problems. His blood pressure on admission was 92/74 mm Hg, serum creatinine was 180 μm/L, plasma [Na$^+$] was 132 mEq/L, and urine volume per 24 hours was 680 ml. Shortly after admission, he developed a cellulitis and was given vancomycin and gentamicin. He became septic and suffered a major GI bleed. Despite adequate antibiotics and transfusions, his blood pressure declined to 60/20 mm Hg, his plasma [Na$^+$] declined to 124 mEq/L, his serum creatinine level rose to 502 μm/L, and he became extremely oliguric. Jaundice supervened 14 days after admission, and he died on the 16th hospital day.

TABLE 11–7. Hepatorenal Syndrome: Laboratory Features

Urine	Marked oliguria
	Low urinary sodium (usually <15 mEq/L)
	Elevated creatinine concentration and osmolality
	Renal failure index (U$_{Na}$/U/P$_{Cr}$ <1.0)
	Slight proteinuria may be present
	Sediment is usually inactive; mild activity compatible with jaundice
	Urine is generally acid
Plasma	Severe disturbance of usual liver function test results
	Marked hyponatremia possible
	Hypokalemia possible
	Rise in serum creatinine level is usually progressive

Approach to the Patient

The constellation of hypotension, hyponatremia, and azotemia suggests relative arterial hypovolemia. The fact that bed rest and diuretics effected disappearance (or decline) of the ascites and improvement confirms this suspicion. Indeed, most examples of HRS are almost certainly examples of prerenal failure due to underfilling of the vascular compartment, the latter circumstance brought about by the sequestration of ascites and edema in the lower extremities. As treatment was given, the azotemia disappeared. Despite this, the creatinine clearance remained impaired. This is a well-documented phenomenon in cirrhosis—that is, the serum creatinine level does not accurately reflect the GFR. This occurs because of the decline in muscle mass, altered secretion of creatinine by the proximal tubule, and decreased methylation within the liver of those amino acids required for creatine synthesis (the precursor of creatinine).

PATIENT NUMBER 4 (continued)

On the second admission, Joe was again hypotensive, hyponatremic, and azotemic, suggesting hypovolemic prerenal failure. However, other problems now supervened, and sepsis, the aminoglycoside antibiotics, and the GI hemorrhage all could explain progressive ATN. Certainly the severe hypotension would complicate the issue and predispose to this problem. In order to diagnose true HRS, the patient should not be hypotensive (a known cause of ATN), should not have evidence of hypovolemia, and should not have other documented causes of ATN (e.g., nephrotoxic antibiotics).

Therapy

The most desirable strategy to follow in dealing with patients who are hospitalized for severe alcoholic cirrhosis and ascites is **a strategy of avoidance.** Based on the features of the cirrhotic process outlined earlier, it is clear that such patients are physiologic time bombs in whom vascular replenishment from the ascitic depot may not keep pace with the many opportunities for vascular emptying. Accordingly, **one should avoid extensive, rapid diuresis; extensive removal of fluid by paracentesis (unless replaced by albumin infusions); rapid and extensive intravenous infusion (unless judged necessary), for fear of expanding and rupturing varices; giving any drug that might cause vomiting or significant diarrhea; or inappropriately reducing the dietary salt intake.**

If tense ascites is present, it should be relieved in an attempt to increase venous return and cardiac output. Normally, the presence of ascites in the peritoneal space increases the intraperitoneal pressure according to the height of the fluid column. In tense ascites, however, because of elastic recoil of the abdominal musculature, the pressure increases beyond what would be expected from the height of the column of fluid, and compression of the vena cava may occur with a resultant decline in venous return.

All fluid losses (e.g., bleeding, diarrhea) should be vigorously replaced. **Diuresis should not be attempted unless the edema and ascites are either extensive or are causing some specific problem** (e.g., respiratory embarrassment or bulging of an umbilical hernia). Diuresis should not be initiated with the potent loop-active diuretics such as furosemide or even thiazides but rather with the less potent diuretics such as spi-

ronolactone or triamterene, which act on the most distal segments of the nephron. These drugs produce a gentle, slow diuresis permitting adequate time for vascular replenishment.

Indeed, spironolactone is the initial diuretic of choice. It should be started in doses of 25 to 50 mg q.i.d. The daily dose should not exceed 100 mg q.i.d. Only if this dose is not producing the required response should a thiazide or furosemide be added. It must be remembered that cirrhotic patients probably can transfer no more than 900 ml/day across the peritoneal membranes. It is probably wise, therefore, to limit diuretic-induced weight loss to 1/2 to 1 pound/day, unless peripheral edema is present to help buffer the diuretic losses. Severe hyponatremia and ARF may be the result of overenthusiastic use of diuretics.

Other than hyperkalemia, the most troublesome complications of spironolactone are RTA painful gynecomastia.

The underlying disorder should be vigorously treated before the advent of HRS.

Treatment of Cirrhosis

For cirrhosis of the liver, treatment focuses on the following areas:

Nutrition. Provide adequate calories and nutrients. If a patient can tolerate it, the daily protein intake should be 80 to 100 g. When encephalopathy is a danger, the daily protein intake should be restricted to 40 g. About half of the calories should be given as carbohydrates. Vitamins should be provided. Salt should not be restricted unless there is clear evidence (24-hour urine collections) that salt retention is present. **Many cirrhotic patients with ascites are able to handle a modest salt intake.**

Electrolyte Abnormalities. Such abnormalities as hyponatremia and hypokalemia should be corrected by reducing free-water intake or by administering a potassium supplement.

Ammonia Levels. These should be kept low by providing gentle cleansing enemas if constipation is present, by giving neomycin (4 to 6 g/day) either by mouth or by a retention enema (2.0 g/200 ml isotonic saline given t.i.d.) or by giving lactulose (10 to 40 g daily).

Infections. Search for and treat infections vigorously. Cirrhotic patients are immunosuppressed and may spontaneously develop infections such as peritonitis. Remember that endotoxemia has been suggested as a cause of HRS.

Treatment of Other Underlying Diseases

For diseases other than cirrhosis, other modalities of therapy should be used (e.g., portacaval fistula for Budd-Chiari syndrome).

Avoid drugs that may compromise renal function (e.g., cyclooxygenase inhibitors such as indomethacin). Current concepts indicate that under conditions that might exist in a cirrhotic patient, such as arterial hypovolemia, the renal vasoconstriction resulting from elevated plasma levels of catecholamines and angiotensin is modulated by the augmented intrarenal generation of prostaglandin E_2, a renal vasodilator. Interfering with prostaglandin production would allow unopposed renal vasoconstriction. Indeed, a reversible form of ARF has been reported in cirrhotic patients after administration of indomethacin.

Treatment of Hepatorenal Syndrome

Once HRS has developed, institute the therapeutic strategies discussed in the paragraphs that follow.

First, ensure that there is no volume contraction because HRS and prerenal failure are almost impossible to differentiate. If there is any question of vascular underfilling, patients should be given large volumes of fluid intravenously, either saline or, preferably, a colloid solution. The dangers of overexpansion are rupture of esophageal varices or augmentation of ascites and edema formation. However, the infusion of colloid sufficient to raise central venous pressure to normal levels, combined with intravenous diuretics, is often rewarded with a brisk diuresis. One of the problems with intravenous infusion is that the abnormal Starling forces tend to force fluid into mesenteric venous channels or into the peritoneal space. Thus, infused fluid may not adequately reexpand the arterial blood volume.

Reinfusion of ascites combined with intravenous furosemide in an attempt to reverse oliguria offers only transient results and is largely a wasted effort. An important advance in the treatment of ARF in liver disease is the availability of the LeVeen peritoneovenous valve. This valve, which serves to pump fluid continuously from the peritoneal space to the venous system, is capable of mobilizing large volumes of ascites within 2 to 3 days. It thus serves as an iatrogenic, synthetic thoracic duct. It not only mobilizes ascites but effectively prevents its reformation. Thus, large volumes of protein-rich saline are quickly returned to the vascular compartment—and stay there. Many patients respond to this maneuver (especially when combined with a diuretic) with a brisk natriuresis. The blood pressure and cardiac output rise, plasma levels of renin and aldosterone decline toward normal, and GFR and renal blood flow may rise dramatically.

The response to the LeVeen valve offers a diagnostic test on pragmatic grounds. A positive response implies that the patient was severely hypovolemic and that the basis of ARF was not HRS. Assuming that the shunt is functioning properly and that ATN has been ruled out, a lack of response suggests true HRS (i.e., ARF because of selective intrarenal vasoconstriction in the absence of hypovolemia). Experience with this device during the past 5 years suggests that many patients with ARF in the setting of cirrhosis and ascites may recover their renal function. This circumstance in turn suggests that many of these patients may not have had true HRS but rather hypovolemic prerenal failure. These shunts may be left in place for many months, and if patients stop drinking, they may enjoy remarkable improvement in both nutritional status and liver function. However, many centers have become disenchanted with the LeVeen valve because of the extensive array of complications that may occur.

A common error made in use of the LeVeen shunt is to wait too long (i.e., until a patient is moribund) before its insertion. If ARF or HRS is advancing and is unresponsive to fluid challenges, good nutrition, diuretics, and other therapies, one should insert the valve early while the patient is well enough to profit from a possible restoration of renal function. Once inserted and functioning, the valve may be left in place as long as required or as long as no complications develop. The common complications are as follows:

1. Disseminated intravascular coagulation
2. Continuous leak of ascites from the abdominal incision
3. Thrombosis of the jugular vein
4. Infection of the shunt and peritonitis
5. Variceal hemorrhage
6. Pulmonary edema
7. Early cessation of shunt function (clotting)

Heart failure, bleeding varices, peritonitis, and severe hepatic encephalopathy are the major contraindications to valve insertion.

The **insertion of a stent between the portal**

vein and a hepatic vein to alleviate portal hypertension has also been used to treat refractory ascites and so-called HRS. In one study, in 28 of 33 patients treated with TIPS for more than 6 months, the mean serum creatinine concentration decreased from 1.5 to 0.09 mg/dl (133 ± 8 μmol/L) to 0.9 ± 0.3 mg/dl (80 ± 27 μmol/L).

This procedure will probably be increasingly used in the future to treat both refractory ascites and ARF in advanced cirrhosis.

> **Hemodialysis or peritoneal dialysis generally has no place in the treatment of HRS.**

Because the underlying problem is severe liver disease, use of these dialysis procedures (which may be problematic in cirrhotic patients) does not add to long-term survival. A possible exception to this statement is in the case of HRS that may accompany severe acute viral hepatitis; here, tiding a patient over while waiting for adequate liver regeneration may be indicated. Use of renal vasodilators or catecholamines to raise blood pressure offers only temporary improvement and is generally not indicated. Considering the high morbidity and mortality accompanying portosystemic shunting procedures, such procedures are to be discouraged.

The recovery rate from true HRS is poor, and the advent of this complication in cirrhosis usually means that death is near.

Hepatorenal Syndrome: A Summary Statement

HRS is a functional or prerenal type of ARF that occurs most commonly in a clinical setting of severe alcoholic cirrhosis of the liver. Because the very nature of the cirrhotic process mandates a tendency toward arterial hypovolemia, prerenal failure is a frequent and expected accompaniment. Indeed, clinical evidence shows that GFR declines in cirrhotic patients as blood volume begins to decrease from markedly expanded levels during the course of the disease. In a consideration of the causes of ARF, HRS cannot be diagnosed unless arterial hypovolemia can be ruled out with certainty. This is not usually possible; therefore, a trial of volume expansion is usually in order. **Strictly speaking, HRS can be diagnosed only if it can be demonstrated that a patient is not responding to intravas-**

cular volume expansion (assuming that ATN is not present). This can most reliably be accomplished using the LeVeen peritoneovenous valve, which mobilizes ascites, expands the plasma volume, and prevents ascites reformation. This procedure has fallen out of favor because of complications; TIPS may become more readily available in the future but will not necessarily have the same effect on ascites removal. Alternatively (and easier to do), it may be feasible, in a monitored bed, to measure central venous pressure, cardiac output, and peripheral vascular resistance in response to volume loading with colloid. In practical terms, most physicians simply administer a trial of isotonic saline or hyperoncotic colloid. Because a diagnosis of HRS should be confined to those patients with isolated intrarenal vasoconstriction in the absence of arterial hypovolemia, a lack of response to a LeVeen valve would, for the moment, appear to be a simple and pragmatic method of differentiating between true HRS and prerenal failure.

The mechanism underlying an increase in intrarenal vascular resistance is unknown, but it may be due to an imbalance between the availability of intrarenal vasodilator prostaglandins (and possibly nitric oxide) and the vasoconstrictor effects of such substances as catecholamines, angiotensin, vasoconstrictor prostaglandins (thromboxanes), or endothelin. HRS augurs poorly for the health of the patient and may proceed to ATN. Death usually follows the advent of ARF in patients with advanced cirrhosis unless a liver transplant becomes available.

SUGGESTED READINGS

Dibona GF: Renal neural activity in hepatorenal syndrome. Kidney Int 25:841, 1984.

Epstein M: Hepatorenal syndrome: Emerging perspective of pathophysiology and therapy. J Am Soc Nephrol 4:1735–1753, 1994.

Epstein M, Lifschitz M: Renal eicosanoids as determinants of renal function in liver disease. Hepatology 7:1359, 1987.

Gordon JA, Anderson RJ: Hepatorenal syndrome. Semin Nephrol 1:37, 1981.

Levy M: The edematous patient. *In* Schrier RW (ed): Manual of Nephrology, 2nd ed. Boston, Little, Brown & Co, 1985.

Levy M: Hepatorenal syndrome. *In* Seldin DW, Giebisch G (eds): The Kidney: Physiology and Pathophysiology, 2nd ed. New York, Raven Press, 1990.

Ochs A, Rossle M, Haag K, et al: The transjugular intrahepatic portosystemic stent-shunt (TIPS) procedure for refractory ascites. N Engl J Med 332:1192–1197, 1995.

Rose B: Clinical Physiology of Acid-Base and Electrolyte Disorders, 3rd ed. New York, McGraw Hill, 1989.

Seldin DW, Alpern RJ: Pathophysiology of edema formation. *In* Seldin DW, Giebisch G (eds): The Kidney: Physiology and Pathophysiology, 2nd ed. New York, Raven Press, 1990.

Staub NC, Taylor AE: Edema. New York, Raven Press, 1984.

Tristani FE, Cohn GN: Systemic and renal hemodynamics in oliguric hepatic failure: Effect of volume expansion. J Clin Invest 46:1891–1894, 1967.

DRUG USE IN RENAL PATIENTS AND THE EXTRACORPOREAL TREATMENT OF POISONINGS

Suzanne K. Swan and William M. Bennett

Normal renal function is required for the metabolism and elimination of many pharmacologic agents. Likewise, pharmacologically active metabolites of many drugs may be dependent on the kidneys for removal from the body. Many compounds, whether excreted by renal or nonrenal means, exert toxic effects in the setting of reduced renal function. Patients with impaired renal function may be maintained within a narrow therapeutic range, avoiding toxicity on one hand and subtherapeutic dosing on the other. In this chapter, basic pharmacologic principles are reviewed and applied to the clinical setting of renal insufficiency. Guidelines for dosage adjustments appear in tabular form, with brief discussions focusing on specific agents. It is important to emphasize that clinicians should not become overreliant on dosing tables or nomograms when treating patients with impaired renal function. Rather, the prescribing physician should maintain a heightened awareness of the pharmacologic alterations that occur in this setting while closely monitoring the patient's clinical course to help guide dosimetry.

PHARMACOKINETICS

Drugs and their active metabolites undergoing renal excretion require dosage adjustments in the setting of renal insufficiency. Dosage modification cannot simply be based on decreased renal excretion because alterations in other pharmacokinetic factors also are involved with drug metabolism (Table 12–1).

Absorption rates of many drugs are altered in patients with renal failure. Uremia-induced vomiting, delayed gastric emptying, and sluggish gut motility secondary to neuropathic changes may contribute to diminished absorption. Aluminum-containing phosphate binders can complex with drugs such as tetracyclines to block absorption by forming insoluble compounds. Phosphate binders can retard gastrointestinal motility. Bowel wall edema, as encountered in nephrotic, cirrhotic, and congestive failure states, may slow drug absorption as well.

Volume of distribution and degree of protein binding for a given agent predict plasma and tissue levels. The volume of distribution is altered by azotemia but not in a predictable way. Most acidic drugs such as penicillins exist in their unbound or pharmacologically active form to a greater degree in patients with renal failure than in persons with normal renal function. Organic acids that accumulate in the uremic milieu are thought to displace acidic drugs from their binding sites or alter the binding proteins themselves. Consequently, a greater proportion of unbound or "free" drug is present in the plasma. This same mechanism also provides higher concentrations of substrate for drug-metabolizing enzymes in the liver. If drug metabolites are excreted by nonrenal means, elevated levels of unbound parent compound may be balanced by increased drug clearance rates secondary to hepatic metabolism. Drugs with decreased protein binding in uremia are listed in Table 12–2.

Biotransformation can be affected by impaired

TABLE 12–1. Pharmacokinetic Factors Altered by Renal Failure

Absorption	Protein binding
Volume of distribution	Biotransformation

TABLE 12–2. Some Drugs in Which Protein Binding Is Decreased in Uremia

Acids	Bases
Barbiturates	Diazepam
Cephalosporins	Morphine
Clofibrate	Triamterene
Dicloxacillin	
Diazoxide	
Furosemide	
Penicillin G	
Phenytoin	
Salicylate	
Sulfonamides	
Valproate	
Warfarin	

renal function. Most drugs are metabolized in the liver by oxidative pathways. Renal failure generally has little effect on these reactions. Exceptions to this involve more rapid oxidation of phenytoin, digitoxin, and propranolol. Quinidine, in contrast, is oxidized more slowly in the presence of renal failure. Other metabolic conversions (e.g., acetylation, hydrolysis, reduction) are normal or modestly slowed in the setting of renal insufficiency. If a drug has active metabolites dependent on renal excretion, significant reductions in dose are necessary to avoid markedly elevated plasma concentrations.

DOSAGE REGIMENS

When GFR is reduced, the elimination of many compounds and pharmacologically active metabolites declines proportionally. Stated another way, the prolongation of a drug's elimination half-life (the time required for the plasma drug concentration to be reduced by half) is proportional to the reduction in GFR. Although drug accumulation may occur at any level of renal insufficiency, such adverse events are relatively uncommon when GFR remains greater than 40 to 50 ml/min. If dosage restrictions are excessive because of fears of toxicity, inadequate therapy may result.

A stepwise process can be used to establish drug dosage regimens for patients with renal failure. This approach aids in achieving therapeutic drug levels while avoiding toxicity (Table 12–3).

Initial Assessment

A history taking and physical examination constitute the first step in assessing dosimetry in pa-

tients with renal impairment. Previous drug toxicity or intolerance should be ascertained if possible. The patient's current medication list (both prescription and nonprescription formulations) must be reviewed to identify potential drug interactions and nephrotoxins. Physical findings suggest the patient's volume status, provide height and weight data used in calculating ideal body mass, and determine whether extrarenal disease states such as hepatic dysfunction exist, requiring additional dosage adjustment.

Calculate Creatinine Clearance

BUN and serum creatinine levels *per se* are insensitive measures of renal function; creatinine clearance (C_{Cr}) is traditionally used to approximate GFR. The fact that lean body mass and age correlate with C_{Cr} directly and inversely, respectively, allows the use of serum creatinine level to estimate the C_{Cr}.[1]

$$C_{Cr} = \frac{(140 - age)\,(body\ weight\ in\ kg)}{72 \times serum\ creatinine\ level}$$

In women, multiply the result by 0.85. It is important to remember that this formula represents only an approximation of renal function. If a patient has acute renal failure, a C_{Cr} of less than 10 ml/min should be assumed for purposes of drug dosage adjustment.

Choose a Loading Dose

For most drugs in the setting of normal renal function, a steady-state concentration is achieved after 3.3 drug half-lives. Because renal failure may prolong an agent's half-life, simply reducing drug doses would be a therapeutic error because such a strategy would delay attainment of a steady-state concentration and therapeutic drug levels. Thus, a loading dose needs to be given for most drugs. This dose usually does not vary from the initial dose given to patients with normal renal function. An exception to this rule is digoxin, for which 50% to 75% of the usual

TABLE 12–3. Establishing Dosing Regimens

1. Initial assessment
2. Assess renal function with creatinine clearance
3. Choose a loading dose
4. Choose a maintenance dose
5. Monitor drug levels

loading dose should be given because of its reduced volume of distribution in renal failure. In patients with significant volume contraction superimposed on renal failure, it may be prudent to lower the standard loading doses of aminoglycosides by 20% to 25% to avoid toxicity.

Choose a Maintenance Dose

Once a loading dose is administered, a maintenance regimen in patients with renal failure may be determined by either one of two methods. First the dosing interval can be lengthened by the following formula:

$$\text{Dosing interval} = \frac{\text{normal } C_{Cr}}{\text{patient's } C_{Cr}} \times \text{normal interval}$$

Alternatively, each individual dose can be reduced and given at standard intervals:

$$\text{Dose} = \frac{\text{patient's } C_{Cr}}{\text{normal } C_{Cr}} \times \text{normal dose}$$

The first or varying interval method can potentially lead to periods of subtherapeutic drug levels. Conversely, the latter or varying dose method allows for more constant drug levels but risks toxicity due to higher trough levels. Thus, the interval method is is preferable for aminoglycosides, whereas the dosage method is more applicable to anticonvulsants and antiarrhythmics.

Monitor Drug Levels

Simply varying the dose or dosing interval is usually not sufficient when adjusting drug regimens for renal failure. Monitoring drug levels when possible may be necessary to ensure therapeutic levels while avoiding toxicity. Drug assays may measure only protein-bound concentrations while significantly underestimating plasma levels of the active form of the drug. An example of this is illustrated by phenytoin. In renal failure, a greater proportion of this drug exists in the unbound or free state. Standard drug determinations do not reflect this increase in physiologically active compound. However, associated with decreased protein binding, a faster rate of clearance may be achieved as a result of increased availability of unbound drug to undergo hepatic metabolism. As a result of these opposing factors, no dose adjustment is generally needed. The therapeutic range, however, is reduced to 4 to 8 μg/ml from 10 to 20 μg/ml, reflecting the increased proportion of active drug present.[2]

For patients receiving hemodialysis, attention must be paid to dose scheduling and the need to give supplemental doses to replace lost body stores. Dialysis clearance of a drug depends primarily on its molecular weight and degree of protein binding. As protein binding increases, dialysis clearance decreases. Likewise, the smaller the compound (<500 daltons), the more drug is removed during a dialysis treatment. In general, scheduled doses should be given after dialysis if possible. Additionally, if a significant portion of a drug is removed, supplemental doses should be given after each dialysis session.

Information compiled from numerous sources is presented in tabular form for dosage adjustments in patients with renal failure (Table 12–4).[3] It must be emphasized that these are general recommendations and thus must be individualized for each patient after considering all the variables affecting a patient's handling of a drug. A few comments on specific drug categories and dosage adjustments for renal insufficiency follow.

Nonsteroidal Antiinflammatory Drugs. Because of their efficacy, over-the-counter accessibility, and numerous clinical indications, nonsteroidal antiinflammatory drugs (NSAIDs) are commanding more attention as nephrotoxic agents. A number of renal syndromes have been associated with NSAID use (Table 12–5). The more common form involves pathophysiologic responses to renal prostaglandin inhibition. Vasoconstriction underlies this response, presents as oliguric acute renal failure, and is generally reversible with discontinuation of the offending agent. Patient risk factors that predispose to this form of drug-induced renal failure have been identified (Table 12–6).

Another form of NSAID nephrotoxicity involves drug hypersensitivity resulting in interstitial nephritis and often nephrotic-range proteinuria. This form of renal failure typically has a protracted course; it is insidious in onset and slow in resolution. Long-term use of NSAIDs and the development of papillary necrosis are clearly linked. Although phenacetin-containing analgesics were viewed as etiologic agents in the past, many NSAIDs have been implicated in the development of papillary necrosis with prolonged use.[4]

Specific recommendations for dose reduction of NSAIDs are not well defined. In patients at risk for developing acute renal failure, NSAID use should be avoided. Sulindac has been sug-

Text continued on page 147

TABLE 12–4. Dosage Adjustments for Patients with Renal Failure

			Adjustment for Renal Failure GFR (ml/min)		Supplement for	
Drug	**Elimination and Metabolism**	**Method**	**10–50**	**<10**	**Dialysis**	**Toxicity Notes**

Antimicrobial Agents

Aminoglycoside antibiotics: Ototoxic, nephrotoxic; rare respiratory paralysis; serum levels to ensure efficacy. Posthemodialysis dose is 2/3 of normal maintenance dose or 1/2 of a loading dose. 50% to 90% absorbed from peritoneum. Volume of distribution larger with obesity, edema, or ascites.

Gentamicin	Renal	D, I	30–70 q 12 hr	20–30 q 24–48 hr	Yes (He, P)	Concurrent penicillins may result in subtherapeutic blood levels.
Netilmicin	Renal	D, I	20–60 q 12 h	10–20 q 24–48 hr	Yes (He, P)	May be less ototoxic than other members of this class.
Tobramycin	Renal	D, I	30–70 q 12 hr	20–30 q 24–48 hr	Yes (He, P)	Concurrent penicillins may result in subtherapeutic blood levels.

Cephalosporin antibiotics: Rare allergic interstitial nephritis; absorbed well when administered intraperitoneally; may cause bleeding in patients with renal failure.

Cefamandole	Renal	I	6–8	12	Yes (He, P)	
Cefazolin	Renal	I	12	24–48	Yes (He, P)	
Cefoxitin	Renal	I	8–12	24–48	Yes (He, P)	
Ceftazidime	Renal	I	24–48	48	Yes (He, P)	
Ceftriaxone	Renal (hepatic)	I	Unchanged	12–24	Yes (He, P)	May raise creatinine by interference with assay.
Cefuroxime	Renal	I	8–12	24	Yes (He), No (P)	
Cephalothin	Renal	I	6–8	12	Yes (He), No (P)	Monitor levels in patients on dialysis.

Miscellaneous antibacterial antibiotics:

Aztreonam	Renal	D	50–75	25	Yes (He, P)	
Chloramphenicol	Hepatic	D	Unchanged	Unchanged	No (He, P)	Half-life markedly prolonged with combined liver and kidney dysfunction.
Ciprofloxacin	Renal (hepatic)	D	50–75	50%	Yes (He, P)	
Clindamycin	Hepatic	D	Unchanged	Unchanged	No (He, P)	Poorly absorbed with antacids or phosphate binders.
Erythromycin	Hepatic	D	Unchanged	50–75	No (He, P)	Ototoxic in high doses in ESRD.
Imipenem	Renal	D	50	25	Yes (He, P)	
Fleroxacin	Renal (hepatic)	D	50–75	50	Yes (He, P)	
Lomefloxacin	Renal	D	50–75	50	No (He, P)	
Metronidazole	Hepatic	D	Unchanged	50	Yes (He)	
Norfloxacin	Hepatic	I	12–24	Avoid	No (He)	
Spectinomycin	Renal		Unchanged	Unchanged	No (He, P)	
Sulfadiazine	Renal	D	25–50	Avoid	?	
		I	8–24	48–72		
Sulfamethoxazole	Renal	I	18	24	Yes (He)	Antifolate activity.
Trimethoprim	Renal	I	18	24	Yes (He)	
Vancomycin	Renal	I or D, I	72–240 500 mg q 24–48 hr	170–240 500 mg q 48–96 hr	No (He, P)	Ototoxic at serum level >50 mg/ml, 40% to 70% absorbed from peritoneum.

Penicillins: Agents in this group cause allergic interstitial nephritis; seizures and coagulopathy at high blood levels.

Amoxicillin	Renal	I	8–12	12–24	Yes (He, P)	
Ampicillin	Renal	I	6–12	12–24	Yes (He, P)	
Dicloxacillin	Renal		Unchanged	Unchanged	No (He, P)	
Mezlocillin	Renal	I	6–8	8	No (He, P)	3 mEq Na$^+$/g
Nafcillin	Hepatic (renal)		Unchanged	Unchanged	No (He, P)	1.9 mEq Na$^+$/g; Coagulopathy
Penicillin G	Renal	D	75	25–50	Yes (He)	Potassium salt has 1.7 mEq/million units; convulsions, false-positive urine protein reactions.
Piperacillin	Renal	I	6–8	8	Yes (He)	1.9 mEq Na$^+$/g
Ticarcillin	Renal	D, I	1–2 g q 8 hr	1 g q 12 hr	Yes (He), No (P)	5.2 mEq Na$^+$/g

Tetracycline antibiotics: Agents in this group potentiate acidosis, raise blood urea nitrogen and phosphorus levels, and increase catabolism. Use of tetracycline should be avoided in renal failure.

Doxycycline	Hepatic		Unchanged	Unchanged	No (He, P)	Group drug of choice for decreased renal function. Not antianabolic.

Antifungal antibiotics:

Amphotericin	Nonrenal	I	24	24–36	No (He, P)	Nephrotoxic, renal tubular acidosis, hypokalemia, nephrogenic diabetes insipidus.
Fluconazole	Renal	D	Unchanged	50–100	Yes (He)	May increase blood cyclosporine levels.
Flucytosine	Renal	I	12–24	24	Yes (He, P)	Hepatic dysfunction, marrow suppression more common in azotemic patients.
Ketoconazole	Hepatic		Unchanged	Unchanged	No (He, P)	

Antimycobacterial antibiotics:

Ethambutol	Renal	I	24–36	48	Yes (He)	Decreased visual acuity, peripheral neuritis.
Isoniazid	Hepatic	D	Unchanged	50	Yes (He)	
Pyrazinamide	Hepatic		Avoid	Avoid	Avoid	
Rifampin	Hepatic	D	50–100	50	No (He)	May cause acute interstitial nephritis, potassium wasting, and renal tubular defects; biologically active metabolite, desacetyl-rifampicin.

Antiviral antibiotics:

Acyclovir	Renal	D, I	5 mg/kg q 12–24 hr	2.5 mg/kg q 24 hr	Yes (He)	Neurotoxic in patients with renal failure, may cause acute renal failure if injected rapidly, intravenously.
Amantadine	Renal	I	48–72	168	No (He, P)	
Didanosine	Hepatic (renal)	I	24	48	Yes (He), No (P)	
Foscarnet	Renal	D	25	10 (avoid)	Yes (He), No (P)	Nephrotoxic; seizures, hypokalemia, hypocalcemia, hypomagnesemia.
Ganciclovir	Renal	I	24–48	48–96	Yes (He), No (P)	

Table continued on following page

TABLE 12–4. Dosage Adjustments for Patients with Renal Failure (*Continued*)

Drug	Elimination and Metabolism	Method	Adjustment for Renal Failure GFR (ml/min)		Supplement for Dialysis	Toxicity Notes
			10–50	<10		

Antihypertensive Agents

In this group, blood pressure is the best guide to dose and interval.

Adrenergic modulators:

Drug	Elimination and Metabolism	Method	10–50	<10	Supplement for Dialysis	Toxicity Notes
Clonidine	Hepatic (renal)		Unchanged	Unchanged	No (He, P)	Rebound hypertension if drug is abruptly withdrawn; tricyclic antidepressants decrease efficacy; potentiates CNS depressant effects of alcohol, sedatives.
Methyldopa	Hepatic (renal)	I	8–12	12–24	Yes (He)	Orthostatic hypotension; retroperitoneal fibrosis; prolonged hypotension due to retained active metabolites; interference with serum creatinine measurement.
Prazosin	Hepatic		Unchanged	Unchanged	No (He, P)	May produce profound hypotension with first dose.

Angiotensin-converting enzyme inhibitors: Hypotensive effect magnified by natriuretic agents or sodium depletion; hyperkalemia; acute renal dysfunction with bilateral or transplant renal artery stenosis. Dry cough 5–10%.

Drug	Elimination and Metabolism	Method	10–50	<10	Supplement for Dialysis	Toxicity Notes
Benazepril	Hepatic (renal)	D	75–100	25–50	Yes (He), No (P)	Rare proteinuria, nephrotic syndrome; dysgeusia, granulocytopenia. Can increase serum digoxin levels.
Captopril	Renal (hepatic)	D, I	75 q 12–18 hr	50 q 24 hr	Yes (He), No (P)	
Cilazapril	Renal (hepatic)	D	25–100	25–50	Yes (He)	
Enalapril	Renal (hepatic)	D	75–100	50	Yes (He), No (P)	Enalaprilat, the active moiety formed in liver.
Lisinopril	Renal	D	50–75	25–50	Yes (He), No (P)	

Beta Blockers:

Drug	Elimination and Metabolism	Method	10–50	<10	Supplement for Dialysis	Toxicity Notes
Atenolol	Renal	D, I	50 q 48 hr	50 q 96 hr	Yes (He), No (P)	Significant accumulation in ESRD.
Betaxolol	Renal	D	Unchanged	50	No (He, P)	
Labetalol	Hepatic		Unchanged	Unchanged	No (He, P)	
Metoprolol	Hepatic		Unchanged	Unchanged	Yes (He), No (P)	
Propranolol	Hepatic		Unchanged	Unchanged	No (He, P)	Metabolites may accumulate; increases bilirubin by assay interference; less frequent doses in some patients with ESRD; hypoglycemia reported in ESRD.

Calcium Blocking Agents

Headache, flushing, and dizziness in patients with renal disease; may increase serum digoxin and cyclosporine levels.

Drug	Elimination and Metabolism	Method	10–50	<10	Supplement for Dialysis	Toxicity Notes
Diltiazem	Hepatic		Unchanged	Unchanged	No (He, P)	Active metabolites; acute renal dysfunction reported.
Isradipine	Hepatic		Unchanged	Unchanged	No (He, P)	Active metabolites; acute renal dysfunction reported.
Nifedipine	Hepatic		Unchanged	Unchanged	No (He, P)	Active metabolites; edema; acute renal dysfunction reported.
Nisoldipine	Hepatic		Unchanged	Unchanged	No (He, P)	Active metabolites; acute renal dysfunction reported.
Verapamil	Hepatic		Unchanged	Unchanged	No (He, P)	Active metabolites; acute renal dysfunction reported.

Cardiac glycosides: Add to uremic gastrointestinal symptoms; serum levels guide to therapy; toxicity enhanced by dialysis potassium and magnesium removal.

Drug	Route of elimination	Method			Dialysis	Notes
Digitoxin	Hepatic (renal)	D	Unchanged	50–75	No (He, P)	Protein binding decreased by dialysis; volume of distribution reduced by uremia.
Digoxin	Renal	D, I	25–75 q 36 hr	10–25 q 48 h	No (He, P)	Radioimmunoassay may overestimate serum levels in uremia; clearance reduced by spironolactone, quinidine, verapamil; hypokalemia, hypomagnesemia enhances toxicity. Volume of distribution decreased in ESRD. Serum level 12 hours after first dose is best guide in ESRD.

Antiarrhythmic Agents

Blood levels most often the best guide to therapy. Half-life may be prolonged in heart failure or with reduced hepatic blood flow.

Drug	Route of elimination	Method			Dialysis	Notes
Adenosine	Hepatic		Unchanged	Unchanged	No (He, P)	
Amiodarone	Hepatic		100%	100%	No (He, P)	Hepatotoxicity. Thyroid dysfunction. Peripheral neuropathy. Pulmonary fibrosis. Active metabolite. Increased plasma digoxin. Increases cyclosporine levels.
Bretylium	Renal	D	25–50%	25%	No (He, P)	Hypotension. Active metabolites.
Cibenzoline	Renal	D, I	100% q 24 hr	66% q 24 hr	No (He, P)	
Disopyramide	Renal	I	q 12–24 hr	q 24–40 hr	No (He, P)	Urinary retention. Protein binding concentration dependent. Volume of distribution decreased in ESRD.
Encainide	Renal	D	75%	50%	?	Encephalopathy. Slow demethylators with long half-life. Active metabolite.
Flecainide	Hepatic (renal)	D	100%	50–75%	No (He, P)	Excretion enhanced in acid urine.
Lidocaine	Hepatic	D	100%	100%	No (He, P)	
Lorcainide	Hepatic	D	100%	100%	?	Active metabolite.
Mexiletine	Hepatic (renal)	D	100%	50–75%	No (He, P)	Increased renal excretion in acid urine.
Moricizine	Hepatic		100%	100%	No (He, P)	
N-acetylprocainamide	Renal	D, I	50% q 8–12 hr	25% q 12–18 hr	No (He, P)	Hemofiltration useful in poisoning.
Procainamide	Renal	I	q 6–12 hr	q 8–24 hr	Yes (He), No (P)	Half-life acetylator phenotype dependent. Active metabolite is N-acetylprocainamide. Lupus-like syndrome. Hemofiltration useful in poisoning.
Propafenone	Hepatic		100%	100%	No (He, P)	Half-life acetylator phenotype dependent. Active metabolite.
Quinidine	Hepatic (renal)	D	100%	75%	Yes (He), No (P)	Active metabolite. Increased plasma levels of digoxin and digitoxin. Excretion enhanced in acid urine. Hemodialysis useful in poisoning.
Tocainide	Hepatic (renal)	D	100%	50%	Yes (He), No (P)	Excretion decreased in alkaline urine.

Miscellaneous Agents

Anticoagulants:

Drug	Route of elimination	Method			Dialysis	Notes
Alteplase	Unknown		100%	100%	?	(Tissue-type plasminogen activator.)
Anistreplase	Unknown		100%	100%	?	
Dipyridamole	Unknown		100%	100%	?	
Heparin	Nonrenal Nonhepatic		100%	100%	No (He, P)	Half-life increases with dose.

Table continued on following page

145

TABLE 12–4. Dosage Adjustments for Patients with Renal Failure (*Continued*)

Drug	Elimination and Metabolism	Method	Adjustment for Renal Failure GFR (ml/min)		Supplement for Dialysis	Toxicity Notes
			10–50	<10		
Miscellaneous Agents (Continued)						
Low-molecular-weight heparin	Unknown	D	100%	50%	?	
Iloprost	Unknown	D	100%	50%	?	
Indobufen	Unknown	D	50%	25%	?	
Streptokinase	Nonrenal Nonhepatic	D	100%	100%	NA	
Sulfinpyrazone	Renal	D	100%	Avoid	No (He, P)	Occasional acute renal failure. Uricosuric effect lost at low GFR.
Sulotroban	Renal	D	30%	10%	?	
Ticlopidine	Hepatic		100%	100%	?	
Tranexamic acid	Renal	D	25%	10%	?	
Urokinase	Unknown	D	Unknown	Unknown	?	
Warfarin	Nonrenal Nonhepatic	D	100%	100%	No (He, P)	Monitor prothrombin time. Decreased protein binding in uremia.
Anticonvulsants: Monitor serum levels.						
Carbamazepine	Hepatic		100%	100%	No (He, P)	May cause inappropriate antidiuretic hormone secretion.
Ethosuximide	Hepatic		100%	100%	No (He)	
Lamotrigine	Hepatic		100%	100%	?	
Oxcarbazepine	Hepatic		100%	100%	?	
Phenytoin	Hepatic		100%	100%	No (He, P)	Measure free and bound levels. Protein binding decreased and distribution volume increased in renal failure. May cause folate deficiency. Interstitial nephritis. Saturable metabolism.
Primidone	Renal	I	q 8–12 hr	q 12–24 hr	Yes (He)	Partially converted to phenobarbital and other metabolites with long half-life. Excessive sedation. Nystagmus. Folate deficiency.
Sodium valproate	Hepatic		100%	100%	No (He, P)	Decreased protein binding in uremia. Concurrent phenytoin, phenobarbital, and primidone shorten half-life.
Trimethadione	Hepatic	I	q 8–12 hr	q 12–24 hr	?	Active metabolites with long half-life. Nephrotic syndrome.
H₂ antagonists:						
Cimetidine	Renal	D	50%	25%	No (He, P)	Increases serum creatinine level and decreases creatinine clearance by inhibition of tubular creatinine secretion. Mental confusion in patients with renal or hepatic disease.
Famotidine	Renal	D	25%	10%	No (He, P)	Acute renal failure reported.
Nizatidine	Renal	D	50%	25%	?	
Ranitidine	Renal	D	50%	25%	Yes (He), No (P)	

ESRD, end-stage renal disease; He, hemodialysis; P, peritoneal dialysis; D, dosage reduction method wherein the percentage of the standard dose is listed; I, interval extension method wherein the number of hours between standard dose is listed.

TABLE 12–5. Renal Syndromes Associated with Nonsteroidal Antiinflammatory Drugs

Sodium retention/edema
Hyperkalemia
Oliguric acute renal failure
Nephrotic syndrome (nil lesion)
Interstitial nephritis
Papillary necrosis

TABLE 12–6. Risk Factors for Developing NSAID-Induced Vasoconstrictive Renal Failure

Congestive heart failure
Cirrhosis
Nephrosis
Sepsis
Shock
Advanced age
Preexisting renal disease
Diuretic use (volume contraction)

gested to be a "nephroprotective" NSAID, but several cases of acute renal failure associated with its use have been reported.[4] If NSAID use is necessary, particularly on a continuous basis, close monitoring of C_{Cr}, as well as urinalysis, should be performed at regularly scheduled intervals.

Diuretics. Patients with impaired renal function often require diuretic therapy to avoid volume overload. Loop diuretics, such as furosemide, bumetanide, and ethacrynic acid, exert their effect from the luminal side of the tubule. As a result of extensive protein binding, most diuretics cannot undergo glomerular filtration and must be secreted by organic anion pumps in the basolateral membrane into the tubular lumen. In azotemic states, organic acids compete with and displace diuretics from these transport channels. As a result, dosage increments are often necessary to achieve the desired diuretic response.[5] An effective dose must initially be established, one that renders a natriuretic response. This is

accomplished by doubling subsequent doses every 30 to 60 minutes until a ceiling dose is reached or diuresis occurs (Fig. 12–1). With the clinically available loop diuretics, ototoxicity is most likely to occur with ethacrynic acid but has also been reported with furosemide and bumetanide.

Aminoglycosides. Widespread use of aminoglycoside antibiotics for life-threatening infections continues. Because of a narrow therapeutic window and GFR-dependent excretion, close attention must be paid to dosage regimens, drug levels, changes in renal function, and concomitant nephrotoxic drug use. As aminoglycosides accumulate, the risk of nephrotoxicity and ototoxicity increases. Bactericidal efficacy of aminoglycosides correlates with therapeutic peak concentrations. Toxicity, on the other hand, corresponds to rising trough levels. Thus, dosage adjustments for these antimicrobial agents should primarily

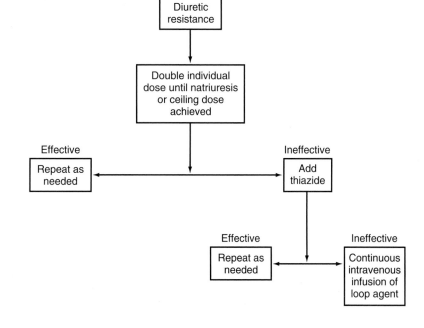

Figure 12–1. Algorithm for treating patients with diuretic resistance.

involve the varying interval format described earlier in this chapter. Individual dose reductions are also occasionally necessary. Assessment of peak and trough aminoglycoside serum levels as well as C_{Cr} is necessary to monitor therapy and avoid toxicity. Concomitant use of loop diuretics, especially ethacrynic acid, greatly increases the risk of ototoxicity. Aminoglycosides also increase the nephrotoxicity of cyclosporine, a commonly used immunosuppressant.

HEMODIALYSIS AND HEMOPERFUSION IN THE TREATMENT OF DRUG OVERDOSE

Hemodialysis, hemoperfusion, and occasionally peritoneal dialysis can be helpful additions to the management of drug overdose or poisoning. In general, it must be emphasized that these measures are not the primary or sole therapy but rather adjuncts to more standard treatments. Conventional measures including cardiorespiratory support, gastric lavage, and activated charcoal can be combined with forced diuresis (either alkaline or acidic) in patients with intact renal function to treat the majority of drug overdoses.

Criteria to be used when considering dialysis or hemoperfusion for drug intoxication treatment include the following:

1. Unstable vital signs despite fluid replacement, mechanical ventilation, and conventional therapy for drug overdose
2. Prolonged coma or prolonged ventilator dependence
3. Progressive deterioration in overall condition despite aggressive care
4. Prospect of delayed toxicity (e.g., paraquat)
5. Overdose with agents known to have toxic metabolites (e.g., methanol, ethylene glycol)
6. Presence of underlying disease that prevents elimination of an offending agent by primary excretory organ
7. Intoxication with an agent known to be readily extractable by either method at a rate greater than that achieved by endogenous elimination

Hemodialysis is the primary route of removal for water-soluble agents with low molecular weights and minimal protein binding. Charcoal hemoperfusion is more effective in removing lipid-soluble drugs that are highly protein bound. The charcoal cartridge competes with plasma proteins by absorbing the drug itself and remov-

ing it from the blood returning to the patient. If dialysis and hemoperfusion are equally effective in removing an agent, dialysis should be used because of a significant incidence of thrombocytopenia (30%) with hemoperfusion. Table 12–7 categorizes agents into those that are effectively removed by hemoperfusion and those that are not.

A fourth type of extracorporeal toxin removal system can be achieved with continuous venovenous hemofiltration or continuous arteriovenous hemofiltration or either of these combined with hemodialysis.[6] Because of the permeable membranes involved, hemofiltration relies on convective transport with elimination of solute (toxin or drug) as solvent is removed. For many solutes, this solvent drag phenomenon often offers equivalent clearance rates when compared with conventional hemodialysis because of its continuous time course. Consequently, posttherapy rebound, which may complicate intermittent regimens such as hemodialysis or hemoperfusion, is avoided with continuous therapies. Unfortunately, relatively little is known about drug or toxin removal with this technique. Further studies are necessary before specific recommendations can be made for the use of this therapy in the treatment of drug toxicity or poisonings.

PATIENT NUMBER 1

Linda, a 50-year-old woman who weighs 55 kg and has chronic renal insufficiency (serum creatinine level 3.0 mg/dl), develops congestive heart failure and atrial fibrillation. Digoxin therapy is indicated. What loading dose would you choose, and at what maintenance dosing regimen?

Calculation of the C_{Cr} is the first step in determining loading and maintenance dosages of drugs excreted by the kidneys. Using Cockcroft and Gault's formula,[1] a significant reduction in C_{Cr} would be calculated for this patient (C_{Cr} = 18.4 ml/min). Administration of 50% to 75% of a normal loading dose of digoxin would be appropriate at this point. If quinidine is added, a further reduction in digoxin clearance should be expected. A maintenance regimen can be tailored for our patient Linda once her condition has stabilized. A standard maintenance dose could be administered every other day if her C_{Cr} is less than 10 ml/min. Conversely, providing 25% to 50% of this standard dose on a daily basis would be an alternative if her C_{Cr} remains

TABLE 12–7. Removal of Drugs and Chemicals by Hemoperfusion

Effective removal from patients already reported:

Acetaminophen	Ethchlorvynol	Mushroom toxins (*Amanita*	Phenobarbital
Acetylsalicylic acid	Glutethimide	*phalloides*)	Phenytoin
Barbiturates	Meprobamate	Paracetamol	Quinine
Carbon tetrachloride	Methaqualone	Paraquat	Salicylates
Chloramphenicol	Methotrexate	Penicillin G	Theophylline
Digitoxin	Methprylon		Thyroid hormone
Digoxin	Methylsalicylate		(T_3 or T_4)

Effective removal probable:

Amphetamine	Diphenhydramine	Quinidine

Effective removal from extracorporeal unit *in vitro*:

Codeine	Isopropyl alcohol	Paraldehyde

Effective removal *in vitro* but highly bound to tissue with a large volume of distribution (and/or highly bound to albumin with low free fraction in plasma):

Amitriptyline	Diazepam	Doxepin	Oxazepam
Chlordiazepoxide	Diquat	Imipramine	Propoxyphene
Chlorpromazine			

Not effectively removed:

Bromide	Ethanol	Lithium	Methanol

Adapted from Winchester JF: Use of dialysis and hemoperfusion in treatment of poisoning. *In* Dagirdas J, Ing T (eds): Handbook of Dialysis. Boston, Little, Brown & Co, 1994, p 579.

---

between 10 and 30 ml/min. Frequent measurement of serum digoxin levels is necessary to ensure therapeutic efficacy while avoiding toxicity.

PATIENT NUMBER 2

Bob is a 79-year-old man who is a nursing home patient and has an indwelling Foley catheter. He develops sepsis and is admitted to the hospital for intravenous antibiotic therapy. His serum creatinine level on arrival is 2.4 mg/dl, and he weighs 60 kg. What loading dose of aminoglycoside would you choose in order to achieve therapeutic serum concentrations (8 μg/ml) rapidly, and at what maintenance regimen, given the patient's fluctuating renal function?

A loading dose can frequently be used to establish therapeutic serum levels of a particular drug. A quick rule of thumb for aminoglycoside loading dose calculations involves multiplying the drug's volume of distribution (L/kg) by the patient's weight (in kg) by the serum concentration desired. In Bob's case, using a volume of distribution of approximately 0.25 L/kg and the patient's weight of 60 kg and a peak serum level for either gentamicin or tobramycin of 8 μg/ml would provide a loading dose of 120 mg, or 2 mg/kg, in our patient Bob (0.25 L/kg × 60 kg × 8 μg/ml). Given the patient's age and presumed intravascular volume-depleted state, it would be prudent to reduce this loading dose by approximately 20% to 25% to minimize toxicity. Drugs may undergo significant alterations in their volume of distribution in the setting of uremia, which must be considered when performing these quick calculations. Likewise, calculations provide a rough estimate of a loading dose for a given patient and must be appropriately tailored to each individual patient. Designing a maintenance regimen for our patient Bob is somewhat more complicated because of his fluctuating renal function. Despite the fact that his creatinine level on admission is 2.4, it will most likely continue to rise on a daily basis for the next several days while his condition is stabilizing. It must always be remembered that serum creatinine level is only a rough estimate of true renal function, and in this particular case, it represents a poor estimate in a very dynamic setting. In adjusting dosage schedules for aminoglycosides because of their significant toxicities, it has generally become standard practice to adjust not only the interval at which a particular dose is administered but the actual quantity of the individual dose as well. For a C_{Cr} of less than 10 ml/min, it would be reasonable to administer 20% to 30% of a standard dose every 24 to 48 hours, depending on peak and trough serum levels as well as the status of the patient's renal function. For a C_{Cr} of 10 to 50 ml/min, providing 30% to 70% of a standard dose approximately every 12 hours would be prudent, again monitoring serum levels closely to ensure therapeutic peak responses and responding to rising trough levels appropriately with further reductions in dose. Finally, administration of the total daily dose of aminoglycoside as a once-daily or once every-other-day infusion is being evaluated in clinical trials.

PATIENT NUMBER 3

Carl, a 22-year-old mechanic, arrives in the emergency room. He is unresponsive. Laboratory studies reveal serum pH 7.0, anion gap 28, lactic acid normal, serum HCO_3 8 mEq/L, and serum creatinine level 2.5 mg/dl. He is not diabetic. A drug screen is negative for salicylates, ethanol, narcotics, and acetaminophen, although family members relate a history of ethanol abuse and suicidal ideation. What differential diagnoses should be considered? When the causative agent of this patient's condition is identified, hemodialysis is instituted. What other therapeutic measures should be taken?

The diagnoses to be considered in Carl's case are those applicable to metabolic acidosis with an increased anion gap. Possibilities include keto-acidosis, uremia, starvation, salicylate overdose, methanol poisoning, ethylene glycol poisoning, lactic acidosis, and paraldehyde overdose. As can be determined from the information provided, many of these possibilities can be ruled out. In this case, ethylene glycol (antifreeze) ingestion should be high on the list, given this patient's alcohol abuse history, occupation, and suicidal ideation. Ethylene glycol is a toxic agent because of its metabolism by the enzyme alcohol dehydrogenase to oxalic acid. This acid is problematic for the kidneys because of precipitation within the tubules, causing obstruction and tubular necrosis, which ultimately delay excretion of this poison. Signs of ethylene glycol toxicity include confusion, seizures, and coma. Later complications that may arise include myositis and myocarditis. If the condition is recognized early, treatment may best be provided with forced diuresis to accelerate renal excretion and to limit oxalate precipitation within the tubules. However, in our patient Carl's case, given his comatose state on arrival and marked acidosis, hemodialysis is in order because of ethylene glycol's readily dialyzable nature. In addition to dialysis, administration of ethanol should be instituted because this substrate competes with ethylene glycol for alcohol dehydrogenase's catalytic effect, ultimately reducing the production of oxalic acid. If ethanol is to be given while the patient is on hemodialysis, it can be administered directly into the dialysis solution to keep the patient's serum ethanol concentration at approximately 100 mg/dl.

REFERENCES

1. Cockcroft DW, Gault MH: Prediction of creatinine clearance from serum creatinine. Nephron 16:31, 1976.
2. Bennett WM: Use of drugs in the patient with renal insufficiency. *In* Rose BD (ed): Pathophysiology of Renal Disease, 2nd ed. New York, McGraw-Hill, 1987, p 577.
3. Bennett WM, Aronoff GR, Golper TA, et al: Drug Prescribing in Renal Failure. Philadelphia, American College of Physicians, 1994.
4. Henrich W: Nephrotoxicity of nonsteroidal anti-inflammatory agents. *In* Schrier RW, Gottschalk CW (eds): Diseases of the Kidney, 4th ed. Boston, Little Brown & Co, 1988, p 1328.
5. Swan SK, Brater DC: Clinical pharmacology of loop diuretics and their use in chronic renal insufficiency. J Nephrol 6:118–123, 1993.
6. Golper TA, Bennett WM: Drug removal by continuous arteriovenous hemofiltration. Med Toxicol 3:341, 1988.

13 ∎ CHRONIC RENAL FAILURE

Kevin W. Finkel and Thomas D. DuBose, Jr.

Programs that provide chronic renal replacement therapy for end-stage renal disease (ESRD) have grown substantially in the past 2 decades. This rapid and unanticipated growth is a result of several factors, including advances in dialysis technology; improved medical care of patients with chronic renal failure (CRF), thus slowing the progression of many forms of chronic renal disease; and a growth in the population of elderly patients with renal disease. As the population of patients with CRF expands, it is necessary that those generalists and specialists providing primary care for these patients, especially as chronic renal disease progresses to end stage, appreciate the diagnostic and therapeutic approach to such patients. Such an approach must consider the principles of the pathophysiologic basis of renal failure and the spectrum of systemic involvement in chronic renal disease. It must also acknowledge when to refer such patients to a nephrologist. In this chapter, an index patient is used to exemplify stages in such a progression, and the clinical course of this patient is used to identify and emphasize those issues pertinent to the development of a core of knowledge that ultimately allows selection of appropriate modalities of renal replacement therapy.

EPIDEMIOLOGY

As reported by the United States Renal Data Systems Annual Report, more than 230,000 people in the United States receive treatment for ESRD. The most common causes of ESRD are diabetes mellitus (26%), hypertension (24%), and glomerulonephritis (19%).

PATIENT NUMBER 1

Martin is a 60-year-old attorney specializing in real estate law. He presents to your office with a 3- to 4-month history of generalized weakness, fatigue, and mild lower extremity swelling. He denies any significant past medical history, although the last time he saw a physician was for a checkup more than 10 years ago. At that time, he was told his blood pressure was "borderline." A follow-up visit had been scheduled, but Martin had not returned because he felt well. Besides, he attributed his blood pressure reading to the stress he was under at work during the time. Martin smokes about one-half pack of cigarettes per day and consumes "six or seven" drinks during the week. He says he has never been one to exercise regularly, but of late he has noted a decreased tolerance to climbing one or two flights of stairs. As a result of his hectic work schedule, Martin has sporadic eating habits and frequently consumes fast foods on the run. His examination is remarkable for a blood pressure of 160/95 mm Hg and trace pedal edema. Laboratory results are as follows: hemoglobin 10 mg/dl, cholesterol 300 mg/dl, potassium 5.5 mmol/L, sodium 138 mmol/L, bicarbonate 18 mmol/L, BUN 40 mg/dl, and creatinine 4.0 mg/dl.

APPROACH TO THE PATIENT

In the initial evaluation of a patient with an increased serum creatinine level, it is important to determine the following: (1) Is the impairment due to an acute or a chronic process? (2) What is the cause of the impairment? (3) Are there any superimposed reversible components? First, documenting the chronicity of the disease determines the prognosis for the patient, because by definition CRF is often an irreversible process. Second, identification of the specific pathologic mechanism influences the short- and long-term therapeutic interventions. Aggressive treatment of the primary process as well as the metabolic abnormalities of CRF may improve patients' symptoms and may slow, to some extent, the inevitable progression to ESRD. Finally, correction of any superimposed reversible factors can restore a level of renal function compatible with a more conservative approach to care and can delay the need for dialysis.

Establishing the Diagnosis

In a patient with an elevated creatinine level, the diagnosis of CRF is confirmed by (1) identifying a disease known to cause chronic renal injury and (2) demonstrating evidence of chronically progressive renal failure.

Diseases Known to Cause Renal Damage

The clinical features of diseases commonly associated with the development of CRF are listed in Table 13–1. Although patients can often provide the clinical information needed to make the diagnosis of CRF, more accurate data demonstrating a slowly progressive rise in the serum creatinine level over time or previously abnormal findings on urinalysis can sometimes be found in old medical records (school, military, insurance, hospital, or former physicians). It is mandatory that these records be routinely searched when evaluating patients with renal failure of unknown cause.

Evidence of Progressive Renal Dysfunction

As already mentioned, one reliable marker of CRF is a previously documented elevation in the serum creatinine level. Unfortunately, in some cases, such information may not be available, and the patient may have an unremarkable past medical history. In these situations, chronicity must be established by other means. As renal failure progresses, renal tubular atrophy and fibrosis usually result in a decrease in renal size. Consequently, assessing kidney size, usually by ultrasonography, to document a reduced renal mass is helpful to establish the diagnosis of CRF. **In most renal diseases, the finding of small kidneys is the most reliable feature of chronicity.** It is important to point out the exceptions to this observation. Normal-sized (or enlarged) kidneys in the presence of advanced CRF can be found in diabetes mellitus, multiple myeloma, amyloidosis, polycystic kidney disease, malignant nephrosclerosis, and rapidly progressive glomerulonephritis.

When renal size is normal or the results of ultrasonography are equivocal, chronicity can be confirmed by demonstrating the presence of secondary hyperparathyroidism (renal osteodystrophy) on bone radiographs. As functional renal mass decreases, hyperphosphatemia, hypocal-

TABLE 13–1. Clinical Features of Diseases Causing Chronic Renal Failure

History

Glomerulonephritis: Macroscopic/microscopic hematuria, proteinuria, renal biopsy, skin rashes, arthralgias/arthritis

Hereditary nephritis: Family history, deafness, lenticular abnormalities (Alport's syndrome)

Diabetes mellitus: Family history, polyuria, polydipsia, retinopathy

Nephrosclerosis: Episodes of accelerated or malignant hypertension, poorly controlled blood pressure for extended periods

Interstitial nephritis: Frequent bladder/kidney infections, enuresis, incontinence, chronic pain, analgesic abuse, gastrointestinal bleeding episodes, macroscopic hematuria, renal colic

Obstructive uropathy: Frequency and/or hesitancy on urination, renal colic, stones, macroscopic hematuria, vaginal bleeding

Cystic disease: Family history, renal colic and stones, macroscopic hematuria

Physical Examination

Glomerulonephritis: Malar rash, arthritis, palpable purpura

Hereditary nephritis: Sensory-neural deafness, ocular abnormalities

Diabetes mellitus: Retinopathy, neuropathy

Nephrosclerosis: Hypertensive retinopathy, elevated blood pressure

Obstruction: Large prostate, palpable bladder and/or kidneys

Laboratory Tests

Chronic glomerulonephritis: Dysmorphic RBCs/RBC casts, oval fat bodies, proteinuria

Diabetes: Hyperglycemia, glycosuria

Interstitial nephritis: Diagnostic intravenous pyelography (IVP) if chronic pyelonephritis

Secondary glomerulonephritis: Positive antinuclear antibody and/or anti-DNA antibody titers, hypocomplementemia

Obstructive uropathy: Dilated renal collecting system on IVP, CT scan, or renal ultrasonography

Hereditary nephritis: Dysmorphic RBCs, RBC casts, abnormal audiogram

Cystic disease: Multicystic kidneys and liver on CT scan, ultrasonography, or diagnostic IVP

Adapted from Miller RB: The patient with chronic azotemia, with emphasis on chronic renal failure. *In* Schrier RW (ed): Manual of Nephrology. Boston, Little, Brown & Co, 1988.

cemia, and deficiency of active vitamin D develop, causing serum parathyroid hormone (PTH) concentrations to rise. The result is subperiosteal resorption of the metacarpals and phalanges on magnified radiographs of the hand, as well as subperiosteal resorption of the distal or medial portions of the clavicles on chest radiography.

A more novel approach to establish chronicity

is measurement of creatinine in the fingernails. Fingernail creatinine level is elevated in CRF and results from increased serum levels some months previously during nail formation. Levels return to normal after a successful renal transplant.

In summary, irreversible renal failure can be established by historic documentation of a previously abnormal serum creatinine level, radiographic demonstration of reduced renal size, or the presence of renal osteodystrophy on skeletal radiographs. Fingernail creatinine determination remains an interesting but infrequently used technique.

Estimation of the Severity of Chronic Renal Failure

Once CRF is diagnosed, the degree of impairment must be determined to guide further therapy. The extent of intervention may range from aggressive treatment of a primary disorder and control of hypertension to more conservative management and preparation for dialysis, depending on the degree of renal dysfunction.

The severity of the renal impairment is determined by the presence of advanced clinical features of CRF (uremia) and by measuring the residual GFR.

The clinical features of advanced CRF are outlined in Table 13–2. An estimate of residual GFR can be obtained by measuring the clearance of endogenous creatinine or radionuclide agents (see the later section on monitoring the progression of CRF).

PATIENT NUMBER 1 (continued)

You perform a careful history evaluation and physical examination on Martin. The only additional information you obtain is that his father and two brothers have hypertension and that one of his brothers is now seeing a kidney specialist. You are unable to gather any information about any blood tests performed during his examination 10 years ago. You obtain a renal sonogram, which shows bilaterally shrunken kidneys. Radiographs of Martin's hands demonstrate subperiosteal resorption of the phalanges, consistent with secondary hyperparathyroidism. These results are highly suggestive that Martin's elevated creatinine level is a result of some chronic process, presumably hypertension, because it is the second leading cause of ESRD.

Identification of Reversible Factors

It is important to identify any potentially reversible factors that contribute to the decreased GFR

TABLE 13–2. Clinical Features of Advanced Chronic Renal Failure (Uremic Syndrome)

Symptoms

General: Fatigue, weakness, lethargy
Skin: Itching, easy bruising, skin discolorations, pallor or frost
Cardiovascular: Dyspnea, orthopnea, edema, pericardial chest pain
Gastrointestinal: Anorexia, early morning nausea, vomiting, dysgeusia, uriniferous breath, early satiety, hiccups
Neuromuscular: Decreased ability to concentrate, restless legs, parethesias, muscle cramps and/or twitching

Signs

General: Bitemporal wasting
Skin: Ecchymoses, excoriations, pallor, hyperpigmentation, hyperkeratoses
Oral: Uriniferous breath, stomatic ulcers
Cardiovascular: Hypertension with retinopathy and/or S4 gallop, murmur, pericardial friction rub, edema, ejection flow murmur
Neuromuscular: Sensory/motor peripheral neuropathy, drowsiness, mental confusion, myoclonus, asterixis, seizures, coma

Laboratory Findings

Elevated BUN and creatinine, decreased GFR
Metabolic acidosis (hyperchloremic or high anion gap)
Normochromic normocytic anemia
Hyperuricemia
Hyperphosphatemia, hypocalcemia
Radiographic evidence of shrunken kidneys and/or early renal osteodystrophy
Proteinuria
Broad granular casts on urinalysis

Adapted from Miller RB: The patient with chronic azotemia, with emphasis on chronic renal failure. *In* Schrier RW (ed): Manual of Nephrology. Boston, Little, Brown & Co, 1988.

in patients with chronic renal disease, because in this situation, the progression to ESRD may be slowed and the initiation of dialysis postponed. Common remedial factors are shown in Table 13–3.

Volume Depletion

Both true and effective circulating volume depletion occur frequently in CRF. As a result of sodium retention, many patients become volume overloaded as renal function deteriorates. These patients may be started on diuretics combined with dietary salt restriction, which can result in ECF depletion. Furthermore, because renal sodium handling is abnormal, any concomitant disturbance such as diarrhea or emesis, which may be mild when renal function is normal, can result in severe volume depletion in patients with CRF. Therefore, close attention to the volume status

TABLE 13–3. Common Reversible Factors in
Chronic Renal Failure

True or effective volume depletion: Vomiting, diarrhea,
    excessive diuresis, congestive heart failure
Urinary tract obstruction: Papillary necrosis, nephrolithiasis,
    bladder outlet obstruction (prostatic hypertrophy or
    cancer, cervical cancer with bladder invasion)
Vascular disease: Uncontrolled, accelerated, or malignant
    hypertension; excessive treatment of hypertension; renal
    artery stenosis; renal vein thrombosis
Infection: Severe bilateral pyelonephritis
Nephrotoxic agents
Metabolic disorders: Severe hypercalcemia,
    hyperphosphatemia, hyperuricemia, potassium depletion,
    metabolic acidosis
Glomerulonephritis or vasculitis: Systemic lupus
    erythematosus, rapidly progressive glomerulonephritis,
    vasculitis, postinfectious glomerulonephritis
Interstitial nephritis: Drugs (allergic interstitial nephritis),
    toxins, and autoimmune diseases (Sjögren's syndrome,
    sarcoidosis)
Pregnancy: Especially with toxemia
Acute renal failure of any cause

---

in patients with CRF is mandatory, particularly
when there is an unexplained rise in the serum
creatinine level.

Urinary Tract Obstruction

Urinary outflow obstruction is common in elderly
men with prostatic hypertrophy and can be corrected by Foley catheterization or transurethral
prostatectomy. In women, obstruction may impli-
cate an invasive cervical or endometrial carcinoma. **Therefore, a rectal examination in
men or a pelvic examination in women is
essential to eliminate urinary tract obstruction as a factor contributing to the renal
impairment.** Renal ultrasonography can usually
detect the presence of obstruction and should be
performed when obstruction is clinically suspected. Urinary tract obstruction can also occur
as a result of bilateral renal stones or renal stone
disease in a solitary kidney. Papillary necrosis
should also be considered, especially in patients
with chronic heavy analgesic abuse, diabetes mellitus, chronic pyelonephritis, or sickle cell nephropathy.

Hypertension

Malignant hypertension, causing both histologic
changes (fibrinoid necrosis) and angiotensin-me-
diated vasoconstriction, decreases renal blood
flow and GFR. Furthermore, if the hypertension
is corrected too vigorously, the injured renal vasculature may be unable to vasodilate appropri-

ately in response to the lowered renal perfusion
pressure, and worsening renal function ensues.
**Therefore, the blood pressure should be
lowered gradually to allow vascular relaxation to occur along with improved control
of hypertension.**

Drugs

Many commonly used medications can compromise renal function either by direct nephrotoxicity (aminoglycoside antibiotics, amphotericin B,
chemotherapeutic agents), by hemodynamic
perturbations (angiotensin-converting enzyme
[ACE] inhibitors, nonsteroidal antiinflammatory
agents) or by inciting an interstitial inflammatory
response (analgesics, penicillin, sulfa-containing
drugs). **Meticulous monitoring of serum levels of any potential nephrotoxic agent,
adjusting the dosage of medications based
on the estimated GFR, and asking patients
to avoid certain medications altogether are
all steps required to avoid worsening renal
function in patients with underlying CRF.**
Many of these agents are found in over-the-
counter preparations and in nonconventional ho-
meopathic agents; thus, a detailed history of all
the medications used by a patient must be obtained.

PATIENT NUMBER 1 (continued)

*Although Martin appears to have chronic renal
disease, you make a meticulous search for any
correctable superimposed factors. He is not taking
any medications, including over-the-counter
antiinflammatory agents. You check his blood pressure
in the supine and upright positions and find no
orthostatic change in the readings. This finding, in
the presence of peripheral edema, makes volume
depletion unlikely. Normal findings on digital rectal
examination, when combined with the results of the
renal sonogram, make obstruction unlikely. Finally,
although Martin's blood pressure is elevated, it is
doubtful that this level of elevation is causing an acute
rise in creatinine level. You therefore inform Martin that
he has CRF secondary to hypertension.*

Toxins

Toxins can cause a decline in renal function in
patients with CRF by various mechanisms, including (1) intratubular precipitation and obstruction, (2) direct tubular toxicity, and (3)
hemodynamic alterations. **Deterioration by intratubular obstruction can often be avoided
by prophylactic volume expansion, which is
one of the rationales for intravenous hydration before administration of parenteral ra-**

diocontrast, in order to avoid the development of contrast nephropathy. Concomitant use of an osmotic or loop diuretic with hydration as a means of increasing the degree of diuresis is controversial. In one report, however, evidence indicated that the use of mannitol or furosemide with hydration was not as effective as hydration alone in preventing contrast nephropathy. Even with intravenous administration of fluids, all attempts should be made to avoid using contrast in patients at high risk of renal failure, such as patients with underlying CRF (serum creatinine level > 1.5 mg/dl, especially if diabetic, elderly, or volume depleted). The ability of newer low-ionic-strength contrast to decrease the incidence of renal failure in high-risk patients is not firmly established, but when radiocontrast examination is necessary in a patient with established renal insufficiency, its use is probably prudent.

Pregnancy

Patients who have CRF and who become pregnant are at increased risk for several complications, including preeclampsia, worsening renal function, intrauterine growth retardation, malignant hypertension, and fetal demise. **The presence of sustained hypertension is the poorest prognostic sign for both a pregnant woman and her fetus.** Generally, women with little or no hypertension and only a moderate decline in renal function (serum creatinine level < 1.5 mg/dl) have an uneventful pregnancy. There are no long-term effects on their renal function. On the other hand, hypertension and more significant renal failure increase the likelihood of a complicated pregnancy and may also result in deterioration of their renal function.

Delaying the Progression of Chronic Renal Failure

Although the agent or mechanism that caused the initial renal injury can often be removed or attenuated, once the kidney has suffered significant damage, **there is an inexorable decline in function that is independent of the initial insult.** It is suspected that regardless of the inciting injury, once enough renal mass is lost, a cascade of common events is triggered, leading to progressive renal failure. Experimental data have implicated several potential progression factors, including hyperfiltration/intraglomerular hypertension, enhanced expression of a series of growth factors, elevated PTH levels, the presence of hyperlipidemia, and complement activa-

tion by increased ammoniagenesis in the remaining nephrons. Furthermore, data demonstrate that modifications of these factors (especially control of intraglomerular hypertension with ACE inhibitors) may delay the onset of ESRD. **Currently, however, only by attenuation of the primary etiologic process, by avoidance of nephrotoxic agents, and by control of hypertension can the progression of CRF be reliably modified.**

Intervention in the Primary Disease

Unfortunately, many primary renal diseases offer no specific therapeutic options or such options have several serious side effects. In general, however, attempts should be made to relieve urinary tract obstruction, control hypertension, correct fluid and electrolyte disorders, treat autoimmune diseases with appropriate immunosuppressant agents, discontinue nephrotoxic drugs, eliminate infection, and correct renal vascular stenosis when appropriate. This therapeutic effort is most often directed by a consulting nephrologist.

Avoiding Nephrotoxins

A comprehensive list of potential nephrotoxins is presented in Table 13–4. Discontinuation of these agents should be routine at the first sign of declining renal function.

TABLE 13–4. Potential Nephrotoxins

Exogenous Nephrotoxins

Antibiotics: Aminoglycosides, tetracyclines, amphotericin, colistin/polymyxin, cephalosporins, penicillin, rifampicin, sulfa-based antibiotics
Anesthetics: Methoxyflurane
Radiographic contrast agents
Heavy metals: Mercury, arsenic, lead, gold, copper, cadmium
Organic solvents: Carbon tetrachloride, ethylene glycol, methanol
Analgesics: Phenacetin, acetaminophen, prostaglandin inhibitors
Antihypertensive agents: Angiotensin-converting enzyme inhibitors, thiazides, loop diuretic agents
Chemotherapeutic agents: Cisplatin, nitrosoureas, methotrexate, mitomycin C
Xanthine oxidase inhibitors

Endogenous Nephrotoxins

Myoglobin
Hemoglobin

Protein Restriction

It has long been recognized that restriction of dietary protein ameliorates the symptoms of CRF. Evidence in animals has shown a clear benefit of protein restriction in decreasing the intraglomerular hypertension associated with a reduction in renal mass. Renal function and the degree of proteinuria also improve. The evidence for a significant benefit of a protein-restricted diet to slow progression of CRF in humans, however, has not been established for all forms of renal disease. The results of a large, national cooperative study on the effects of a low-protein diet on the progression of CRF were recently reported by the Modification of Diet in Renal Disease study group. The overall results after 2 years of follow-up failed to demonstrate an overall benefit. However, the rate of progression of renal failure in all groups of patients, including controls, was very slow, and it is hoped that with more prolonged follow-up a significant benefit will be identified. **In anticipation of such results, it has become common practice to initiate a protein-restricted diet in patients with CRF (0.8 g/kg body weight of dietary protein per day).**

Control of Hypertension

The correlation between systemic hypertension and progressive renal failure was observed many years ago. It was recognized that transmission of systemic pressure to the glomerulus, with the resultant intraglomerular hypertension, has a significant role in the progression of CRF. Therefore, control of blood pressure emerges as a paramount issue in the preservation of renal function.

Animal studies have shown that ACE inhibitors are more effective in slowing the evolution of renal failure than other classes of antihypertensive medication, presumably because of their preferential vasodilatory effect on the efferent arteriole. This efficacy of ACE inhibitors has now been demonstrated in selected human populations. Patients with diabetic nephropathy were randomized to placebo or an ACE inhibitor while continuing other blood pressure medications. Although no differences in blood pressure control were noted between the two groups, those patients who received the ACE inhibitor experienced a 50% reduction in the incidence of death, dialysis, and transplantation. The results of other studies suggest that ACE inhibitors may also be beneficial in the nephropathy associated with sickle cell disease, as well as IgA nephropathy,

the most common cause of glomerulonephritis internationally. **Patients on ACE inhibitors should be closely monitored for changes in renal function and hyperkalemia, because a decline in renal function and hyperkalemia represent the most significant side effects of these agents in patients with CRF.** Consequently, caution should be exercised when treating patients with disorders that are associated with the development of hyperkalemia, such as diabetes mellitus or tubulointerstitial nephritis. **Given the current evidence, an ACE inhibitor should be considered the primary choice as an antihypertensive agent in patients with CRF if there are no other contraindications to its use. Absolute contraindications include (1) bilateral renal artery stenosis or stenosis in a solitary kidney or renal allograft and (2) advanced renal failure (GFR < 20 ml/min).**

Metabolic Control

Type 1 diabetes mellitus is associated with a 30% chance of developing CRF. Until the results of the Diabetes Control and Complications Trial were published, whether tight control of serum glucose levels had any effect on the microvascular complications of the disease was controversial. In that trial, patients were randomized to either usual control or tight control (three or more injections each day or use of an insulin pump). After a follow-up of more than 6 years, intensive glycemic control was found to decrease significantly the incidence of nephropathy, neuropathy, and retinopathy. **Intensive control of hyperglycemia in patients with type 1 diabetes mellitus slowed or delayed the development of nephropathy, although the incidence of severe hypoglycemic episodes was significantly increased.** The long-term effects of repeated hypoglycemia and ways to implement such glucose control in a less select and larger group of patients remain issues currently under consideration.

Besides the known deleterious effects on the kidneys of sustained hyperglycemia, evidence also suggests that hyperlipidemia may cause progression of CRF. Many kidney diseases are associated with hypercholesterolemia. In several models of renal disease in animals, feeding a low-cholesterol diet or treatment with a cholesterol-lowering agent results in improvement of renal function and a reduction in the degree of proteinuria. Whether this benefit accrues in renal failure in humans is unclear. However, it seems wise to recommend lowering elevated serum cholesterol levels in patients for its proven cardiovascular benefits.

PATIENT NUMBER 1 (continued)

You have a long conversation with Martin about the implications of your diagnosis. He is quite dismayed that there is "nothing else you can do" to cure his renal disease except make recommendations about therapies that may only slow its progression. Furthermore, he feels that many of these recommendations are unduly restrictive on his current lifestyle. He does not like to take medications. He is a meat-and-potatoes man and finds a dietary restriction of salt, protein, cholesterol, and potassium unpalatable. He does not know where he can find the time to incorporate regular exercise into his day. Finally, he is frightened by the loss of personal control and autonomy that accompanies the development of ESRD and the need for dialytic therapy.

You patiently discuss all these issues with Martin and make it clear that you understand his position and that he is not alone in his feelings. You tell him you will make arrangements for him to attend meetings sponsored by the local Kidney Foundation, where he can meet and talk with other people in similar circumstances. In addition, in consultation with a nephrologist, you make several therapeutic recommendations:

1. *Control blood pressure. Although an ACE inhibitor should be considered, he already has hyperkalemia, which can become significantly worse with this agent. In this case, you instead recommend a calcium channel antagonist.*
2. *Add a diuretic. This will improve his symptoms of edema, improve blood pressure control, and decrease the hyperkalemia. You will need to monitor his fluid balance closely in subsequent visits.*
3. *Sodium-, protein-, cholesterol-, and potassium-restricted diet.*
4. *Regularly scheduled walks. If diet and exercise do not lower his cholesterol adequately, you will add a cholesterol-lowering agent.*

You should recognize that this patient has a hyperkalemic hyperchloremic (non-anion gap) metabolic acidosis. The degree of acidosis is mild, so you choose not to start alkali therapy immediately. Furthermore, you are about to treat the hyperkalemia, which alone can improve the acidosis (see the later section on metabolic acidosis).

Monitoring the Progression of Chronic Renal Failure

The rate of progression of CRF is highly variable in individual patients; therefore, frequent follow-up is necessary. Furthermore, because the symptoms of early uremia can be nonspecific, monitoring patients with CRF for changes in subjective complaints, physical findings, and laboratory data, especially an estimation of GFR (such as creatinine clearance) and a urinalysis, should be routine. The accuracy of the tests commonly used to evaluate renal function has been much criticized, however.

Limitations in Creatinine Measurements in Chronic Renal Failure

Time-honored laboratory methods for monitoring renal function include determinations of serum creatinine and endogenous creatinine clearance and the Crockcroft-Gault calculation of creatinine clearance based on age, weight, and gender.*

Some also advocate the use of the reciprocal of the serum creatinine level (1/Cr) plotted against time.

The serum creatinine level is dependent on the balance between generation and excretion. As CRF progresses, the creatinine generation rate and the route of creatinine excretion may change, leading to alterations in creatinine levels or clearance totally independent of the effects of GFR. **It is apparent that GFR can decline to a significant degree with little change in the serum creatinine level in some circumstances. Thus, serum creatinine determination is an imprecise means of assessing renal function, especially on a one-time basis without knowledge of a previously established value.**

Total Muscle Mass

Serum creatinine is directly proportional to muscle mass. Any change in muscle mass affects the serum creatinine level independent of GFR. Women and elderly patients typically have lower muscle mass and hence lower serum creatinine values. In a patient with significant muscle wasting, a serum creatinine level in the normal range may represent a significant reduction in GFR. **Therefore, a serum creatinine value must always be interpreted with a consideration of the patient's age, gender, and muscle mass. In other words, a normal serum creatinine level does not ensure that the GFR is normal.**

---

*$C_{Cr} = (140 - age) \times weight (kg)/P_{Cr} \times 72$ (men)
$C_{Cr} = [(140 - age) \times weight (kg)/P_{Cr} \times 72] \times 0.85$ (women)

Protein Intake

The most important dietary source of creatinine is meat. Consuming a low-protein diet can result in a decrease of the serum creatinine level by 10% to 30%. **Therefore, when a patient with CRF is placed on a protein restricted diet to slow the progression of the disease, the serum creatinine level may initially improve, although there has been no real change in renal function.**

Mode of Creatinine Excretion

Creatinine is normally eliminated by glomerular filtration (90%), with a small amount appearing in the urine by tubular secretion (10%). As renal function deteriorates, however, tubular secretion becomes responsible for a larger proportion of creatinine excretion (up to 50% in some diseases). Because creatinine clearance is a measure of both filtration and secretion, it follows that as creatinine secretion increases in progressive CRF, GFR can fall significantly with little change in serum creatinine level or creatinine clearance. **Therefore, creatinine clearance overestimates GFR as renal disease progresses to near end stage.**

Just as filtration can decrease without a significant change in serum creatinine levels, these levels can increase when the GFR is stable. Drugs that compete with creatinine for tubular secretion raise the serum creatinine level without affecting filtration. Two commonly used medications that have this effect are cimetidine and trimethoprim. In advanced renal insufficiency, the cimetidine-creatinine clearance relies on this effect to decrease creatinine secretion and is considered a more reliable index of GFR in patients with values less than 20 ml/min. Standard doses of cimetidine are given 3 days before and on the day of performance of a routine creatinine clearance test.

Finally, some substances not normally found in the serum can react as creatinine in a colorimetric assay, leading to a false elevation in the serum creatinine value. The most common substances are ketoacids and some cephalosporin antibiotics. **Changes in levels of serum creatinine and creatinine clearance must be considered with the knowledge of changes in muscle mass, diet, accompanying illness, and medications.**

The Crockcroft-Gault equation has similar limitations because it depends on the serum creatinine value. In addition, because this formula uses body weight in the calculation, it overestimates GFR in states of obesity or edema, in which weight gain is not associated with an increased muscle mass.

The use of the reciprocal of creatinine (1/Cr) plotted against time for monitoring the progression of CRF is based on the expectation that the rate of decline will parallel the decrement in GFR over time. In such a case, a linear decline establishes the rate of progression. An abrupt increase in the slope of the line would indicate a superimposed secondary process, and a decrease in the slope would suggest stabilization of the disease. Because 1/Cr is based on a measured value, it is also subject to the same inconsistencies previously mentioned. For example, some studies have suggested that the progressive decline in 1/Cr is not linear in CRF, especially when nearing end stage, thus questioning its utility in monitoring the progression to ESRD.

PATIENT NUMBER 1 (continued)

After initiation of your therapy, Martin returns for a follow-up visit. He is in much better spirits after attending the Kidney Foundation program and has been adhering to his diet. He feels better. Evaluation at this time shows his blood pressure to be 135/75 mm Hg. His serum potassium level is 4.0 mmol/L, and his bicarbonate level has risen to 24 mmol/L. His serum creatinine level has fallen to 3.2 mg/dl. You recognize this is not due to an improvement in GFR; rather, it reflects Martin's adherence to a protein-restricted diet. With an understanding of its numerous flaws, you determine 24-hour creatinine clearance, which is measured as 30 ml/min. You plan to see Martin in follow-up every 2 months to monitor him closely for signs and symptoms of progressive renal failure. It is also appropriate to obtain assistance from a consulting nephrologist to help care for Martin.

TREATMENT

Metabolic Acidosis

Normal acid-base homeostasis is maintained by a balance between acid production and net renal acid excretion. Net renal acid excretion is composed of two components, reabsorption of filtered bicarbonate and excretion of acid in the form of titratable acidity and ammonium.

As renal failure progresses, ammonium production declines largely because of a loss of renal mass. Hyperkalemia can be a contributing factor because it inhibits renal ammonium production and excretion. In CRF, hydrogen ion secretion by the collecting duct may also decrease. This secretion of acid is under the control of aldosterone and is also influenced by systemic acid-base balance, tubular flow rate, distal sodium delivery, and potassium balance (hyperkalemia decreases acid secretion). Some patients with CRF, especially those with diabetes mellitus or tubulointerstitial nephritis, may acquire a syndrome of selective aldosterone deficiency that results in a hyperchloremic (non-anion gap) metabolic acidosis by two mechanisms: (1) a direct decrease in acid secretion in the collecting duct and (2) hyperkalemia-induced suppression of ammoniagenesis. **Early in CRF, metabolic acidosis is typically characterized as hyperchloremic acidosis and is attributed to a decrease in ammonium production and net acid secretion. As renal failure progresses to end stage, the accumulation of organic acids causes an elevation in the anion gap.**

It is necessary to treat the acidosis to prevent the deleterious effects of long-standing acidemia on bone and muscle. Acidosis increases the catabolism of muscle and may play a part in the wasting and malnourishment of CRF. Retained acid is also buffered by bone salts, resulting in progressive demineralization, and can be additive to the effects of secondary hyperparathyroidism. Alkali should be administered in quantities sufficient to return the systemic pH to normal. In hyperkalemic hyperchloremic metabolic acidosis associated with selective aldosterone deficiency, correction of the potassium level alone (diuretics or Kayexalate) may attenuate the acidosis. Sodium bicarbonate tablets are the preferred source of alkali replacement because sodium citrate (Shohl's solution) increases aluminum absorption from the gut in patients receiving aluminum-containing phosphate binders and antacids.

Volume Disorders

Patients with advanced CRF have a relatively fixed amount of sodium excretion impairing their ability to regulate salt balance precisely. As a result, they are prone to both volume depletion and volume overload, depending on the clinical circumstances. **Consequently, it is important to monitor volume status frequently in patients with CRF, especially during an intercurrent illness or with a change in a therapeutic intervention.** Clinical parameters such as body weight, jugular venous pressure, and clinical signs of congestive cardiac failure are the most reliable markers of volume status. On the other hand, laboratory findings such as fractional excretion of sodium, urinary sodium concentration, and urinary osmolality may not be accurate

because of the relatively fixed sodium excretion that accompanies CRF.

In states of volume overload, sodium intake should be restricted. If necessary, sodium excretion can also be augmented with the use of diuretics. When choosing the diuretic agent, keep in mind that thiazides are ineffective once the GFR falls below 30 ml/min. In that case, a loop diuretic is the appropriate drug selection. Close monitoring of the volume status, serum potassium level, and renal function is absolutely critical in these patients. The use of potassium-sparing diuretics should be avoided. In states of volume depletion, diuretics should be withheld and any underlying disorder (diarrhea, emesis) corrected. Depending on the degree of volume depletion as determined by orthostatic blood pressure, weight loss, pulse, and skin turgor, judicious administration of intravenous saline is advised. **The fundamental principle is to maintain euvolemia.**

Potassium Disorders

Regulation of potassium balance by the kidneys is accomplished primarily by the regulation of potassium secretion in the cortical collecting tubule. As CRF progresses, potassium excretion falls because of a decline in the GFR and a defect in tubular secretion. The serum potassium level typically does not usually rise until GFR is less than 15 ml/min. However, certain renal diseases are associated with the development of selective aldosterone deficiency (diabetes mellitus and tubulointerstitial nephritis), in which case hyperkalemia can occur at a much higher GFR. As renal excretion of potassium declines, the gastrointestinal (GI) tract, in particular the colon, increases the fecal excretion of potassium. Handling of potassium loads after a meal is also dependent on the movement of potassium into the cell interior. This process is facilitated by insulin, beta-adrenergic stimulation, and a functioning sodium-potassium triphosphate. **Therefore, in CRF or in the presence of aldosterone deficiency, beta-blocker therapy, diabetes, and digitalis can cause severe hyperkalemia.** Prompt treatment of hyperkalemia is mandatory when myocardial toxicity is detected by ECG. In this situation, intravenous calcium is given to directly oppose the cardiac effects of potassium. Intravenous insulin is used to drive potassium intracellularly, usually given with glucose to avoid hypoglycemia. The effectiveness of parenteral bicarbonate administration to increase cellular uptake of potassium is more variable but is probably most useful when there is an accompanying metabolic acidosis. Inhaled beta agonists have also been found useful in driving the intracellular accumulation of potassium in CRF. All of these maneuvers are temporizing because potassium eventually leaks out of the cells. **Thus, the definitive treatment of hyperkalemia is removal of potassium to reduce total body potassium content.** In mild cases, potassium can be removed from the body with an ion-exchange resin (Kayexalate) given either orally or as a rectal enema. It exchanges a sodium ion for a potassium ion in the colon and can therefore result in volume overload. Cases of severe hyperkalemia are treated with dialysis. However, the temporizing measures described earlier should be performed *immediately* to protect the patient until dialysis can be arranged.

Water Balance

As renal function declines, patients lose the ability to both dilute and concentrate the urine. As a consequence, patients with CRF are at risk for water intoxication (hyponatremia) and dehydration (hypernatremia). Patients with high circulating arginine vasopressin levels (volume depletion, congestive cardiac failure, postoperative pain) are at increased risk for developing hyponatremia when given hypotonic fluids; thus, this practice should be avoided. The treatment of asymptomatic hyponatremia is simple fluid restriction. When the disorder is symptomatic (stupor, coma, or altered mental status), it is treated with hypertonic saline, often combined with a loop diuretic to avoid sudden volume overload and osmotic shifts.

Hypernatremia is less often a problem because most patients have an intact thirst mechanism. Therefore, hypernatremia is typically encountered in elderly or debilitated patients who may have an impaired thirst response (stroke or dementia) or limited access to free water (nursing home patients on high-osmolar gastrostomy tube feedings). Euvolemia is established with saline infusion, and any free-water deficit is replaced with half-normal saline or 5% dextrose in water.

Correction of both hyponatremia and hypernatremia should be gradual (not to exceed 0.5 to 1 mmol/L/hr or 12 to 24 mmol/day) to avoid the complications of central pontine myelinolysis or cerebral edema, respectively.

Magnesium

In severe CRF, magnesium excretion by the kidneys begins to fall. However, intoxication is unusual unless a magnesium load is given, typically in the form of a magnesium-containing antacid (Mylanta, Maalox) or laxative (magnesium citrate, milk of magnesia). **Magnesium-containing agents should not be prescribed in patients with a GFR less than 30 ml/min.**

Calcium and Phosphorus Disorders (see also Chapter 14)

The kidneys have a pivotal role in the control of serum calcium and phosphorus levels. As a result, patients with CRF can develop a bone disease associated with elevated PTH levels. With a progressive decline in GFR, serum phosphorus level rises, causing hypocalcemia by directly complexing with calcium and by inhibiting the production of active vitamin D. The hypocalcemia and low vitamin D levels cause an increase in serum PTH levels, which stimulate bone resorption. **Thus, secondary hyperparathyroidism represents an attempt to normalize serum calcium levels as renal function deteriorates.** Renal osteodystrophy is a relatively early event in CRF because elevated serum PTH levels can be detected when the GFR falls below 60 ml/min. Treatment consists of control of serum phosphorus levels with dietary restriction and orally administered calcium-containing phosphate binders, as well as active vitamin D replacement. Aluminum-containing phosphate binders (Amphojel, Alu-Caps) should be avoided. Aluminum accumulation in CRF can result in bone disease, anemia, and dementia. The combination of aluminum-containing phosphate binders and sodium citrate (Shohl's solution) is absolutely contraindicated because this has been reported to cause acute and severe chronic aluminum toxicity.

PATIENT NUMBER 1 (continued)

Despite numerous telephone calls, Martin has missed several appointments and finally returns 8 months later. He feels very weak, has early morning nausea, and bruises easily, and his skin is very itchy. He has continued to take his blood pressure medicine and diuretic, but his edema has returned, and he is no longer adhering to any kind of diet. He has taken a leave of absence from the law firm. Blood tests reveal creatinine 8 mg/dl, BUN 80 mg/dl, hemoglobin 7.5 g/dl, calcium 6.5 mg/dl, phosphorus 8 mg/dl, potassium 5.6 mmol/L, and bicarbonate 15 mmol/L.

TABLE 13–5. Laboratory Characteristics of the Anemia of Chronic Renal Failure

Normochromic normocytic anemia
Echinocytes (burr cells)
Normal or high serum iron concentration, normal or low iron-binding capacity
Normal or high serum ferritin
Decreased reticulocyte index
Normal platelet count, possibly increased bleeding time
Decreased ^{51}Cr RBC survival
Decreased hemoglobin-oxygen affinity (increased 2,3-diphosphoglycerate)

TABLE 13–6. Primary Causes of the Anemia of Chronic Renal Failure

1. Decreased erythropoietin production
   Loss of viable renal parenchyma
   Decreased hemoglobin oxygen affinity (increase in 2,3-diphosphoglycerate from acidemia)
2. Inhibitors of erythropoiesis (uremic toxins)
3. Hemolysis (uremic alterations of RBC membrane)

SPECIFIC ORGAN DYSFUNCTION IN CHRONIC RENAL FAILURE

Hematologic Abnormalities

Anemia

As CRF progresses, anemia eventually develops in all patients. The laboratory features of this anemia are presented in Table 13–5. The principal cause of the depressed erythrocyte count is decreased erythropoietin (EPO) production by the diseased kidneys, although other factors are involved (Table 13–6). Recombinant EPO is now widely used to correct the anemia of CRF. In many cases, it is administered parenterally three times per week during dialysis. It can also be given by a subcutaneous route, which often requires lower doses and less frequent injections. **The most common complication of EPO administration is the development or exacerbation of hypertension. Increases in blood pressure with EPO are usually mitigated if the hematocrit rises slowly.** Other potential complications include accelerated thrombosis of hemodialysis vascular access and decreased dialysis efficiency because of hyperviscosity. EPO administration to patients with CRF improves their sense of well-being and may have beneficial cardiac effects, such as decreasing left ventricular hypertrophy. Therefore, it should be given to anemic patients with CRF to maintain the hematocrit above 33%.

Platelets

Patients with CRF have a bleeding tendency manifested mainly by ecchymoses, purpura, epistaxis, and prolonged bleeding from venipuncture sites. This condition is a result of impaired platelet function, evidenced by a prolonged bleeding time. Various treatment regimens to correct this bleeding diathesis are available (Table 13–7). Selection of which therapy to use is based on the desired time of onset of action and duration of effect. Cryoprecipitate and DDAVP are used in emergent situations (active bleeding, before a percutaneous renal biopsy). When immediate action in unnecessary, treatment with conjugated estrogens and consideration of initiation of dialysis are appropriate measures.

Leukocytes

In advanced CRF, the neutrophils from patients may demonstrate impaired chemotactic function and lymphocyte numbers may show an absolute decrease. Functional effects on cellular immunity are demonstrated by a depressed delayed-type hypersensitivity response. These immunologic abnormalities increase the susceptibility to infection and decrease the immunogenicity of vaccinations. Nevertheless, various vaccinations are recommended for patients with CRF (Table 13–8). Response is variable, especially to vaccination for hepatitis B.

TABLE 13–7. Treatment of Bleeding Abnormalities in Chronic Renal Failure

Agent	Dosage	Duration of Action
Cryoprecipitate	10 units IV every 12–24 hr	12–18 hr
1-Deamino-8-D-arginine vasopressin (DDAVP)	0.3 µg/kg IV in 50 ml saline given over 15–30 min	4–8 hr; tachyphylaxis after 1–2 treatments
Conjugated estrogen	0.6 mg/kg/day IV for 5 days	2 wk
Dialysis	1–3 treatments	Variable; peritoneal dialysis may be better than hemodialysis

TABLE 13–8. Recommended Immunizations in Chronic Renal Failure

Vaccine	Dosage	Frequency of Administration
Influenza A and B	0.5 ml (15 μg) via single IM injection	Annually
Pneumococcus	0.5 ml (575 μg) via single SC or IM injection	Booster depending on antibody response and levels
Hepatitis B	2 ml (40 μg HbsAg) at 0, 1, 5, and 6 months; 1 ml IM in each deltoid	Booster depending on antibody response and levels
Tetanus toxoid	0.5 ml single IM injection	Booster every 10 years

Dermatologic Disorders

Patients with CRF may develop several skin disorders such as discoloration (iron overload), xerosis (dry skin), or irregular pruritic papules (Kyrle's disease), but the most common condition is chronic severe pruritus. The cause of this pruritus is unknown, and it is often resistant to any form of therapy. In the skin, elevated levels of calcium, phosphorus, and magnesium, as well as elevated plasma histamine levels, all have been implicated as etiologic factors. Treatment consists of administration of antihistaminic agents and application of soothing skin lotions. EPO has also been reported to decrease pruritus, possibly by lowering plasma histamine levels. Consistent improvement has not been noted after parathyroidectomy or lowering of the serum phosphorus level.

Nervous System Disorders

Nervous system dysfunction is common in CRF. Before the initiation of dialysis, the disorder is typically a neuropathy or encephalopathy. Once dialysis is begun, the neurologic disturbance may be related to dialysis disequilibrium or dialysis dementia.

Uremic Encephalopathy

Uremic encephalopathy can occur with either acute or chronic renal failure, typically when the GFR falls below 10 ml/min. The signs and symptoms of the disorder have a vast range of severity, from anorexia and nausea to seizures and coma (Table 13–9). The more severe manifestations usually complicate acute renal failure. Symptoms resolve after dialysis is started. **Narcotic analgesics, particularly meperidine and its metabolite normeperidine, lower the seizure threshold and accumulate in the plasma of patients with CRF. These agents should be used sparingly in patients with advanced renal failure.**

Uremic Neuropathy

Patients with CRF can develop a mononeuropathy or, more commonly, a polyneuropathy. **Uremic polyneuropathy is manifested by bilaterally symmetric impairment of both sensory and motor function.** The sensory changes typically occur in a glove-stocking distribution in the lower extremities and can be easily confused with the polyneuropathy of diabetes mellitus. Sensory symptoms usually develop first. Motor disturbances are a late finding and cause muscle wasting and weakness in the arms and legs. Physical findings include the loss of deep tendon reflexes and impaired vibrational, pain, light touch, and temperature sensation. **Dialysis is the treatment of choice for uremic neuropathy, but its success is dependent on the condition of the patient at the time it is started.** If the neuropathy is severe, especially if motor function has already been impaired, dialysis may only partially improve the symptoms even after several years. **Consequently, initiation of dialysis is indicated in patients with documented uremic neuropathy because clinical disability may not be reversible if therapy is delayed.**

Dialysis Disequilibrium

Dialysis disequilibrium is a neurologic disorder often associated with characteristic electroencephalogram (EEG) findings. It occurs either during or shortly after initiation of dialysis. Mild

TABLE 13–9. Signs and Symptoms of Uremic Encephalopathy

Early:	Anorexia, nausea, insomnia, restlessness, decreased attention span, decreased sexual interest
Moderate:	Vomiting, sluggishness, easy fatigue, drowsiness, sleep inversion, decreased sexual performance
Severe:	Itching, disorientation, bizarre behavior, myoclonus, asterixis, convulsions, stupor, coma

manifestations include nausea, emesis, restlessness, and headache. More serious complications such as seizures, obtundation, and coma can result. The cause of the syndrome is still in dispute, although evidence of brain swelling on head CT scans in affected patients implicates increased brain water content as the cause. Whether this cerebral edema results from the previous accumulation of so-called idiogenic osmols or from acute changes in cerebrospinal fluid pH is unsettled. Mannitol infusion during the initial dialysis may prevent the syndrome. Severe dialysis disequilibrium was more common in the past, when acutely uremic patients with very high BUN levels were dialyzed for prolonged periods. **Dialysis disequilibrium is prevented by initiating dialysis gradually in patients with markedly elevated BUN levels.**

Dialysis Dementia

Dialysis dementia, rarely encountered today, is a progressive, frequently fatal neurologic disease almost exclusively encountered in patients on long-term dialysis. The initial symptoms include dysarthria, apraxia, and speech disturbance. Patients may manifest personality changes, psychosis, seizures, and a characteristic EEG pattern. In most cases, the disease progresses to death in 6 months. **It has been reported that this disorder is caused by accumulation of aluminum in the brain from aluminum-containing antacids or aluminum-contaminated dialysis water. Aluminum intake should be avoided by patients with CRF.**

Gastrointestinal Disorders

GI disorders are common in patients with CRF, although whether they occur in greater frequency than in the general population remains controversial. However, it is certain that increased morbidity and mortality due to hemorrhage are present in ESRD. Two broad categories of disturbances can be identified in CRF, functional disorders and specific anatomic lesions.

Functional Disorders

GI symptoms are common in progressive CRF and include early morning nausea, anorexia, early satiety, and taste disturbances (dysgeusia). These may result from uremia itself or from medications used medically to treat the complications of progressive renal failure. Constipation is a common malady and may result from medications, dietary changes, fluid restriction, and inactivity. Gastric emptying can be delayed in patients with ESRD, resulting in early satiety and emesis. The cause is unknown, but dialysis amyloidosis due to accumulation and deposition of β_2-microglobulin may have a causative role.

Specific Anatomic Lesions

Various lesions of the GI tract that occur in CRF are outlined in Table 13–10. Upper GI hemorrhage is frequently reported in patients with CRF. On endoscopic examination, gastritis is noted in virtually all patients and may account for significant bleeding in more than 20% of patients. Likewise, erosive esophagitis is a common cause of bleeding (5% to 20%). **Telangiectasias (angiodysplasia) have been observed throughout the GI tract in CRF and are the most common cause of bleeding in patients.** The pathophysiologic basis of angiodysplasia is unknown, but it has been suggested to be an acquired lesion of aging. These lesions should be localized endoscopically and either cauterized or photo/cryocoagulated. Many of these lesions, however, are not visible or are beyond the reach of conventional endoscopic procedures. In these circumstances, therapy with combined estrogen-progesterone preparations may reduce the incidence of bleeding episodes. Surgical resection remains the final therapeutic option.

Lower GI tract lesions associated with severe renal failure include angiodysplasia, diverticulosis (the incidence is increased in patients with polycystic kidney disease), and colonic ulcers. Colonic perforation has been described in patients given Kayexalate retention enemas mixed with sorbitol. **In the diagnostic evaluation of the GI tract of symptomatic patients with CRF, endoscopy is recommended because radiologic procedures are less sensitive in detecting many of the lesions.**

TABLE 13–10. Gastrointestinal Lesions in Chronic Renal Failure

Oral: Stomatitis, parotitis
Esophageal: Esophagitis, Mallory-Weiss tear
Gastric: Gastritis, peptic ulcer, telangiectasias
Small bowel: Pepic ulcer (duodenum), duodenitis, telangiectasias
Large bowel: Cecal ulcers, stercoral ulcers, diverticulosis/diverticulitis, telangiectasias
Pancreatic: Pancreatitis
Hepatic: Congestive hepatomegaly, hepatitis C, cytomegalovirus

Skeletal Disorders

In advanced CRF, four forms of bone disease can be discerned: (1) secondary hyperparathyroidism (osteitis fibrosa cystica), (2) osteomalacia due to aluminum intoxication, (3) adynamic bone disease, and (4) β_2-microglobulin amyloidosis. **Maintenance of the integrity of the skeleton in CRF is achieved through (1) strict control of serum calcium and phosphorus levels, (2) administration of active vitamin D, (3) control of metabolic acidosis, and (4) avoidance of aluminum-containing products.**

Dialysis-associated amyloidosis is an often incapacitating complication for patients on dialysis. Deposits composed of β_2-microglobulin are predominantly localized in joints and periarticular bone. The principal manifestations are chronic arthralgia, carpal tunnel syndrome, and eventually destructive arthropathy, especially of the shoulders and hips. Cases of cervical spine deposits causing spinal cord compression, paralysis, and death have been described. **Accumulation of β_2-microglobulin is due to decreased renal clearance of the substance and possibly its increased generation when the blood comes into contract with material (cuprophane) used to manufacture certain types of dialysis membranes.**

Cardiovascular Disorders

Cardiovascular disease is the most common cause of death of patients with CRF. This most likely reflects the fact that heart disease and CRF share common risk factors such as hypertension and diabetes mellitus. Evidence suggests, however, that uremia itself may exacerbate heart disease. Patients with type I diabetes and nephropathy have a much higher risk of cardiac death than do those without nephropathy. Likewise, the hemodynamic stress of dialysis and the anemia and hyperlipidemia associated with CRF may adversely affect cardiac disease.

Hypertension in Chronic Renal Failure

More than 80% of patients have hypertension at the start of dialysis. This is typically the result of salt and water overload and responds well to the initiation of dialysis. Blood pressure medications often can be decreased or stopped after dialysis is started. In other patients, the hypertension is driven by increased vascular tone due to elevated systemic or local vasoconstrictor substances. In these cases, dialysis does not adequately control the blood pressure and an antihypertensive agent must be given.

Initially, euvolemia should be restored by imposing sodium restriction and increasing sodium excretion with the use of a diuretic. **Poorly controlled hypertension in a patient with CRF, despite high doses of conventional antihypertensive medications, often responds to the addition of a diuretic, demonstrating the volume dependence of the hypertension.**

If the blood pressure remains elevated after establishing euvolemia, medication should be started. Initial therapy may consist of a calcium channel antagonist, an ACE inhibitor, or an adrenergic blocker. Particular attention should be paid to the route of excretion, because some agents accumulate in renal failure, possibly causing severe hypotension. Also, the effects on serum potassium excretion should be considered when choosing an agent such as an ACE inhibitor or a beta blocker. Should this medication fail to control blood pressure adequately, an agent from one of the other two classes can be added to the regimen or a direct vasodilating agent such as hydralazine can be used. **Finally, if hypertension remains uncontrolled, minoxidil, the most potent vasodilator available, should be substituted. This agent causes reflex tachycardia and avid sodium retention, however, so a beta blocker and a diuretic should be used concomitantly.** Hirsutism and pericardial effusion are potential side effects of treatment with minoxidil. Bilateral nephrectomy is an infrequently used method for blood pressure control.

Ischemic Heart Disease

Ischemic heart disease develops frequently in patients with CRF. As previously discussed, hypertension is common in this population. Hypertension, along with anemia of CRF, results in left ventricular hypertrophy. Lipid abnormalities also are associated with CRF, particularly hypertriglyceridemia and depressed high-density lipoprotein levels. Finally, the most common cause of ESRD is diabetes mellitus, which also influences the development of ischemic heart disease.

The clinical manifestations of ischemic heart disease are no different in patients with CRF than in the general population. Similarly, medical management with nitrates, beta blockers, calcium channel antagonists, and anticoagulants is the same. However, the diagnosis of ischemic heart disease may be more difficult in CRF. **Levels of creatine phosphokinase (CK)-MB isoen-**

zymes and results of exercise and radionuclide stress testing may be altered in CRF.

Elevation in total CK can be found in 10% to
50% of patients with advanced CRF, usually less
than 3 times the upper limits of normal, although
levels 5 to 10 times greater are occasionally
found. Also, 5% to 30% of patients with advanced CRF without evidence of ischemia have
been reported to have an elevated percentage of
CK-MB in their sera. **In patients who have
CRF and who are suspected of having myocardial infarction, it is the pattern of change
in CK and CK-MB levels rather than absolute values that are diagnostic.**

Results of ECG exercise stress testing are frequently equivocal in patients with CRF because
of poor exercise capacity resulting from polyneuropathy, chronic anemia, and poor physical con-
ditioning. Thallium stress testing with the vasodilating agent dipyridamole produces a regional
hyperemia in proportion to the blood flow reserve of each coronary vessel, and results may be
inaccurate in CRF. The vasodilating effect of
dipyridamole is mediated by adenosine, levels of
which have been shown to be raised in CRF.
Abnormally elevated resting adenosine levels
may produce reduced vascular responsiveness to
dipyridamole, resulting in falsely negative responses in patients with CRF. **Consequently,
coronary angiography should be considered
in symptomatic patients who have a high risk
of ischemic heart disease and are acceptable
candidates for invasive therapies.**

Heart Failure

Congestive heart failure is common in CRF. It
may be due to depressed systolic function associated with a dilated left ventricle (60%) or due to
diastolic dysfunction related to a thickened and
stiff left ventricle with impaired diastolic filling
(40%). **Because treatments for these forms
of heart failure are different, cardiac function in symptomatic patients should be evaluated with echocardiography.**

Therapy of typical systolic heart failure includes decreasing the preload by establishing euvolemia and initiating appropriate medications
such as nitrates and diuretics.

Afterload reduction is accomplished by normalization of blood pressure. In this case, beta
blockers are generally avoided because they can
further impair compromised ventricular function.
The addition of digoxin to enhance ventricular
performance may also be necessary.

In patients with diastolic dysfunction, therapy
is aimed at reducing the degree of left ventricular

hypertrophy, controlling blood pressure, slowing
the heart rate to increase ventricular filling time,
and improving ventricular compliance. These
goals are achieved by correction of anemia and
administration of beta blockers, calcium channel
antagonists, and/or ACE inhibitors. In this patient population, the use of digoxin is not only
ineffective but can result in further cardiac decompensation.

PATIENT NUMBER 1 (continued)

*You again perform a detailed history taking and
physical examination of Martin and identify no
superimposed reversible process. He has not been
taking any new over-the-counter medications. No
physical findings suggest either volume overload or
depletion. You obtain a renal sonogram, which does
not show any evidence of urinary tract obstruction. A
repeated creatinine clearance determination is 10 ml/
min. In consultation with a nephrologist, you tell Martin
he will need dialysis in the very near future. At this
point, it is appropriate to inform Martin of his options
for treatment of ESRD. These include hemodialysis,
peritoneal dialysis, and, if medically fit,
transplantation. Through the local Kidney Foundation,
you supply him with written materials and videotapes
that review each of these modalities. The choice
ultimately is Martin's, and you should address his
questions and concerns openly and offer support when
you can during this difficult time. Until dialysis is
necessary, you will see him on a monthly basis. In the
meantime, in consultation with a nephrologist, you can
begin several therapeutic measures:*

1. *Continue the blood pressure medication and
   change his diuretic to furosemide.*
2. *Resume dietary restrictions.*
3. *Start calcium carbonate as a phosphate binder
   and to increase serum calcium levels.*
4. *Begin oral vitamin D (1,25-
   dihydroxycholecalciferol).*
5. *Add sodium bicarbonate tablets for the acidosis.*
6. *Administer subcutaneous EPO twice a week for
   anemia.*
7. *Avoid magnesium- and aluminum-containing
   products.*
8. *Schedule an appointment for Martin with a renal
   social worker, who will guide him through the
   multiple, often confusing steps necessary for
   patients with ESRD to receive health care
   benefits.*

DEFINITIVE TREATMENT FOR END-STAGE RENAL DISEASE

Preparation

As CRF progresses, patients should be informed
about the impending need for dialysis and be

given information about the various options available, including hemodialysis, peritoneal dialysis, and transplantation. This discussion should be started early in the course of the disease and should involve a social worker who is familiar with the problems unique to patients with CRF. The choice of treatment modality is typically personal and involves many factors such as family support, finances, living situation, eyesight, and patient motivation.

Access

Hemodialysis

Permanent access to the blood compartment must be created in patients. Two general types exist. Creation of an endogenous arteriovenous fistula (AVF) and anastomosis with a graft made of polytetrafluoroethylene (AVG). The most desirable method is the formation of an AVF. Compared with AVGs, AVFs have a much longer lifetime and are much less prone to thrombosis or infection. **To give a patient the best chance of receiving an AVF, the nondominant arm should not be used for blood pressure measurements or venipuncture.** An AVF typically takes 2 to 6 months to mature for use; thus, appropriate timing of surgery is necessary. Synthetic grafts, on the other hand, require only 2 to 3 weeks to mature. However, given the much higher complication rates, grafts are the less desirable form of vascular access.

Peritoneal Dialysis

A cuffed Tenckhoff catheter should be placed 2 to 3 weeks before initiation of dialysis to allow for peritoneal membrane closure and healing of the catheter tract.

Indications for Dialysis

In acute renal failure, dialysis is initiated to prevent life-threatening complications (Table 13–11). In CRF, however, the indications are often less firm. Dialysis is initiated when conservative management no longer maintains a patient's quality of life and productivity. The symptoms of CRF typically develop once the creatinine clearance falls below 10 ml/min, although they can occur earlier in diabetic patients. After chronic dialysis is initiated, patients usually note an improved sense of well-being, may consume a more liberal diet, and may require fewer medications, especially antihypertensives.

TABLE 13–11. Indications for the Initiation of Dialysis

Acute Indications
　Uremic syndrome
　Volume overload unresponsive to diuretics
　Hyperkalemia uncontrolled with therapy
　Severe metabolic acidosis
　Major bleeding episode

Chronic Indications

　Creatinine clearances <0.10–0.15 ml/min/kg lean body weight (GFR <8–10 ml/min). In diabetic, creatinine clearance <0.15–0.20 ml/min/kg (GFR <10–15 ml/min)

PATIENT NUMBER 1 (continued)

Martin returns in a month. He is feeling better and has chosen hemodialysis. He has made arrangements at the law firm to work around his dialysis schedule, including doing some work at home. He does not feel comfortable about doing "medical procedures," so he does not want peritoneal dialysis. He also does not want his girlfriend to see him with a tube in his stomach. Not now, but in the future, he'd also like to be evaluated for a kidney transplant. He admits that he now recognizes how important compliance with therapy is in order to maintain his sense of well-being. Repeat laboratory studies reveal creatinine 8 mg/dl, BUN 80 mg/dl, hemoglobin 9 mg/dl, calcium 9 mg/dl, phosphorus 5 mg/dl, potassium 4.9 mmol/L, and bicarbonate 22 mmol/L.

At this point, Martin should be observed monthly and monitored for any signs of uremia that would necessitate initiation of dialysis. Also, now is the time to schedule an appointment with a vascular surgeon to create vascular access, preferably an endogenous AVF.

SUMMARY

1. Determination of the chronicity of renal failure should be made by review of old medical records, assessment of renal size, and demonstration of renal osteodystrophy on bone radiographs.

2. Serum creatinine levels and calculated creatinine clearances are inaccurate measures of actual renal function because creatinine is affected by various factors including the degree of tubular secretion, amount of muscle mass, gender, diet, medications, and intercurrent illnesses.

3. A careful search should be made for superimposed reversible processes such as volume depletion, new medications, or urinary tract obstruction when renal function declines in a patient with CRF.

4. Meticulous control of hypertension, particularly with the use of ACE inhibitors, strict gly-

cemic control in diabetic patients, and dietary protein restriction are currently the methods used to slow the progression of renal failure.

5. The integrity of the skeleton in CRF is maintained by controlling serum calcium and phosphorus levels with the use of a low-phosphate diet and administration of calcium-containing phosphate binders and active vitamin D compounds, as well as correction of metabolic acidosis.

6. Cardiac disease is the leading cause of death in ESRD. Ischemic disease is treated medically or surgically in the usual way. Treatment of heart failure is dependent on determination of the type of dysfunction present (diastolic or systolic) by echocardiography.

7. Creation of an endogenous AVF is the preferred method of vascular access for hemodialysis because of its lower incidence of thrombosis and infection when compared with access created with a synthetic graft.

8. Dialysis may be initiated for life-threatening complications, particularly in the setting of acute renal failure, but in CRF it more often is started when conservative management no longer maintains a patient's quality of life and productivity.

SUGGESTED READINGS

Appeal G: Lipid abnormalities in renal disease. Kidney Int 39:169, 1991.

Brenner BM, Rector FC (eds): The Kidney, 4th ed. Philadelphia, WB Saunders, 1991.

Daugirdas JT, Ing TS (eds): Handbook of Dialysis, 2nd ed. Boston, Little, Brown & Co, 1994.

Elser AR: Gastrointestinal bleeding in maintenance dialysis patients. Semin Dialysis 1:198, 1988.

Eschbach JW, Egrie JC, Downing MR: Correction of the anemia of end stage renal disease with recombinant human erythropoietin. N Engl J Med 316:73, 1987.

Fraser CL, Arieff AI: Nervous system complications in uremia. Ann Intern Med 109:143, 1988.

Ma KW, Greene EL, Raij L: Cardiovascular risk factors in chronic renal failure and hemodialysis populations. Am J Kidney Dis 19:505, 1992.

Parfrey PS, Harnett JD, Griffiths SM, et al: Congestive heart failure in dialysis patients. Arch Intern Med 148:1519, 1988.

Schrier RW (ed): Manual of Nephrology. Boston, Little, Brown & Co, 1988.

Sherrard DJ, Hercz G, Pei Y, et al: The spectrum of bone disease in end-stage renal failure—an evolving disorder. Kidney Int 43:436, 1993.

United States Renal Data Report. Bethesda, MD, The National Institutes of Health, The National Institutes of Diabetes and Digestive and Kidney Diseases, Division of Kidney, Urologic and Hematologic Diseases, 1994.

14 | RENAL BONE DISEASES AND ALUMINUM TOXICITY IN RENAL PATIENTS

Jack W. Coburn, William G. Goodman, and Isidro B. Salusky

The kidneys maintain the body's external balance of calcium, phosphorus, and magnesium. They synthesize calcitriol (1,25-dihydroxycholecalciferol, or $1,25(OH)_2D_3$), the active form of vitamin D. They are a major target organ for parathyroid hormone (PTH) action and the site of its clearance and degradation. They are the major route of excretion for aluminum that enters the body, and they are responsible for the degradation and metabolism of the β_2-microglobulin that is synthesized in the body. Therefore, it is not surprising that mineral metabolism and the integrity of the skeletal system are altered as nephron function is lost.

Some degree of bone disease, collectively called *renal osteodystrophy,* nearly always accompanies chronic renal failure. Because several different disorders of bone can develop, they should be called the *renal bone diseases* or the *renal osteodystrophies,* as it is necessary to identify the predominant problem. Renal bone diseases are of several types, and a number of different pathogenic mechanisms are involved (Table 14–1). The first general type is normal- or high-turnover bone disease, which arises in large part from the action of excess PTH. A second general type is the low-turnover disorders; aluminum toxicity is a major pathogenic factor, and it produces either osteomalacia or "aplastic" or adynamic bone without excess osteoid. Another condition of low bone turnover lacks significant aluminum accumulation. The latter arises primarily from oversuppression of PTH action. Finally, a condition termed *dialysis amyloidosis* is not really a metabolic bone disease but affects bones, joints, and tendons and produces symptoms and findings that must be distinguished from the problems arising from altered mineral metabolism.

TABLE 14–1. Types of Disorders Affecting Bone in Renal Failure

High (or normal) bone turnover
  Osteitis fibrosa
  Mild hyperparathyroidism
Low bone turnover
  Aluminum toxicity
    Osteomalacia
    Aplastic bone disease with aluminum toxicity
    Adynamic bone without aluminum
Mixed bone disease
  Osteitis with marked hypocalcemia (unusual with modern therapy)
  Transition between lesion of osteitis fibrosa and osteomalacia
  Dialysis amyloidosis (β_2-microglobulin amyloid)

> **PATIENT NUMBER 1**
>
> Connie, a hemodialysis patient, presents with severe left leg pain. She is a 47-year-old secretary with end-stage renal disease (ESRD); she has undergone regular dialysis for 7 years. She has fared relatively well and has worked full time. She now presents with severe pain in the left pretibial area. The pain is aggravated by weight-bearing but gradually eases when she sits to relax at night. She has suffered no trauma, and she denies other pain. She has a full range of motion; the only finding on examination is minimal localized tenderness over the left upper pretibial area. Specific questioning reveals that she is less able to climb stairs without using a handrail and to rise to a standing position after sitting on a low couch; she must sit in a chair with armrests and push herself up with her arms. Her medications include long-acting diltiazem for hypertension, calcium carbonate tablets (500 mg, four with each meal), and a multivitamin.

SYMPTOMS AND CLINICAL FEATURES

Several symptoms or specific syndromes occur in association with the various renal bone diseases. However, the symptoms are vague and poorly defined and develop insidiously. Because few objective findings are noted, the nature of the problem is often overlooked until the condition is advanced. The symptoms are rarely specific to any particular disorder. The pain of hyperparathyroidism is typically worsened by weight-bearing activities. Most commonly, patients with severe secondary hyperparathyroidism have no symptoms at all.

Our patient Connie also has symptoms of proximal myopathy. This most commonly affects the lower extremities, causing difficulty climbing stairs or rising from a low chair. These symptoms are usually not mentioned by patients unless they are specifically asked about this weakness. Proximal myopathy can arise as a consequence of secondary hyperparathyroidism or aluminum toxicity and can occur in the absence of calcitriol even when PTH is not elevated. Why severe proximal myopathy is not observed more frequently in ESRD is unclear.

PATIENT NUMBER 1 (continued)

Connie was discovered to have renal disease at age 35 years. Her serum creatinine level was 220 μmol/L (2.5 mg/dl), and a renal biopsy showed interstitial nephritis. She failed to keep appointments with her physician until 8 years ago, when she became weak and tired easily. She was found to have severe renal insufficiency and was started on hemodialysis. Her symptoms improved, and she was able to continue working.

A review of the last year's predialysis monthly blood chemistry panels reveal serum calcium levels of 2.3 to 2.5 mmol/L (9.2 to 10.0 mg/dl) and serum phosphorus levels of 2.9 to 3.5 mmol/L (9.0 to 10.9 mg/dl). Connie states that she follows the prescribed doses of calcium carbonate given as phosphate binders. Her alkaline phosphatase level is 380 IU/L (normal 20 to 115 IU/L) with a GGT level of 20 U/L (normal 15 to 45); her serum aluminum value is 1.2 μmol/L (32 μg/L; normal < 0.3 μmol/L). The intact PTH value is 120 nmol/L (1240 pg/ml), normal 1.5 to 6.5 nmol/L; 1 year ago, the intact PTH was 90 nmol/ L (910 pg/ml). Skeletal radiographs show no abnormalities of her left tibia and no subperiosteal erosions. A bone scan reveals increased uptake throughout her skeleton, particularly in the skull and ends of the long bones; also noted is local increased uptake over the proximal left tibia.

Effect of Dialysis

In patients with advanced renal failure and ESRD, hyperphosphatemia is usual and metabolic acidosis is common. Patients dietary intake of calcium is often low, and they may have subop-

timal intake of vitamins, including vitamin D. The initiation of dialysis affects these parameters: The serum calcium level often rises, in part because of the use of dialysate calcium of 3.0 to 3.5 mEq/L, which leads to the net flux of calcium from dialysate into the patient. In patients undergoing continuous ambulatory peritoneal dialysis (CAPD), a tendency to hypoalbuminemia is commonly associated with normal total calcium levels despite an abnormally increased level of ionized calcium. Hyperphosphatemia is nearly universal in patients with ESRD, and initiation of dialysis affects levels of serum phosphorus less than serum calcium; it is often worse in those undergoing hemodialysis than CAPD. Thus, 90% to 95% of patients undergoing hemodialysis require phosphate-binding agents to reduce their predialysis serum phosphorus levels of 1.4 to 1.9 mmol/L (4.3 to 5.9 mg/dl), which are considered optimal levels in patients with ESRD. Acidosis improves with dialysis, but the serum bicarbonate levels are commonly subnormal when measured just before hemodialysis.

Alkaline Phosphatase

Bone alkaline phosphatase originates from osteoblasts, and the levels rise slowly and progressively as osteitis fibrosa develops. However, the levels often remain within the normal range; hence, alkaline phosphatase determination is not sensitive for detecting severe osteitis fibrosa in many patients. When the serum alkaline phosphatase level is elevated, the serum GGT or 5′ nucleotidase level should be determined to preclude a hepatic cause of the elevated level. Fractionation of alkaline phosphatase can be carried out, but it is costly and not readily available. For practical purposes, an elevated level of alkaline phosphatase with normal GGT activity defines bone alkaline phosphatase.

Parathyroid Hormone Levels

PTH levels are above normal in most patients with ESRD, but the degree of elevation is modified by PTH metabolism, the PTH antiserum used for the assay, and the degree of secondary hyperparathyroidism. Because of differences in PTH assays, a brief consideration of PTH metabolism is needed. Thus, PTH is secreted as the intact 84-amino-acid molecule that is quickly degraded into midregion and C-terminal fragments. With the midregion and certain C-terminal PTH assays, the magnitude of PTH elevation in renal failure is markedly accentuated because the clearance of these PTH fragments from the plasma is substantially reduced in renal failure. In patients with ESRD and moderate to severe osteitis fibrosa, the midregion PTH value exceeds the upper normal limit by at least 15 to 20 times, whereas the N-terminal or intact hormone assay values are at least four to five times normal. The two-site immunoradiometric (IRMA) or immunochemilucence (ICMA) intact PTH assays combine two antibodies, and both are more sensitive and more specific over a very wide range of values than are other types of PTH assays. A large population study of dialysis patients from Toronto (treated with either CAPD or hemodialysis) found that the intact PTH value must exceed threefold the upper normal before osteitis fibrosa occurs and must be seven times normal before all patients with significant osteitis fibrosa are included.

Connie's PTH levels are elevated to a level suggesting that she has marked secondary hyperparathyroidism.

Other Diagnostic Studies

For Connie, **bone radiographs** would be useful to preclude a local process affecting the tibia and causing the pain. A metabolic bone survey may reveal features of osteitis fibrosa (severe secondary hyperparathyroidism) and extraskeletal calcification. Subperiosteal erosions, the most sensitive radiographic feature of osteitis fibrosa, are most readily seen on the radial surfaces of the phalanges (Fig. 14–1). Very rarely, erosions occur in the sacroiliac joints, along the pubic rami, or along the lateral scapulae when hand films are negative. Brown tumors of osteitis fibrosa are rare in renal hyperparathyroidism. It should be remembered that the radiographic findings of erosions do not date their appearance unless an earlier radiograph is available for comparison. Also, a radiographic finding of erosions is not very sensitive, and the absence of erosions, as in Connie, does not rule out the presence of severe secondary hyperparathyroidism. Radiographs were useful for precluding extraskeletal calcifications in our patient. Indeed, such calcifications are common in patients such as Connie when the serum Ca × P product exceeds 6.0 (mmol × mmol) (>75 in mg/dl × mg/dl) (see Fig. 14–1).

A **bone scan** in patients with marked secondary hyperparathyroidism commonly shows increased isotope uptake in a diffuse and symmetric pattern. This scintiscan also detects extraskeletal calcifications, such as those in the lungs,

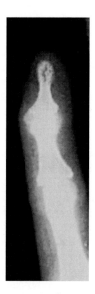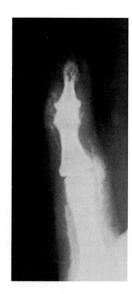

Figure 14–1. The patient is a 31-year-old woman who has end-stage renal disease managed with continuous ambulatory peritoneal dialysis. She developed pain, swelling, and warmth of her right index finger. She had recently become less compliant with the prescribed aluminum hydroxide, and her serum phosphorus level increased from 1.9 to 2.9 mmol/L (5.9 to 9.0 mg/dl), with a serum calcium level of 2.4 mmol/L (9.6 mg/dl). Radiographs showed the development of periarticular and soft-tissue calcifications during a 6-week period. Her pain responded to indomethacin treatment, and the swelling decreased after she had resumed her phosphate-binding agents. Parathyroidectomy was ultimately done because her serum phosphorus level remained elevated.

that are too diffuse to be detected by radiographs. Connie's scan revealed increased local uptake at the site of the leg pain. The mechanism by which this process is accentuated at some specific local area is unknown.

PATIENT NUMBER 1 (continued)

Connie is prescribed calcitriol, 1.0 and then 2.0 μg, with each hemodialysis; also, she is more compliant in adhering to her low-phosphorus diet. Her leg pain decreases and finally disappears. She can climb stairs more easily, and she rises from a chair with less difficulty. Her alkaline phosphatase level fell over 3 months to 150 IU/L, and her intact PTH to 550 pg/ml. Her serum phosphorus level fell to 2.2 mmol/L (6.8 mg/dl) but later rose to 2.8 mmol/L (8.7 mg/dl); her serum Ca level was 2.8 mmol/L (11.2 mg/dl) and later was 2.9 mmol/L (11.6 mg/dl).

MANAGEMENT

The appropriate treatment of our patient Connie can be considered for the various stages of her renal failure. During the earlier period, when she had a serum creatinine level of 220 μmol/L (2.5 mg/dl), several treatment options might delay or even prevent the development of secondary hyperparathyroidism. Several placebo-controlled studies document the safety and effectiveness of daily oral therapy with low doses of calcitriol or 1-α(OH)-vitamin D in patients with stable renal disease and creatinine clearances of 15 to 45 ml/min. In these trials, various features of secondary hyperparathyroidism observed in bone biopsy specimens improved, serum PTH levels were reduced, and no worsening of renal function occurred in comparison with placebo-treated patients. Reliable data indicate that dietary phosphate restriction or appropriate administration of oral calcium carbonate or calcium acetate as phosphate binders also retards the development of secondary hyperparathyroidism. However, no controlled trials document the effectiveness of these therapeutic maneuvers. One major problem is that most asymptomatic patients with mild to moderate renal insufficiency do not seek medical care until they reach more advanced renal failure, or patients may be unwilling to follow complex therapeutic regimens, as was the case with Connie. Nonetheless, these therapeutic measures should be considered, particularly for individuals who have greater risk factors for developing high-turnover bone disease, as in our patient Connie (Table 14–2).

Several aspects of management of secondary hyperparathyroidism are appropriate in **ESRD.** These include **control of hyperphosphatemia,** choice of **proper dialysate calcium,** the use of **vitamin D sterols,** and, when needed, **parathyroidectomy.**

TABLE 14–2. Factors Predisposing to High/Normal- Versus Low-Turnover Bone Disease

High/Normal Turnover	Low Turnover
Children; young adults > older patients	Diabetes mellitus
Long duration of renal insufficiency	Prior parathyroidectomy
Long duration of dialysis	Prior renal transplant (steroids)
Female > male patients	Aluminum exposure (dialysate, oral)
Tubulointerstitial diseases > glomerular diseases	Binephrectomy
Hyperphosphatemia (via increased PTH)	Calcitriol therapy, CaCO$_3$ or Ca-acetate therapy
	High Ca in CAPD solutions

Phosphate control, ineffective in Connie's case, is one of the most important and yet difficult aspects of management in patients with ESRD. The maintenance of proper serum phosphorus levels in such patients involves **(1) dietary phosphate restriction, (2) proper use of phosphate-binding agents,** and **(3) adequate phosphate removal by dialysis.** The difficulties in preventing hyperphosphatemia arise because of poor compliance with phosphate-restricted diets (particularly in the United States and Canada, where the diet is high in phosphate content), the high efficiency of phosphate absorption by the gut, the low "potency" of phosphate-binding agents so that very large doses are required, and the relatively small quantities of phosphate removed by most dialysis procedures. Dialysis is ineffective in the removal of phosphate because only a small fraction of phosphate is present in plasma and the ECF compartment and because of the relatively poor permeability of most dialysis membranes to phosphate itself.

Dietary phosphate should be lower than 900 to 1000 mg/day; this can be accomplished by eliminating dairy products and restricting foods prepared with dairy products. Nonetheless, more than 50% of ingested phosphate is absorbed by many patients with ESRD, while the net removal of phosphate by thrice-weekly dialysis rarely exceeds 400 mg/day when the net removal is extrapolated over 7 days per week. Simple mathematics indicates the need for phosphate binders. It is our **strong recommendation** that only the calcium-based phosphate binders, calcium carbonate or calcium acetate, be prescribed except in very rare situations. The dose required may be quite high and is usually adjusted empirically. When a patient such as Connie increases her phosphate intake, much larger doses of binders are required. A small fraction of the calcium may be absorbed, thus increasing the risk of hypercalcemia. This risk of hypercalcemia can be largely avoided by reducing the **dialysate calcium** to 2.5 mEq/L (1.25 mmol/L). In rare circumstances, dialysate calcium concentrations as low as 2.0 mEq/L (1.0 mmol/L) are needed. The choice between calcium carbonate and calcium acetate must be made for individual patients. Calcium carbonate is available in many forms and is considerably cheaper; some patients are able to control their serum phosphorus levels only with calcium acetate. Calcium citrate should not be used because the citrate markedly augments the absorption of aluminum (see the later section on patient 2).

Using adequate dialysis for the removal of phosphate is also important. The presence of a very small fraction of exchangeable phosphate in the ECF and its relatively slow flux out of other compartments limit the net phosphate removal during hemodialysis. Within the first 30 to 45 minutes of dialysis, serum phosphorus concentrations fall strikingly to values about one third of the predialysis value; thereafter, the levels remain relatively stable at 0.65 to 1.0 mmol/L (2.0 to 3.1 mg/dl). Thus, the gradient for net transfer of phosphate from the plasma to dialysate falls, further reducing the amount of phosphate removed during the later hours of hemodialysis. Peritoneal dialysis, which is considerably less efficient than hemodialysis in removing solutes such as urea and creatinine, leads to better phosphate removal than hemodialysis because the gradient between plasma and dialysate always remains high with the former. For this reason, patients undergoing CAPD often require lower doses of phosphate-binding agents than those on hemodialysis.

Calcitriol therapy is an important tool for the control of secondary hyperparathyroidism in patients with ESRD. The disappearance of Connie's localized bone pain provided strong evidence that this pain had osteitis fibrosa as its basis. A significant decrease in PTH levels was noted, although the levels were still high. The persistent hyperphosphatemia and hypercalcemia precluded the continued use of vitamin D. Whether it might have been possible to reduce the dialysate calcium even lower, use larger doses of calcium carbonate to lower the serum phosphorus level, and increase the dose of calcitriol to produce greater PTH suppression is conjectural. Current evidence suggests that pulse therapy with either intravenous or oral calcitriol is equally effective in reducing PTH levels; moreover, pulse therapy is probably more effective than continuous low daily oral doses. Hyperphosphatemia is one factor that prevents adequate suppression of PTH levels by pulse-dose calcitriol. Our inability to control Connie's hyperphosphatemia was a major factor predicting that calcitriol therapy would ultimately fail.

PATIENT NUMBER 1 (continued)

Because of the rise in serum Ca and P, calcitriol is discontinued. A bone biopsy shows features of osteitis fibrosa with negative aluminum staining. Parathyroidectomy is recommended, and Connie agrees.

Parathyroidectomy

A decision was finally made to remove Connie's hyperplastic parathyroid glands surgically. Sec-

ondary hyperparathyroidism sometimes requires parathyroidectomy. Aluminum-related bone disease must be ruled out, and severe secondary hyperparathyroidism must be documented by biochemical, roentgenographic, and bone histologic criteria. The indications include (1) the appearance of calciphylaxis, (2) severe skeletal pain and myopathy, (3) progressive extraskeletal calcifications and refractory hyperphosphatemia, (4) persistent hypercalcemia (serum calcium level > 2.9 to 3.0 mmol/L, or 11.6 to 12.0 mg/dl), and (5) pruritus intractable to dialysis or other medical treatment. When hypercalcemia does develop, other causes of hypercalcemia, including sarcoidosis, hypercalcemia of malignancy, and the excess intake of calcium and vitamin D, must be considered and ruled out. An algorithm to follow in reaching a decision for parathyroidectomy is shown in Figure 14–2.

Our patient Connie had symptomatic hyperparathyroidism with bone pain and proximal myopathy. She had mild hypercalcemia and hyperphosphatemia, with a serum Ca × P product exceeding 6.0 (>75 in mg/dl); the latter precluded the continued administration of calcitriol.

PATIENT NUMBER 1 (continued)

At Connie's surgery, three very large parathyroid glands are easily located; the fourth gland (the right superior) is much smaller. A fifth parathyroid gland, weighing 2.8 g, is removed with the thymus. The first three large glands (weighing 2.4, 3.5, and 4.5 g, respectively) are removed; the right superior gland, which is most normal in gross appearance, is transected, leaving one fourth behind; the excised portion weighs 800 mg. The four largest glands are irregular and nodular, showing pseudoadenomatous changes.

The optimal surgical procedure (e.g., subtotal parathyroidectomy, total parathyroidectomy plus forearm transplantation of parathyroid fragments, or total parathyroidectomy) depends in part on the operative findings. The choice of a surgeon with broad experience with parathyroid surgery in patients with ESRD is critical. Recurrence of hyperparathyroidism from hyperplasia of remnant parathyroid tissue (either in the neck or in transplanted tissue in the forearm) versus induction of aplastic bone because of subnormal PTH levels is a factor to consider in a decision about the type of surgery. If only three glands are found, they should all be removed under the assumption that a fourth gland has not been located.

Our surgeon chose to excise totally the three largest glands, leaving a portion of the smallest

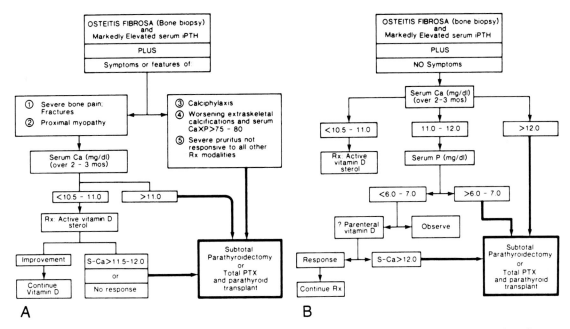

Figure 14–2. Algorithm showing an approach to decision-making for parathyroidectomy in secondary hyperparathyroidism in a patient with end-stage renal disease with symptoms (A) or without symptoms (B). (Reprinted from Salusky IB, Coburn JW: The renal osteodystrophies. *In* DeGroot LJ, et al (eds): Endocrinology, 2nd ed. Philadelphia, WB Saunders, 1989.)

and most normal-appearing gland in the neck. As noted, other surgeons choose to remove all the parathyroid glands and to transplant small portions of the gland to the forearm muscles.

PATIENT NUMBER 1 (continued)

Postoperatively, serum Ca and phosphorus are measured every 8 hours. By 24 hours after surgery, Connie's serum Ca level fell to 1.85 mmol/L (7.4 mg/dl) and her phosphorus to 1.55 mmol/L (4.8 mg/dl). An infusion of calcium gluconate is prepared with 100 ml of 10% Ca gluconate added to 200 ml of 5% dextrose in water; this is infused at 30 ml/hr and delivers approximately 2.5 mmol (100 mg) of elemental calcium per hour. The patient is also given oral calcitriol, 1.0 μg twice daily; calcium carbonate is given orally in doses of 4.8 g every 4 hours. After the calcium gluconate infusion is started, serum Ca is measured every 4 hours to be certain that hypercalcemia does not ensue. Twenty-four hours later, the calcium gluconate infusion is discontinued when serum Ca level rises to 2.25 mmol/L (9.0 mg/dl). During the next few days, Connie's serum Ca level ranges from 2.1 to 2.2 mmol/L and her serum phosphorus level is 1.2 to 0.71 mmol/L. Four weeks later, her serum Ca level increases to 2.4 mmol/L; calcitriol is discontinued, but the calcium carbonate is continued at 2.4 g with each meal. Her serum phosphorus level stabilizes at 1.7 to 1.8 mmol/L (5.2 to 5.6 mg/dl). Her muscle strength improves, and she climbs stairs normally.

Postoperative Management After Parathyroid Surgery and the Hungry Bone Syndrome

Preoperatively, patients should receive calcitriol, 1 to 2 μg/day for 2 to 3 days before surgery to raise intestinal calcium transport to a high level immediately after surgery. When the serum calcium level decreases below 1.9 to 2.0 mmol/L (7.6 to 8.0 mg/dl) postoperatively, intravenous calcium gluconate should be prepared to provide 2.5 mmol of calcium per hour (100 mg/hr of elemental calcium). If the serum calcium level continues to fall, the rate of the infusion should be doubled. Intravenous infusion of calcium may be necessary for as briefly as 24 to 48 hours until the net intestinal absorption of calcium increases appropriately. If the postoperative fall of serum Ca is less than 0.4 to 0.5 mmol/L (<1.6 to 2.0 mg/dl), it is likely that a large parathyroid gland has not been discovered and thus remains in place or that the skeletal histology was not that of osteitis fibrosa.

Connie developed substantial hypocalcemia as well as a fall in serum phosphorus levels after parathyroidectomy. These are features of the hungry bone syndrome, which results from rapid remineralization of bone with deposition of calcium, phosphorus, and magnesium into the bone. The hypocalcemia can be profound and can lead to tetany and major seizures; the latter can be very violent and can cause major fractures and rupture of tendons. For this reason, it is critical to monitor serum calcium and phosphorus levels frequently after surgery and to treat hypocalcemia with intravenous calcium in adequate amounts and begin therapy with large doses of calcitriol and oral calcium. If the serum magnesium level falls to subnormal levels, supplemental magnesium should be given.

In Connie, the hungry bone syndrome was relatively short lived, probably because of the long period of calcitriol therapy before the parathyroidectomy. In patients with markedly elevated alkaline phosphatase levels, hypocalcemia can persist as long as 2 to 3 months. Initiation of oral calcium replacement and large doses of calcitriol hastens the recovery. Such patients ultimately do not need calcitriol and require oral calcium salts only as a phosphate-binding agent. Serum phosphorus levels fall as well; hypophosphatemia does not require treatment unless the levels fall below 0.60 mmol/L (1.8 mg/dl). Administration of any phosphate markedly aggravates the tendency to profound hypocalcemia; thus, phosphate replacement should be avoided unless the hypophosphatemia is quite severe. Hypomagnesemia occasionally develops with the hungry bone syndrome, and supplemental magnesium is also needed. Aluminum-containing gels should be avoided postoperatively because of the risk of aluminum-related bone disease (see the later section on patient 2). The finding of five parathyroid glands, present in about 1% of the population, indicates the importance of a skilled and highly experienced parathyroid surgeon who is familiar with the varied parathyroid anatomy.

General Discussion

Our patient Connie developed severe and symptomatic secondary hyperparathyroidism. She eventually developed symptoms that required parathyroidectomy. Increased secretion of PTH probably began several years before she started dialysis and when her serum creatinine was "only" 220 μg/L. The processes that contribute to the development of secondary hyperparathyroidism include (1) phosphate retention (but often with little or no initial rise in serum phosphorus level), (2) reduced renal synthesis of calcitriol, (3) reduced responsiveness of bone to the calcemic effect of PTH, and (4) a fall in the ionized Ca level in the blood (Table 14–3). As parathyroid hyperplasia develops, changes in the

parathyroid glands *per se* often occur so that higher concentrations of calcium are needed to suppress the PTH secretion by individual parathyroid glands. This is termed a *shift in the setpoint* for calcium-mediated PTH suppression. When this occurs, a higher serum calcium level is needed to reduce PTH secretion. In advanced renal failure, true hyperphosphatemia is prevalent, hypocalcemia is more common, and the intestinal absorption of calcium is reduced. The parathyroid glands undergo changes, with diffuse hyperplasia being replaced by areas of adenomatous hyperplasia. The parathyroid cells from the areas of adenomatous hyperplasia have reduced numbers of receptors for vitamin D; hence, suppression of PTH secretion during calcitriol therapy is less. Other cellular changes may occur, with a specific chromosome loss, and the cells can exhibit monoclonal behavior. As a result of the marked hyperplasia that occurs with enlargement of the glands, the secretion of PTH is greatly amplified.

Interactions among these regulatory factors are complex. For example, phosphate retention, perhaps at an intracellular level and without a perceptible change in serum phosphorus level, can inhibit calcitriol synthesis; this reduced calcitriol synthesis can lead to less normal feedback suppression of PTH by an elevated calcium level. Despite increased PTH secretion, the diseased kidneys' synthesis of calcitriol is not adequate to reverse the process; hence, even more PTH is required.

Vitamin D Metabolism

The kidneys are the major organs responsible for maintaining the normal serum levels of calcitriol, the most active form of vitamin D. Calcitriol synthesis is stimulated by PTH, hypocalcemia *per se,* and a reduced dietary intake of phosphate. Calcitriol synthesis is inhibited by the opposite changes and by calcitriol *per se*. The actions of calcitriol include stimulating the intestinal absorption of both calcium and phosphorus (slightly less for the latter) and suppression of PTH secretion, both by a direct effect of PTH to inhibit the message for synthesis of prepro-PTH, an initial step in PTH synthesis, and indirectly by raising the serum calcium level. Calcitriol also affects the metabolism of bone cells and modulates the function of the immune system.

It was initially believed that reduced calcitriol synthesis was the major factor causing osteomalacia in renal failure; however, the abnormal vita-

TABLE 14–3. Factors Contributing to High Serum PTH Levels in Renal Failure and Responsible Pathogenic Mechanisms

Cause of Increased PTH	Pathogenic Mechanisms
Hypocalcemia	Hyperphosphatemia, low serum calcitriol levels, skeletal resistance to PTH action on bone
Low calcitriol levels	Phosphate retention, nephron destruction, metabolic acidosis, altered transtubular phosphate flux
Shift of parathyroid set-point (higher calcium needed to suppress PTH secretion per cell)	Phosphate retention, low calcitriol level, ? other
Nodular parathyroid hyperplasia	Decreased density of vitamin D receptors
Diffuse parathyroid hyperplasia	Reduced serum calcitriol, phosphate retention, ? other
Chromosome loss in parathyroid cells	Unknown: results in autonomous PTH secretion
Skeletal resistance to PTH action	Down-regulation of PTH receptors, hyperphosphatemia, low calcitriol
Reduced PTH degradation—interpretation of PTH assay	Reduced renal clearance of PTH fragments (midregion, C-terminal)

min D metabolism does contribute in a major way to the development of secondary hyperparathyroidism. Phosphate retention (even without an increase in serum phosphorus level) is of importance in reducing calcitriol synthesis in early renal failure. Increased extrarenal synthesis of calcitriol can occur when the plasma levels of 25(OH)D are raised markedly during treatment with pharmacologic doses of vitamin D_3 or 25(OH)D_3. Abnormal vitamin D metabolism rarely causes osteomalacia in patients with renal failure; such an occurrence is likely limited to patients with coexistent vitamin D deficiency, as indicated by subnormal serum levels of 25(OH)D, the circulating form of vitamin D. It is likely to occur before ESRD is reached, and it presents in patients who do not have significant hyperphosphatemia.

When did secondary hyperparathyroidism develop in Connie? We don't know for certain, but it is likely that serum PTH levels were significantly elevated when her serum creatinine level was 220 μmol/L (2.5 mg/dl). A review of her early dialysis records shows that her serum calcium level was 2.15 to 2.20 mmol/L (8.6 to 8.8 mg/dl) during the first 3 months of starting dialysis; thereafter, her serum Ca level rose to 2.4 mmol/L (9.6 mg/dl). Consuming large doses of calcium carbonate as a phosphate binder contributes to normal or even slightly elevated serum calcium levels among patients undergoing dialysis. A long duration of slowly progressive renal failure, the presence of tubulointerstitial disease, and an increased duration of dialysis are risk factors for development of progressive and significant secondary hyperparathyroidism. Younger patients and females are also at greater risk.

A bone biopsy, performed after double tetra-cycline labeling and with the preparation of un-decalcified specimens, provides precise identification of the nature of the bone disease present. Surface staining for aluminum is important to preclude the presence of significant aluminum loading; very rarely, iron localization can be the cause of osteomalacia. Most hospital pathology laboratories are not able to prepare histologic sections of undecalcified bone or to use the special stains required; hence, the samples must be sent to specialized laboratories. Tetracycline (0.5 g b.i.d. for 2 days) is given over two periods separated by a specific interval (usually 12 to 18 days) for double labeling. This permits the measure of bone formation rate and the distinction of low-, normal-, and high-turnover states. A bone biopsy can be easily performed in an outpatient setting with local anesthetic combined with intravenous analgesia similar to that used for gastrointestinal endoscopy (e.g., intravenous low-dose midazolam and meperidine). In general, a bone biopsy is needed only for problem cases, for making decisions about parathyroidectomy, to rule out aluminum toxicity, or to identify the cause of hypercalcemia.

Severe hyperparathyroidism leads to peritrabecular fibrosis (osteitis fibrosa) and high bone turnover, as noted in Connie's bone biopsy specimen. The osteoid seams may be wide, as occurs with osteomalacia; however, the presence of increased bone formation permits a clear distinction between osteitis fibrosa and osteomalacia. The absence of aluminum staining is useful to preclude the rare coexistence of aluminum loading and hyperparathyroidism (see the later section on patient 2). Patients occasionally show mixed renal bone disease, with features of both osteitis fibrosa and osteomalacia with impaired

TABLE 14–4. Clinical Features of the Renal Bone Diseases and the Associated Etiologic Factors

Clinical Feature	Pathologic Process
Bone pain	Aluminum, β_2-M-amyloid, osteitis fibrosa
Acute periarthritis, joint pain	β_2-M-amyloid, high PTH, periarticular calcifications
Proximal myopathy	Aluminum, high PTH, reduced vitamin D
Pruritus	High PTH, high serum P, hypercalcemia (any cause), uremia itself
Fractures	Aluminum, β_2-M-amyloid, osteitis fibrosa
Skeletal deformities	Aluminum > osteitis fibrosa (except in children)
Bone cysts	β_2-M-amyloid >> osteitis fibrosa
Osteopenia	Aluminum, β_2-M-amyloid
Extraskeletal calcifications	Phosphate excess, high PTH, low serum Mg, high calcitriol
Tendon rupture	High PTH; β_2-M-amyloid

Aluminum, aluminum accumulation; β_2-M-amyloid, β_2-microglobulin amyloidosis.

mineralization. These most often represent a transition from one disorder to another.

SYMPTOMS AND CLINICAL SYNDROMES ASSOCIATED WITH SECONDARY HYPERPARATHYROIDISM

Several symptoms or specific syndromes occur in association with secondary hyperparathyroidism.

Symptoms are often vague and poorly defined, and they develop insidiously. Because there are few objective findings, the clinical condition is often overlooked until it is advanced. Similar symptoms can result from totally different pathogenetic processes (Table 14–4), yet the management must be tailored to the specific cause.

Muscle weakness affects the proximal muscles of the lower extremities, making it difficult to climb stairs or to rise from a low chair. Bone pain may or may not be present. Vague, deep pains in the back, hips, legs, and/or knees are often related to weight-bearing or a change in position. The pain, particularly with dialysis amyloidosis, is worse at night. Hyperparathyroidism can occasionally cause localized, severe bone pain (e.g., involving a pretibial area, ankle, or hip), as occurred in our patient Connie. Localized bony tenderness may or may not be a feature. Skeletal deformities are much more common in children than in adults but can occur in adults as a result of altered bone remodeling or osteomalacia.

Connie's improvement of her pain during treatment with calcitriol provided support for the view that secondary hyperparathyroidism was the cause of her localized tibial pain, which is an unusual feature of hyperparathyroidism. Connie lacked certain features of secondary hyperparathyroidism. She did not have pruritus, which is often severe in patients with marked hyperparathyroidism. Also, she did not have obvious extraskeletal calcifications ("metastatic" calcifications), which can be profound in patients with ESRD (Fig. 14–1 and Table 14–5).

Pruritus can occur with uremia *per se*, with

TABLE 14–5. Types of Extraskeletal (Metastatic) Calcifications, Pathogenic Factors, and Their Management

Type/Location	Pathogenic Factor	Consequences	Management
Conjunctival	High pH of eye High Ca × P product	Acute: "red eye" Chronic: "white eye" with calcific plaque	Reduce Ca × P Product
Periarticular	High Ca × P product	Acute "arthritis" or periarthritis	PO$_4$ control, PTX
Tumoral	High Ca × P product	Periarticular masses, restricted motion Local pain, inflammation minimal	PO$_4$ control, PTX
Pulmonary	Unknown°	Pulmonary insufficiency, pulmonary hypertension	Unknown
Cardiac	Unknown°	Arrhythmias, cardiac failure	Unknown
Vascular	?, low serum magnesium *Plus* high PTH and high serum P	Often no symptoms Calciphylaxis (rare)	None known PTX for calciphylaxis

°The chemical composition of these visceral calcifications differs from that of other extraskeletal calcifications.

PTX, parathyroidectomy.

Modified from Coburn JW, Slatopolsky E: Vitamin D, parathyroid hormone, and the renal osteodystrophies. *In* Brenner BM, Rector FC Jr (eds): The Kidney, 4th ed. Philadelphia, WB Saunders, 1990.

secondary hyperparathyroidism, with marked hyperphosphatemia, and with hypercalcemia *per se*. If hypercalcemia is present, lower-calcium dialysate may be needed; if hyperphosphatemia exists, efforts at phosphate restriction should be vigorous. **Parathyroid surgery should be performed for pruritus only when evidence of marked hyperparathyroidism is unequivocal.**

Acute periarticular inflammation or true arthritis can develop as a consequence of extraskeletal calcifications or pseudogout. Symptoms and signs can appear over 1 to 2 days, and radiographs often show periarticular calcifications (see Fig. 14–1). Acute symptoms often respond to therapy with antiinflammatory agents. If hyperphosphatemia develops, it should be treated. Patients undergoing dialysis rarely develop acute gouty arthritis.

Spontaneous tendon rupture occurs not infrequently in patients on dialysis; the Achilles, quadriceps, and digital tendons are most often involved. The cause is unknown, but its association with evidence of overt secondary hyperparathyroidism and its occurrence in primary hyperparathyroidism suggest that high PTH levels predispose to the process.

Calciphylaxis is an unusual syndrome characterized by peripheral ischemia, skin necrosis, and vascular calcifications. It evolves in dialysis patients with a history of uncontrolled hyperphosphatemia and hyperparathyroidism (Fig. 14–3). It may progress quickly and be fatal; at times, its

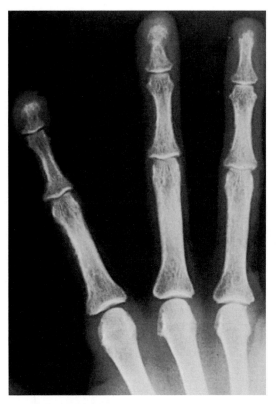

Figure 14–4. Right hand of a 32-year-old woman with juvenile polycystic disease and congenital hepatic fibrosis. During 4 years of hemodialysis, the midregion parathyroid hormone rose slowly from 24,000 to 79,000 pg/ml and alkaline phosphatase increased to 744 IU/ml. She had a ruptured quadriceps tendon in the past, but she otherwise lacked musculoskeletal symptoms. Radiographs show subperiosteal erosions on the radial surfaces of the second and third digits; there were also erosions and bulbar deformities of the distal phalanges, producing pseudoclubbing.

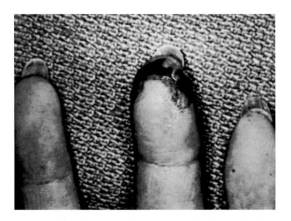

Figure 14–3. This hemodialysis patient developed painful ischemic lesions of his fingers; his serum calcium level had been 2.4 mmol/L (9.6 mg/dl), serum phosphorus level 3.4 mmol/L (10.5 mg/dl), alkaline phosphatase level 335 IU/ml, and parathyroid hormone level 12 times normal with an "intact assay." Because of the progression of the lesion, parathyroidectomy was done, with disappearance of pain within 4 to 5 days and healing of the lesion by 6 weeks.

course is often reversed by parathyroidectomy. Patients with diabetes mellitus can show similar features, but the course is little affected by such surgery.

Overt secondary hyperparathyroidism is defined by the presence of markedly elevated PTH levels and bone biopsy specimens showing severe osteitis fibrosa. These patients may have no bone pain or any of the symptoms or signs noted above. Biochemical observations include normal or increased serum calcium levels, serum phosphorus levels that are often elevated and refractory to phosphate binders, and bone alkaline phosphatase levels that show a progressive increase over time. Radiographs commonly show subperiosteal erosions and extraskeletal calcifications (see Figs. 14–1 and 14–4).

PATIENT NUMBER 2

Bobby is referred because of azotemia, skeletal deformities, bone pain, and hypercalcemia.

Bobby is a 10-year-old boy who is referred from a town in Arizona for evaluation regarding bone pain, poorly healing fractures, and an inability to walk.

At age 4, he had been seen with a 2-year history of polydipsia, polyuria, and enuresis associated with retardation of growth. He had not been ill except for repeated urinary tract infections. He was smaller than his siblings, but his ability to walk and his neurologic development were normal. He was found to have increased levels of serum creatinine and blood urea. Serum P level was normal, and serum Ca level was low. He had metabolic acidosis with a serum bicarbonate value of 14 mmol/L. A cystourethrogram disclosed a large bladder without obstruction or ureteral reflux. Aortography showed absence of the left kidney and a small dysplastic right kidney.

He was treated with dihydrotachysterol, 0.2 mg/day, aluminum hydroxide gel, 10 ml q.i.d., and sodium citrate solution (Bicitra) to treat his metabolic acidosis.

When Bobby was 5 years old, he had a fracture of his right forearm, which healed with closed treatment. He developed seizures, which various medications, including phenobarbital, valproic acid, and carbamazepine, failed to control. A fall when he was 6 resulted in a pathologic fracture of the left femur that failed to heal after immobilization for 7 months; he did not regain the ability to walk. Serum C-terminal PTH level was elevated to 10 times normal, and he had hypercalcemia. On the basis of these findings, a subtotal parathyroidectomy was performed. His parathyroid glands were enlarged to approximately two to three times the normal size, and histologic findings showed parathyroid hyperplasia.

Approach to the Patient

Bobby presented with hypercalcemia and certain radiographic features of secondary hyperparathyroidism that represented earlier erosions that had not mineralized when aluminun-related bone disease replaced the osteitis fibrosa. These manifestations of aluminum-related bone disease have been termed *pseudohyperparathyroidism*; other causes of hypercalcemia are listed in Table 14–6. In the past, the findings of hypercalcemia, symptomatic bone disease, and radiographic features of earlier hyperparathyroidism led to parathyroid surgery that was often not indicated.

TABLE 14–6. Causes of Hypercalcemia in Patients Undergoing Dialysis

1. Secondary hyperparathyroidism (usually severe)
2. Aluminum-related bone disease
3. Low bone turnover without aluminum (adynamic bone) with calcium salts as PO_4 binders
4. Therapy with calcitriol or other vitamin D sterol
5. Large doses of $CaCO_3$ or Ca-acetate (particularly with 1 or 2 above)
6. Dialysate Ca > 3.0 to 3.5 mEq/L (particularly CAPD)
7. Extrarenal nonrenal calcitriol synthesis (sarcoidosis, tuberculosis, or other granulomatous disorder)
8. Immobilization (particularly in patients with 1, 2, 3, or 6 above)
9. Malignancy: Renal cell carcinoma; neoplasm of lung or gastrointestinal tract; multiple myeloma
10. Marked hypophosphatemia

Modified from Coburn JW, Slatopolsky E: Vitamin D, parathyroid hormone, and the renal osteodystrophies. *In* Brenner BM, Rector FC Jr (eds): The Kidney, 4th ed. Philadelphia, WB Saunders, 1990.

PATIENT NUMBER 2 *(continued)*

Postoperatively, Bobby's C-terminal PTH levels were within the normal range, and his serum phosphorus was maintained at normal levels with aluminum hydroxide. However, the poor healing of bone persisted; he subsequently developed additional fractures of the long bones. He led a bed-to-chair existence.

Examination when Bobby was first seen at UCLA disclosed evidence of marked growth retardation with severe angulation of the right arm due to malunion of a humeral fracture and bilateral angular deformities of both lower extremities. He was unable to walk because of bone deformities and pain.

His serum creatinine and urea nitrogen levels had remained stable, and his creatinine clearance was 25 ml/min/1.73 m². His serum phosphorus level was 1.2 to 1.4 mmol/L (3.7 to 4.3 mg/dl), and serum calcium level was 2.8 mmol/L (11.2 mg/dl). A midregion PTH value was 1380 pg/ml (normal 80 to 330 pg/ml). His alkaline phosphatase level was 140 IU/L; GGT, 14 U/L. His serum electrolyte determinations included sodium 144 mmol/L, potassium 3.6 mmol/L, chloride 116 mmol/L, and bicarbonate 18 mmol/L. His plasma aluminum level was 8.8 μmol/L (255 μg/L); normal <0.3 μmol/L (<8 μg/L). Twenty-four hours after the infusion of deferoxamine (DFO), 40 mg/kg, his serum aluminum level rose to 44.5 mmol/L (1200 μg/L).

Serum Aluminum

Plasma or serum aluminum levels are often above normal in patients with ESRD (normal range <0.3 mmol/L or <10 μg/L), but the levels are usually below 1.5 mmol/L (40 μg/L) unless there is an exogenous source of aluminum (oral aluminum gels or aluminum-contaminated dialysate). Evidence of aluminum toxicity is common when plasma levels exceed 3 mmol/L (80 μg/L), but values of 1.5 to 3 μmol/L (40 to 80 μg/L) can be found in aluminum-intoxicated patients when aluminum exposure has been withdrawn for longer than 3 to 6 months.

PATIENT NUMBER 2 (continued)

An iliac crest bone biopsy, performed after double tetracycline labeling, showed patchy osteomalacia and "absent" bone formation; 75% of the trabecular surface stained positive for aluminum using the aurin tricarboxylic stain (normally there is no aluminum). Aluminum-related bone disease with low bone turnover was diagnosed.

Bone biopsy is the only certain way to diagnose aluminum-related bone disease. Very rarely is the potentially risky therapy with DFO justified without biopsy proof of aluminum toxicity.

PATIENT NUMBER 2 (continued)

The aluminum gels and the Bicitra were discontinued. Bobby then received DFO by subcutaneous injection, 1 g each week for the next 6 months. Clinically, he became more alert and showed marked improvement in his weakness and bone pain; his seizures became very infrequent. Radiographs after 6 months of treatment showed normalization of the physes, new endosteal bone formation, and healing of his fractures.

Bobby returned to UCLA Medical Center for corrective orthopedic surgical procedures performed in three stages over a 1-year period. Two years after the first operation, he was able to walk to school and was independent in his activities of daily living. He returned to school for the first time in 4 years. His renal function has remained stable, with no need for dialysis.

Bobby had osteomalacia, one of the conditions with low bone turnover that are found among patients with ESRD and that sometimes occur in those with stable but advanced renal insufficiency. In Bobby's situation, the osteomalacia is caused by **aluminum accumulation.**

Before considering the diagnosis and management, it is important to consider briefly the **metabolism of aluminum.** Normally, the intake of aluminum is 2 to 4 mg/day, and only a minute fraction of this ingested aluminum is absorbed and then excreted in the urine of a person with normal renal function. When renal function is reduced, the absorbed aluminum cannot be excreted readily and the aluminum is retained in the body, where it is deposited in bone, the liver, the central nervous system, and other tissues, including the parathyroid glands. Aluminum loading can arise from aluminum-contaminated

dialysis solutions or from repeated administration of aluminum-contaminated intravenous solutions, such as casein hydrolysate or albumin. It also occurs when the oral intake of aluminum is markedly increased (e.g., during long-term therapy with large doses of aluminum hydroxide, aluminum carbonate, or sucralfate).

Intestinal absorption of ingested aluminum is enhanced 10- to 20-fold by citrate ingestion, and other factors have relatively trivial effects on its absorption. Significant amounts of citrate are found in several over-the-counter preparations, such as Bicitra (citric acid/sodium citrate or Shohl's solution), calcium citrate, Alka-Seltzer, and even in large amounts of orange juice. When aluminum enters the body of a patient with ESRD being treated with dialysis, the aluminum is removed by dialysis rather slowly because most plasma aluminum is bound to the protein transferrin. Aluminum affects bone formation in several ways: It impairs osteoblast proliferation and/or function, it alters the solubility of calcium phosphate crystals, and it directly inhibits the secretion of PTH by the parathyroid glands.

Manifestations of Aluminum Toxicity

In the past, aluminum accumulation was the most important cause of either osteomalacia or highly symptomatic aplastic bone disease in patients with renal failure.

Aluminum-related bone disease, also called *fracturing osteomalacia,* can present with severe bone pain, fractures, and proximal muscle weakness. Bone biopsy shows either osteomalacia or aplastic bone disease. Laboratory features include normal or elevated serum calcium levels, PTH levels that are often lower than expected, and plasma aluminum levels that generally exceed 3 μmol/L (81 μg/L). After infusion of the chelating agent DFO, 40 mg/kg, plasma aluminum level increases, often by more than 6.0 μmol/L (165 μg/L). When aluminum-loaded patients are withdrawn from aluminum for several months, histologic features of aluminum toxicity can persist, with plasma aluminum levels as low as 0.8 μmol/L (22 μg/L) and an increment of plasma aluminum after DFO that is far less. Features that often help separate aluminum-related bone disease from secondary hyperparathyroidism are listed in Table 14–7. Radiographs may show demineralization, fractures (which at times may heal), pseudofractures (particularly involving the ribs of afflicted adult patients), or evidence of prior erosions, or they may be nondi-

TABLE 14–7. Features That Help Differentiate Aluminum-Related Bone Disease from Hyperparathyroid Bone Disease

Feature	Hyperparathyroid Bone Disease	Aluminum-Related Bone Disease
Fractures	Not characteristic	Common
Proximal muscle weakness	Occurs	Common
Acute periarthritis	Occurs	Uncommon
Tendon rupture	May occur	Not characteristic
Extraskeletal calcifications	Common	Not characteristic
Serum calcium	Low to high; often > 2.5 mmol/L	Often high, often > 2.7 mmol/L
Serum phosphorus	Variable, may be > 2 mmol/L	Variable, may be < 1.8 mmol/L
Alkaline phosphatase	80% to 800% of normal	40% to 300% of normal
Serum PTH:		
Intact assay	Most > 3-fold normal°	< 3- to 7-fold normal°
Midregion assay	Most > 10–15 times normal°	< 10 to 15 times normal°
Serum/plasma aluminum	Rarely > 5 µmol/L	Generally > 3 µmol/L†
	Often < 3-fold normal	Rarely < 1.5 µmol/L
Increment in serum Al after DFO‡	Rarely > 14 µmol/L	Generally > 6 µmol/L; rarely < 3 µmol/L
Microcytic anemia	Unusual	Common in epidemics (dialysate Al high)
Risk factors	Young age, noncompliance	Diabetes, prior PTX, prior transplant, prior binephrectomy, Al^{3+} exposure

°Increment above PTH level of normal subjects.
†Basal serum aluminum reflects exposure to aluminum (oral or via dialysate).
‡Less predictable after patient has had no exposure to aluminum for 6 months or more.

agnostic. The bone scan may be nonrevealing, may show diminished generalized uptake, or may reveal pseudofractures that cannot be detected on radiographs.

Severe aluminum loading can also cause altered brain function (dialysis encephalopathy) and was likely the cause of Bobbie's seizures. Aluminum toxicity can cause proximal myopathy, microcytic anemia (despite normal iron stores), and perhaps abnormal myocardial function. Factors other than aluminum can also lead to a condition with low bone formation (see Table 14–2). Patients lacking aluminum and iron usually have no symptoms.

Management of Aluminum Loading or Aluminum Toxicity

The management of aluminum loading or toxicity is reviewed, particularly for patients who have ESRD and who require treatment with dialysis. When patients with renal failure have biochemical evidence of aluminum loading, they should be treated by withdrawing all aluminum-containing drugs and using aluminum-free dialysate (e.g., <0.3 µmol/L (<8 µg/L). Patients with ESRD and serum aluminum levels exceeding 3.0 µmol/L (>80 µg/L) have evidence of recent exposure to aluminum. Whether chelation therapy with DFO

is indicated depends on the symptoms and the evidence for true toxicity of aluminum. If a patient has symptomatic bone disease or encephalopathy, the symptoms commonly improve after chelation therapy with DFO. When encephalopathy is present, the chance of improvement or even survival is less when treatment is restricted to the withdrawal of aluminum exposure. When chelation therapy is indicated, DFO doses should not be given more frequently than **once weekly,** and the lowest possible doses should be used (e.g., 0.25 to 1.0 g/wk). After DFO is given, 8 to 12 hours is required before optimal chelation occurs; after the dose of DFO is given, dialysis should be done using a high-flux dialysis membrane to facilitate removal of the DFO chelates of both aluminum and iron, as well as the non-chelated DFO. Plasma aluminum levels should be monitored 8 to 24 hours after first giving the DFO; if the serum aluminum level after the first DFO dose exceeds 18.5 µmol/L (500 µg/dl), the DFO dose should be reduced because of the risk of precipitating acute aluminum neurotoxicity with the DFO treatment.

Mucormycosis, which is commonly fatal, is the most important risk of DFO therapy in patients with renal failure. Mucormycosis is believed to occur because DFO chelates iron (as well as aluminum) and therefore acts as a siderophore that stimulates both the growth and pathogenicity of certain microorganisms, including the fungus causing mucormycosis. The optimal duration of DFO therapy is unknown, but a patient's clinical status and a repeat bone biopsy after 6 to 12 months may provide a guide to a need for further treatment. Hypocalcemia and an increase in PTH levels are common during DFO therapy; some patients develop overt secondary hyperparathyroidism and require parathyroid surgery. Therapy with calcitriol is indicated when the serum calcium level declines. Bobby received a larger dose of DFO than we would give if we encountered such a patient today.

PATIENT NUMBER 3

Roberta, a 52-year-old divorced woman with insulin-dependent diabetes mellitus and end-stage diabetic nephropathy, is hospitalized with confusion, inability to walk, and a presumed new stroke.

Roberta has had insulin-dependent diabetes for 35 years. Her diabetic control has been excellent for the past 15 years, but it had been erratic before that time. She developed progressive renal failure and has required hemodialysis for the past 4 years. She had hypertension in the past and suffered an earlier cerebrovascular accident with minimal residual deficit. She has been able to walk only a short distance, and she is very depressed. Three months ago, she had a slightly elevated serum calcium level of 2.65 mmol/L (10.6 mg/dl). Her serum P level is 2.1 mmol/L (6.5 mg/dl), and alkaline phosphatase level is 55 IU/L. An intact IRMA PTH level is 7.5 pmol/L (75 pg/ml). A bone biopsy reveals 10% surface staining for aluminum but little or no uptake of tetracycline and no double labels (i.e., bone formation is near zero). Her aluminum gels are discontinued (Alucaps, two with each meal), and she is given calcium carbonate, 650-mg capsules, two with each meal.

Two months later, Roberta has confusion, lethargy, and reduced ability to walk when she is brought to the dialysis unit. She is hospitalized with a tentative diagnosis of a new stroke. Laboratory findings reported 6 hours later include levels of serum Ca of 3.2 mmol/L (12.8 mg/dl), phosphorus 2.0 mmol/L (6.2 mg/dl), and albumin 33 g/L (3.3 mg/dl). She showed no improvement after a standard hemodialysis that used dialysate with a calcium concentration of 3.5 mEq/L. When the hypercalcemia was recognized, Roberta had a repeat hemodialysis treatment the next day with the dialysate Ca lowered to 2.0 mEq/L. After this, her mental and neurologic symptoms quickly resolved. The next week, the intact PTH result, obtained at the time

of hospital admission, was reported to be 3.0 pmol/L (30 pg/dl).

Roberta had mild and asymptomatic hypercalcemia that prompted a bone biopsy. The latter showed a low bone turnover state with minimal or insignificant aluminum staining. This condition is termed *adynamic* or *aplastic* bone; it represents a condition with subnormal bone turnover without significant aluminum staining. Most evidence indicates that this is a condition of oversuppressed PTH levels, even though the values of PTH are often normal or slightly above. Most patients with this condition have intact PTH levels below 10 nmol/L (100 pg/ml), and the finding of hypercalcemia combined with a PTH level less than 15 pmol/L (150 pg/ml) strongly supports this diagnosis.

This condition is associated with few if any symptoms. However, patients who have low bone turnover and who are exposed to aluminum loading are very susceptible to the development of symptomatic aluminum-related bone disease. For this reason, dialysis recipients with low PTH levels (< 10 pmol/L) should not be treated with aluminum-containing gels. Also, patients with aplastic or adynamic bone are more susceptible to the development of hypercalcemia when they are given calcium carbonate or calcium acetate as phosphate binders. Such susceptibility to hypercalcemia is thought to arise because bone turnover is very low and bone has a limited capacity to act as a buffer for the added calcium entering the body from the gut. This susceptibility to hypercalcemia may explain why many recommend the routine use of dialysate with 2.5 mEq/L calcium in dialysate. When such dialysate is used, hypercalcemia is rare in patients taking calcium-based phosphate binders. When hypercalcemia does develop in a patient with low bone turnover, the serum calcium level is quickly lowered after dialysis using a dialysate calcium of 2.0 to 2.5 mEq/L; the latter permits the removal of excess calcium during dialysis. This contrasts with the partial correction of hypercalcemia or only transient improvement by the use of low-calcium dialysate in a patient with hypercalcemia and a condition with high bone turnover. Preliminary evidence suggests that routine dialysis for patients with low bone turnover but lacking aluminum, with the dialysate calcium concentration lowered to 2.0 mEq/L, is followed by a modest rise in intact PTH and an increase in bone formation rate to normal.

PATIENT NUMBER 4

Roger, a 63-year-old retired salesman who has undergone regular hemodialysis for 12 years, is evaluated for pain in his neck, shoulders, and hips.

Twelve years ago, Roger began regular hemodialysis for ESRD due to biopsy-proven glomerulonephritis. He fared quite well for the first few years and because of this would not consider a renal transplant. His only problems have included surgical revision of the Cimino arteriovenous fistula of his left forearm, 3 years ago, and carpal tunnel release surgery, also on the left side, 2 years ago. His medications include folic acid, 1 mg daily, calcium acetate, 4 tablets with each meal, and one multivitamin daily. During the past 12 months, he has noted progressively severe aching pain in his shoulders, hands, and hips. He also has aching in his neck. The pain is worst at night and during hemodialysis. He finds that walking about the room when he awakens during the night provides relief, but he often awakens 1 to 2 hours later with the same problem. His symptoms are unaffected by the weather.

Laboratory results for the previous few months include serum levels of urea of 68 to 75 mg/dl, creatinine 13.5 to 15 mg/dl, calcium 9.9 to 10.2 mg/dl, phosphorus 5.2 to 6.5 mg/dl, albumin 42 g/L (4.2 g/dl), aluminum 24 µg/L, intact PTH 15 nmol/L (150 pg/ml), and alkaline phosphatase 65 IU/L. Urea reduction ratios, determined with his monthly laboratory values as indices of adequate dialysis, were 69% and 71% with the last two measurements.

Pain that is worse with inactivity is characteristic of most patients with **dialysis amyloidosis.** The pain can be quite severe, and it most commonly involves the shoulders and hands; however, it can also occur in the hips and knees. Carpal tunnel syndrome is often the first manifestation of this syndrome, and most adults who have undergone dialysis for more than 10 to 15 years have symptoms of carpal tunnel syndrome.

PATIENT NUMBER 4 (continued)

Results of Roger's physical examination are generally unremarkable except for the typical urochrome pigment of a long-term dialysis patient. Roger has some reduction in the flexibility of his fingers and slight numbness of the thumb and first finger of his right hand. He climbs stairs well and has no problem rising from a low chair.

As with most disorders affecting the bones and joints in patients undergoing dialysis, physical

findings with the initial appearance of symptoms were scarce. Neurologic manifestations of carpal tunnel syndrome or a positive Tinel's sign may be present. When this disease advances, patients may have trigger fingers, decreased flexibility of the fingers, and tendon sheath cysts, which can be quite large. Patients with **dialysis amyloidosis** can also have features of secondary hyperparathyroidism, and **dialysis amyloidosis** can coexist with the more typical forms of the renal bone diseases. As the disease advances, patients may have limited motion of the shoulders and cervical spine. Dialysis amyloidosis can predispose long-term dialysis recipients to hip fracture, as well.

PATIENT NUMBER 4 (continued)

Roger's skeletal radiographs show (1) moderate degenerative changes of the cervical spine, (2) multiple thin-walled cysts involving both proximal humeri, both hips, and the metacarpals, and (3) mild sclerosis of the end plates of the lumbar vertebral bodies. The radiologist interprets the cysts as being possible brown tumors and the overall findings as consistent with renal osteodystrophy.

These radiographic features are quite typical of **dialysis amyloidosis**; the development of thin-walled cysts at the ends of the long bones often represents amyloidomas that develop at the site of tendinous insertions, where they enlarge to replace the trabecular bone. These cysts are most commonly seen in the ends of the long bones (humerus, femur) or in the metacarpals (Fig. 14–5). They somewhat resemble brown tumors that arise with osteitis fibrosa. However, brown tumors are quite uncommon with the osteitis fibrosa that develops in patients with ESRD. Also, when brown tumors occur, they are most often single and involve sites such as the jaw or ribs. Lesions of **dialysis amyloidosis** also affect the spine, and the cervical spine is involved earlier and more extensively than the thoracic or lumbar spine. Involvement of tendon sheaths of the hands can produce limitation of motion and the inability to open jars or unlock doors.

AMYLOIDOSIS DUE TO β₂-MICROGLOBULIN

In adults undergoing dialysis for more than 5 years, a unique type of amyloidosis develops and causes symptoms affecting the bone and joints. β₂-Microglobulin is the major constituent of this type of amyloidosis, termed **dialysis amyloidosis.** Normally, β₂-microglobulin, a protein with MW 13,000, is a normal protein constituent of plasma that is filtered at the glomerulus and degraded by the renal tubules. With end-stage renal failure, the degradation of β_2-microglobulin is halted and its blood levels are increased more than 40- to 50-fold above normal. For uncertain reasons, several years pass before the amyloid deposits of β_2-microglobulin form; the amyloid deposits appear sooner in patients starting dialysis after age 50, and they are unheard of in pediatric patients on dialysis. This amyloid has a predilection for deposition around tendons, joints, and the periosteum; deposits in visceral organs are unusual. Data suggest that the syndrome may be less common or may appear later in patients who undergo dialysis using certain highly permeable membranes; however, no data indicate that changing to the use of such a membrane leads to improvement of symptoms or reverse of the lesions.

PATIENT NUMBER 4 (continued)

A review of the dialysis parameters of our patient Roger indicates that he has received dialysis for 4 hours thrice weekly, using a highly permeable Fresenius F80 dialyzer (polysulfone) for the past 6 years. Before that he had dialysis for 3.5 hours per session and he used a dialyzer with a standard cellulosic membrane. Shoulder ultrasound examination is performed. This discloses enlargement of the supraspinatus and biceps tendons to about twice the maximum range of normal. Roger receives indomethacin regularly, with partial relief of his symptoms. He is encouraged to be a candidate for a cadaveric renal transplant when it becomes available.

Management of this syndrome is difficult. Nonsteroidal antiinflammatory drugs may provide partial relief of the symptoms. Also, the symptoms usually improve quickly or disappear after receipt of renal transplant, with good function. However, skeletal radiographs obtained under these circumstances show no evidence of resolution of the deposits. Once the syndrome has appeared and become symptomatic, there is little evidence that the use of larger or more permeable dialyzers affects the patient's symptoms. A specific diagnosis is usually made clinically based on a patient's specific symptoms. The finding of cystic lesions on radiographs or enlarged tendons on shoulder ultrasonography provides diagnostic support for this diagnosis. Until a specific therapy for this disorder is available, there is little justification for highly invasive biop-

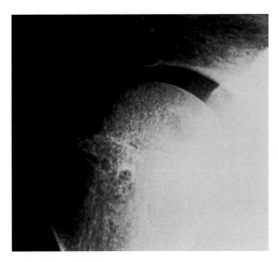

Figure 14–5. The patient is a 56-year-old man who had undergone hemodialysis for 14 years. He had pain in his shoulders, much worse at night; radiographs showed thin-walled cysts of both shoulders and the metacarpals as well. He had had numbness and pain in his hands, with relief of symptoms following carpal tunnel release surgery. The tissue removed showed birefringence characteristic of amyloid, and an immunoperoxidase stain revealed β_2-microglobulin. The pain in his shoulders improved after intraarticular steroid therapy.

sies to provide a tissue diagnosis. A bone biopsy is occasionally useful to preclude the coexistence of aluminum toxicity or severe osteitis fibrosa.

SUGGESTED READINGS

Coburn JW, Frazao J: Calcitriol in the management of renal osteodystrophy. *Seminars Dialysis* 9:316–326, 1996.

Coburn JW, Goodman WG: Risk factors for aluminum toxicity and its prevention. *In* De Broe ME, Coburn JW (eds): Aluminum and Renal Failure. Dordrecht Kluwer Medical Publishers, 1990, pp 345–367.

Goodman WG, Coburn JW: The use of 1,25-dihydroxyvitamin D_3 in early renal failure. *Annu Rev Med* 43:227–237, 1992.

Goodman WG, Coburn JW, Ramirez JA, Slatopolsky E, Salusky IB: Renal osteodystrophy in adults and children. *In* Favus MJ (ed): Primer on the Metabolic Bone Diseases and Disorders of Mineral Metabolism. 2nd ed. Kelseyville, California: American Society of Bone and Mineral Research, 1993, pp 304–323.

Goodman WG, Coburn JW, Slatopolsky E, Salusky IB: Renal osteodystrophy in adult and pediatric patients. *In* Favus M (ed): Primer on the Metabolic Bone Diseases and Disorders of Calcium Metabolism. Kelseyville, American Society for Bone and Mineral Research, 1990, pp 200–212.

Hercz G, Pei Y, Greenwood C, et al: Aplastic osteodystrophy without aluminum: The role of "suppressed" parathyroid function. *Kidney Int* 44:860–866, 1993.

Koch KM: Dialysis-related amyloidosis. *Kidney Int* 41:1416–1429, 1992.

Malluche H, Faugere M-C: Renal bone disease 1990: An unmet challenge for the nephrologist. *Kidney Int* 38:193–211, 1990.

Pei Y, Hercz G, Greenwood C, et al: Risk factors for renal osteodystrophy: A multivariant analysis. *J Bone Miner Res* 10:149–156, 1995.

15 | NUTRITIONAL CONCERNS FOR PATIENTS

WITH KIDNEY DISEASE

James L. Bailey and William E. Mitch

PATIENT NUMBER 1

Terrence, a 72-year-old man, is sent to you from a nursing home because of "abnormal labs." He wants to see you to find out "when can I have this operation on my knees to take care of this arthritis." He has severe osteoarthritis of his knees and ambulates only short distances with the help of a walker. Because of his inability to walk, he sold his house and moved into a nursing home 6 months ago. He has been to a number of surgeons, none of whom want to operate on his knees because of his renal disease. "I feel pretty good except for this damn pain in my knee. I figure if I have me this operation I'll be fine."

He also relates a long-standing history of renal disease. Twenty years ago, he was told that he was spilling protein in his urine, and his doctor considered performing a kidney biopsy but finally decided not to. Except for a "blood pressure pill," he takes no medication and otherwise has been well. On examination, Terrence appears well. His blood pressure is 145/85 mm Hg, his lungs are clear, his heart rhythm is regular with an S4 gallop, and his abdomen is benign. He has swelling in his distal interphalangeal joints consistent with osteoarthritis, and he has some crepitus on flexion and extension of the knees, but they are not swollen. He has good peripheral pulses and trace pedal edema. An adequate 24-hour urine collection done 2 months ago revealed a creatinine clearance of 15 ml/min. His urinary sediment shows an occasional WBC, rare granular casts, and 2+ protein. Other laboratory results are remarkable for a serum potassium level of 6.5 mmol/L, bicarbonate of 17 mmol/L, a creatinine level of 5.8, and a BUN of 64 mg/dl. His serum calcium level is 7.1 mg/dl, phosphorus level is 8.2 mg/dl, and serum albumin is 3.5 g/dl with a normal WBC count and a hematocrit of 30%. His ECG shows a normal sinus rhythm, a left axis, and tall peaked T waves.

Impression. This 72-year-old man has chronic renal failure (CRF), most likely secondary to chronic glomerulonephritis, and presents with signs and symptoms of advanced renal disease including anemia, metabolic acidosis, hyperkalemia, and secondary hyperparathyroidism.

Any chronic disease presents a dilemma for the practicing physician, especially whether or not to treat. A natural tendency is to treat every aspect of the disease process, but this may ultimately do more harm. The beneficial effects of therapy often have to be weighed against the side effects of treatment. Moreover, a patient may have little insight into the underlying disease and may harbor false expectations, wrongly focusing on one aspect of treatment; this may be not only inappropriate but unnecessary.

Many nutritional concerns are related to the treatment of a patient with renal disease. These include the requirement to achieve fluid, electrolyte, and mineral balances as well as to reduce azotemia. Dietary modifications to accomplish these goals can seem contradictory to patients if they appear to be at variance with traditional nutritional recommendations. Moreover, such dietary modifications often create a bland or even unpalatable diet, contributing to a patient's noncompliance, especially if the patient has adapted to a chronic disease. **These considerations make education by a skilled dietitian an integral aspect of the care of any patient with renal disease. Patient education facilitates compliance and minimizes the need to prescribe extra medicines; it can decrease morbidity and often forestall the need for dialysis.** To take advantage of a patient's favorite foods and ensure an adequate intake of nutrients, a skilled dietitian is critical for successful therapy.

184

As we delve into this first case, it is apparent from the laboratory results that Terrence has advanced renal disease, but he has few overt symptoms of uremia. This combination can make attempts to modify the diet difficult. **Ironically, a feeling of wellness can be deleterious by promoting a false sense of security and self-denial.** If medications or other medical causes of hyperkalemia (e.g., hypoaldosteronism) are excluded, dietary potassium restriction should be the mainstay of preventing hyperkalemia in chronic renal disease. In the absence of dietary potassium restriction, hyperkalemia can cause cardiac arrhythmias and sudden death. Dietary potassium restriction involves avoiding brightly colored fruits and vegetables, chocolate, and potatoes (Table 15–1). It is essential that patients be counseled in the nuances of a renal diet by a trained nutritionist. Counseling is helpful in avoiding more aggressive therapy such as diuretics or potassium exchange resins, which can create additional morbidity.

Dietary protein restriction has traditionally been a mainstay of therapy for chronic renal disease (Table 15–2). Protein restriction can reduce anorexia, nausea, and vomiting and other symptoms of uremia that otherwise might prompt the initiation of dialysis. Patients who consume large amounts of protein are also eating considerable amounts of potassium, phosphorus, and calcium, because the content of these minerals is invariably high in protein-rich foods. Interestingly, metabolism of proteins generates phosphates and sulfates, which contribute to the acid that must be excreted by the kidneys. Excess

acid is detrimental because it increases protein degradation and amino acid oxidation, thereby increasing the requirement for protein. Restricting dietary protein improves a patient's acid-base status.

Nutritional studies in the 1950s determined that the minimum daily protein requirement for normal adult men and women is approximately 0.6 g/kg ideal body weight, with the bulk consisting of high-quality protein that is rich in essential amino acids. A dietary intake below this amount induces malnutrition unless supplemented with essential amino acids. Any dietary protein restriction must take into account several factors—first, the degree of renal insufficiency. Patients with mild CRF and a GFR $\geq$ 60 ml/min have not been shown to benefit from a low-protein diet.

However, in a patient such as Terrence, with more advanced renal failure and a GFR < 25 ml/min, there are clear advantages to a protein-restricted diet.

- First, the accumulation of nitrogen-containing waste products (e.g., urea, guanidine, and so on) is less, forestalling uremic symptoms.
- Second, a more favorable nitrogen balance results with decreased acid accumulation, and thus metabolic acidosis improves.
- Third, dietary phosphorus is lower, necessarily limiting the requirements for phosphate binders.
- Fourth, protein restriction can have a favorable effect in retarding the progression of renal insufficiency.

TABLE 15–1. Foods High in Potassium

Fruits	Vegetables	Miscellaneous
Avocados	Baked potatoes	Chocolate
Bananas	French fries	Gingerbread
Cantaloupe	Potato chips (high sodium)	Ginger snap cookies
Honeydew melon	Instant potatoes	Molasses
Coconut, dried	Dried beans and peas:	Nuts of any kind
Grapefruit	baked beans, black beans, black-eyed peas,	Orange Crush soda
Grapefruit juice	cowpeas, butter beans, chick peas, kidney	Postum grain beverage
Oranges	beans, lentils, lima beans, field peas	Lite Salt
Orange juice	Parsnips	Salt substitutes
Nectarines	Pumpkin	
Dried fruits:	Raw carrots	
dates, figs, prunes, raisins, coconut,	Raw mushrooms	
apricots	Raw spinach	
Prune juice	Tomato products:	
Mangos	tomato sauce, catsup, tomato juice, spaghetti	
Papayas	sauce	
Persimmons	Winter squash	
Plantain	Yams	

TABLE 15–2. Recommended Dietary Protein and Energy Intake for Patients with Chronic Renal Failure

Glomerular Filtration Rate (ml/min/1.73 m²)	Protein	Energy (kcal/kg/day)	Carbohydrate % Total Calories	Fat % Total Calories
≥70 without apparent progression	0.8–1.0 g/kg/day	Sufficent to maintain desirable body weight	As recommended for normal adults	As recommended for normal adults
25–70 with apparent progression	0.60 g/kg/day of high-biologic-value protein	≥35	50% primarily complex carbohydrates	The remaining nonprotein calories
5–25	0.55–0.60 g/kg/day (≥0.35 g/kg/day of high-biologic-value protein)	≥35	50% primarily complex carbohydrates	The remaining nonprotein calories
<5 (hemodialysis)	1.0 g/kg/day	≥35	50% primarily complex carbohydrates	The remaining nonprotein calories
<5 (peritoneal dialysis)	1.2–1.4 g/kg/day	≥35	Same	Same

Once again, a dietitian skilled in planning a diet will have a favorable impact, but careful consideration of the extent of protein restriction must include factors such as a coexisting catabolic illness, whether the patient is taking drugs that can affect protein metabolism such as glucocorticoids, or whether the patient has significant proteinuria. For our patient Terrence, we are not told how much urinary protein he is losing each day. This value should be quantified with a 24-hour urine collection, and the quantity of proteinuria should be factored into the protein-restricted diet. Specifically, the daily protein requirement should be increased by an amount equal to the protein lost daily in the urine.

Dietary protein restriction should have a favorable effect on phosphorus metabolism because foods rich in protein are generally rich in phosphorus (Table 15–3). This is important because it helps prevent secondary hyperparathyroidism and because phosphorus restriction may retard the progression of renal disease. Normal adults have 600 to 700 g of phosphorus in the body, of which 35% is extracellular. When renal function declines to a GFR < 30 ml/min, phosphate retention and hyperphosphatemia occur. As GFR declines, the fractional excretion of urinary phosphate per remaining nephron increases because circulating levels of parathyroid hormone (PTH) rise. This occurs because the high phosphorus and low vitamin D levels lead to a low circulating calcium level. The lower levels of vitamin D occur because of reduced production of $1,25(OH)_2D_3$ in the remaining proximal tubules, which catalyze the 1α-hydroxylation of cholecalciferol to create the most active form of vitamin

D. Interestingly, vitamin D not only increases the absorption of calcium and phosphates from the gut but also suppresses the production of PTH. Excess PTH stimulates the release of calcium from bone, resulting in osteopenia; it may also hasten the progression of renal disease.

Poor control of serum phosphorus levels can potentiate symptoms associated with rheumatologic disease, including osteoarthritis, as in Terrence. Patients or physicians often mistakenly attribute the symptoms of "arthritis" to a primary joint disease instead of recognizing that secondary hyperparathyroidism may have a primary role. Therapy of hyperphosphatemia hinges on a two-pronged approach that includes dietary phosphorus restriction (5 to 10 mg/kg/day) and the use of an appropriate phosphate binder to facilitate excretion of excess phosphorus through the gut. It should be emphasized that the main source of dietary phosphorus is protein-rich foods; thus, dietary protein restriction is generally sufficient to achieve the needed phosphorus restriction. Unfortunately, adherence to protein and phosphorus restriction can result in an inadequate intake of calcium; this condition can be aggravated because intestinal absorption of calcium is low in patients with renal disease. To meet calcium requirements, 1.5 g calcium per day is needed. Calcium carbonate can be given as a phosphate binder to raise calcium intake to 1.5 g/day. However, the use of calcium carbonate as a phosphate binder should be avoided if the serum Ca × P product exceeds 60 mg/dl because of a high risk of soft tissue calcification. If the serum calcium product is too high, short-term therapy with an aluminum binder is safe.

TABLE 15–3. High-Phosphorus Foods

Food Group	Food Name	Serving Size	Phosphorus (mg)
Dairy	Milk	1 cup	250
	Yogurt	1 cup	350
	Cream	1 cup	230
	Cheese	1 piece	300
	Ice cream	1 cup	190
	Pudding	1 cup	250
	Custard	1 cup	310
	Cottage cheese	1 cup	340
	Cream pies or desserts	1 slice	130
Fruits/vegetables	Baked beans	1 cup	264
	Beans (kidney, red, navy)	1 cup	280
	Dried beans (white, navy, pinto)	1 cup	250
	Dried peas, blackeyed peas, split peas	1 cup	180
	Soybeans and soy foods	1 cup	300
	Dried fruit	1 cup	180
Bread and cereals	Waffles	1 item	257
	Oat-bran muffin	1 item	160
	Cornbread	1 item	152
	Biscuits	1 item	100
	Pancakes	1 item	90
	Whole wheat bread	1 slice	98
	Cereal—All Bran	1 cup	794
	Cereal—Granola	1 cup	380
	Cereal—raisin bran	1 cup	250
Protein foods	Liver	1 slice	390
	Sausage	1 item	300
	Meats	3 ounces	250
	Egg	1	150
	Peanut butter	1 Tbsp	80
Beverages	Beer	1 cup	62
	Colas	1 cup	61
Miscellaneous	Nuts	2 Tbsp	80
	Chocolate	1 ounce	115

In contrast, long-term therapy with an aluminum salt (i.e., for months) increases the risk of aluminum toxicity.

A vitamin D supplement is occasionally useful for patients with osteomalacia and a low serum calcium level but should never be used when the serum phosphorus level is high because vitamin D increases intestinal phosphate absorption. With appropriate instruction and compliance with a well-planned diet, vitamin D is seldom necessary in a predialysis patient.

One of the hallmarks of advanced renal disease is metabolic acidosis. An adult eating a normal diet generates 1 mEq acid per kilogram of body weight per day, and this must be excreted by the kidneys. In renal failure, the ability to excrete acid is compromised and patients develop metabolic acidosis, which stimulates catabolism of body protein. Negative nitrogen balance develops, and patients experience generalized weakness and fatigue. Correction of acidosis with bicarbonate supplements has both objective and subjective beneficial effects and should be pursued. Acidosis also increases the transcellular shift of potassium, leading to hyperkalemia. With proper therapy including dietary protein restriction and sodium bicarbonate supplements, most patients do not have to restrict dietary potassium rigorously.

PATIENT NUMBER 1 (continued)

Terrence was interviewed by a renal dietitian, who found that because of his long-standing history of hypertension, he was attempting to limit his dietary sodium and used a salt substitute liberally. In addition, he ate two or three bananas a day as well as an orange. *He also reported that he could not resist having chocolate cake for dessert.* The dietitian instructed the nursing home and the patient about a new dietary plan restricting protein to 0.6 g/kg and phosphorus to 800 mg. Appropriate modifications were made to limit dietary potassium by eliminating the bananas and fruit, and the patient understood the dangers of using a salt substitute. In addition, a mild salt restriction (2000 mg sodium per day) was instituted, and 1.5 g of $NaHCO_3$ was given with each meal. When serum phosphorus was <5.5 mg/dl, calcium carbonate was started. A serum intact PTH level was drawn.

It should be obvious that not all patients need severe dietary potassium restriction and that each patient's diet must be individually designed. In normal adults, the kidneys readily excrete excess potassium, but with renal insufficiency, the ability to regulate serum potassium becomes increasingly less effective. This is especially true when an abrupt change in potassium intake occurs. The gut can and does excrete a portion of daily intake, and thus constipation can aggravate a tendency toward hyperkalemia. With advanced renal insufficiency, the gut cannot excrete enough potassium to match normal intake, thereby necessitating dietary potassium restriction.

PATIENT NUMBER 1 (continued)

Several weeks later, Terrence was seen in follow-up. His blood pressure was 130/80. His serum potassium level was 4.5 mmol/L, serum bicarbonate level was 25 mmol/L, phosphorus level was 4.5 mmol/L, and serum calcium level was 9.6 mg/dl. The intact serum PTH level obtained previously was 428 µm/ml. This high level slowly decreased over the next 6 months, and the patient's arthritic symptoms gradually abated. Both the patient's weight and renal function remained stable, and he was able to return to living in an apartment.

As the clinical course of our patient Terrence illustrates, mild sodium restriction potentiates the efficacy of antihypertensive medications and should always be a mainstay of therapy for hypertension. Furthermore, vigorous control of blood pressure is likely to be effective in slowing the progression of renal insufficiency. Because the ability to excrete sodium is altered in patients with kidney failure, dietary restriction (Table 15–4) could achieve these beneficial effects. Nutritional measures may not be glamorous, but they are simple to implement and cost-effective, and compliance is relatively easy to assess. To monitor changes in sodium levels, body weight should be measured. A 24-hour urinary measurement for urea nitrogen excretion can be used to assess compliance with the dietary protein restriction, provided that renal function is stable.

PATIENT NUMBER 2

Eileen, a 54-year-old woman with non–insulin-dependent diabetes mellitus, comes to your office complaining that her feet are swollen. She and her husband used to love dancing, but she has become very self-conscious of her appearance and has stopped dancing. She was diagnosed as having diabetes some 15 years ago, and she has always had difficulty controlling her blood sugar until recently. She notes that she "tries" to avoid candies and foods with sugar. Her favorite foods are canned soups. Six months ago, she noted that her feet were swollen when she went to bed each night, and last month she noted that her "belly" began to swell. A neighbor noted that her face looked a little puffy, and Eileen decided to visit you, her doctor. She denies any chest pain or shortness of breath and is not aware of any liver disease. She was told by her eye doctor that diabetes had affected her vision and that she might require laser treatments in the near future. He was concerned because her blood pressure was high. She also notes that her urine "foams" and that she has been urinating quite frequently. On examination, Eileen has anasarca with a blood pressure of 190/100 in both arms; it does not change when she stands. Funduscopic examination shows background proliferative retinopathy with dot and blot hemorrhages. Her neck is supple, and her neck veins are not distended, but dullness is noted over each lung base. Her heart rhythm is regular, and she has an S4 gallop. Her abdomen is distended, and she has marked abdominal wall edema as well as sacral and thigh edema 4+. Laboratory studies reveal normal electrolyte values and a serum creatinine level and BUN of 2.4 and 22 mg/dl, respectively. Her serum albumin level is 1.5 g/dl, serum cholesterol level is 339, and blood sugar value 145 mg/dl. ECG shows left-axis deviation with evidence of left ventricular hypertrophy. Chest radiography shows bilateral pleural effusions and an enlarged heart. A 24-hour urine collection reveals a creatinine clearance of 32 ml/min and contains 440 mEq of sodium, 12 g of nitrogen, and 11 g of protein. In summary, this is a 54-year-old woman who has long-standing non–insulin-dependent diabetes and who develops anasarca as part of the nephrotic syndrome. Her salt intake is very high. **Her lifestyle has become very circumscribed, and she is ashamed of her appearance.**

Unfortunately, this is not an uncommon case. More than 25% of patients treated by dialysis have end-stage renal disease because of diabetic nephropathy. About 40% of these patients initially present with features of the nephrotic

TABLE 15–4. Foods High in Sodium

Canned meats	Meat sauces
Cured meats	Soy sauce
Hot dogs	Salad dressing
Luncheon meats	Gravies
Sausage	Dips
Bacon	Cheese
Canned foods (except fruit)	Dehydrated soups
Salt-covered snacks	Canned soups
Pickles, olives	Bouillon
Mustard	Salted spices
Catsup	Meat tenderizers
Barbecue sauce	Seafood seasoning
Peanut butter	Table salt
Frozen dinners	Salt substitutes (some)
Buttermilk	Fast foods

syndrome, which is characterized by edema, proteinuria > 3.5 g, hypoalbuminemia, hyperlipidemia, and lipiduria. Edema reflects inappropriate retention of sodium by the diseased kidneys and is synonymous with an overload of sodium in the body. The serum sodium level is usually low, reflecting an even greater overload of water. Treatment of the edema has therapeutic ramifications because vigorous blood pressure control can slow progression of renal insufficiency. Blood pressure control is always easier to achieve if ECF is reduced. Assuming that the 24-hour urine collection was performed properly, diuretic therapy alone will not be sufficient to reduce the edema because she is consuming 10 g of sodium per day! Diuresis achieving a net loss of ECF always requires dietary salt restriction, which necessarily entails a drastic modification of the diet. In particular, our patient Eileen must become knowledgeable about the salt content of various foods, and she should be educated to use appropriate flavorings and seasonings that can enhance the palatability of food and encourage dietary compliance. She should understand how foods with a high salt content prevent her from losing edema and increase morbidity and mortality. By understanding the relationship between salt in the diet and edema formation, she will be able to grasp the need for dietary compliance. Simply adding additional antihypertensive medications is generally counterproductive unless dietary salt is restricted, because additional medications are not effective in blood pressure control. Another factor is the cost of medications, and it should not come as a surprise that simply adding medicines fosters noncompliance because patients becomes disheartened and lose confidence in the physician.

The symptom that often brings a patient to a doctor is the cosmetic effect of edema, **and a physician can and should take advantage of such legitimate patient concerns to foster dietary compliance.** Patients often become compliant with dietary restrictions when they see positive results, in this case, a decrease in unsightly edema or a decrease in abdominal girth. The initial approach to our patient Eileen's problem entails dietary sodium restriction to 2 g/day or less, coupled with the institution of loop diuretics. Thiazide diuretics are ineffective in patients with renal insufficiency and can increase the serum creatinine level.

Management of a patient's proteinuria presents additional dilemmas. Simply increasing dietary protein does not effectively treat low plasma and tissue protein pools. Indeed, excess dietary protein can be harmful because a high-protein diet is associated with an increase in proteinuria that exceeds a secondary increase in albumin synthesis. In fact, the increase in proteinuria because of excess dietary protein can actually worsen nitrogen balance, whereas a low-protein diet can cause a significant reduction in albumin excretion and a modest increase in serum albumin level. With less dietary protein, albumin synthesis can decrease, but any decrease is more than offset by a larger decrease in both albumin catabolism and excretion. Residual renal function may be preserved as a result of dietary protein restriction, because the prognosis of most renal diseases worsens as proteinuria increases. This relationship may simply reflect the severity of the underlying renal disease and greater damage to the glomerular basement membrane, but it has been argued that proteinuria *per se* may be injurious to the kidneys.

What constitutes the appropriate degree of dietary protein restriction is not established. In practice, we recommend that the total amount of protein consumed by patients with nephrotic-range proteinuria equal the amount of protein lost in the urine each day plus 0.8 g/kg of a patient's ideal body weight. The increase in dietary protein above the minimum requirement (0.6 kg/day) is recommended because studies suggest that dietary protein requirements are somewhat increased by the nephrotic syndrome, in part because dietary protein is not used with 100% efficiency to synthesize body protein. Coupling a regimen of dietary protein restriction with an angiotensin-converting enzyme (ACE) inhibitor could prove useful in decreasing the degree of proteinuria and favorably altering protein and lipid metabolism.

Although an ACE inhibitor has been shown to retard the progression of renal disease in insulin-dependent diabetic nephropathy, this benefit in non–insulin-dependent diabetic nephropathy has not been established. Because hyperkalemia is a serious side effect of ACE inhibitor therapy, close monitoring is needed and early institution of dietary potassium restriction should be considered.

PATIENT NUMBER 2 (continued)

Eileen is instructed in a 2-g sodium, 70-g protein diet, and diuretic and ACE inhibitor therapy is initiated. Within a month, she has a diuresis and loses more than 40 pounds. Her 24-hour urinary sodium excretion is now 100 mEq/day, and protein excretion has decreased to 7 g/24 hr. She is much more positive about her appearance, has begun to exercise regularly, and has started dancing again.

It is often difficult to balance the nutritional concerns of diabetic patients with their nutritional concerns about the renal diet because it usually includes an increase in complex carbohydrates to replace lost calories when protein is restricted. A diabetic diet generally restricts sugars, but complex carbohydrates do not cause a major change in insulin requirements or in the degree of diabetic control. Dietary education is crucial in achieving compliance and neutral nitrogen balance and includes training in meal planning and the nutritional contents of various foods. Compliance with a low-protein diet can be measured by a 24-hour urine collection for urea nitrogen as long as proteinuria is less than 5 g/day (Table 15–5). When proteinuria exceeds this amount, the nitrogen in this excess (protein is 16% nitrogen) should be added to the average nonurea nitrogen excretion of 0.031 g/kg ideal body weight. Dietary protein restriction also makes sodium restriction easier, and with a modest increase in the serum albumin level, a more effective diuresis may ensue. Diuretics must be used judiciously, paying careful attention to the physical findings, including the presence or absence of neck vein distention and changes in orthostatic blood pressure to detect early signs of excessive diuresis. Evaluating the BUN relative to the creatinine concentration can also prove helpful, but caution is urged because a BUN-to-serum creatinine ratio > 10:1 can also occur because of gastrointestinal bleeding. Other options for mobilizing edema include bed rest or the use of support hose.

Information provided about our patient Eileen does not indicate if the serum bicarbonate is decreased. If it were, then sodium bicarbonate supplements should be given if the salt- and protein-restricted diet coupled with diuretics does not correct metabolic acidosis. Again, our

TABLE 15–5. Estimation of Protein Intake for Patient Number 2

Eileen weighs 70 kg, and her 24-hour urinary collection is as follows:
    Total volume = 2400 ml
    Total creatinine = 1100 mg
    Total protein = 7 g
    Urinary urea nitrogen = 7.9 g

$$
\begin{aligned}
\text{Nitrogen balance } (B_N) &= \text{ nitrogen intake } (I_N) - \\
&\quad \text{urea nitrogen appearance (U)} - \\
&\quad \text{nonurea nitrogen excretion} \\
&\quad \text{(NUN)}^* \\
&= I_N - U - NUN
\end{aligned}
$$

If the patient is in steady state, nitrogen balance is zero and thus input equals output. The above equation can be rearranged as follows:

$$
\begin{aligned}
I_N &= U + NUN \\
&= 7.9 \text{ g N/day} + (70 \text{ kg} \times 0.31 \text{ g N/kg/d} + 7 \text{ g} \\
&\quad \text{urinary protein} \times 0.16) \\
&= 7.9 \text{ g N/day} + (2.17 \text{ g N/kg/d} + 1.12 \text{ g N/kg/d}) \\
&= 11.19 \text{ g N/day}
\end{aligned}
$$

Assuming that protein is 16% nitrogen, we can divide by 0.16 and obtain

$$
= 70 \text{ g protein/day}
$$

Therefore, our patient Eileen is adhering to her protein restriction

---

*Nitrogen in feces, urine creatinine, uric acid, other unmeasured nitrogen-containing compounds and urinary protein > 5 g.

concern about acidosis derives from stimulation of protein and amino acid degradation stimulated by acidosis.

Hyperlipidemia in the nephrotic syndrome results from increased synthesis of lipids and apolipoproteins as well as a reduction in their catabolism. Levels of very-low-density lipoproteins and intermediate-density lipoproteins are increased, whereas levels of high-density lipoproteins tend to be unchanged or decreased. Hypoalbuminemia or changes in the composition of plasma proteins are thought to contribute to the genesis of the hyperlipidemia, but whatever the cause, whether the hyperlipidemia associated with the nephrotic syndrome should be treated is controversial. Most investigators agree that treatment is required in patients with other risk factors yielding heart disease, such as hypertension, diabetes, or obesity. Our patient Eileen has multiple risk factors for heart disease, and her high serum cholesterol level warrants therapy. Initial treatment always entails a reduction in dietary fat, especially saturated fat and cholesterol. The loss of calories should be made up using nonsaturated fats and complex carbohydrates. Every effort should be made to treat the underlying disease, but barring curative therapy, dietary manipulation remains the cornerstone of treatment. In some instances, dietary protein re-striction coupled with an ACE inhibitor may be all that is required, because this combination can reduce proteinuria; hyperlipidemia may resolve, obviating the need for further reduction in di-etary fat and cholesterol beyond that associated with a low-protein diet. When the primary dis-ease is not easily amenable to therapy, as in Eileen's case, dietary protein and lipid restriction is needed. Dietary fat should constitute no more than 30% of the available calories, and no more than 33% of fat calories should be composed of saturated fats. In most instances, diet alone is not effective and the clinician must resort to lipid-lowering agents. Bile acid–binding agents are resins that can lower low-density lipoprotein cholesterol but usually not to the degree needed for this patient. In addition, these agents can cause abdominal bloating as well as constipation. **For patients with more severe renal insuffi-ciency being treated with phosphate bind-ers, bile acid–binding agents also bind to the phosphate binders, effectively neutralizing the action of both drugs.** Nicotinic acid has a good safety record, but many patients tolerate it poorly because the drug causes flushing. The hydroxymethylglutaryl coenzyme A (HMG CoA) inhibitors have revolutionized therapy and do correct serum lipid levels. Cost is usually the most important factor in determining efficacy of this class of drugs.

PATIENT NUMBER 3

Luke, a 54-year-old man, presents with vomiting and inability to keep food down. He notes that he has had a low-grade fever at home and comes to you because he developed shaking chills. On examination, the patient is diaphoretic and has a temperature of 100.8°F. His blood pressure is 140/90 mm Hg and pulse is 110. The examination is remarkable for guarding and tenderness on palpation in the right upper quadrant. Laboratory studies reveal normal findings on chest radiography and ECG, but his WBC is 16.2/mm³ with a left shift to more polymorphonuclear leukocytes. His alkaline phosphatase level is elevated, and his total bilirubin is slightly increased. An abdominal ultrasound examination reveals a dilated common bile duct containing stones. The patient is given cefoxitin and an aminoglycoside and later undergoes surgery, when an inflamed gallbladder is removed. Blood cultures subsequently grow enterococci. On the 10th hospital day, Luke's serum creatinine level begins to rise without any diminution of urine output. The patient is not orthostatic, and renal ultrasonography shows his kidneys to be normal size with normal parenchyma. No obstruction is noted. The urinary sediment demonstrates numerous granular pigmented casts and some WBCs and 1 + protein. Luke continues to have good urine output, but his BUN and creatinine levels rise each day. His urinary sodium level is greater than 20 mEq/L, and the calculated fractional excretion of sodium is > 2. In summary, this 54-year-old man presents with acute cholecystitis. His hospital course is complicated by the development of acute renal failure (ARF) that is high output in character and is most likely secondary to aminoglycoside use.

ARF occurs in approximately 2% to 5% of all hospitalized patients and has a mortality rate of at least 50%. The risk of ARF is higher in pa-tients with comorbid conditions including sepsis, trauma, hypoalbuminemia, and multisystem or-gan failure, as well as those who have recently undergone surgery. Our patient Luke has acute tubular necrosis, ostensibly from aminoglycoside toxicity. The time course after institution of the antibiotics and surgery and the high urinary out-put are consistent with this diagnosis, as is the presence of granular pigmented casts.

The clinician has some difficult management decisions to make. Unlike the previously de-scribed cases, in which renal function is fairly stable, Luke's function is in a state of flux, neces-sitating closer follow-up and careful adjustment of medicine doses plus monitoring of minerals and electrolytes on a daily basis. In ARF compli-cated by increased catabolism due to sepsis, sur-gery, and the severity of the underlying illness, nitrogenous waste products are rapidly gener-ated, outstripping the capacity of the residual renal function. Even without sepsis and surgery, excessive protein catabolism and sustained nega-tive nitrogen balance are characteristic of ARF. ARF increases the release of amino acids from skeletal muscle and impairs the use of amino acids for protein synthesis. Hormonal factors may be responsible for some of these changes, includ-ing resistance to the anabolic effects of insulin and increased circulating levels of PTH, gluca-gon, catecholamines, and corticosteroids. Circu-lating inflammatory mediators such as tumor ne-crosis factor and interleukins may also have a role. Because the kidneys have a major role in amino acid catabolism, various nonessential amino acids (e.g., arginine and serine) that are synthesized in the kidneys become essential in ARF.

The optimal dietary protein requirement for

patients with ARF is not known. Influencing factors include the type of underlying illness, the catabolic state of the patient, and the need for dialysis. **In most cases, it is impossible to keep a patient in positive or even neutral nitrogen balance because comorbid factors such as sepsis, burns, or trauma contribute to the hypercatabolic state of the patient.** Simply increasing nitrogen intake is not a solution, because the diet is quickly reflected in a rising serum urea level and accelerated urinary nitrogen appearance. These changes often prompt the need for dialysis, which by itself can stimulate muscle protein catabolism and may create problems including hypotension with further renal parenchymal damage, infection, bleeding, and even death.

With high-output ARF, patients may not have edema; the more usual presentation is with uremic symptoms. Timely intervention can forestall and may even obviate the need for dialysis. With respect to Luke, patient 3, dietary protein restriction should be instituted immediately for two reasons: First, increasing dietary protein beyond the minimum daily requirement has not been shown to be efficacious in producing protein anabolism; several studies suggest it might even be harmful. Second, a high-protein diet would simply promote accumulation of nitrogenous waste products, resulting in more uremic symptoms and a higher serum urea concentration plus a higher acid load. By restricting dietary protein, the degree of uremia can be reduced, the acidosis may be corrected, and the serum phosphorus level can be better controlled. Reports indicate some possible benefit to supplementing the diet with essential amino acids while minimizing intake of nonessential amino acids. On the other hand, aggressively providing large supplements of amino acids early in the course of ARF may be counterproductive, especially in ischemic tubular necrosis. Metabolic demands caused by increased renal blood flow and sodium reabsorption related to a high-protein diet can compromise oxygen supply, leading to more kidney damage. Thus, it is prudent early in the course of ARF to limit dietary protein until the degree of renal failure has stabilized. If it appears that the episode of ARF will not resolve within 4 or 5 days, then the amount of protein intake can be varied. For patients able to eat, the gut should always be used because of the many advantages over parenteral nutrition. Our patient Luke suffered a toxic insult to his kidneys, and this form of renal damage generally causes less catabolism than does an ischemic insult, and the patient can be treated conservatively. If dialytic intervention is required, protein or amino acid intake should be increased to 1 g/kg/day to compensate for substrate losses during therapy and the protein catabolic effects of dialysis.

Besides alterations in protein metabolism, ARF changes carbohydrate metabolism. Hyperglycemia is common secondary to insulin resistance, and increased hepatic gluconeogenesis is accelerated as a result of the conversion of amino acids released during protein catabolism. Both factors contribute to hyperglycemia. In most patients, insulin resistance and increased hepatic gluconeogenesis cause minimal changes in serum glucose, but in diabetic patients blood glucose levels may be more difficult to control.

Control of electrolyte values is a critical goal in treating patients with ARF because the damaged kidneys and other organs have not adapted to the changes in potassium, phosphorus, acid, and so on caused by ARF. Diet alone is usually sufficient to control hyperkalemia, but it is important to monitor other sources of potassium, including medications (e.g., penicillins or drugs that interfere with ion exchange such as trimethoprim), blood transfusion, and potassium in intravenous fluids. Minuscule amounts of intravenous potassium can cause dramatic changes in serum potassium levels in patients with ARF, and intravenous fluids with potassium should be discouraged. **A patient's ability to participate in such restrictions must not be underestimated, especially for a patient instructed in the goals of therapy and reassured that the restrictions are temporary.** For example, early dietary instruction and planning can be very helpful in avoiding draconian measures such as potassium-binding resins (e.g., Kayexalate) or dialysis. **As with CRF, much of the catabolism associated with renal failure can be attributed to acidosis, and if a patient can tolerate the sodium load, then every effort should be made to correct acidosis with sodium bicarbonate.** If a patient is being treated by intravenous hyperalimentation, acetate can be added to the fluid because it is converted to bicarbonate by the liver. Obviously, the patient must not have liver disease that would prevent metabolism of the acetate.

In many cases of ARF, sodium restriction is a mainstay of therapy because the ability to excrete salt is compromised. The goal of restricting sodium intake is to avoid fluid overload and the need for dialysis. The tendency for fluid overload is easily monitored by simply measuring changes in body weight. A loop diuretic can often be used to manage changes in extracellular volume, but if dialytic intervention is required, judicious fluid management can curtail how often it is required, can facilitate volume removal at the time of the treatment by avoiding large volume shifts, and theoretically can stave off further ischemic insults to the renal parenchyma. Avoiding large swings in extracellular volume with hemodynamic stability could lead to a more rapid return in renal function. **From a practical standpoint, the pharmacy should be asked to concentrate all medicines in dextrose/water solutions (i.e., D_5W).** Salt in the diet should be limited to 2 g, and a dietitian should be consulted to facilitate education and to coordinate dietary changes. A skilled dietitian can also make suggestions about seasonings to make the diet more palatable. It is important that patients have fluid restricted to avoid overload (monitored as an increase in weight), especially if they are oliguric or anuric. In patients such as Luke, fluid restriction is probably not necessary and may even be detrimental, especially if they begin to lose weight, signaling a loss of extracellular volume.

If a patient requires dialysis, a vitamin supplement should be given because water-soluble vitamins are removed by dialysis. Supplementing vitamin C above 250 mg/day should be avoided because it is metabolized to oxalic acid, which can induce renal damage from secondary oxalosis. Trace element toxicity can be a problem if a patient receives daily intravenous infusion of these elements, bypassing the selective absorptive process that occurs in the gut. Because diseased kidneys are unable to remove the excess amounts infused, toxicity occurs.

Hypocalcemia often occurs with ARF. The causes include high circulating levels of phosphorus, which suppress the serum calcium level, but vitamin D levels are also low. Serum PTH levels tend to be high and can cause hypercalcemia during the resolving stage of ARF. Dietary protein restriction tends to correct the hyperphosphatemia, but a phosphate binder may also be necessary. When hyperphosphatemia is corrected, the serum calcium level becomes normal. The physician should wait for this to occur, because calcium supplements given to correct hypocalcemia can lead to systemic calcifications. They should be avoided unless a patient has tetany.

PATIENT NUMBER 4

Bob is a 63-year-old man who received a heart transplant 8 years ago. He has fared quite well, but 4 years ago he developed renal failure, which was thought to be secondary to the immunosuppressive therapy used to treat his heart transplant. Eighteen months ago, he was started on peritoneal dialysis and fared very well initially. He reports that he was able to play 18 holes of golf a day and continue his job as a salesman, although it required extensive traveling. About 6 months ago, he noted increasing fatigue and weakness. His physical stamina declined. He tires easily now, can no longer play golf, and had to give up traveling. His employer thought that Bob had just been working too hard and gave him some time off, but he has noted no improvement in the past week. In fact, he notes shortness of breath with minimal exertion. He also has developed very loose stools and notes that food just doesn't taste good anymore. Over the past 3 or 4 days, he has developed nausea, cannot keep any food down, and has lost 15 pounds.

Bob states that he continues his usual peritoneal dialysis regimen, doing four 2-L exchanges four times a day. When he started dialysis, he was urinating frequently, but now he goes only once a day and has scant urine. He takes a vitamin and states that he sometimes remembers to take his calcium supplements. He has recently seen a cardiologist, who admitted him to the hospital for cardiac catheterization and heart biopsy and told him, "It's not your heart that's the problem." On examination, the patient appears cachectic. He weighs 66 kg, and his height is 6 ft. His blood pressure is 130/70 mm Hg and pulse is 67. He has temporal muscle wasting. His neck is supple; he has no jugular venous distention. His lungs show some decrease in breath sounds at the bases, and his heart seems normal. Bob's abdomen is benign, and the Tenkhoff peritoneal catheter site is not infected. He has ankle edema. Laboratory studies reveal a serum sodium level of 137 mmol/L, chloride level of 103 mmol/L, bicarbonate of 18 mmol/L, and potassium of 2.9 mmol/L. His BUN is 45 mg/dl, and he has levels of serum creatinine of 25 mg/dl, phosphorus 2.5, and calcium 6.9 mg/dl. His liver function test results are unremarkable, but his serum albumin level is 2.3 g/dl and serum proteins are 6.2 g/dl, with an alkaline phosphatase level of 147 IU/L. His hematocrit is 25%, and his WBC count is 4.5. He asks you, **"What can I do to feel better, Doc?"**

In summary, Bob is a 63-year-old man who has ESRD after a heart transplant and is being treated by dialysis. After initially faring well, he develops uremic symptoms over 18 months. His physical findings are remarkable because of evidence of malnutrition and excessive extracellular volume. His laboratory results, in particular the low BUN and high serum creatinine, suggest that he is starving because of his uremic symptoms.

Bob illustrates some of the sequelae that can

occur if a patient is inadequately dialyzed. It is obvious that the patient is not well: He is cachectic and has a constellation of complaints, all of which can be attributed to uremia. These include nausea, vomiting, diarrhea, fatigue, and loss of endurance. The laboratory values confirm that Bob is suffering from malnutrition, because both the serum albumin and protein values are low, and the BUN is low, suggesting that the patient is not eating. What is more striking is that both the serum phosphorus and potassium levels are too low for a patient with ESRD, again suggesting that he is not eating.

Nearly one third of patients undergoing peritoneal dialysis suffer from malnutrition, as indicated by low serum levels of protein and albumin. Loss of protein and albumin in the peritoneal fluid is variable; some patients may lose more than 20 g/day, but most lose between 4 and 8 g/day, necessitating a more liberal protein intake. This often proves difficult even in the most compliant of patients for a number of reasons. The peritoneal dialysate fluid compresses the stomach and other digestive organs, creating a feeling of satiety. Moreover, dextrose in the dialysate can contribute up to 1000 kcal/day of calories, and the carbohydrate is often converted to fat, producing a clinical situation not unlike marasmus. Efforts to improve the nutritional status of a patient undergoing peritoneal dialysis rely on several strategies. First, it should be ascertained if the patient is a suitable candidate for peritoneal dialysis. Suitability may change when residual renal function declines, when the effectiveness of the peritoneum as a dialysis membrane deteriorates, or when the patient's interest in peritoneal dialysis wanes. Any of these problems could alter the dialysis prescription or prompt a switch to hemodialysis. However, if the dialysis prescription is satisfactory and it is ascertained that the patient is getting the prescribed amount of dialysis, then alterations in the patient's diet should be pursued. **Because of protein losses in the peritoneal dialysate fluid, the dietary protein restriction is generally liberalized to 1.2 to 1.4 g/kg ideal body weight.** Foods with high biologic value (rich in essential amino acids as a percentage of weight) may be useful in patients with severe protein malnutrition. For example, boiled egg whites can be sprinkled on the food. They are economical and have the added advantage of being low in phosphorus content.

In our patient Bob, it is not apparent why he has become uremic if the history is correct and the patient was faring well until 6 months ago. First, it must be determined that the dialysis is adequate. Because he is seeking medical advice, it is likely that it is. Next, it must be determined why dialysis is not working sufficiently well to prevent uremia. One striking difference is noted between the initial period of successful therapy and the current unsuccessful period: Urinary output has declined. This suggests that residual renal function has declined, and this appears to be the most likely reason for the gradual onset of uremic symptoms. Initially, the combination of dialysis and residual renal function provided the patient with sufficient clearance of uremic toxins, but the patient's dialysis prescription was not adjusted to compensate for the gradual loss of residual renal function, and uremic symptoms appeared. A similar scenario can occur in elderly patients with chronic renal disease. Uremia often appears in a subtle form. Elderly patients often have other medical problems or are taking medicines that contribute to anorexia and inanition, resulting in loss of muscle mass and a lower level of creatinine production. Subtle changes in serum creatinine values in a thin patient may signify a marked decrement in renal function. The patient's response to the accumulation of unexcreted waste products can be maladaptive because his or her dietary intake of protein falls sharply, leading to a further decline in body mass. It behooves the clinician to recognize that **a mildly elevated serum creatinine level in a slim elderly patient may actually signify severe loss of renal function.** Improving the nutritional status in these patients can entail more than simply increasing caloric intake.

PATIENT NUMBER 4 (continued)

Attempts were made to increase the volume of dialysate used per dialysate infusion, but Bob tolerated this change poorly. A peritoneal dialysis automatic cycler was tried at night, but the patient could not sleep and was switched to hemodialysis. His nausea and vomiting quickly resolved, and his appetite improved. Within 2 months, Bob had gained 10 pounds. His edema resolved, and his albumin level increased to 4.0 mg/dl. He resumed his golf game after 6 weeks. He no longer travels for his job, but he likes it better that way.

Besides inadequate dialysis, it is worth remembering that severe secondary hyperparathyroidism can contribute to anorexia and weight loss in patients undergoing dialysis. Elevated phosphorus, alkaline phosphatase, and PTH levels in a patient such as Bob should prompt aggressive measures to control serum phosphorus levels in conjunction with vitamin D therapy. Successful therapy can result in a return of appetite and an improvement in nutritional status.

SELECTED REFERENCES

Drum W: Nutritional support in acute renal failure. *In* Mitch WE, Klahr S (eds): Nutrition and the Kidney. Boston. Little, Brown & Co, 1993, pp 314–345.

Gilmour ER, Hartley GH, Goodship THJ: Trace elements and vitamins in renal disease. *In* Mitch WE, Klahr S (eds): Nutrition and the Kidney. Boston, Little, Brown & Co, 1993, pp 114–131.

Kopple JD, Monteon FJ, Shaib JK: Effect of energy intake on nitrogen metabolism in nondialyzed patients with chronic renal failure. Kidney Int 29:734–742, 1986.

Maroni BJ: Requirements for protein, calories, and fat in the predialysis patient. *In* Mitch WE, Klahr S (eds): Nutrition and the Kidney. Boston, Little, Brown & Co, 1993, pp 185–212.

Maroni BJ, Steinman T, Mitch WE: A method for estimating nitrogen intake of patients with chronic renal failure. Kidney Int 27:58–65, 1985.

Mitch WE, Walser M: Nutritional therapy of the uremic patient. *In* Brenner BM, Rector FC (eds): The Kidney. Philadelphia, WB Saunders, 1991, pp 2186–2222.

16 | PSYCHIATRIC ASPECTS OF RENAL CARE

Norman B. Levy

The patients described in this chapter illustrate the major psychiatric manifestations of renal care: uncooperativeness, depression and suicide, anxiety, problems of rehabilitation, and sexual dysfunctions. The discussion of these problems deals with the potentially curative and ameliorative measures that may be taken by medical professionals.

UNCOOPERATIVENESS

PATIENT NUMBER 1

Billie is a single 23-year-old African-American inner-city woman. She entered the dialysis unit with a pastrami (spiced meat) sandwich in hand and proceeded to eat it in an exhibitionistic manner while cursing out the nursing and physician staff. She was confronted by a no-nonsense nurse who refused to start the patient on dialysis until she was able to conduct herself with reasonable decorum. After some time elapsed and the patient was being dialyzed for a while, the nurse asked the patient how things were going in her life. This question brought on tears and the statement, "Life is shit!" She said that her boyfriend Kenny had just broken up with her because he had heard that women on dialysis cannot have babies.

Background information on this patient includes the fact that she is a product of a severely emotionally deprived childhood and was able to liberate herself from her home when she became pregnant at the age of 15 (before renal failure). Although a high school dropout, she is a person of superior intelligence and is street smart. She had been able to establish some economic stability in her life as a salesperson. However, minor skirmishes with the law because of petty theft, including two arrests but no imprisonment, have impaired her. In general, she is well liked by the staff because of her quick wit and her concern about the feelings of others. Her relationship with Kenny, a tough African-American of about the same age, had been quite stable despite his own minor problems with the law

connected with his selling marijuana. She attained a fair degree of social stability in the past year in part because of her relationship with him.

This case illustrates some of the causes of uncooperative behavior and addresses the issue of what to do about it. As exemplified by the actions of the no-nonsense nurse, setting and enforcing reasonable guidelines can be an important way of dealing with this problem. Medical professionals who permit uncooperative patients to engage too freely in their behavior enable disruption of the dialysis unit and give patients the wrong message of passive permission by the staff. In this case, the nurse set limits and enforced them by not permitting Billie to be dialyzed unless she could act reasonably appropriately. Further, the nurse attempted to find out what was underlying this behavior by asking the patient about recent events in her life at the appropriate time. Here, Billie's frustration and depression resulted in anger that was displaced onto the dialysis unit and staff.

Causes of Uncooperativeness

Frustration Tolerance

Children and infants have great difficulty tolerating frustration. As one gets older, one should gain the ability to delay immediate gratification in favor of longer-term gains. Adults vary greatly in their attainment of this aspect of maturity. Immature adults usually feel angry about not getting what they want when they want it. **Virtually every form of medical treatment involves a delay in gratification and some frustration, and its benefits are not usually immediately realized.**

Depression

Depression may be viewed as anger expressed inwardly. However, some of the inward expression of anger may also be seen in its outward manifestations.[1] In the case previously cited, Billie's sadness at losing her boyfriend resulted in her expressing her frustration and anger in a displaced manner. Severely depressed patients with poor self-esteem may have major difficulty mobilizing sufficient energy to be constructive in their lives. Their self-destructiveness may be at odds with the positive effects of medical treatment and may outweigh the benefits. The ultimate reflection of this problem is suicide (discussed later).

Slower forms of self-destruction may be manifested by not adhering to diet and missing dialysis runs.

Anger at Being Sick

Good health is often taken for granted, and when one recovers from illness, one expects that good health will continue. Although we acknowledge our mortality, each of us harbors a combined wish/fantasy that we will somehow continue life and good health indefinitely. The news media tend to promote such an attitude by announcements of medical and surgical "cures." The public has almost begun to believe that major diseases have been or soon will be cured. Recognizing and accepting having a serious illness are major tasks for every patient. Expectation and feelings of entitlement to good health may result in anger when we become sick. The anger is often connected with a sense of injustice, rationalized around ideas such as, "I'm a married woman with two children. It's not fair that I have kidney disease and the nurse over there is single and has normal kidney function."

Authority Intolerance

A hierarchy of authority figures exists in the medical establishment. **Physicians, nurses, and other medical personnel all are authority figures, and patients react to medical personnel as they do to other authorities.** This attitude at times shows up by slips of the tongue. For example, I have on many occasions been called "Father" by my Catholic patients. Many patients cope well with dependent situations. They may derive satisfaction from the regression involved and look to a parental figure for guidance, comfort, and protection. However, for a significant minority, physicians and other medical personnel are the focus of their anger as other authority figures have been in the past.

DEPRESSION AND SUICIDE

PATIENT NUMBER 2

Kevin, a single 27-year-old white man who had been diabetic for 15 years, developed renal failure 3 months before I initially saw him. He had additional complications of diabetes in being legally blind, although he was able to read large print after laser treatment and had progressive neuropathy, from which he anticipated becoming wheelchair bound shortly. He was an only child of two diabetic parents who died of complications of their illness 2 and 4 years before the patient's renal failure. Unemployed, blind, and alone, he saw dialysis as the last straw. When I saw Kevin in consultation, he told me that he had given up on life. He said that he didn't know why he continued to permit himself to be dialyzed. He refused antidepressant medication and psychotherapy, which I offered him. **Two weeks after my interview, he was found dead. He had hung himself.**

Although this is an extreme case of depression that led to suicide, it well illustrates some aspects of this disorder. As previously mentioned, depression may be described as anger reflected inwardly and often occurs in response to loss.[2] Our patients sustain many losses. Two thirds of patients undergoing dialysis never return to full-time work activity. Job loss results in loss of income and possibly loss of self-esteem and gender identity. Among these patients, losses are many and extend beyond employment. Patients with renal failure, especially those on dialysis, may lose their freedom, longevity, and sexual function. Although we are all depressed at certain times, a relatively small percentage of the population has a true syndrome of depression. This involves more than just a depressed mood and includes somatic concomitants of it, such as an eating disorder, a sleeping disorder, feelings of poor self-esteem, feelings of being better off dead, and indeed even suicidal wishes and acts. **A significant percent of patients with renal failure are clinically depressed and should be treated for it.**[2] Our patient Kevin lost his eyesight, physical freedom, and ability to ambulate and suffered constraints and restrictions connected with being on dialysis. We know nothing about his sexual function, but we may be correct to speculate that it may have been significantly compromised. His response was extreme but not unusual in patients on dialysis. We do know that suicide is more common in dialyzed patients than in the general population.[3, 4] It is not known whether patients on dialysis have a greater incidence of suicide than persons with other chronic severe illnesses. This may well be so, because patients on dialysis, unlike many others, have the avenue for their demise readily at hand, although not exemplified in Kevin's case. It is not uncommon for suicidal patients undergoing dialysis to miss dialysis runs and go on a potassium binge. In days past, when external shunts were used, patients were readily able to exsanguinate. Perhaps having an easy way to commit suicide predisposes dialysis patients to it. About 1 in 1000 patients on dialysis actually commits suicide. A larger number engage in other forms of behavior that are self-destructive and may lead to death, such as severe dietary indiscretion. **It is urgently important for physicians and other professionals to identify clinically depressed patients who are prone to suicidal behavior so that adequate measures may be instituted.** Little is known about depression and suicide in renal transplant recipients.[5] No studies have investigated suicide and depression in this population. Suicide is probably no more prevalent among renal transplant recipients than among other groups medicated with prednisone, the most common psychologic complication of which is depression. Therefore, professional personnel should carefully monitor depression in these individuals, especially during periods in which they are receiving large doses of steroids.

ANXIETY

> **PATIENT NUMBER 3**
>
> Robert was a 21-year-old college student who showed all behavioral signs of anxiety while undergoing dialysis and expressed the feeling that being on hemodialysis was "like watching a Dracula movie." He attempted to diminish his anxiety by operating his radio and television set while writing letters during hemodialysis.[2]

The process of hemodialysis is more anxiety provoking than peritoneal dialysis because it involves greater immediate potential threat to life and well-being. Although mishaps on dialysis are rare, they do occur. Virtually all patients on hemodialysis for any reasonable period of time have seen others in such situations.

Anxiety may be manifested in a number of different ways. Some people experience it directly and are able to identify it as anxiety. Others experience it indirectly. In the past, when hemodialysis runs took several hours and patients usually stayed overnight on their units, anxiety was commonly encountered as insomnia. Masturbation, especially among men, is common in patients on hemodialysis. Although experienced as a sexual phenomenon, it is essentially a method of reducing anxiety.

Anxiety is also encountered in renal transplant recipients. Having a transplant and awaiting organ rejection is equated to having the Sword of Damocles hanging over one's head.[6] However, patients tend to acclimate themselves to the situation. They do become anxious when and if early signs of rejection occur. Anxiety is also a side effect of prednisone.

PROBLEMS IN REHABILITATION

> **PATIENT NUMBER 4**
>
> Arnold is a 30-year-old carpenter who felt that physicians and nurses in his dialysis unit would strongly disapprove of him if he did not reestablish himself in his work after being on dialysis for several weeks. When he went out for the first time since being sick to subcontract for a major carpentry job, he developed a medical problem. When asked how he felt about returning to work, Arnold said, "I didn't know whether I could do it . . . I felt down in the dumps . . . I am willing to try . . . You never known until you try . . . I'll have to try again." He continued to have medical problems several months after this. In the 5 years that he has been monitored since then, he never returned to carpentry and worked only intermittently as a bartender.

It is unfortunate that "full rehabilitation" is usually measured by full-time return to work, household, or school activity. This model is not really feasible for patients on dialysis. As we all know, patients on dialysis often do not have a feeling of well-being, caused by the treatment itself as well as its sequelae. Unlike people who have normal kidney function and have continuous removal of wastes from their body, patients on dialysis receive this intermittently. It is important to keep in mind that the artificial method of replacing kidney function probably does not replicate in many ways the normal functioning of the kidneys, much of which is not fully understood. Although erythropoietin has increased quality of life, we do know that it has had little or no effect on increasing dialyzed patients' employment rate, which, as previously mentioned, is about only one third of the dialysis population. Other reasons for diminished vitality include secondary hyperparathyroidism and renal osteodystrophy, to mention just two. Manual workers have more difficulty returning to work than white collar workers, professionals, and business people because their work tends to be less time flexible, is more physical, and is less likely to be adaptable to the requirements of life on dialysis. **Because rehabilitation tends to be seen as a function of work activity, it therefore favors those occupations connected with higher socioeconomic status, such as business and the professions.**

Our current economic system, in an attempt to diminish the "punishment" of illness, provides monetary and other compensations to those it considers to be unable to work because of sickness. Therefore, to an extent it encourages partial or full retirement, especially among those for whom work has never been a highly prized activity. Healthy manual laborers and blue collar workers tend to retire at a younger age than individuals in business and in the professions.

Men and women differ in respect to rehabilitation, and work for most is a significant factor in self-esteem. Even in these days of greater gender equality, women who are married still have greater flexibility (but less so than their mothers did) than others in terms of outside work versus home-oriented activities. Such an option is not available to men and single women. Married women on dialysis are more likely to be able to leave the outside work force and become homemakers, which may be more compatible with life on dialysis.

SEXUAL PROBLEMS

PATIENT NUMBER 5

Martin, a 44-year-old physician who had been known to be diabetic for 10 years, had been on dialysis for 2 years when he developed further progression of diabetic retinopathy, which made it necessary for him to retire from his specialty practice. Because he complained of depression, I was asked to see him in psychiatric consultation.

He was clearly depressed and had a mood, eating, and sleeping disorder and feelings of poor self-esteem. He was not suicidal and did not have thoughts about being better off dead. As part of every history, I ask about sexual function. He reported that he had some difficulty getting erections during the past 2 years since being on dialysis, but he said that he has been totally impotent since the onset of his depression several weeks ago. I saw him in once-weekly supportive psychotherapy and placed him on a tricyclic antidepressant, nortriptyline. About 4 weeks after initiation of treatment, his depression began to lift and be reported marked improvement in his sexual function. After 8 weeks of treatment, he resumed his usual predepression sexual function.

People on dialysis of both genders suffer more loss in sexual functioning than most patients with other chronic physical illnesses. Before systematic investigation of the sexuality of patients with renal failure, clinicians observed that men on dialysis had more problems with impotence than can be explained on the basis of their apparent medical findings such as fatigue, anemia, and intermittent azotemia. When inquiries were made about the sexual function of these patients, it was discovered that both men and women had marked diminution in the frequency of sexual intercourse in comparison with that before renal failure. **About 70% of men on dialysis and 43% of renal transplant recipients are partially or totally impotent.**[7] Both men and women on dialysis and recipients of renal transplants have a diminution in sexual function as measured by frequency of sexual intercourse. Women on dialysis also have a diminution in frequency of orgasm during sexual intercourse. Investigations into the origins of these sexual functions largely incriminate organic as opposed to psychologic causes. The main method of ascertaining this differential is by measures of nocturnal penile tumescence, based on the fact that men normally have erections during phase 1 rapid-eye-movement (REM) sleep. This method is based on the assumption that those who complain of impotence but have erections during the night have psychologic causes of this problem, whereas those who are impotent and show no ability to get an erection during the night have an organic cause. The precise organic reason for impotence in patients on dialysis as well as in renal transplant recipients is not fully understood. A number of metabolic and other factors have been incriminated. These include high levels of prolactin, low levels of testosterone, diminished ability to produce sperm, cessation of menstruation, and hyperparathyroidism. One psychologic cause of sexual dysfunction is depression, in which diminution of the libido is common. Our patient Martin illustrates this. It also shows that the combination of diabetes and end-stage renal disease has concomitant somatic reasons for sexual dysfunction. The sexual dysfunction of diabetic patients is probably based on a peripheral neuropathy.

Compromise in the sense of gender identity is another cause of impotence. Men who have total cessation of urination may perceive this as a loss of function of the penis, which is the organ for urination as well as sexuality. Cessation of menstruation as well as a less attractive appearance may be perceived by women as defeminizing. **Failure to continue work and reversal of family roles may be interpreted by both sexes as compromise in their gender identity.** Also, organic causes may produce secondary psychologic impotence. If an organically caused episode of impotence is felt to be a major blow to an individual's sense of masculinity, he may withdraw from sexual situations and feel less manly, leading to further deterioration in his sexual function. Treatment of sexual dysfunction of these patients is directed at the underlying cause. For example, depression may be treated by an antidepressant as cited earlier. Hyperprolactinemia may be treated with bromocriptine, hyperparathyroidism may require surgical therapy, and psychologic difficulties should be appropriately treated as discussed in the later section on treatment.

PSYCHIATRIC FITNESS FOR TRANSPLANTATION

PATIENT NUMBER 6

Lisa, a 25-year-old patient with a history of anorexia nervosa, developed kidney failure and was placed on a cadaveric waiting list. A suitable organ was found 2 years later, and transplantation was successful. However, because of persisting anorexia and bouts of severe starvation, her transplanted organ was essentially starved to death. It was removed, and she was returned to dialysis.

Although it is difficult to prognosticate human behavior, one of the few semireliable indicators is past performance. The variables are great, and

either an individual's maturity or his or her regression can lead to variations from past behavior patterns. However, this was not the case for Lisa, who, despite her severe anorexia nervosa, somehow managed to convince a transplant surgeon that her previous illness would not affect subsequent treatment. Unfortunately, this was not the case.

Transplantation should be avoided in individuals who are seriously depressed or psychotic or who have a history of medical noncompliance. Steroids may be unsettling in any of these patients and can produce a very stormy course. Surgeons know from their own experience and that of their colleagues that it is inadvisable to operate electively on individuals who predict their own demise or who do not expect to survive after the intended operative procedure.

Another relative indicator of adaptation is the nature and strength of support systems provided by family and friends. If such a system is strong, it helps patients work through the adversities of the situation. Lack of such a strong system may leave patients with little to rely on.

The presence or absence of deviant personalities or of mild or moderate psychologic syndromes is not a reliable predictor of adaptation and should not be used to determine fitness for transplantation.

TREATMENT OF PSYCHIATRIC PROBLEMS

Preventive Therapy

Many measures may diminish or minimize the incidence of psychologic problems among patients. Such maneuvers include careful assessment of patients before a specific renal therapy is selected so that the treatment can be tailored to an individual's psychologic needs.

More independent patients should be on forms of self-therapy or should undergo transplantation. It is also important to identify individuals who are at greater risk for psychologic difficulties, based on their past history and their current presentation. These patients should be monitored more closely than others, especially by psychologically trained practitioners, so that if problems arise they may be treated early.

Group Therapies

The most successful group therapies have been those in which the major focus has not been on psychologic aspects. A psychologic focus tends to scare participants away. The groups that have been able to attract relatively consistent attendance have been characterized by their emphasis on coping, their limited number of sessions, their location in centers in which patients are dialyzed, their inclusion of partners of patients, and their educational aspects. These characteristics may be achieved by inviting guest professionals such as dietitians, social workers, nephrologists, and transplant surgeons to offer useful information.

Environmental Manipulations

These comprise relatively simple to more complex activities that sensitive physicians initiate to ameliorate conflicts, avoid difficulties, and otherwise promote a patient's coping with illness and treatment. Included are such activities as setting up days and hours with compatible fellow patients and compatible staff, engaging in reasonable compromises concerning dietary restrictions, and offering sound advice, when appropriate, about activities outside the medical situation.

Psychotherapy

Renal patients, as a group, tend to resist formal psychotherapy. They already feel "overdoctored" and as a group use denial extensively in facing their psychologic problems. However, selected well-motivated patients may be suitable for psychotherapy and may be greatly helped by it. This treatment, although usually the domain of psychiatrists or psychologists, may also be performed by adequately trained social workers and nurses. Generally, both dialysis and transplant recipients respond to supportive therapies that are focused on particular syndromes and tend to use psychoactive medications. A few patients have undergone extensive psychoanalysis requiring a few visits each week for a year or longer. There are psychologically minded, younger, and very well-motivated individuals with kidney disease who should be carefully identified.

Pharmacotherapy

The symptoms associated with anxiety, depression, mania, and psychosis can usually be either eradicated or markedly ameliorated by the use of psychoactive medications. Fortunately, most of these medications are not removed by the kidneys and are not dialyzable. The exceptions are the barbiturates, which should be avoided, and lithium, which involves special considerations, mentioned later. **All major tranquilizers, all antidepressants, and the benzodiazepines pass the blood-brain barrier, are fat soluble, are metabolized by the liver, are not excreted by the kidneys, and are not dialyzed.**[8] The general rule is to use no more than two thirds the maximum dose that would be given to persons with normal kidney function. The reasons are discussed in Chapter 12 and include such considerations as absorption, distribution in the body, and protein binding in patients with renal failure. Lithium, a relatively simple salt, is removed by the kidneys and is dialyzable. It can be used by giving a single dose after each dialysis run. Without kidney function, relatively little of it is removed until the next dialysis. Blood levels of lithium can easily be monitored.

Behavioral/Sexual Techniques

A method of treating sexual dysfunction that was originally described by Masters and Johnson and modified by Helen Singer Kaplan and others has potential wide use in patients on dialysis. The basis for its efficacy lies in the fact that people who have sexual dysfunction tend to withdraw from intimate contact with their partners. Behavioral sexual therapy is practiced by trained social workers and other professionals and involves the use of sensate focusing, which is a method of sexual stimulation, and the setting of sexual goals that are feasible and that do not necessarily include actual intercourse. It favors a progressive, relaxed intimacy that can be successful in markedly improving the sexual function of patients—even those with the severest degree of organically caused sexual dysfunction.

CONCLUSIONS

It is important for medical professionals to be cognizant of the stresses and psychologic complications experienced by patients undergoing dialysis and renal transplantation. Although prevention may be an important aspect, a number of treatment modalities offer patients cure or improvement.[9, 10]

REFERENCES

1. Burton NJ, Kline SA, Lindsay RM, et al: The relationship of depression to survival in chronic renal failure. Psychosom Med 48:261, 1986.

2. Reichsman F, Levy NB: Problems in adaptation to maintenance hemodialysis: A four-year study of 25 patients. Arch Intern Med 130:850, 1972.
3. Abram HS, Moore GL, Westervelt FB Jr: Suicidal behavior in chronic dialysis patients. Am J Psychiatry 127:1199, 1971.
4. Haenel T, Brunner F, Battegay R: Renal dialysis and suicide: Occurrence in Switzerland and in Europe. Compr Psychiatry 21:140, 1980.
5. Steinberg J, Levy NB: Psychiatric factors in renal transplantation. *In* Chaterjee SN (ed): Manual of Renal Transplantation. New York, Springer-Verlag, 1979, pp 167–173.
6. Levy NB: Renal transplantation and the new medical era. *In* Guggenheim F (ed): Psychological Aspects of Surgery. Basel, S Karger AG, 1986, pp 167–179.
7. Levy NB: Sexual adjustment to maintenance hemodialysis and renal transplantation: National survey by questionnaire. Trans Am Soc Artif Intern Organs 19:138, 1973.
8. Levy NB: Psychopharmacology in patients with renal failure. Int J Psychiatry Med 20:303–312, 1990.
9. Levy NB, Blumenfield M, Beasley CM Jr, et al: Fuoxetine in depressed patients with renal failure and in depressed patients with normal kidney function. Gen Hosp Psychiatr 18:3–13, 1996.
10. Brown TH, Brown RLS: Neuropsychiatric consequences of renal failure. Psychosomatics 36:244–253, 1995.

17 | SELECTED ETHICAL ISSUES IN CARING FOR THE RENAL PATIENT*

Ronald Baker Miller

INTRODUCTORY COMMENTS

This chapter begins by describing how the history of nephrology and that of bioethics are interconnected and offers a few comments on the purpose of the chapter. It then provides a summary of the principles, concepts, and methods of clinical bioethics that are applicable to medicine generally, not just to nephrology. After a brief overview of the range of ethical issues in nephrology follows an analysis in greater depth of selected ethical issues in chronic renal failure, end-stage renal disease (ESRD), and dialysis. These are illustrated by descriptions of ethical dilemmas that I faced with a number of beloved patients who taught me more about the practice of medicine and more about life than I cared to admit I did not know (when I met them).

We follow Elizabeth Baldwin from her childhood fears caused by observing her father's slow uremic demise due to polycystic kidney disease (leading to her vow never to marry or to have children), to the symptomatic onset of her disease as a young adult (and the reaffirmation of her vow), and to renal failure beginning with the birth of her own two children.

We then agonize over the withholding of dialysis from Rodney, a high school junior with cystic fibrosis, and from Rose, a middle-aged housewife with analgesic nephropathy. Rose presented in renal failure before the term ESRD entered our lexicon and when one had to be not only young and otherwise healthy but also an outstanding member of society to be accepted for long-term dialysis.

We meet Melissa, a 3-year-old who was refused long-term hemodialysis (in the days when dialysis was rationed as a scarce commodity) because of "mental retardation," which "miraculously disappeared" after a successful renal trans-

plant, insisted on by her devoted nephrologist. Then we skip ahead in time to the present to discuss a concern that the expansion of "acceptance criteria since the enactment of Medicare entitlement" and perhaps other factors such as fear of litigation or economic gain have led nephrologists to inappropriately dialyze "patients with limited survival possibilities and relatively poor quality of life," as described by the Institute of Medicine. We then recommend guidelines for accepting patients for ESRD treatment.

In discussion of advance directives, we describe Dimitrios, a self-employed married businessman who requested (before he or his physician ever heard of a living will) that his nephrologist stop dialysis should Dimitrios become too ill to make decisions for himself and be a burden on his wife, whom he wished to spare the agony of making such a decision. We also review the distress of a family and a physician who decided to forgo continued treatment of a housewife who was on home dialysis and who became critically ill and delirious. Her treatment preferences under desperate circumstances were unknown to her nephrologist of 15 years. In considering do-not-attempt-resuscitation (DNAR) orders, we present the plight of Fleetwood and his family, who requested that his preference not to be resuscitated (should cardiac arrest occur) not be temporarily suspended when we thought it appropriate to do so.

In the final section on withdrawal of dialysis, we consider whether we should withdraw treatment of an incompetent patient, Theodore Phoenix, who had no surrogate or advance directive. He appeared to be suffering from the effects of a devastating dementing illness, and we admitted that in his present condition would not be considered for initiation of long-term dialysis. The final patient, Heather, had renal failure from accelerated hypertension and an organic brain syndrome that did not improve on even daily

---

*This chapter is copyrighted by Ronald Baker Miller.

203

dialysis. She competently elected to discontinue dialysis despite reservations of her family and her physician.

After recommending guidelines for the withdrawal of dialysis, we offer a few concluding remarks.

THE INTERCONNECTED HISTORY OF NEPHROLOGY AND BIOETHICS

The historical developments of nephrology (particularly the care of patients with ESRD) and of bioethics are parallel. Nephrology developed as a result of extraordinary growth in understanding the physiology of the kidneys and the biochemistry of fluid and electrolytes. It also evolved as a result of the application of new technologies: the pH meter, the flame photometer, the electron microscope, radioimmunoassay, and radiographic and other imaging techniques. The subdisciplines of long-term dialysis and renal transplantation similarly grew from new knowledge and new technology: The excretory and metabolic functions of the kidneys and the immunologic basis of transplant rejection became better understood, and new technologies included the artificial kidney, the biocompatible arteriovenous shunt, and the application of adrenal corticosteroids and azathioprine for engrafted patients.

Bioethics developed a decade or two later than nephrology. It emerged in the context of the civil rights movement, which facilitated the notion of the right to self-determination in medical decisions. In preceding centuries, these decisions had been made by paternalistic pronouncements. Bioethics was, at least in part, a response to the new dilemmas posed by the extraordinary technologies of acute and long-term dialysis, mechanical ventilation, cardiopulmonary resuscitation (CPR), and abrogation of transplant rejection. Indeed, some say that long-term hemodialysis gave birth to bioethics in Seattle in the early 1960s, when patients came from all over the world to be treated and when so few human and machine resources were available that decisions had to be made about who should live and who would die. To make these heart-wrenching decisions, a multidisciplinary patient selection committee was formed. It became known pejoratively as the "God Committee," a name conceived in obvious social discomfort with the job at hand. Although bioethics committees developed independently nearly two decades later, patient selection committees may have set the

stage for the acceptance of multidisciplinary ethics committees, which became a powerful means for analyzing and resolving ethical dilemmas in clinical medicine.

THE PURPOSE OF THIS CHAPTER

The purpose of this chapter is to review the application of bioethics (which evolved from philosophic and religious roots) to clinical nephrology. Clinical medical ethics is a discipline for a systematic approach to the identification, analysis, and resolution of moral dilemmas that arise in the care of patients. How did doctors and patients get along before the development of this new discipline? Some say there were fewer questions about what *should* be done because there were fewer options for what *could* be done. Others note that medicine is inherently ethical, and although decisions were made paternalistically ("parentalistically," to be politically correct), they were always intended to be in the best interests of patients. Bioethics has enriched our care of patients. For example, it has helped us to understand that what nephrologists believed to be in the best interests of their patients was not always what patients believed to be in their own best interests. This perspective is exemplified by the mnemonic of a thoughtful bioethicist, WILTBURN: What's It Like To Be You Right Now? This bioethicist, Ruth Purtilo, also noted that the intellectual accomplishment of resolving a clinical ethical dilemma is emotionally exhausting, just as it was in the days before we had heard of bioethics, self-determination, informed consent, advance directives, DNAR, persistent/permanent vegetative state (PVS), Quinlan, Cruzan, and Kevorkian. The majority of ethical decisions in caring for renal patients should *not* be easy; they are not decisions between right and wrong, virtue and vice. They are decisions between two goods, between two principles (both correct but in conflict), or between the same principle (or the same right) from the differing perspectives of two individuals (or of one individual and of society).

Finally, by way of introduction, I should note that bioethics, like medicine generally, is best learned from patients. We in the health care professions have the enormous privilege of being involved in the lives of our patients. The care of a patient with chronic disease allows us to get to know the patient as a person. **As Peabody said in 1927, "the secret of the care of the patient is in caring for the patient."**[1] Indeed, the privilege of the practice of medicine involves a sacred trust—the bond between patient and physician—which we must respect and must never violate.

THE PRINCIPLES, CONCEPTS, AND METHODS OF CLINICAL BIOETHICS

The ethical issues of nephrology for the most part are qualitatively the same as those of medicine generally, but many of the issues are quantitatively more intense. This is in no small measure a result of the ingenuity and success of nephrologists and transplant surgeons in having developed multiple treatments for renal failure. The diversity of alternative treatments requires careful weighing of the benefits, risks, and burdens of all options so that the nephrologist and the patient care team may inform and advise patients and their families. The intensity of decision making was substantially greater when dialysis was less able to relieve uremic symptoms and more likely to cause unpleasant symptoms and when transplantation was more likely to be complicated by lethal infection. Although successful transplantation was better able to restore health and well-being, transplant recipients were more likely to die than if they remained on dialysis.

Before we can deal with specific ethical issues of renal patients, we should review the principles, concepts, and methods of clinical ethics. These enable informed medical decision making (including refusal of interventions), planning for serious illness and for the potential loss of decision-making capacity, and resolution of ethical dilemmas and conflicts.

Principles of Bioethics

First- and Second-Order Principles

The first-order principles of biomedical ethics have been enunciated by the Kennedy Institute of Ethics at Georgetown University (and thoroughly examined by Beauchamp and Childress[2]). **The principles are respect for autonomy (the right of self-determination), nonmaleficence (doing no harm), beneficence (doing good or what is in the best interest of patients), and justice (fairness in the allocation of resources and in treating like individuals in like circumstances in like ways).**

Secondary principles of bioethics include confidentiality and privacy, integrity and veracity (honesty and truth telling), fidelity (promise keeping), respect for persons and for the sanctity of life, the golden rule (the rule of reciprocity), and proportionality (decision making by weighing the benefits and burdens of any given action).

Conflicts of Principles: Ethical Dilemmas

Bioethical dilemmas are conflicts of values in which any single resolution is rarely unequivocally right and others absolutely wrong. These dilemmas may result from the varied perspectives of the patient, the health care professional, and society. Ethical concerns from a patient's perspective include the need for confidentiality, privacy, respect as an individual (and as a member of a cultural, religious, or philosophic group), justice (with access to affordable, effective health care), and the right to make decisions for oneself and to be helped (as well as not to be harmed). Health care professionals need the right to practice according to professional and personal ethical standards, respect for selfless provision of care, and reasonable reward (particularly in the form of personal satisfaction) for the care of others. Society needs the goals of medicine to be met in the context of an equitable and affordable allocation of health care resources. The allocation needs to be balanced with other societal needs and with respect to allocation of one form of health care versus another and with respect to one group of individuals versus others. The goals of medicine are to restore, maintain, promote, and teach health; to prevent or cure illness; to reduce impairment and restore function; to preserve the quality as well as the extent of life; to prevent suffering and relieve pain; and to provide comfort, care, and hope always.

Another way to think about bioethical dilemmas is to categorize the essential questions of medicine. The first of these are medical questions to be answered by physicians: What is wrong? What can be done? The second are value questions to be answered by patients: What should be done? Who should decide? And on what basis? The third are allocation questions to be answered by society: What patients, conditions, or treatments will or will not be covered? And for those that will not be covered, why not?

The Terms and Concepts of Ethics and Morality: Moral Theories and Traditions

Although the adjectives *ethical* and *moral* are interchangeable, the corollary nouns *ethics* and *morality* are not—at least conceptually they are not. **Ethics is the philosophic discipline that systemically examines what is right, good, or just in human conduct. Morality is a social, religious, or professional tradition of values about what is right, good, or just.**

Utilitarianism is a consequence-based theory that defines *good* as that which promotes happiness and *right* as that which produces the greatest good. Some speak of utility as the concept in which the end justifies the means or as a calculus of the greatest good for the greatest number.

Common morality is often principle based. Primary principles include autonomy (which is a libertarian approach), nonmaleficence and beneficence (which are utilitarian approaches), and justice (which is egalitarian).

Casuistry is a case-based approach in which reasoning is by analogy with paradigm cases and their associated maxims and precedents. The circumstances of particular cases are relevant, often even determinative. Judgments are tentative and presumptive, more or less probable, and thus rebuttable and subject to challenge. The four steps in casuistic analysis are discernment of the facts (grounds) of the case; comparison with paradigm cases (perceiving differences and similarities); consideration of arguments, maxims, and warrants (justifications); and making judgments, realizing that they have only probable certitude.

Kantian deontology is an obligation- or duty-based approach emphasizing the fundamental importance of human dignity. Deontologic theories are not consequentialist or utilitarian. They include divine law, natural law, natural rights, contractarian theories, the virtues approach, and the categorical imperative of Kant. A categorical imperative admits of no exceptions (i.e., is absolutely binding), states how morally one must act, and holds that maxims must be valid for everyone. Kant's imperatives, then, require unconditional conformity with universalizable obligations of conscience by rational beings to treat all individuals with respect and as ends, never as means only.

Individual libertarianism is an individual's rights-based approach or tradition, whereas *communitarianism* is community based. *Character ethics* is virtue based; the *ethics of care*, relationship based. The latter holds that obligations are dependent on relationships. Another approach is to invoke the ethics of a vocation—that is, a *professional oath or code.*

Finally, we should mention the *pluralistic casuistry of Baruch Brody*, who appreciated that none of the foregoing approaches is invariably best in analyzing an ethical problem.[2a] Thus, he would use a combination of these approaches or would use different approaches for different problems, whichever seemed more appropriate.

Practical Approaches to Ethical or Moral Problems in Medicine: The Methods of Clinical Ethics

Essential Steps in Analyzing a Medical Ethics Problem

Because we intend this chapter to be practical, the following list of questions may be useful in analyzing problems:

- **What are the medical facts (the diagnosis, prognosis, and treatment options)? Does the patient have decision-making capacity, and if not, does he or she have an advance directive or a surrogate decision maker?**
- **What are the values, concerns, and preferences of the patient (and of the health care team)? What is the patient's assessment of his or her quality of life?**
- **Is there a conflict of values (i.e., an ethical dilemma), or is there simply a communication problem?**
- **What are the contextual, cultural, religious, financial, institutional, legal, and societal circumstances?**
- **What are the possible solutions, and what are the benefits and burdens of each?**
- **Is more information required? Who should obtain it?**
- **To whom should the analysis and recommendations be communicated?**

Shared Medical Decision Making: Informed Consent and Refusal

The doctor-patient relationship is a fiduciary, covenantal alliance best served by shared decision making. **All members of the health care team have the right to inform the patient. The physician has the responsibility to make recommendations, and the patient (or patient's surrogate) has the right to make decisions.**

Informed decision making is advisable whenever a question arises about the purpose of a procedure or whenever a procedure is intrusive or has significant risk. It requires decision-making capacity, disclosure of all material information, understanding of that information, and voluntariness

of decision. The medical information required includes the nature of the illness (and its expected consequences), the therapeutic options and their risks, and expected outcomes. Informed voluntary decision making encourages rational and acceptable decisions (by respecting patients' rights to information and to self-determination) and helps to maintain trust between physicians and patients.

Informed decision making is difficult to accomplish when patients are anxious or frightened or when problems are new, unfamiliar, emotionally laden, or socially stigmatizing. Decisions are difficult when treatments are multiple or complex and when outcomes are uncertain, benefits are marginal, and risks are substantial.

Nondisclosure is permissible when the patient waives the right to information, when an emergency arises and the patient lacks decision-making capacity, and possibly when disclosure would be harmful to the patient, a concept called *therapeutic privilege.* Placebo therapy is no longer thought acceptable except under conditions understood to be investigational with advance, uncoerced approval by the subject (who is also a patient).

Involuntary treatment is legal only for children when parents consent to the treatment and for mentally disordered individuals who are a danger to themselves or others—and even then, only temporarily. Laws governing involuntary treatment vary somewhat from jurisdiction to jurisdiction.

To determine lack of decision-making capacity, a primary care physician (or nephrologist) should engage the patient in ordinary conversation while observing the patient's behavior and mood (as well as his or her answers to relevant questions). One may need to ask the patient's family or friends their opinion of the patient's capacity or may need to consult a psychiatrist or neurologist. **Criteria for lack of decision-making capacity are inability to understand one's circumstances or disclosed information, inability to analyze risks and benefits, or inability to state a preference.** An irrational or unreasonable decision suggests that the patient lacks decision-making capacity, but it is not by itself sufficient to judge that an individual lacks decision-making capacity. Note that incapacity may be temporary or fluctuating and may be the case for some decisions but not for others. Incompetence is a legally (judicially) determined lack of decision-making capacity. A person should be presumed competent unless proved or adjudicated not to be.

Competent individuals have a fundamental or constitutional right to make decisions about their health care. They have the right to refuse life-sustaining treatment, including enteral and parenteral nutrition and hydration. However, states have the right to demand clear and convincing evidence of the individual's choice (although only a few states have this high an evidentiary standard). The patient's right includes the option to make health care decisions—even decisions that others believe are not in the individual's best interests, even if life forsaking.

Previously competent individuals have the same right, which may be exercised through an advance treatment directive (commonly known as a *living will*) or by a surrogate who expresses a substituted judgment for the individual based on knowledge of the patient's values or previously expressed judgments. If such values or judgments are unknown, a previously competent patient (like a never-competent individual) may have decisions made by a surrogate who judges what is in the best interest of the patient (based on conjecture of what the patient would judge was in his or her best interest were he or she able).

To plan for the treatment of incompetent individuals, one should anticipate the development of incompetence and should encourage the patients to make advance directives and to discuss them with their proxy and physician. Physicians should emphasize the desired and achievable goals of therapy. When treatment cannot achieve benefit for a patient, the physician should recommend comfort care only. That is, rather than asking whether life-sustaining treatment should be discontinued, the physician should make a recommendation to do so. Otherwise, the guilt may be overwhelming for relatives "forced" to make a decision to end the life of their loved one.

Morally valid surrogates have significant involvement with the patient and ideally are chosen by the patient. Surrogates should have no conflicts with the patient, should have knowledge of the patient's values and wishes, and should be willing to express them.

Legally valid surrogates are defined by statute in most states, which usually give priority to a proxy appointed by the individual or to a conservator or guardian. Thereafter, priority is given to the spouse, a parent or adult child, siblings, and other relatives or friends, especially those who are or will be health caretakers of the individual.

Minors may be morally appropriate decision makers for themselves but are rarely granted that privilege legally except in a few specific circumstances. These circumstances include living independently (or in the military), being married or pregnant, having a contagious disease or substance abuse, or having been sexually abused.

Planning for Serious Illness and the Possibility of Loss of Decision-Making Capacity: Advance Directives and the Values History

THE NEED FOR PLANNING AND COMMUNICATION

Serious illness and the loss of ability to make decisions for oneself could befall any of us, at any time, without warning. Thus, we should all prepare for such an eventuality, but few of us do. Just as only a minority of individuals have a testamentary will, few have a living will (a treatment directive) or a durable power of attorney for health care (even though one or both are legal in every state). Knowing the value of such advance directives, physicians have a responsibility to discuss them with patients and to strongly encourage that they be executed and periodically reviewed. Advance directives are especially advisable for patients with ESRD because their chance of needing one is considerably greater than that of average patients. Not only do dialyzed patients have a substantial risk of life-threatening illness (approximately 25% per year), but they may need to change from one form of renal replacement therapy to another, and decision-making capacity may be lost. Furthermore, as many as 10% of dialyzed patients discontinue dialysis each year because the burdens of illness and treatment outweigh the benefits. Perhaps half of such individuals are no longer able to make decisions for themselves and should thaerefore have an advance directive.

Thus, primary care physicians who care for patients with advancing renal insufficiency, and especially nephrologists who care for patients during long-term dialysis and after renal transplants, should ensure that no patient lacks an advance directive because of failure to understand what it is and how helpful it can be to relatives and health care professionals who otherwise are burdened with making decisions for seriously ill persons unable to speak for themselves. Advance planning calls for frank, open discussion of the patient's condition and prognosis. It is most important to discuss serious illnesses (including death and disability) that could develop and impair ability to decide what should be done. All these matters are difficult to consider in our culture. In a private setting with the patient's loved ones or friends present, the physician should speak compassionately but plainly and honestly about such matters. The physician must not be rushed, must be willing to listen, and should ask the patient what he or she has understood so that misconceptions can be corrected. A lack of trust, confidence, or respect can doom such discussions. Differences in cultural beliefs or values and uncertainty about prognosis (or about the outcomes of different treatment options) all complicate decision making but are not usually insurmountable barriers. Even if no document is produced, such discussion goes a long way toward clarifying patients' goals and ensuring the likelihood that their preferences will be honored. Furthermore, many patients are relieved when they have had an opportunity to communicate about such difficult matters.

ADVANCE DIRECTIVES (INCLUDING CPR/DNAR)

Advance directives are formal, written, legal means of documenting one's preferences for treatment (or for forgoing treatment) and of appointing a proxy or surrogate to make decisions on one's behalf should one become unable to do so. An advance directive that states treatment preferences is commonly called a *living will.* It is most often used to specify treatments that one would want to limit or that one would not want to have under specific circumstances, but it can also be used to indicate treatment one would want. An advance directive to appoint a health care proxy to make decisions with one's physician in most states is called a *durable power of attorney for health care.* These directives are durable and remain legal for a number of years (or indefinitely) unless rescinded by the individual.

In contrast, a *do-not-resuscitate (DNR) order,* which is a directive to forgo CPR should one sustain a cardiac or pulmonary arrest, is usually not durable. When written as a DNR order or more properly as a *do-not-attempt-resuscitation* (DNAR) order, it usually lasts only for that hospitalization or for that nursing home admission and has to be rewritten at the time of a future admission. Thus, DNAR orders usually are not considered advance directives, although their function (like that of most treatment directives) is to limit or forgo treatment that the individual judges inappropriate or burdensome. Prehospital DNR policies have been developed in recent years in many cities and a few states. These policies allow paramedics not to perform CPR in the home or in long-term care facilities. Although these prehospital directives are usually durable, they are usually not called advance directives; however, there is no reason why a patient's preferences about CPR could not be included in an advance treatment directive. Until the day when CPR preferences are queried for all patients and documented in their charts, the preference for a CPR attempt is likely to be presumed for all patients. The preference for CPR has been assumed for many years despite the fact that its overall success is far less today than in early years, when it was applied selectively to patients with myocardial infarction, electrocution, or drowning. Indeed, the success of CPR in patients with ESRD is so poor that questioning all dialysis patients about their preferences is increasingly advised.

Except in jurisdictions that require clear and convincing evidence of one's treatment preferences, the need for an advance directive to be written and witnessed and to be a legal document is not great because the overwhelming majority of physicians and hospitals wish to respect the rights of patients to make their own health care decisions and to appoint their own surrogates. Furthermore, in any jurisdiction, the critically important aspect of advance directives is that they be considered and (whether documented or not) that one's values, beliefs, and treatment preferences be clarified in one's own mind and be communicated to those in a position to see that they are carried out if the individual loses decision-making capacity. That means communicating these matters to one's physician and to the person one wishes to have make decisions. It is important not only to understand and communicate one's values and preferences but also to select a proxy who will express one's preferences (not those of the proxy if they differ) and to advocate one's best interests as the individual (not the proxy) would judge them. The proxy should be able to communicate effectively with the physician and should be available and accessible to the physician, the hospital, and the patient's family.

Patients benefit from formulating a treatment directive by having considered their health, potential illness, and treatment options in relation to their values, goals, and preferences. Patients' discussions with their physician and loved ones may further clarify their position on such matters as well as communicate their preferences to ensure that they are carried out. The physician and loved ones are thus relieved of the burden of struggling with uncertainty when making decisions if patients are too ill to do so for themselves. The physician and the proxy are afforded legal protection so long as they follow the wishes in good faith.

A shortcoming of advance treatment directives is that they are not automatically updated and might no longer reflect one's current preferences. A potential disadvantage of having an advance directive is that its content may not be known yet its existence may be presumed to indicate a preference not to be treated—even when the opposite is the case. A similar misunderstanding may occur if the directive uses standard but vague phrases (such as extraordinary treatment, "heroic measures," "artificial means," or "dependence on machines," which are subject to highly variable interpretation) or if the directive is inadequately reviewed by patients with their physician or proxy.

Opinions about what constitutes a good advance directive differ. That is, what is a good advance directive for one individual may differ from a good directive for another. Some believe that one should have only a proxy directive and not a treatment directive because it is so difficult to predict the specific illness and all its nuances that one will develop, as well as all the contextual circumstances, events, and persons that influence appropriate decisions. They hold that it is best simply to name the person in whom one has the confidence to entrust complex, serious, life-and-death decisions.

Others believe that treatment directives are helpful as long as they are general enough to guide the physician and proxy but not so specific that they constrain or restrict their making decisions that the patient, if competent, would make differently. Still others believe that treatment directives should be as specific as possible and should state not only the goals for treatment but also the values by which one would wish to be treated, as well as specific preferences in various hypothetical circumstances. One should also indicate how much leeway, if any, he or she wishes to give the proxy and the physician to override stated treatment preferences if they both thought the stated treatment preferences were no longer in the patient's best interests.

Finally, some believe there is no such thing as a good treatment directive because no one can be sure what he or she would choose were he or she to develop a serious health problem. Those who espouse this position place emphasis on the fact that many people change their minds. For example, few people who say they'd rather be dead than blind or quadriplegic actually commit suicide or request euthanasia when blindness or quadriplegia occurs. Most, however, believe that even an imperfect advance directive is better than no directive in most circumstances.

With regard to the components of a good advance directive, most are discussed in detail in the writings of the Emanuels.[3, 3a, 3b] The need for flexibility or leeway in advance directives was discussed in a study of dialysis patients by Sehgal and colleagues.[4] Some of the suggestions of both groups of researchers follow.

Goals of treatment may be specified, as suggested by Emanuel,[3] by having the patient check one of the following statements:

- Prolong life and treat everything.
- Attempt cure but reevaluate often.
- Value the quality of life more than the duration of life.
- Provide comfort care only.

Alternatively, patients may write their goals in their own words for their advance directives.

The Emanuels developed scenarios or vignettes that are examples of very serious conditions that patients might develop. It is suggested that patients check the goal and a number of treatments they would wish to forgo for each of the following scenarios:

- Coma or permanent unconsciousness with no hope of recovery
- Coma with a small chance of recovery, a greater chance of brain damage, and a still greater chance of not recovering
- Inability to recognize people, speak meaningfully, or live independently, and a terminal illness
- The same but without a terminal illness
- Chronic illness with mental disability or physical suffering and development of an acute life-threatening but reversible illness
- One's current state of health and development of an acute life-threatening but reversible illness

One could also indicate where he or she would wish to be treated: in an acute care hospital, a nursing home, a hospice institution or program, or at home. The Emanuels also suggest that one indicate which conditions would be so unendurable that one would wish to withhold or withdraw life-sustaining treatment such as dialysis. Conditions that the person could check include untreatable pain, severe loss of higher mental function, inability to share love, dependence on others, or being a severe burden on one's family.

It is wise for patients to specify the leeway to override stated treatment preferences that they would wish to grant their proxy and physician if both thought the patient's stated preference was no longer in his or her best interests (e.g., because of a change in circumstances or because the patient developed an additional serious illness or because a new treatment became available).[4] One might indicate no leeway, a little, a

lot, or complete leeway. An example of a particularly difficult decision that 17 leading bioethicists could not agree on was the following[4a]:

A patient stated in his or her advance directive, "If I should ever become severely disabled by incurable dementia, I would not wish life-sustaining treatment." But when the patient became severely and irreversibly demented, he or she no longer seemed to be the same person, and furthermore, he or she seemed quite happy. What should be done? What would you want done? Why?

Making an advance directive can be as difficult as answering all of the foregoing questions for these or additional scenarios, or it could be as simple as stating whom one wishes to make decisions should one become unable to make or express decisions oneself.

If an advance directive is formulated— whether as a formal, legal, written document or as an informal oral statement—it should be communicated to the chosen proxy and, with the patient's permission, to others who are seriously concerned with the patient's welfare and who would respect his or her preferences. It should also be communicated to his or her physician(s). If written documents are available, they should be provided to the proxy, the patient's family, the physician, the hospital, and the dialysis unit.

Advance directives can be changed or rescinded at any time. One should reconsider treatment preferences and update his or her advance directive (write a new one or change, suspend, or cancel the old one) whenever one's circumstances change (or whenever one wishes to do so). If changes are made, one should inform the proxy, the family, the physician, the hospital, and the dialysis unit, preferably in writing. If an advance directive is rescinded, each page should have a line drawn through it and the word *rescinded* or *superseded* written on it. This should be signed, dated, and preferably witnessed.

The Patient Self-Determination Act, a federal law in the United States, requires that hospitals, long-term care facilities, hospice programs, home health agencies, and prepaid health plans inform patients at the time of admission of their rights, under state law, to accept or refuse therapy and to formulate advance directives. Dialysis units are not so mandated, but the End-Stage Renal Disease Data Advisory Committee suggested they be required to provide this information to patients at the time of admission. Furthermore, an important initiative of the National Kidney Foundation encourages the use of advance directives. The National Kidney Foundation has written a guide for patients and their families and guidelines for dialysis facilities on implementing advance directives.[4b, 4c] The National Kidney Foundation has drafted guidelines for the initiation and withdrawal of dialysis.[4d–f] Patients may wish to indicate under what circumstances they would wish dialysis treatments to be discontinued and they be allowed to die. Although they could always make such decisions at the time if they were capable, their loss of ability to make decisions, if anticipated to be permanent, might itself be a condition for which they would wish treatment to be stopped.

THE VALUES HISTORY

Gibson and colleagues,[5] at the University of New Mexico, studied how public guardians might be trained to be effective health care decision surrogates for patients who had no morally valid surrogate. They developed what they called a *values history* which consisted of questions that public guardians could ask friends of the patient to gain insight into the patient's values, beliefs, attitudes, and preferences in order to make health care decisions appropriate for the individual (i.e., to make substituted judgments for the patient rather than surmising what was in the patient's best interest).

Topics that might be included in a values history questionnaire are

- The patient's religious or philosophic beliefs
- The patient's attitudes toward life in general, independence and control, health, doctors and illness, death and dying, finances, and health care
- The patient's wishes about artificial ventilation, artificial nutrition and hydration, dialysis, organ transplantation, surgery, amputation, autopsy, and the funeral, eulogy, and obituary

In the course of this project, Gibson and colleagues discovered that the questions that they had developed could also help anyone to gain insight into his or her own values, to clarify them, to articulate them, and ideally to document them in writing. This could be helpful in preparing one's own advance directive.

Ethics Consultation, Ethics Committees, and Patient Care Conferences

Ethical concerns, issues, and dilemmas that arise in the care of a patient warrant reflection, consideration, and often discussion in order to make appropriate decisions about a patient's care. Traditionally, problems beyond the expertise of the attending physician are referred to an expert consultant who makes recommendations to the attending physician or patient. In many instances, this approach is effective as well as efficient, and it is generally preferred by physicians. It permits direct contact with patients and families and allows for follow-up reevaluation. It is applicable to ethical as well as medical problems.

In some cases or issues, however, referral to a hospital ethics committee may be more appropriate. The multidisciplinary committee has diverse expertise and multiple points of view that increase the likelihood that the concerns of all stakeholders will be considered and that more options for resolution of the problem will be conceived and considered. Unlike the individual consultant approach, which suggests that ethics is a matter for an expert, the committee model suggests that moral discourse is a community enterprise. Furthermore, nonphysician health care personnel may be more comfortable referring their ethical concerns about the care of a patient to a multidisciplinary committee than to a physician ethics consultant. Whenever the case raises issues that might have policy implications for the hospital (or for a dialysis unit or renal center), discussion and review by a committee may be particularly appropriate.

Nephrologists are generally comfortable with multidisciplinary committees because the care of dialyzed patients is a multidisciplinary team enterprise (e.g., in developing life plans for and with patients) and because they are familiar with patient selection committees in the past and with the medical review boards of local ESRD networks. Nephrologists, like other physicians, may, however, be offended or intimidated if the care of "their" patient is referred to an ethics committee. The misconception of a judgmental "God squad" and the perceived political or moral power of an institutional ethics committee may make a patient care conference more appealing.

A conference including the patient's primary caretakers (e.g., attending physician, primary nurse, nurse manager, social worker, chaplain, consultant physician) can consider ethical as well as medical and communication problems quite effectively and without the concern or stigma attached to an ethics committee discussion. Such conferences can be as informal or as formal as the circumstances warrant. They can be attended by the patient, family members, and even an ethicist, if appropriate. This discussion itself raises two questions. Should an ethics committee discussion of a case be called a *consultation*? I submit that it should not be unless the committee obtains information directly by meeting with the patient and primary caretakers and by reviewing the chart or whatever clinical information is relevant. The ethics committee too often obtains all of its information from one primary caretaker who "presents the case." Even then, the creativity of a dispassionate group of individuals with diverse viewpoints and expertise is extremely valuable in conceiving options and solutions that might otherwise never be considered. However, because the deliberations are based on hearsay or second-hand information, they should not in themselves be determinative in the care of the patient and should be called *case* or *committee discussion* or *case* or *committee review,* not *consultation.* Furthermore, such recommendations should be considered tentative.

Second, to whom should the recommendations of an ethics committee case review or discussion be communicated? They should most often be communicated to the attending physician (if he or she was not present at the meeting, as would have been preferable) and to the patient (or, if the patient lacks decision-making capacity, to the patient's surrogate). It may at times be appropriate for a representative of the committee to inform the patient directly, but this can often be done by the attending physician, especially if he or she was present at the discussion. The same considerations apply to documenting the recommendations in the patient's record (as well as in the minutes of the ethics committee meeting). At other times, it is inappropriate to inform the patient (and inappropriate to place a note in the patient's record). A dispute between two members of the health care team about the proper care of the patient represents such a circumstance. In this case, the ethics committee may be serving a peer review function rather than a patient care function, and the proceedings may best be documented in the minutes of the committee meeting only and may preferably not be communicated to the patient or family unless they already know of the disagreement or unless the disagreement leads to a change in patient care that would not otherwise have occurred. In the peer review mode, it may not be necessary or appropriate to have requested permission of the patient or surrogate for the discussion to take place, whereas this is mandatory for ethics consultations and ethics committee case reviews undertaken in the patient care mode. In one other circumstance, informed consent for discussion and communication of the results of the discussion may not be necessary: when the discussion is retrospective and intended solely for educational purposes or for institutional policy development (not for care of the individual patient).

Dispute or Conflict Resolution: Discussion, Arbitration, Mediation

Although many of the landmark cases in bioethics were decided in the courts, all would prefer more efficient, more proximate, more medically informed and less litigious avenues for resolution of disputes about the care of patients. The overwhelming majority of disputes are misunderstandings and are resolved simply by discussion or effective communication (sometimes at the behest of a third party). If not dealt with promptly, however, even simple misunderstandings may result in contentious polarization, which may then require more than discussion between the two parties most directly involved. Such matters in hospitals often come to the bioethics committee and may be resolved by suggestions of the spokesperson for the committee, and thus the need for even calling a meeting of the committee is obviated. If the committee is convened, however, its deliberations and pronouncements often solve the problem in a manner justifying the term *arbitration* (i.e., the moral authority of the committee is imposed on the disputants, who accede to the wisdom of the committee). The goal of ethics committee review, however, should be to facilitate ethical consideration by the stakeholders or disputants themselves rather than to impose a recommendation that they must follow. Indeed, this is the methodology of mediation, a form of dispute or conflict resolution in which the third party, the mediator, simply facilitates communication between the disputants and the parties themselves propose the solution. **Mediation seems particularly well suited to disputes in health care ethics and may more often lead to lasting resolution of conflicts than would arbitration or committee dictum.**

AN OVERVIEW OF ETHICAL ISSUES IN NEPHROLOGY

Our discussion thus far has been relatively straightforward. Although a number of moral theories and traditions can be applied to specific cases by various approaches or methods and by individual health care professionals, ethics consultants, or committees, the real challenge is their successful application in the routine clinical setting. An analogy can be made with clinical medicine: Although medical science is complex and ever evolving, it can be learned and understood more easily than it can be applied in making correct diagnoses and selecting appropriate and effective therapies.

The next section of this chapter deals with the art of analyzing clinical ethical problems and resolving them in satisfactory ways. It does so by presenting cases in my experience and by discussing some of the issues that might be encountered in the selected circumstances of renal failure and dialysis. Were I to expand the chapter to a disproportionate length, I would review the ethical issues in suspected or incipient renal disease, in acute renal failure, in critically ill, terminally ill, and dying patients, and in the use of patients for teaching and research.

Most importantly, I would discuss the innumerable ethical issues in renal transplantation (which, like those in dialysis, contributed significantly to the development and maturation of the field of bioethics). These include issues in obtaining donor organs (procuring kidneys for transplantation), issues in the allocation of donor organs (the selection of recipients), donor issues, recipient issues, and issues in xenotransplantation of nonhuman organs to humans.

I might also have discussed the ethical problems faced by medical students, residents, and fellows. I would have liked to address topics such as home care, hospice, medically futile interventions, allowing patients to die, physician assistance in suicide or death (active, voluntary euthanasia), and difficult and challenging patients (those who are unpleasant or a nuisance, those who are a danger to themselves [noncompliance] or a threat or danger to others, those who are demanding, and those who suffer iatrogenic complications).

Finally, I would wish to discuss health care financing and delivery, including the lessons of the Medicare–ESRD Program, the Health Care Financing Administration's global capitation demonstration project, the status and prospects of managed care, and the need for a single-payor system should managed care fail (because there is no prospect for a return to indemnity insurance with fee-for-service reimbursement).

The cases will raise many more questions than will be answered. Furthermore, the apparent answers (i.e., the way the patients' problems resolved or were resolved) are not to be construed as the only ethically appropriate resolution and certainly not as the best resolution but rather the resolution I chose at my stage of inexperience or immaturity (or chosen by the patients and their surrogates with my consent or assent).

The listing of ethical issues that might be and indeed often are encountered in these categories of patients and in society's provision of care to them will necessarily be incomplete but may serve as a guide to those who wish to think or read further about the ethical problems of clinical nephrology (i.e., the ethical problems in caring for the renal patient).

ETHICAL ISSUES IN CHRONIC RENAL FAILURE, END-STAGE RENAL DISEASE, AND DIALYSIS

This section is organized according to the usual chronologic progression of the patient, from conservative management of progressive renal insufficiency, to preparation for definitive management (usually first by dialysis and often thereafter by transplantation), to dialysis, and sometimes to discontinuation of dialysis. I hope that the case presentations inform and illuminate, if not elucidate, the didactic concepts to be considered.

Progressive Renal Insufficiency

PATIENT NUMBER 1

Elizabeth Baldwin was a child in a conservative, undemonstrative family when her father, a professor of theology at a New England university, was discovered to have impaired function of polycystic kidneys. In the early 1950s, little could be done other than to treat hypertension and urinary infection, which were often present, and to avoid instrumentation when patients had episodes of gross hematuria in order not to introduce infection. For the most part, physicians were helpless bystanders as renal dysfunction progressed, able only to treat acidosis and, in patients with iron deficiency, anemia. The symptoms of uremia could be ameliorated only in early stages. Polycystic disease progressed very slowly and allowed some pathophysiologic adaptation, which delayed the onset of symptoms or at least the patient's appreciation of the symptoms. What unfortunately followed was often a long, unpleasant, symptomatic uremic phase before death.

So it was for Elizabeth's father. He was unable to concentrate mentally and became easily fatigued so that he could no longer teach and write. Thus, he was at home, where Elizabeth, now a schoolgirl, and his other children witnessed his gradual decline. At first the professor just had less stamina, poor appetite, and occasional itching. As time progressed, he was frequently nauseated, lost weight, and scratched himself incessantly to the point of ecchymoses and excoriation. To his chagrin, he became increasingly irritable and short-tempered with the children. They tried to understand, but it was hard no longer to be told stories or to be read to, and it was worse to be reprimanded for the least transgression. They hardly noticed that he had become sallow, pale, and almost ashen, but they were aware that he now dragged his feet when he walked and seemed less stable than before (because of neuropathy) and that he had developed peculiar jerks and twitches. One night when the family doctor came to visit because Professor Baldwin was exhausted from vomiting nearly all day long, Elizabeth overheard Dr. Scranton say to her mother that the end might be approaching, and he reminded her to "have the children checked since they could have it too." Needless to say, at age 8, after nearly 3 years of watching her father's progressive and now accelerating deterioration, Elizabeth was frightened. She kept her fears to herself and just sobbed herself to sleep night after night. She vowed never to get married and never to have children because "if she had it too," they would suffer terribly. These vows became a nightly ritual as a defense against her fear and sadness in the final weeks of her father's illness. First he developed painful pericarditis, which made him sleep sitting up in bed hunched over his pillow, and then convulsions, and finally coma, with a peculiar frost over his grim countenance.

At the age of 13, Elizabeth was sent off to board at finishing school. She became quite independent and excelled in her schoolwork. Tomboy no more, she loved the monthly Sunday afternoon dances and the chance to socialize. By the time she was ready for college, she was maturing into a young woman and began to reexamine her often repeated vows. She came to think of marriage as one of life's great experiences that she should not deny herself so long as whomever she married agreed not to have children. Sure enough, at age 19, her worst fears were confirmed by an examination after an unexpected and frightening episode of gross hematuria. Not long thereafter, she developed the first of many urinary tract infections and was prescribed prophylactic sulfisoxazole and chlorothiazide for mild hypertension.

Perhaps again as a paradoxic defense against her fear of following in her father's footsteps, she broke not only her vow not to marry but also her pledge not to have children. By the time she was finally referred for nephrologic evaluation, she had had two difficult pregnancies—severe pyelonephritis in the first and poorly controlled hypertension and an increase in serum creatinine level from 1.8 mg/dl to 3.6 mg/dl late in the second. Fortunately, her children were healthy, although the second was born at only 34 weeks.

> I have had the privilege of getting to know Elizabeth, her husband (a minister), her younger brother (who also has polycystic disease), and her children (one of whom has the disease). Elizabeth felt quite well for 5 years on conservative therapy. Then she developed uremic symptoms, which disappeared on a strict low-protein diet. She followed it religiously because she was stubbornly insistent on continuing to teach school as long as possible before acceding to dialysis. Elizabeth's saga will continue in the next section of the chapter, but for now I should explain why I've gone into such detail in her narrative.

Elizabeth's story is long and detailed because I learned it paragraph by paragraph during the 6 years I monitored her before dialysis, first at 2- or 3-month intervals, and, by the time she was to start dialysis, at 2- to 3-week intervals. Indeed, I almost had to extract the details from Elizabeth, who was herself surprised by the childhood and teenage memories she had apparently repressed. As they became known, Elizabeth changed from a frightened, recalcitrant patient (who often refused to have laboratory tests or to fill prescriptions) to a model, albeit stoic, patient whose personal fortitude is not only to be admired but may well explain her overall exceptional course to date. She enjoyed general good health on dialysis for some years as well as after a cadaveric renal transplant. She also reared accomplished teenagers and practiced her own innovative school teaching, to which she returned after adjusting to late afternoon dialysis at the center.

The ethical challenge in caring for patients like Elizabeth during the slow progression of renal insufficiency is knowing for each patient when to initiate various therapies, how to share decision making, and when to begin planning for definitive therapy. In the early days of long-term hemodialysis, this technology was so scarce that many patients died without ever receiving it, and many others developed severe complications such as malnutrition and neuropathy due to excessive protein restriction of excessive duration while waiting for a dialysis position to become available. Physicians vowed that when there were sufficient dialysis machines and nurses to run them, we would start patients on dialysis early, before they even had uremic symptoms, in order to spare them the suffering of the patients of an earlier time.

This was a double-edged sword, however: Patients who started on dialysis before developing uremic symptoms might intellectually understand why they had been started, but they rarely accepted it emotionally. This was particularly true in days when patients had more symptoms (headaches, nausea, itching, hemodynamic instability, muscle cramps, new cell syndrome, and the like) during and shortly after each dialysis than the day after dialysis or the day before the next dialysis.

Thus we came to see the judgment pendulum (regarding how long to sustain patients on conservative therapy before initiating dialysis) swing back. Similarly, we had to learn that malnutrition and neuropathy were extremely difficult to reverse, and although aluminum-containing phosphate binders might prevent periarticular calcifications and slow the development of hyperparathyroidism, they sometimes caused brain and bone disorders that were far worse. We had to learn that transfusions for symptomatic anemia not only did not doom a patient to reject a transplant but, paradoxically, improved the success of transplantation. Nevertheless, we had once again to severely restrict transfusion for anemia when human immunodeficiency virus became prevalent, and this, unfortunately, was before the availability of erythropoietin. Perhaps most important of all, we had to learn through personal experience to share decision making with patients because bioethics (with its emphasis on patient autonomy, informed consent, and the central importance of goals based on patient values, beliefs, and preferences) was just coming of age at the same time and was not sufficiently known to guide us in these matters.

We sometimes learned the hard way to listen to patients' responses to open-ended questions about treatment options rather than to tell them paternalistically what to do. Indeed, **patients fared better when they were part of the solution.** We learned to take the time to participate personally in teaching and to discuss treatment preferences with patients rather than, for our own convenience, pass authority to the dietitian, social worker, dialysis nurse, and transplant surgeon. As is obvious in Elizabeth's case, with an autosomal dominant disorder (but also true of patients with acquired renal disorders), we have to be sensitive to how the illness and its treatment affect the entire family, not just the patient. Also, we must take the time (the constraints of managed care notwithstanding) to involve the family as well as the patient in education and advance planning.

Predialysis, Pretransplant: Preparing for Dialysis and/or Transplantation

PATIENT NUMBER 1 (Continued)
Elizabeth was glad to be alive, to have married, and to be an exceptionally talented school teacher, but her family was more important to her than anything else, especially her preteen children. As her serum creatinine level rose, she overcame her fears by talking of her father's illness. This was very painful for her. She realized that today he could have been on dialysis or have a transplant, and so could she. She also realized that by the time her children might need it, treatment will be even better, and thus perhaps she need not feel guilty for knowingly bringing them into this world. She began to ask all sorts of questions: What was it like to be on dialysis? Could it be done at home? How much more risky was a transplant? What were the side effects and risks of medications to prevent transplant rejection? How long would a transplant last?

Elizabeth's long-term goal was to be as healthy as possible and to be able to travel with her husband, a national leader in his church and a widely sought speaker on church doctrine and modernization. For this she wanted a transplant. Her children were not yet in their teens, however, and she didn't want to risk dying, a chance that, in her mind, more than outweighed the improved sense of well-being she would have from a successful transplant. To be sure of seeing her children at least enter high school, preferably college, Elizabeth decided she would undergo dialysis when conservative therapy would no longer suffice.

She lived at some distance from the center and wished to be able to readjust her treatment schedule to accommodate her children's needs and her own desire to return to teaching when they were a little older and when she had more stamina. She therefore decided to perform home peritoneal dialysis. At that time, the machine to produce and deliver peritoneal dialysate was large, and dialysis was performed nightly during sleep. Continuous ambulatory peritoneal dialysis, continuous cycling peritoneal dialysis, and dialysate in bags were not yet available. Elizabeth and her husband had their bedroom enlarged and equipped with electric outlets and with plumbing (at considerable personal expense) months in advance of her starting dialysis.

Much of the planning was done with the nurses and technicians of the home training unit, but Elizabeth had not wanted to take the time (as they had suggested she do) to visit a patient undergoing peritoneal dialysis because of her children's busy schedules and, perhaps, because she wasn't feeling as well as she professed to her nephrologist. The surgeon who was to implant the dialysis catheter insisted that Elizabeth observe a patient actually connect herself to dialysis so that Elizabeth would appreciate the importance of aseptic technique and what was involved in the proper care of the catheter and the exit site. When she did, only the day before her own surgery was planned, Elizabeth suddenly realized this was not for her. The thought of a catheter in her own abdomen and the possibility that it would jeopardize her marital relationship were more than she could bear. Thus the surgery was changed to construction of a hemodialysis vascular access, and Elizabeth began center hemodialysis.

Perhaps I failed by never having discussed her sexuality; I only discussed the fact that a peritoneal catheter would not preclude sexual intercourse. I also failed by not having Elizabeth visit a patient on home peritoneal dialysis earlier. Perhaps I also failed because she is so intelligent and seemed so confident in her choice of home peritoneal dialysis that I did not discuss the plan and its implications as thoroughly as I might have with another patient.

Perhaps Elizabeth would have fared very well on peritoneal dialysis, and perhaps it would not have alienated her husband. Knowing Elizabeth, the independence and ability to control her schedule of home dialysis would have made sense. Perhaps she would have done it if I hadn't given in so easily and had dissuaded her from switching to hemodialysis at the last minute. Elizabeth had to have a second hemodialysis access, an upper-arm fistula, because the first access, a radiocephalic fistula, never matured adequately. Perhaps that also was my mistake: not insisting on construction of vascular accesses for patients who planned peritoneal dialysis (or planned transplantation without preceding dialysis) but knowing that intractable peritonitis (or other complications of peritoneal dialysis or of a transplant) might require hemodialysis at a later date and that it would be wise to be prepared for such an eventuality.

These ruminations may sound like the wailings of an insecure nephrologist. More generously, they are expressions of humility of one appreciative of the imperfect art of informing and advising patients without manipulating or coercing them, and of one wishing to learn from his own mistakes in order to do better next time with the same patient and with other patients.

Although I speculate what might have been, I am not discontent, because Elizabeth did achieve her goals of seeing her children succeed in high school and of returning to work as a teacher before deciding after 6 years of dialysis to have a transplant. The graft is now in its second year without rejection, although Elizabeth has some Cushingoid features despite a reduction to low-dose prednisone.

Elizabeth has fortunately fared very well overall, and ethical problems have been few. What are the usual predialysis and pretransplant ethical concerns? Many of the most serious issues are addressed in subsequent sections on withholding dialysis and on accepting patients for ESRD therapy (i.e., for dialysis or transplant). Less distinctive and less conspicuous but equally important issues are those of the practice of medicine generally: knowing the patient as a person, respecting the person as an individual, sharing decision making, facilitating informed consent (or refusal) and advance planning, protecting confidentiality, and promoting patients' interests and advocating for their needs in the medical marketplace.

In order to do all these things, the primary care physician and the nephrologist need to work together and to involve all members of the team in the care of the patient: the vascular and transplant surgeon, other medical consultants as indicated, the dialysis and transplant-coordinating nurses, the dietitian, the social worker and chaplain, the dialysis technician, and the patient, his or her family and friends, and, when appropriate, other patients.

When a patient presents late (renal insufficiency can be an amazingly asymptomatic condition) or is referred late, the patient and the nephrologist are strangers. The primary care physician (if there is one) must not abandon the patient. This physician, who often knows the patient as a person and sometimes as a member of a family or a community, has an obligation to continue in the care of the patient at least until a smooth transition has allowed the nephrologist to become the patient's primary physician. The original primary care physician can often assist the patient in expressing his or her goals, values, beliefs, and preferences. If the patient is too ill to speak for himself or herself, the primary care physician along with the patient's proxy may be able to clarify the patient's previously expressed wishes or, by substituted judgment, the likely choice of the patient. Do not minimize the importance or complexity of these choices, which include not simply definitive renal replacement therapy versus palliative, symptomatic, temporary treatment but also the appropriate modality (hemodialysis, peritoneal dialysis, cadaveric or living donor transplant). If dialysis is chosen, the appropriate setting (center or home) must be considered.

Dialysis

Withholding Dialysis

In this day of extreme emphasis on patient autonomy (often without regard for what might be appropriate constraints or limits on autonomy), it is difficult to imagine a patient with renal failure not being referred to a nephrologist, at least in the United States. Nonreferral is an extremely important issue in some countries, however, and an issue of uncertain magnitude here in the United States. It is one thing to withhold dialysis or transplantation at the informed and voluntary request of a patient but quite another for a nephrologist to withhold dialysis surreptitiously or for a primary care physician not to refer a patient to a nephrologist without explaining to the patient or surrogate why this is the case. It is no secret that clandestine withholding of dialysis occurs, but the extent of the practice is unknown. Equally important, the basis for decisions to withhold dialysis is unknown and should be studied. One report from Canada[6] listed reasons why patients were advised to forgo dialysis: nonuremic dementia; metastatic or refractory malignancy; irreversible, end-stage heart, lung, or liver failure; irreversible neurologic disease with impaired activities of daily living; terminal illness or multisystem failure; and the need to restrain or sedate patients in order to dialyze them. Other criteria listed by Moss[7] include permanent unconsciousness, inability to relate to others, refusal by the patient concurrently or (if no longer competent) in an advance directive, and failure of a trial of dialysis.

Ask any clinician, and he or she will tell you that it is far easier to withhold than to withdraw a treatment. Ask any ethicist, and he or she will tell you that should not be and that ethically withholding and withdrawing are the same. I will return to this matter when I discuss the withdrawal of dialysis, but for the present, three points are worth making. First, if a treatment that a patient might want but does not know about is withheld surreptitiously, the patient cannot request it. Second, if the nephrologist would refuse to stop dialysis once started, unless the patient is certain that he or she would or would not want dialysis, he or she is forced to make a decision without the benefit of a trial of therapy. The same is true if the patient believes that it is morally wrong to stop a treatment once it has been initiated. Third, if a patient's condition and circumstances are such that it would not be acceptable to withdraw therapy, then it is not acceptable to withhold therapy from that patient.

Except in an emergency or when it would endanger a third party, a competent adult may refuse any treatment, at any time, at any place, for any reason (or for no reason) and arguably need not be informed (i.e., may waive that right) and, so long as not incompetent, may express a reason that is not rational. This is also true for an incompetent patient who expressed his or her preference in an advance directive (although the U.S. Supreme Court in the Cruzan decision allowed states to require clear and convincing evidence of the patient's preferences). It is nevertheless emotionally daunting for a health care provider to have a patient forgo a treatment that the health care provider believes would benefit the patient. Even more difficult was the case of Rodney.

PATIENT NUMBER 2

Rodney was a 19-year-old high school junior who looked only 12 because of cystic fibrosis. He had serious renal insufficiency from taking aminoglycoside antibiotics, which had been used repeatedly for respiratory tract infections. Rodney knew that if his renal insufficiency progressed to end stage, he would not be allowed a renal transplant because of his propensity for respiratory tract infections, which would be aggravated by the immunosuppressive medications necessary for a renal transplant (pulmonary transplantation had not yet been performed for patients with cystic fibrosis). Rodney decided he would not undergo long-term dialysis because he judged it would be a "straw-that-broke-the camel's-back" burden added to the frequent hospitalizations for pneumonia despite thrice-daily thoracic thumping and postural drainage after inhalation therapy, which had lately become unpleasant chores.

Each new health care professional who met Rodney at first questioned his decision not to be dialyzed and was sad to know it. As one got to know Rodney, however, one had great respect for how bravely he faced his illness, including the gradual worsening of renal function, and for his maturity far beyond his years. Rodney had visited both a pediatric and an adult dialysis unit and, having considered the matter many times, seemed resolute in his decision. He never showed a hint of ambivalence or uncertainty, which mystified even his parents.

On his final admission, azotemia progressed rapidly. His primary physician, a pulmonologist, consulted a new nephrologist "just to be sure." He in turn found no remediable condition and discussed the need for dialysis with the patient and his parents. The nephrologist described several scenarios of what might occur during the week or two after urine production became minimal if dialysis were not provided. After talking with the pulmonologist who had monitored the patient for a decade, the nephrologist decided not to try to talk the patient into dialysis. He recommended that the patient stay in the hospital so that whatever symptoms developed could be treated.

Rodney's nausea was controlled with Compazine and his itching with Benadryl, both of which made him somewhat drowsy. On the final day of his life, he developed circulatory overload and required morphine to lessen his awareness of dyspnea. As nightfall approached, Rodney became anxious that dyspnea would recur, and he requested dialysis. The nephrologist felt uncertain and called the pulmonologist. A morphine drip was started, and the patient expired in his sleep.

To this day, the nephrologist asks, Was this right? Which was authentic for Rodney—the prior decision not to be dialyzed or the final request to be dialyzed? And why did Elizabeth have the right to change her mind but not Rodney? I have come to learn that life and the decisions a physician must make are rarely easy: At least the big decisions are often discomfiting and leave one with the quandry, What might have been? I remember Rose, about whom I debated whether I should even inform her that dialysis could save her life, and later I agonized because I had.

PATIENT NUMBER 3

Rose was a 53-year-old housewife married to a carpenter. Seven years previously she had an episode of flank pain and hematuria, which led to discovery of an enlarged kidney. The kidney was removed and found to contain an angiomyolipoma. Anemia and a BUN of 30 mg/dl and creatinine level of 2.5 mg/dl postoperatively were neither investigated nor monitored. In 1966, Rose felt extremely fatigued, had lost 10 pounds, and was found to have severe anemia with a hematocrit of 15% and renal insufficiency. She had a creatinine level of 16 mg/dl and a BUN of only 125 mg/dl (probably relatively low because of an aversion to meat). Her remnant kidney was small (not large, as it should have been after removal of the other) and had several calyceal stones or medullary calcifications. The intern learned she had had headaches for 20 years, and she stated that to combat them she had taken 3 to 5 Empirin compound tablets per day. Her husband was convinced that this was a gross underestimate, because he found two or three empty bottles in the trash every week or two when he discarded sawdust from his workshop. Note that phenacetin had not been removed from Empirin compound at that time.

Remember that the year was 1966. Rose's city had only two dialysis units, and only 1 woman in 20 was accepted for dialysis. The only woman we could recall having been accepted was a 23-year-old with chronic glomerulonephritis and three young children. Furthermore, Rose's health insurance through her husband's union didn't cover this "experimental" new treatment. Rose and her husband had scrimped and saved a little each week for 25 years. Their life savings of $18,300 would be quickly exhausted if they had to pay for dialysis.

I thought it unlikely that Rose would be accepted for long-term dialysis even though one of the units in town was planning to train patients to dialyze at home on a Kiil dialyzer with a Sweden Freezer dialysate tank. But who was I to "play God" and not inform Rose of the possibility? I did tell her, but she was not accepted even though her cousin, a congressman, phoned to put pressure on the hospital, which depended in part on public funds. Rose died a miserable uremic death, doubly distraught because she knew others were being saved.

For those of us in dialysis, this seems far away and long ago. But what would happen today if Rose were in a health maintenance organization, had metastatic, chemotherapy-resistant breast cancer, and I recommended a bone marrow transplant?

Initiating Dialysis: The Acceptance (or Selection) of Patients for ESRD Therapy (with an Emphasis on Dialysis Rather Than Transplantation)

Just as it is crucial that primary care physicians not fail to refer patients who might benefit from definitive ESRD therapy (i.e., dialysis or transplantation) and that nephrologists not withhold therapy on arbitrary grounds (especially without discussion with the patient, the family, and the primary care physician), so too is it increasingly accepted that nephrologists not accept patients for dialysis who either cannot benefit from dialysis (e.g., a patient who is in a permanent vegetative state and who develops ESRD) or who would be harmed by dialysis (e.g., a patient who has unrelievable pain or suffering due to metastatic malignancy and who would prefer not to live and who develops ESRD). Rather than pressure such patients or their families to accept definitive renal replacement therapy, primary care physicians and nephrologists should allow such patients to die of their renal failure, albeit with compassionate, palliative treatment of unpleasant or intolerable symptoms and with assent of the patient or, if the patient is incompetent, the surrogate.

An increasing concern is that for a significant number of patients who are undergoing dialysis, the burdens substantially outweigh the benefits. The optimal way to avoid manipulation or coercion of patients to be selected for (or to remain on) dialysis inappropriately is a subject now under active consideration by the nephrology community. The National Kidney Foundation has drafted guidelines for the initiation and withdrawal of dialysis.[4d–f]

Before considering guidelines that may help the nephrology community in making appropriate decisions for individual patients in terms of whether to forgo, try, or start permanent renal replacement therapy for ESRD, let us briefly review the history of patient selection for such therapy, present a case illustrative of the difficulty of making prospective selection decisions, and review the consequences of laissez-faire decision making. Presented thereafter are results of surveys that suggest that nephrologists, in the absence of professional guidelines, may accept patients for dialysis who cannot benefit. Next, procedural and substantive guidelines are proposed, and a trial of dialysis recommended for all patients (or at least for patients who are ambivalent about starting dialysis).

SELECTION COMMITTEES AND MELISSA'S CASE

The Quinton-Scribner shunt (Teflon cannulas in a forearm artery and vein connected by a separable, spliced Silastic tube that allowed the patient's blood to shunt from artery to vein when not connected to the artificial kidney) was conceived by Belding Scribner of the University of Washington. Overnight, a condition with 100% mortality (ESRD) was converted to one with a 95% 2-year survival. Many times more patients were referred or presented for care than could be treated. Scribner and colleagues elected to refer patients who could benefit medically (in those days, it was not appreciated that young children and patients with serious extrarenal illnesses such as diabetes or cardiovascular disease could benefit) to an Admissions and Policy Committee, a committee with seven lay members and two physician advisors appointed to serve anonymously by the King County Medical Society and the Seattle Hospital Council. The committee selected patients after considering factors including age, gender, marital status, number of dependents, education, occupation, income, future potential, capacity to accept treatment, and ability to dialyze at home.

Although Fletcher's foundational book *Morals and Medicine* was published in 1954,[8] some say that the 1991 appointment of the lay committee (to select from medically suitable candidates those who would receive treatment at the Seattle Artificial Kidney Center, later the Northwest Kidney Center) was the defining event marking the entrance of bioethics into clinical medicine.[8a] It may also account, in part, for bioethics' preoccupation with life-sustaining technology, with issues of life and death, and with end-of-life decision making. Others recall an interest in the other extreme of life by André E. Hellegers and

the patronage of the Kennedy family in founding the Joseph and Rose Kennedy Institute for the Study of Human Reproduction and Bioethics (now the Kennedy Institute of Ethics) at Georgetown University in 1971. Still others note the founding of the Hastings Center in New York in 1969 by Daniel Callahan, a philosopher, and Willard Gaylin, a psychiatrist, and suggest that the new discipline of bioethics would have developed even without the events in Seattle. Many might agree that the multicentric genesis of the field demonstrated that a need for such a discipline existed and that the time was right both for philosophic reflection in medicine and for selection committees to select from an abundance of patients with renal failure those few who would receive a scarce and prohibitively expensive therapy.

PATIENT NUMBER 4

Melissa was 3 years old when she was discovered in 1965 to have ineradicable urinary tract infection with renal insufficiency due to severe chronic pyelonephritis—all presumably complications of reflux nephropathy that progressed despite urologic correction of reflux. She was thought to be mentally as well as physically retarded, and some questioned the propriety of renal replacement therapy. However, the attending nephrologist had developed a strong bond with Melissa during the 6 months she followed a conservative regimen of a Giordano-Giovannetti diet, bicarbonate, Amphojel, and dihydrotachysterol. The nephrologist was at a university that had received federal funds to establish one of six demonstration hemodialysis centers in the country. It had a patient selection committee that rejected Melissa for hemodialysis because two other children without mental retardation were waiting for the only hemodialysis opening at the center. The committee did not, however, have authority over transplantation or peritoneal dialysis. Melissa's nephrologist insisted she be on the waiting list for a renal transplant and initiated peritoneal dialysis even though he knew peritonitis might supervene and, if active at the time a donor kidney became available, would preclude transplantation. Fortunately, a transplant was performed before any complication of peritoneal dialysis occurred. Even more important, the mental retardation "miraculously" disappeared during the first 2 months as uremia abated with an excellently functional renal transplant.

One wonders how many patients like Melissa with remediable medical problems (in her case brain dysfunction related to renal failure) were denied treatment in the days of selection committees or, for that matter, in subsequent years when selection committees were no longer necessary or required. In any event, selection based on social criteria came in for harsh criticism (to some, surprisingly harsh in view of the commonality of the values used in Seattle). Some preferred a first-come, first-served policy or a lottery. The latter was considered but decided against by the Seattle committee. Truly no one was happy with having to ration dialysis (i.e., to deny beneficial care). Rather than facing the problem of how to select patients when resources (machines, nurses to run them, and money to pay for both) were inadequate, the nephrology community focused on the demon of scarcity and how to find funds to provide the extraordinary, life-saving, but expensive new therapies of dialysis and transplantation.

As might be expected, American ingenuity succeeded: Industry mass-produced dialyzing membranes and dialysate delivery systems; doctors, nurses, social workers, dietitians, and technicians were attracted to the field; and a combination of publically funded units, private insurance, Medicaid, and eventually (with the passage of Public Law 92-603 in 1972) Medicare made dialysis available to most who needed it. No longer did one have to select the patient for the treatment (at first only long-term hemodialysis and, for a few, transplantation). Now one could select the proper treatment from a growing diversity of treatments (home and center hemodialysis, home peritoneal dialysis, and living-related and cadaveric transplantation).

LAISSEZ-FAIRE INITIATION OF DIALYSIS

With public entitlement for the vast majority of patients with renal failure and with the opulence of cost-plus reimbursement of hospitals, a philosophy developed that no one should be denied care. Thus, the acceptance of patients for renal replacement therapy broadened substantially, largely for good but perhaps in small measure for suspect reasons. As both younger and older patients were accepted and as nephrologists experimented with accepting patients with diabetes and cardiovascular disease, the medical contraindications of earlier days were found to be relative, not absolute. Dialysis of patients at home was initially undertaken to expand the number of patients who could be cared for in limited facilities and without public funding. It proved successful, and dialysis units moved out of hospi-

tals, and some became for-profit units of individual physicians or of a new industry fueled by entrepreneurial motivations. This industry was given exemption from previously strict regulation, perhaps because of the increasing federal and state cost of ESRD care. Currently, 60% of dialysis patients in the United States are treated in freestanding, for-profit dialysis units.

The incidence of new patients with ESRD in the United States (as of the most recent data, those for 1993) is 219 per million population. This is 10% higher than in Japan, twice as high as in Canada, three times as high as in Europe, and four times as high as in the United Kingdom. The U.S. incidence is 5 to 10 times that initially imagined, as is the cost of the Medicare ESRD Program despite very substantial efforts to increase the efficiency of dialysis and a more than 50% decrease in per-patient reimbursement. The primary factor in the rising cost of the U.S. ESRD Program ($8 billion in 1993) is the increase in the total number of patients, numbering, as of 1993, 218,000 patients (compared with 16,000 patients in 1974, when the program cost $230 million annually).

THE INSTITUTE OF MEDICINE STUDY OF THE MEDICARE ESRD PROGRAM

Data of this sort and other concerns led the U.S. Congress to request a study of the Medicare ESRD Program by the Institute of Medicine (IOM), which issued its report in 1991.[9] With regard to ethical issues, the IOM Committee focused on the acceptance of patients for treatment, the termination of treatment, and the ethical difficulties of dealing with problem patients. The first of these three concerns is discussed in this section, and the second concern is discussed in a subsequent section of the chapter. Space constraints preclude discussion of noncompliant, disruptive, and abusive patients.

The IOM Committee noted, "Some concern has been expressed that patient acceptance criteria have expanded since enactment of the Medicare ESRD entitlement, resulting in an increasing number of patients with limited survival possibilities and relatively poor quality of life. The Committee, recognizing this concern, believes that patient acceptance criteria should be medical, not economic, and based on concern for the best interests of individual patients. . . . Age was considered and explicitly rejected by the Committee as a patient acceptance criterion, as it does not measure the ability of an individual to benefit from treatment. Comorbidities—at any age—are the primary determinants of quality of life and of survival. . . . Decision-making about the initiation of treatment should result from informed discussion among the patient, the family, the physician, and other care givers."

The committee then noted that "ESRD patients usually rate their quality of life higher than do 'objective' observers" and further stated, "This emphasizes the need to respect patient preferences very highly in decisions about their care." Although wise and articulate, the committee recommendations up to this point largely reflected the practice of the majority of nephrologists (certainly the practice of the best nephrologists) and were not controversial or likely to change practice. These recommendations, however, might not have reassured Congress and the Health Care Financing Administration that nephrologists were to be trusted to follow the recommendations.

The Committee went on to say, "Physicians should recognize that the existence of a public entitlement does not mean that they are obligated to treat all patients who present with kidney failure. Clinical judgment and patient-family preferences will sometimes indicate terminal palliative care rather than life-extending care. Thus, the choice is not between treatment and abandonment, but rather between different goals of treatment." This important recommendation has been the catalyst for much introspection by the nephrology community and is likely to result in the development of guidelines that the committee itself recommended: "The Committee recommends that patients, clinicians in adult and pediatric nephrology, and bioethicists develop guidelines for evaluating patients for whom the burdens of renal replacement therapy may substantially outweigh the benefits. . . . These guidelines should be flexible and encourage the physician to use discretion in assessing an individual patient."

My response at the time to this (and to other pleas for nephrologists to develop selection criteria not unlike those of the early Seattle experience) was that guidelines were not necessary. I suggested that the ethical response to the technologic imperative that "Whatever can be done, should be done" should be "Yes, but only if it is appropriate and of benefit, and if a competent informed patient (or surrogate) wishes it to be done, and if doing it does not have substantial, unjustified adverse or unjust consequences for others." I believed that "the considered judgment of a competent patient who has been informed (by a non-conflicted, knowledgeable nephrologist of good judgment who knows the patient well and has explained the patient's condition and prognosis, treatment options and their expected consequences, and the risks of the alternatives including those of no definitive treatment) suffices for the overwhelming majority of patients."[10]

I argued thus at a national meeting of nephrology nurses who found me naïve, stating on the one hand that some patients undergoing dialysis were not benefiting and on the other hand that nephrologists were benefiting at the patient's expense or at the government's expense. I did not and do not believe their claim (which they obviously exaggerated for emphasis) that "nephrologists will dialyze the dead for dollars" applies to more than an extremely rare nephrologist. However, the underlying assumption of their hyperbole is worthy of the attention of nephrologists: When there is a potential conflict of interest such as personal financial gain, when a patient is accepted for dialysis, it may be misconstrued as the basis if the acceptance is questionable. I believe there are more likely explanations for accepting patients who may benefit only marginally, if at all, and will discuss them shortly.

Despite the fact that there is no *a priori* or inherent requirement for acceptance or selection guidelines, the extremely compelling empirical data of Moss and colleagues[11] have convinced me that guidelines are necessary and very likely to be helpful in making appropriate decisions with patients about the initiation of dialysis.

SURVEYS AND THE ACCEPTANCE OF PATIENTS

In 1990, Moss sent a questionnaire (and two follow-up mailings) to a random sample of medical directors of the 1897 adult dialysis units in the United States. Of 524 questionnaires, 318 were returned (a 61% response rate). One question related to the initiation of dialysis: "If your unit was requested to begin dialysis of a permanently unconscious patient (e.g., persistent vegetative state or multiple strokes), what would usually be done (begin or withhold dialysis)?" Surprisingly, 17% responded that they would provide dialysis! The investigators speculated that "some physicians may place an unqualified value on the preservation of human life" and that "some physicians may misunderstand the ethical and legal aspects of making decisions for such patients." With regard to responses to a question whether or not to withdraw dialysis of a patient with severe, permanent dementia, "some respondents indicated that they would be afraid to stop dialysis . . . if there was the potential for litigation."[11] This could conceivably be a partial explanation for the surprising number who would start permanently unconscious patients on dialysis.

Although other questions in this study related to withdrawal of dialysis are discussed later, their results are presented now to support the notion that guidelines may be necessary and would be helpful to nephrologists.

The medical directors were asked, "If a competent patient (i.e., one with decision-making capacity) asked to stop dialysis, how would your unit usually handle the request (stop or continue dialysis)?" Ninety-two percent "indicated that their units would usually honor a competent patient's request to stop dialysis." When asked, "If a patient receiving dialysis in your unit who had not previously expressed wishes for future care becomes permanently and severely demented (e.g., Alzheimer's disease or multi-infarct dementia), what would usually be done (stop or continue dialysis)?" 32% would stop, but a surprisingly large 68% would continue.

These data are demonstrated in Table 17–1, which shows that 15% of nephrologists would both initiate dialysis on a patient in a persistent vegetative state and continue dialysis on a patient who developed severe, irreversible dementia (actions that most ethicists would judge inappropriate). Only 30% would both withhold dialysis from a patient in a persistent vegetative state and withdraw dialysis from a patient who developed severe, irreversible dementia (actions that most ethicists would judge appropriate).

It is unlikely that these responses reflect what nephrologists really believe ought to be done or what they would elect for themselves were they the patient. Unfortunately, Moss and colleagues' questionnaire did not provide answers about why the dialysis directors would do what they stated they would do, but one can conjecture that fear

of litigation by patients' families was an important factor. In addition, I suspect that many nephrologists believe it is not their right to deny someone treatment for which they have entitlement to Medicare benefits, even though the IOM report emphasized that Medicare entitlement does not obligate treatment.

This study convinced me that even though guidelines for the acceptance of patients for therapy of ESRD should not be necessary in the ideal world, they are necessary in the real world. I believe that guidelines are necessary not so much to inform nephrologists about what other nephrologists believe should be done under various circumstances but rather to reassure nephrologists that their own intuitive responses and judgments are appropriate. Guidelines would give them the courage of their convictions because they would provide the support of professional opinion if a nephrologist were challenged by a dissenting relative or attorney.

GUIDELINES FOR THE ACCEPTANCE AND REJECTION OF PATIENTS

It is, nevertheless, with trepidation that I come to the conclusion that guidelines should be developed. My concerns are several. First, I fear that guidelines may be used by some without discretion (i.e., without what Aristotle called "practical wisdom"). Second, I believe that guidelines, which should be flexible and optional, may be interpreted to be rigid policies or standards of practice and thus misused as a basis for judging the behavior of nephrologists (e.g., in litigation). Third, I fear that guidelines may become Procrustean criteria for judging entitlement, insurance coverage, or reimbursement for dialysis or transplantation.

Guidelines may be procedural or substantive or both. Procedural guidelines are less likely to be controversial, but even they must be considered at length and approved by potential patients and the public as well as by nephrology professionals if they are to be accepted and used.

Procedural Guidelines

Procedural guidelines for acceptance of patients for ESRD therapy might include the following:

1. All patients who could conceivably benefit from ESRD therapy (even if only palliative therapy) should be evaluated by a nephrologist and, whenever appropriate, by a transplant physician or surgeon.

2. Patients should be referred to nephrologists early enough in the course of progressive renal failure that they can be evaluated and treated

TABLE 17–1. How U.S. Dialysis Directors Stated They Would Treat Permanently Unconscious Patients Who Developed ESRD and ESRD Patients Who Developed Severe, Permanent Dementia

		If a permanently unconscious patient developed ESRD, % of directors who would:	
		Start Dialysis	Withhold Dialysis
If a chronic dialysis patient developed severe, permanent dementia, % of dialysis directors who would:		17%	83%
	Continue dialysis 65%	15%	53%
	Withdraw dialysis 32%	2%	30%

Data from Moss AH, Stocking CB, Sachs GA, Siegler M: Variation in the attitudes of dialysis unit medical directors toward decisions to withhold and withdraw dialysis. J Am Soc Nephrol 4:229–234, 1993.

medically and can learn about the various therapeutic modalities and settings for renal replacement therapy before they are so ill that such consideration is difficult. There should be adequate time to allow maturation of a radiocephalic arteriovenous fistula or peritoneal access should either hemodialysis or peritoneal dialysis be appropriate for the patient.

3. All therapeutic modalities and settings that are not medically contraindicated should be available to all patients. That is to say, patients should be informed of the pros and cons and indications and contraindications of dialysis and transplantation, hemodialysis and peritoneal dialysis, home dialysis and center dialysis, and living donor and cadaveric transplantation.

4. If the patient has decision-making capacity, decisions are to be made by the patient after being informed of the benefits and risks of all treatment options, including that of symptomatic therapy only. The patient should be informed of the consequences, course, and support to be expected if definitive treatment is declined. In addition to discussion with the nephrologist, the patient should be encouraged to visit the renal treatment or dialysis center and to discuss treatment options with other health care professionals and other patients. If appropriate, the patient should see a transplant physician or surgeon. Before making a final decision, it would be wise for the patient to review his or her understandings, concerns, and preferences with his or her primary care physician.

5. If the patient lacks decision-making capacity, decisions may be made on the basis of an advance directive if the patient has one. A prior treatment directive (i.e., living will), if it covered the current situation, would allow decisions to be based on the express wishes of the patient. A proxy directive (i.e., a durable power of attorney for health care) would allow the agent-in-fact under a durable power to make decisions based on substituted judgment (i.e., what the patient would have wanted, if it can be surmised) or, if such information is not available, based on the best interests of the patient.

6. Whenever there is uncertainty about whether to institute therapy, a trial of dialytic therapy should be undertaken. To do so ethically requires that the attending health care professionals have the courage to discontinue dialysis should the trial result in a state of health unacceptable to the patient.

7. Even when a trial seems unnecessary, whenever peritoneal dialysis or hemodialysis is undertaken (rather than palliative care or renal transplantation), the first month of dialysis should

be considered a trial. After 1 to 3 months, the decision to initiate therapy should be reconsidered. That is, the benefits and burdens of dialytic therapy should be assessed from the patient's perspective, and the treatment regimen should be modified to improve the balance of benefits over burdens or discontinued if that is the competent patient's informed preference.

8. If procedural guidelines are supplemented by substantive guidelines, the latter are to be flexible and are to be applied to individual cases with discretion appropriate to the particular circumstances and exigencies of that unique case. Furthermore, exceptions and exemptions are to be expected and should not automatically trigger officious or bureaucratic oversight.

Substantive Guidelines of Three Types

Substantive guidelines are more controversial and debatable than procedural guidelines. If they are to be widely applied (and particularly if they might achieve such recognition that they were used as standards of care for judging professional competence or for decisions about reimbursement), they must be acceptable to patients with ESRD and to the informed public as well as to nephrology professionals (including nurses, social workers, and transplant physicians and surgeons).

In an effort to be reasonably comprehensive and particularly for the purpose of stimulating discussion, I suggest three types of substantive guidelines. The first are guidelines for the acceptance of patients; the second and third are for the refusal of patients. The first set lists criteria for ability to benefit from ESRD therapy. The second set is for recommending against dialysis of an individual patient because the burdens are expected, with reasonable certainty, to outweigh the benefits. The third set includes guidelines for rationing—that is, for denial of therapy that could benefit the individual patient but that society might decide not to offer.

TYPE 1 SUBSTANTIVE GUIDELINES: CRITERIA FOR THE ABILITY TO BENEFIT FROM ESRD THERAPY

1. The patient should have severe, symptomatic, and irreversible (i.e., truly end-stage) renal failure (with neither a remediable underlying cause of the renal failure nor remediable factors contributing to the renal dysfunction) requiring dialysis or transplantation to prevent disabling

or life-threatening complications and to sustain health. Such renal failure usually is clearly evident from azotemia and the uremic syndrome, but the renal failure occasionally is primarily manifested by the retention of salt and water. This clinical state of intolerable circulatory overload can occur without severe intrinsic renal disease when a patient has severe cardiac disease and only moderate renal dysfunction except for extreme resistance to diuretics. The edematous state sometimes is markedly improved by a short course of dialysis, which, by ultrafiltration, restores salt and water balance and improves cardiac function and responsiveness to diuretics. At other times, intractable heart failure is judged to be a contraindication to continuing dialysis, but at times even extreme heart failure seems to resolve dramatically with intermittent long-term dialysis, which may have to be continued indefinitely. I suggest that patients who have end-stage heart failure and who are not candidates for cardiac reduction surgery or cardiac transplantation be considered for a trial of dialysis.

2. The patient should have no untreatable illness making life unbearable from his or her perspective. That is, the patient may have problems of health other than the renal failure, but none (nor a combination of such conditions) so severe that it makes life (after correction of the renal failure) unbearable. If, in the patient's informed and considered opinion, death is preferable, dialysis should not be undertaken (or if it has been initiated, it should be discontinued).

3. Before initiating dialysis, informed, voluntary consent should be given after full disclosure of the burdens and benefits of treatment and explicit explanation that the patient has the right to refuse dialysis or to discontinue dialysis at any time (irrespective of whether it was understood to be a trial when initiated). This criterion is included in the list of substantive as well as procedural guidelines in order to emphasize that the ultimate basis for deciding whether or not a patient can benefit from dialysis is his or her own opinion.

4. The patient should be able to benefit from ESRD therapy. If benefit cannot be predicted with reasonable assurance, the patient (or if he or she is unable to indicate his or her wishes, the patient's surrogate) may be willing for the patient to undergo a trial of dialytic therapy. For dialysis to continue beyond the trial, the trial must be successful or purposely extended. It is reasonable to request the treatment team, the patient, and the patient's family all to agree, in advance, on criteria to judge success or failure of the trial, but flexibility should be allowed in both the crite-

ria and the duration of the trial (or its extension because of an indeterminant outcome).

5. The patient's referring physician (particularly when he or she is also the patient's primary physician of long standing or of a particularly close relationship) should explore with the patient (and with his or her extended family if that is the patient's preference) and with the nephrologist the various modalities and settings of therapy available to the patient, their benefits, their risks, and their burdens. The patient (and, if he or she wishes, his or her close family and friends) should have an opportunity to obtain advice not only from the primary physician and nephrologist but also from other members of the ESRD treatment staff (dialysis and renal transplant nurses, social workers, dietitians, technicians, and chaplains) and from other patients with ESRD. The patient should see not only patients on peritoneal and hemodialysis but also patients who have successful renal transplants and those whose transplant failed and who are back on dialysis. The patient should also be told survival statistics of patients on dialysis and after transplantation.

The reason to include the previous guideline in the substantive rather than the procedural group is to list the details that the patient needs to consider in deciding whether or not dialysis will be of benefit. Early discussion should include consideration of common complications (e.g., failure of vascular or peritoneal access) as well as those that are uncommon or that may not be anticipated by the patient (e.g., life-threatening illness, physical debility or disability, bone disease, dementia, severe depression, and cardiopulmonary arrest). Patients should be asked what care they would want under such circumstances and should be informed of their right to make formal advance directives. The latter may be as simple as appointing a proxy to serve if the patient becomes incompetent or as detailed as explaining therapeutic approaches that the patient would wish to be followed under various circumstances and goals the patient might hope could be achieved.

TYPE 2 SUBSTANTIVE GUIDELINES: CIRCUMSTANCES THAT MIGHT PRECLUDE BENEFIT FROM ESRD THERAPY

1. The renal insufficiency is reversible or is not severe enough to cause disabling or life-threatening complications or to prevent health to be sustained without dialysis or transplantation (i.e., dialysis or transplantation is not yet indicated).

2. Extrarenal illness is so severe and so resistant to treatment that the patient does not wish to live and therefore prefers no definitive treatment of the renal failure. Particular care must be taken to detect treatable psychologic depression, especially in the elderly, in whom it is notably underdiagnosed.

3. Death is imminent because of a condition other than renal failure. Interpretation of imminence should be flexible to allow weighing the burden of the symptoms of the nonrenal disorder plus the burden of initiating dialysis against the benefit of prolonging life (or delaying death).

4. The patient is permanently unconscious (i.e., in a persistent or permanent vegetative state or in a coma from which the patient is not expected to recover).

5. The patient has such severe, irreversible (i.e., end-stage) dementia that the patient is suffering or is unable to experience pleasure or to relate meaningfully to other people (although the individual might still have the ability to respond purposefully to some environmental stimuli).

6. The patient lacks decision-making capacity but has previously, when competent, explicitly refused therapy for ESRD or has indicated that he or she would not wish life-sustaining treatment of any sort under circumstances such as those that have at present befallen the patient.

7. The patient underwent a trial of dialytic therapy and the patient (if the patient lacks capacity, the patient's surrogate) concluded that the burdens outweighed the benefits and elected to discontinue dialysis.

TYPE 3 SUBSTANTIVE GUIDELINES: PATIENTS FOR WHOM SOCIETY MIGHT CONSIDER RATIONING ESRD THERAPY

Unlike the previous category of guidelines (whom not to dialyze), which is surprisingly less controversial among nephrologists than the first category (whom to dialyze), this category (guidelines for rationing therapy) is extremely controversial at the present time in the United States. Listed next are possible groups of patients (for whom society might elect not to provide public funds for ESRD therapy) in decreasing order of acceptability (i.e., in increasing order of controversiality).

1. The first group is currently excluded from ESRD therapy or more properly from the Medicare ESRD Program in the United States. This group comprises approximately 7% of patients who have ESRD and who are undergoing dialysis

(and doubtless an additional number who elect to—or have to—forgo dialysis because they are not eligible for Medicare benefits). Although Public Law 92-603 provided categoric entitlement for ESRD regardless of age, individuals are not entitled to benefits if they are not eligible for Social Security benefits (or are not spouses or dependents of eligible individuals). This was an unintentional result of the technical, bureaucratic way the congressionally mandated benefits were enacted. This group includes some public employees, some in covered occupations who fail to apply for benefits, and some who have never worked. Thus, the group includes many who are poor or minorities. The IOM Committee recommended entitlement be extended to all U.S. citizens and resident aliens with ESRD.

2. For transplantation—so long as donor organs continue to be scarce—patients who are so noncompliant after psychotherapy (or who refuse psychotherapy) that they can reasonably be expected to reject a transplant because of failure to take prescribed posttransplant medications dependably on their own (or if they have a reliable family member, when the medications are presented for them to take). If such noncompliant patients do receive a transplant, they should be warned, in writing, that if they reject the graft for failure to take prescribed medications, they will not receive a second and certainly not a third transplant.

3. Patients for whom ESRD therapy can be expected to be of marginal benefit or who failed a reasonable trial of dialysis (by criteria they agreed to before the trial) but who now request dialysis (or a transplant).

4. Hostile, abusive, contumacious patients who are dangerous and harm other patients or staff and who refuse or fail to respond to psychotherapy or supervised isolation. Before such patients are refused dialysis, serious efforts must be undertaken to understand the reasons for their behavior and to modify it. Due process procedures may be needed in such cases as well.

5. Seriously ill newborns with renal failure and severe neurologic damage or major physical, disabling handicap or other serious and disabling illness that will be lifelong. This most arguable of the groups of patients for consideration of rationing by society might be considered by some to be included in the preceding category of substantive guidelines (i.e., circumstances that might preclude benefit from ESRD therapy). Although some interpret inclusion of severely neurologically or physically disabled newborns as ageism or as discrimination against the disabled, my primary concern is the suffering of the infants

themselves over a lifetime and the suffering of their families and others who attend them.

Who Should Develop Guidelines?

If guidelines are to be developed, who should develop them? Were guidelines for acceptance of patients for ESRD therapy to be used only to assist patients and health care professionals in making informed, appropriate decisions, it would not matter who developed them so long as they were good and were helpful. Appreciating, however, that guidelines are likely to be used for other purposes and to have potential impact on many different groups of individuals in the nephrology community, it seems wise to involve all sufficiently interested parties in the development of the guidelines. This is not to suggest that there be equal representation of all groups or that all groups should necessarily participate in the development of guidelines but, rather, that all interested parties should be invited to do so. The list of organizations that might have an interest in developing ESRD guidelines is substantial and in the United States might include a minimum of 20 professional and patient groups. The presidents of the American Society of Nephrology, the National Kidney Foundation, and the Renal Physicians Association ("representing practicing and academic nephrologists, health care delivery professionals and patients with kidney disease") issued a joint statement of principles basic to the development of practice guidelines.[12] They stated that the "process must be an interdisciplinary endeavor." They gave "examples of public policy issues that may be affected by practice guidelines: Quality and utilization review criteria, physician licensing and accreditation, determinants of tort liability, regulations regarding reimbursement, guidance for medical insurance benefit decisions, development of cost-containment initiatives, and development of information and decision support systems."

Toward Consensus and Follow-up

We presented the three categories of substantive guidelines not only to be complete and to stimulate thought and discussion but also to demonstrate guidelines some may think unnecessary (type 1, or criteria of ability to benefit from ESRD therapy) or may judge inappropriate at this time (type 3, or rationing guidelines). Indeed, it was the type 2 guidelines "for evaluating patients for whom the burdens of renal replacement therapy may substantially outweigh the benefits" that were proposed by the IOM Com-

mittee. In an excellent review, Moss stated that he believes that the nephrology community has an emerging consensus about the presumption to forgo dialysis (to the type 2 list he would add "patients who are unable to cooperate with the dialysis process").[7] He also lists arguments for and against guidelines. My list of benefits of guidelines to forgo dialysis (informed by Moss's list) is as follows: improved medical and ethical decision making by reducing physicians' fear of arbitrary, discriminatory judgments and fear of liability and litigation; reduction of professional and patient anxiety and distrust; reduction of inappropriate, arbitrary variations in practice; prudent use of a societal resource; and realization of professional and public consensus and understanding.

When guidelines are developed, how should they be evaluated and by whom? If they are found valid and effective, how should they be promulgated, how should they be used, and should they be enforced? And importantly, when should they be reevaluated and revised?

Advance Directives

An overview of the need to plan for serious illness and the possibility that one might lose decision-making capacity, and an overview of advance treatment and proxy directives and the values history were presented earlier. This section presents cases to illustrate the clinical importance of advance directives and the formidable challenges they pose for patients, proxies, and physicians.

PATIENT NUMBER 5

Demetrios was 7 years older than his physician and ever so much wiser. He was always ahead of his time. At age 17, during World War II, he enlisted in the Seabees to see the world and to defend his country. He not only had to lie about his age to get in, but when he was found to have protein in his urine, he had to get a friend to "lend" him a specimen, which he submitted as his own. At the end of the war, when he was anxious to be discharged, he had forgotten about the protein in his urine. It was rediscovered and would have detained him for medical evaluation had he not again obtained a buddy's specimen. Only later would he wish the kidney condition were "service connected."

Demetrios, or Mitsos, as he preferred to be called, probably had chronic pyelonephritis, perhaps reflux nephropathy. At a famous New York hospital, he had been found to have pyuria and left ureteral reflux as an infant, and his parents were told he had chronic pyelonephritis when he was age 9. He was unaware of this and had even forgotten the proteinuria on Seabee examinations until he was found to have a creatinine level of 2.8 mg/dl and hypertension on a routine examination at age 40. He was referred to a world famous nephrology group in another city for further evaluation. A percutaneous renal biopsy was performed and interpreted to show "latent glomerulonephritis." Two weeks later, he went to the nephrologist's office with his wife, Sophia, to learn the findings on biopsy. Rather than talking with them together, the senior nephrologist spoke with each of them separately. Each was told that Mitsos had only 2 years to live. Neither knew the other had been told this prognosis, and each was shocked and profoundly depressed, but neither told the other (wanting not to burden each other with such ominous news). It was only after Mitsos had outlived the nephrologist's prognosis and when long-term dialysis and renal transplantation had become available that they shared their experiences.

Renal insufficiency did progress despite control of hypertension, and Mitsos was referred for my evaluation and for me to consider dialysis as uremic symptoms had appeared. For several months, symptoms were minimal on a protein-restricted diet, and the patient agonized whether or not he would accept dialysis because he wished not to be a burden on Sophia and his high school–age children. Unbeknownst to us, he visited another dialysis unit. He asked the nurse in charge if he could speak with the patients because he might need to start dialysis in a month or two. She introduced him to a man his age. The gentleman said he tolerated dialysis reasonably well and was pleased to be alive, but he stated he was destitute. He, like Mitsos, had been a self-employed businessman, and he and his wife had saved $50,000 to send their children to college and to use for their own retirement, but now it was gone. Before he could qualify for Medicaid, he had had to spend all but $2000 of his savings. He advised Mitsos to liquidate his savings, put the cash in a coffee can, and bury it in the backyard.

Mitsos was frightened by this story, but forewarned, he and Sophia prepared. She had been a homemaker. Now she would return to the work force to seek employment that provided group health insurance without preexisting illness exclusion. Ironically, she went to work for a large insurance company whose health insurance benefit covered family expenses up to $50,000. This was unfortunately to become exhausted after a year of hemodialysis and an unsuccessful cadaveric renal transplant.

The transplanted kidney was rejected despite antilymphocyte globulin and high-dose adrenal steroids. Steroid therapy was in turn complicated by a bleeding duodenal ulcer, which had to be oversewn. Vagotomy and pyloroplasty were also performed.

Because insurance benefits were dissipating, Mitsos transferred all of his financial assets to his wife as personal property and made the most difficult decision of his life. He divorced Sophia, although he absolutely adored her. He did so in order that their savings and assets would not be depleted by medical expenses and would be available for their children's college education and for Sophia's support when he was gone (he was exceptionally objective without being depressed or unduly pessimistic). Although he divorced primarily for Sophia's benefit, Mitsos was old fashioned and felt guilty as well as bereft. Two years later, the divorce would have been unnecessary because the U.S. Congress then passed Public Law 92-603, which provided Medicare benefits for ESRD therapy.

As was true for many patients on dialysis in the late 1960s and early 1970s, dialysis sustained Mitsos's life but not his health. He was anephric because his native kidneys had been removed to prepare for the transplant (as was common in those days, particularly if the patient had had urinary tract infection or had poorly controlled hypertension), and the transplant was removed due to pain and inflammation complicating exuberant rejection. Because of his anephric state, Mitsos had severe anemia, requiring transfusions to the point of hemosiderosis, and he developed symptomatic bone disease with disabling hip pain. Despite the usual control of blood pressure by ultrafiltration, Mitsos had a subarachnoid hemorrhage. Although he recovered quickly, he was fearful of a recurrence or of other neurologic impairment. He had witnessed the development of organic brain syndrome in two men his age and feared this disorder might disable him as well. Although we did not then know the etiology, Mitsos's fear was probably quite appropriate because he used more than average amounts of aluminum-containing medication not only to control phosphorus but also because of his ulcer and intermittent melena.

Mitsos knew his only hope for regaining health was a successful renal transplant. However, he had developed so many antibodies from transfusions that he realized it was unlikely that a match would be found. Furthermore, he remembered what a toll the first transplant had taken on him. He grew increasingly philosophic, resigned to his own fatality, and requested an appointment to see me in the office, not in the dialysis unit.

Mitsos brought Sophia with him. He asked me to tell them my honest evaluation of his health and to give as realistic a prognosis as I could. Mitsos reminded me that he and Sophia had learned the hard way that doctors are not infallible in giving prognoses, but he nevertheless requested my best guess so that he and his wife could plan their remaining time together and could prepare their children for the inevitable.

Mitsos conceded that his greatest fear was that he could lose the ability to think and communicate and thus lose control of his health care and of his own destiny. In that event, he told me and Sophia, he wished that she not be burdened with decisions on his behalf. He requested that I, his physician, make the hard decisions so that if he were suffering or if he had become a burden to his family, dialysis was to be discontinued in order that he might die. I agreed to his poignant plea, although I hoped he would have a better course than either he or I anticipated and that he would not lose decisional capacity.

Mitsos seemed relieved by our agreement, made long before I knew about a living will or the appointment of a health care proxy other than the next of kin. Our agreement made sense, however, particularly for Mitsos, because it was clearly an authentic expression of his devotion to his family, his concern that Sophia not have to make an emotionally wrenching decision to let him die (or worse yet to stop the treatment that kept him alive), and his desire not to be a burden. His trust in me to make decisions for him further strengthened our bond and mutual respect.

The next—that is, the last—6 months were not easy. Mitsos had thoracic and hip pain so severe that nerve blocks were performed and nerve section considered. He had a brief period of suicidal depression. He then developed a febrile illness with intensified hip pain. I think he knew the end was near, and he refused hospitalization for 2 days, but he could stand the pain no more and was admitted. *Escherichia coli* was growing in his blood sample and in a left hip aspirate, and antibiotic therapy was modified according to sensitivities. Nevertheless, he became semicomatose and tachypneic and appeared moribund. I ordered that resuscitation not be attempted if an arrest occurred. Then, not atypically for Mitsos, he improved for some days but remained stuporous and noncommunicative. He was obviously malnourished and catabolic, and he now developed a decubitus ulcer over his right hip. I feared that even if he recovered from the infection, he would be bedridden, and this would be—from his perspective—a fate worse than death. Thus, after consultation with two physicians who knew him well, all treatment was discontinued except for analgesics given to lessen grimacing and moaning when he rolled onto his left hip. One day later, Mitsos had an arrest and no resuscitative attempt was made. How difficult it is to honor the death request of an inspirational patient who has truly become a friend.

Although I had practiced and taught medicine for 20 years, I had no idea how little I knew about (1) the place of honest communication with seriously but not necessarily terminally ill patients; (2) the benefit for them, their loved ones, and the physician of advance treatment and proxy directives; and (3) the indebtedness of physicians to patients for education and emotional reward.

PATIENT NUMBER 6

Charlene was a housewife and mother of three teenage sons. Her older sister and mother treated her like a child. Thus, she was spoiled and used to getting her way—often at the expense of her husband, an accountant. Charlene was referred in 1973 at the age of 38 for renal insufficiency (creatinine level 15.6 mg/dl) and poorly controlled hypertension. We elicited a history of pyelonephritis at ages 7, 23, and 32 and found consistent calyceal abnormalities on an IVP that had been performed before her last pregnancy at age 24. At the time of referral, her kidneys were atrophic and unobstructed and her urine was sterile. With control of hypertension, renal function worsened and uremic symptoms developed and forced initiation of dialysis.

Charlene was not happy on dialysis and opted for a cadaveric renal transplant, which she received in the summer of 1974. Unfortunately, primary nonfunction ensued and she had no response to intravenous steroid therapy. The graft had to be removed for a *Staphylococcus aureus* wound infection, and the wound was allowed to close by secondary intention. During the next year, repeated "stitch abscesses" were a great annoyance but at the time seemed minor. In retrospect, they were the harbinger of future decline.

Charlene returned to hemodialysis but had access problems. Her radiocephalic arteriovenous fistula, which had never functioned well, thrombosed shortly after the transplant, and a bovine interposition graft was placed in the other forearm. Next she developed an eczematous dermatitis overlying the bovine fistula. We thought it might be due to the iodine-containing antiseptic used to prepare the skin before cannulating the fistula for dialysis. However, the dermatitis persisted despite removing the iodine promptly after application with copious amounts of alcohol and even despite omitting iodine from the skin preparation altogether. We constructed a second access in her other forearm, never used iodine on the overlying skin, and the dermatitis occurred there as well—always most severe overlying the forearm fistula but truly involving much of both forearms. It waxed and waned without clear relationship to therapy (she saw several dermatologists and tried myriad remedies) or to her state of chronic anxiety. Indeed, the dermatitis persisted for the rest of her life.

Charlene was never happy on center dialysis and fought with the nurses to the point of mutual aggravation and tears. She was very particular about access care, blood flow rate, and ultrafiltration pressure, and she frequently had calf cramps or vomiting when hypotensive and requested early conclusion of dialysis. Even the head nurse and her nephrologist (who mediated innumerable disputes) lost patience and one day suggested to the patient that if no one could run her dialysis acceptably at the unit maybe she should dialyze herself at home. To our pleasant surprise, she not only accepted our suggestion that she and her husband train to perform hemodialysis at home but she became a model patient.

We had to walk a tightrope in listening to the patient both at her monthly office visits and at the time of intermittent telephone calls. On the one hand, we had to tune out and not be annoyed by her plaintive whining about minor nuisances, and on the other hand had to pay prompt attention to concerns that were somehow communicated in a different tone of voice and represented serious medical problems. She was an astute observer, and once we learned to distinguish when she was calling about a genuine concern, we found she never cried wolf.

Charlene's husband, Norman, was attentive, incredibly patient, and loyal and was present throughout every dialysis. He had a modest income, but he and Charlene loved to travel with their boys. They modified a camper to accommodate a sorbent dialysis system, which they used during vacations and travel to national parks. However, Norman always had trouble cannulating her fistulas, and Charlene had to have one access surgery after another. In part, revisions were performed because of the persistent dermatitis, which was always most severe immediately overlying the fistula and thus caused speculation that she might have an allergic reaction to the material of the interposition graft. Bovine carotid artery was changed to Gore-Tex (polytetrafluroethylene) to endogenous saphenous vein. The other problem necessitating fistula revisions was intermittent *S. aureus* infection, sometimes superficial in the skin but on five occasions over the next 10 years involving the fistula or graft itself and causing septicemia.

After the first two episodes of staphylococcal sepsis, the patient and her husband were discovered to be nasal *Staphylococcus* carriers, and antibiotics were given for a prolonged time. In addition, the patient, who had never cared for the discomfort of another person's inserting her dialysis needles, learned to cannulate her own fistulas. She wore a face mask, scrubbed her forearm with antiseptic for 5 minutes by the clock, and was meticulous in needle placement. Nevertheless, perhaps because bacteria could not be totally eliminated by preparing the skin (because of the dermatitis), Charlene had three more episodes of staphylococcal sepsis.

Charlene had more than her share of other medical problems as well: an episode of hepatitis, chronic metabolic acidosis more severe than in other patients but never explained, an episode of upper gastrointestinal bleeding, hyperparathyroidism uncontrolled medically and for which she underwent subtotal parathyroidectomy, episodic bronchitis with asthma, and anemia with iron deficiency but intolerance of oral and intravenous iron such that she requested periodic transfusions. Nevertheless, Charlene was vigorous and active in family and social life, and she convinced the transplant surgeon to put her on the list for a second transplant.

As she had on the two prior occasions, Charlene diagnosed her fifth and final episode of staphylococcal sepsis. On each occasion, 12 to 24 hours before she had fever and before any local inflammation over the fistula, Charlene had severe generalized pain that was difficult to localize in muscle or bone. It occurred in her trunk and flank as well as her extremities and did not localize to joints. It was typical for her, however, and on each of the last three episodes we drew blood cultures even though she had not yet developed fever, and on each occasion the results were positive.

In retrospect, we should have empirically started antibiotics while awaiting the blood culture results, because with the fifth episode she not only had septic pulmonary emboli as she had had with the first episode but she also developed endocarditis with emboli to her brain, liver, and spleen. Charlene was critically ill and responded poorly to intensive therapy with multiple antibiotics under the direction of an infectious disease consultant. She was encephalopathic, ventilator dependent, jaundiced, and severely anemic (hematocrit declined from 31% to 23%). After 3½ weeks of antibiotic therapy, she had a temperature of 104.4°F and a pulse of 160.

If I did not see the patient's husband in the hospital, I phoned him each evening, and during the hospitalization I had several conferences with him and his sons. Because there was no condition from which Charlene could not theoretically recover to her prehospital state, no one questioned the aggressive therapy despite its failure to improve her condition. I decided empirically to remove surgically both dialysis fistulas even though neither had overlying inflammation or abnormality on ultrasonography or gallium scan. If Charlene's condition failed to improve a week after removal of the dialysis fistulas, I planned mitral valve replacement. Just before it was to be done, her temperature was still over 104°F, her abdomen became distended (and she grimaced to palpation of the right upper quadrant where her gallbladder could not be palpated, although it was mildly distended on ultrasonography), and she became hypotensive. The cardiac surgeon refused to consider mitral valve surgery but recommended cholecystostomy. A general surgeon was willing to operate if the family and I insisted, but he believed that Charlene should be allowed to die without further intervention.

I held a conference with the patient's husband, her eldest son, and her older sister, who had always been close to Charlene and was very protective of her. We were joined by the three consulting physicians, a chaplain (the patient was very religious), and the social worker from the dialysis unit, who knew the patient well. The patient's mother was invited but was too upset to attend. However, she surmised we would recommend discontinuation of all but comfort therapy, and she told her older daughter that Charlene had told her (just before she entered the hospital) that she would never stop dialysis under any circumstance (even though other patients she had known had done so).

Indeed, to our great embarrassment, when the question was asked "What would the patient want us to do?" we learned that not a single one of us (the primary nephrologist, the renal social worker, the husband, the sister, or the son) had ever discussed such matters with Charlene. Although state law provided both a natural death act and a durable power of attorney for health care, neither had been explicitly discussed with the patient. They had only been presented at a quarterly educational program for patients to which home patients were invited. Of greatest importance, the nephrologist (who had known the patient for 15 years) had never discussed Charlene's preferences for care should she become critically ill and had never asked what to do should she become decisionally incapacitated. Although everyone at the conference (except for the consulting physicians and surgeons) thought they knew the patient very well, none could predict what she would tell us to do under the present circumstances. Indeed, we had conflicting notions of this substituted judgment approach and even questioned what the patient might have meant in telling her mother she would "never stop dialysis." Some thought she might simply be reassuring her mother that she wasn't a quitter and that the statement might not apply to circumstances in which she was dying. She did indeed die en route to have a CT scan of the gallbladder and abdomen, but what if she had been able to live another week or two or three?

I learned a very valuable lesson, which I really should have known intuitively. Unfortunately, I did not learn it in time to help Charlene and particularly her family, who suffered greatly during the 7 weeks of her final hospitalization. The final 2 weeks were especially difficult, when we repeatedly asked ourselves what was the right thing to do and would Charlene want us to do it.

Do Not Attempt Resuscitation (DNAR) Orders

Resuscitation of patients with cardiopulmonary arrest became a practical possibility in the 1960s with demonstration of the efficacy of closed-chest cardiac massage and the development of mechanical ventilators and cardiac defibrillators. Success was initially frequent because CPR was performed on otherwise healthy individuals with witnessed arrests due to such conditions as electrocution, near-drowning, anesthetic overdose, and acute myocardial infarction. It became accepted practice to attempt resuscitation for all patients who suffered cardiopulmonary arrest on the grounds of presumed consent (assuming no one wished to die). Thus, it became the only major intervention routinely initiated without explicit consent.

In the 1970s as CPR was provided to virtually all patients, it was less frequently successful, and it became apparent that it was sometimes inappropriate because it prolonged the suffering of dying patients or left some patients with severe neurologic impairment (individuals who might be sustained indefinitely with mechanical ventilation and intensive care). Physicians began to omit CPR for patients for whom they thought it would be harmful or futile, at first without informing patients or families and often without adequate discussion with nurses. Later, of course, DNR orders (or more properly DNAR orders in view of the decreasing frequency of successful resuscitation) were recommended to improve honest prospective communication with patients, families, and health care professionals, especially nurses.

During the 1980s, the many meanings and the multiple implications of DNAR orders became apparent. Two categories of communication difficulties deserve mention. The first to be clarified were problems of communication between the physician and the patient (or when the patient was unable to communicate, between the physician and surrogates of the patient). As Tomlinson and Brody wrote,[13] the rationale for a DNAR order might be that the likelihood of medical benefit or success was nil or that the quality of life before (or anticipated after) CPR was so poor that CPR was inappropriate. For the latter circumstance, the patient's values and the patient's evaluation of his or her quality of life and preferences were determinative in decisions to forgo CPR. If the quality of life before an arrest were so poor that the patient would not want resuscitation to be attempted, implications for other treatments (e.g., whether or not the patient would want treatment of hypotension, arrhythmia, infection, or renal failure) probably should be discussed. This points out the desirability of advance discussion between physician and patient and the fact that a DNAR order is really an advance treatment directive even though it is not usually durable, and the order requires rewriting on the patient's readmission to the hospital.

The second category of communication difficulties is that between physician and nurse (or other health care provider). Although DNAR orders, like advance directives generally, are frequently interpreted without careful discussion with the patient or without careful reading of the chart to know the patient's reasons for requesting (or the physician's rationale for writing) one, a DNAR order should never in itself be interpreted to apply to anything other than a cardiopulmonary arrest. The DNAR order does not indicate what should be done if the patient develops an arrhythmia, hypotension, or respiratory distress, nor does it reflect whether or not the patient should be cared for in an intensive care unit or should be dialyzed, transfused, or given antibiotics. The first group of disorders (arrhythmia, hypotension, respiratory distress) often presage cardiopulmonary arrest, and thus their treatment might be called *prearrest interventions.* It is extremely helpful to nurses for physicians to write which prearrest interventions should be provided and which should not whenever a DNAR order is written. The second group of interventions (intensive care unit care, dialysis, transfusion, antibiotic therapy, and so on) has been called *concurrent care concerns* and may be addressed in advance or as they arise because they usually do not have the same need for urgent decision as for prearrest interventions.

In the late 1980s and early 1990s, attention shifted from DNAR orders back to orders for CPR because of health care professionals' increasing attention to outcomes data showing the infrequent success of indiscriminate application of CPR and because of the public's increasing fear of being sustained "by machines" in states they would not wish. For hospital patients, only about a third survive CPR; of those, only about a third survive a month or more after hospital discharge; and of those, only about half survive without significant neurologic impairment. For patients who are elderly or who have major organ

dysfunction (and this includes renal failure as well as cardiac or pulmonary dysfunction), the results are significantly worse.

Thus, some propose a presumption to not attempt resuscitation on patients in a permanent vegetative state or who are dying or have major organ failure without a specific order and a written justification. Were this to be an institution's policy, it would need to be made known to prospective patients because most people are aware that the standard practice in the United States is to attempt resuscitation on anyone who has cardiopulmonary arrest and does not have a DNAR order.

Others propose that CPR be discussed with *all* patients because even young, healthy patients may unexpectedly suffer cardiopulmonary arrest. If health care professionals can tell patients that they discuss patients' preferences of this sort (and also who they would wish to make medical decisions for them if they became unable) with *all* patients, those who might otherwise assume that health professionals were withholding information about an ominous or fatal illness might feel less anxious. If this approach is undertaken, patients' preferences should also be routinely reviewed whenever a significant, relevant change occurs in a patient's condition or circumstances.

Although readers may find these considerations just matters of common sense, it may be helpful to consider a case in which a difference of opinion arose between physician and family in terms of what the patient would want.

PATIENT NUMBER 7

Fleetwood, or Fleet, as he preferred to be called, was a happily married salesman with five children. He was pleasant and well liked, although the immature plaintive whine with which he expressed his very low tolerance for pain or inconvenience grated on one's nerves. Fleet was sometimes pitied for his unmanly timidity, but it was convenient that he rarely objected to recommended therapy or tests.

Fleet was referred for mild but progressive azotemia when he was 44 years old. At age 34, he had been found to have hypertension, which led to the discovery that he had only one kidney, proteinuria, and microscopic hematuria. He was found to have a nephritonephrotic urinary sediment, and in the absence of evidence of a systemic disorder, it was assumed that Fleet's primary disease was chronic glomerulonephritis. With control of hypertension, the progression of renal insufficiency was slow, but Fleet agonized over having to have renal replacement therapy.

He was frightened of the risks of a transplant and began evening center hemodialysis in 1977 at age 49. He continued to work during the day and drove throughout southern California as a computer salesman. Fleet was very reluctant to increase dialysis from twice to three times a week, which we advised because of poor control of fluid and potassium balance. On several occasions, Fleet had to have an extra dialysis for circulatory overload with congestive heart failure. In 1979, Fleet had to be hospitalized for staphylococcal sepsis complicating vascular access infection. He had a pulmonary lesion (which resolved without surgery), pericarditis, atrial fibrillation, and a brief episode of ventricular tachycardia.

On two occasions in 1980, Fleet had episodes of extreme muscle weakness due to hyperkalemia while he was driving in Los Angeles. On each occasion, emergency dialysis in Los Angeles was arranged because Fleet could not safely drive to his dialysis center in Orange County. It was this danger to others that finally convinced Fleet he should accept the advice to increase to thrice-weekly dialysis.

Fleet had lost weight and stamina during his hospitalization, and with the increase to thrice-weekly dialysis, he found it increasingly difficult to do his job. His boss wanted him to retire, but Fleet felt he could not provide for his family on disability income. He requested transfusions, more frequently than we thought wise, and hoped to have the endurance his job required. He developed neurosensory hearing loss requiring a hearing aid, and his renal disease was speculated to be Alport's hereditary nephritis. He also developed cataracts, which made it difficult to drive at night, and a peripheral neuropathy with some loss of balance. With further malaise consequent to an episode of hepatitis B, Fleet had to quit his job, and he became depressed. He had an episode of ventricular tachycardia during dialysis and was referred for cardiac evaluation. He became anxious about his health and saw himself failing—and not so slowly. Thus, Fleet finally agreed that a transplant should be performed in the hopes of substantial improvement of overall health.

Because of having many transfusions, Fleet had antibodies to multiple HLA antigens, but in June 1982, a cadaveric donor with whom he had a negative crossmatch finally became available. To our great disappointment, a rejection episode was evident on the fifth posttransplant day. It failed to respond to high-dose intravenous steroids or to plasmapheresis, and a swollen, tender graft with a large hematoma was removed on the 19th day when Fleet was rapidly becoming dangerously thrombopenic. His hospital course was complicated by E. coli urinary tract infection, bladder bleeding, gastrointestinal infection, two more episodes of ventricular arrhythmia, an episode of congestive

heart failure after two transfusions, and, understandably, depression.

After Fleet's discharge, his condition did not improve. He was as weak and inactive after a month as he had been the day he went home. His diet was liberalized in hopes of improving his nutritional state. Nutritional supplements were prescribed, and a dietitian worked with Fleet and his wife to allow favorite nutritious foods. To accommodate this and to avoid fluid overload, Fleet was dialyzed four times a week. A cardiologist who had gotten to know Fleet rather well during the preceding 3 years prescribed a supervised exercise program in the outpatient cardiac center. Group psychotherapy was arranged, as well as frequent pastoral care visits. Despite all of this and the constant attendance and encouragement of his wife, Elaine, Fleet continued to lose ground, albeit slowly. Despite quinidine, he had another episode of ventricular tachycardia on dialysis. His cardiac rhythm was thereafter monitored throughout every treatment. Fleet had premature ventricular contractions (PVCs)—isolated, in couplets, and occasionally in bursts. Watching them on the monitor, he came to appreciate that they were the cause of his palpitations, which he had previously ignored. Now knowing our concern over his PVCs, Fleet became increasingly anxious. He whimpered each time he had a palpitation. By the time his cardiac neurosis was recognized, it was too late: He now knew a palpitation was due to a PVC and that multiple PVCs could be lethal. Painful peripheral neuropathy failed to respond to vitamins, analgesics, or anticonvulsants. It appeared that the only treatment that could improve Fleet's condition was a successful renal transplant, and I was pleased that the transplant surgeon was willing if a compatible cadaveric donor could be found. A daughter volunteered to be a donor but was blood type incompatible (to my relief, because I felt conflicted about her offer: wanting the best for Fleet but judging his chance for success sufficiently poor not to justify putting a living donor at risk).

In June 1983, Fleet was readmitted in congestive failure with recurrent ventricular tachycardia. Needless to say, Fleet and Elaine were very depressed. His psychiatrist and the chaplain who knew him best (as well as his cardiologist) were consulted and agreed with Fleet's preference that he not be resuscitated should a ventricular arrhythmia occur. We asked if he wished to discontinue dialysis, and he did not. The cardiologist, having failed to control the arrhythmias with quinidine and procainamide, tried two experimental drugs, but PVCs continued to occur periodically, occasionally in runs. Despite control of fluid balance, congestive failure continued and I elected to increase the dose of digoxin while monitoring blood levels. To be able to fine-tune the dose, he was switched from tablets to the pediatric elixir. Two days after the first increase in dose, a blood level (which had been 1.2 ng/ml 3 days previously) was reported to be 8 ng/ml (the therapeutic level is 0.8 to 2.9 ng/ml)! I was actually reviewing Fleet's daily laboratory test results when this report came in. I surmised it was a laboratory error (as did the cardiologist to whom I phoned the result) but ordered that a new sample be obtained and the test be repeated immediately.

I feared that this patient, predisposed as he was to ventricular arrhythmia, could not tolerate digitalis toxicity and wondered how, if by chance the laboratory result were not an error, he might have developed such a toxic level. I couldn't imagine that large a dosage error and deduced it would have to result from an intentional overdose. I knew Fleet was sufficiently depressed that were he another patient, he might have intentionally taken an overdose. If that were the case, I almost wished I had not discovered the high blood level because I appreciated how much the patient was suffering—he cried frequently and openly—and how little benefit he had received from psychotherapy. I didn't think Fleet would have had the guts to commit suicide, however, and I knew of his staunch religious beliefs as well. Thus, I came to speculate that one of his children might have been so upset by Fleet's plight and suffering that he or she might have given Fleet an overdose. Aghast at this possibility, I wrote an order to rescind the DNAR order and went to tell the patient's wife. Fleet was so ill and so depressed that I had found him incapable of understanding anything of this magnitude in recent days. Furthermore, in the spirit of therapeutic privilege, expecting that within an hour or two I would receive a report that the extreme digoxin level had been a laboratory error, I did not wish to upset the patient.

Meanwhile, the nurse manager of the unit had called a pharmacist to investigate whether a dosage error had been made. The patient's wife was upset with me for having rescinded the DNAR order because she believed Fleet was suffering terribly and that death would be a blessing—despite the fact that we were still hoping we could get the patient strong enough to go by wheelchair to the wedding of his oldest son just 10 days hence. While I was talking with Elaine, along came Sister Mary Frances, who was a chaplain and who knew the patient and his wife very well. Both she and I were members of the hospital's bioethics committee, and we knew each other and each other's perspectives quite well. She, too, was upset to hear that I had rescinded the DNAR order. Rather than argue in front of the patient's wife, I took her aside. I admitted this was an interesting conflict and might be educational for the bioethics committee to review at some future time. She immediately said, "Ron, how about tonight? We could call an emergency meeting of the committee." I agreed, never imagining the case could become even more complex, but it did.

First, the repeat digoxin level was reported to be 8.4 ng/ml. Second, the pharmacist discovered that the patient had been given 10 times the prescribed dose by a nurse newly graduated from nursing school. This occurred despite the fact that being unfamiliar with the pediatric elixir, she had asked a senior nurse to check her calculation and the dose she had measured for oral administration. Third, the patient's wife and the chaplain believed we should ask the patient what he would want even though I told them he was not now competent. I arranged to meet at the patient's bedside with them and with two of the patient's children shortly before the bioethics committee meeting. We asked the patient a number of questions, and all agreed he was not only incapable of abstract thought but also unable to understand the details of what had transpired. However, when asked if he was suffering sufficiently that he would prefer to be dead, he said "No," and when asked whom he would want to make decisions for him, he said "Elaine."

The family preferred not to attend the bioethics committee meeting but asked that I phone them after the meeting no matter how late. The nurse who had given the medication was too upset to attend, but we invited the director of nursing. The only person who could not attend the meeting was the one member of the committee with actual graduate education in ethics. At the meeting, Sister Mary Frances and I presented the social, psychologic, spiritual, and medical aspects of Fleet's case and answered many questions. The committee concluded that although it was most unfortunate that the overdose might be on the nurse's conscience—and forever, were the patient to die of an arrhythmia (which might or might not be attributable to the overdose, because potentially lethal arrhythmias were occurring long before the overdose)—nevertheless, the DNAR order should be reinstituted. The rationale was as follows: (1) If an arrest were to occur, the patient had indicated—when he had decision-making capacity on admission—that he would not wish resuscitation (and he definitely had understood that the consequence could be death). (2) To rescind the DNAR order until the digoxin level returned to a therapeutic range (i.e., until an arrest due to an arrhythmia could no longer be attributed to the overdose) was to put the welfare of the nurse above that of the patient. (3) A matter that I had not taken into account in rescinding the DNAR order was that the hospital's liability for negligence (under the *res ipsa loquitur* rule of evidence) did not justify suspending the DNAR order.

I left the meeting depressed that my conviction (that the DNAR order should be suspended until the digoxin level declined to a therapeutic level) was not shared by a single other individual on the committee. Like a tune you can't get out of your mind, I kept repeating the expression, "Fifty thousand Frenchmen can be wrong."

Only an hour later, when telling my bioethicist mentor and friend (who had been unable to attend the meeting) what had transpired, did I come up with a justification for my position that the order should be suspended. I am convinced that the patient himself would have wished to suspend the order so that his death would not be on the conscience of the nurse, whom he had gotten to know and like. If by any chance that were not the case, I am convinced that I could have persuaded Fleet (were he to have regained the ability to think and reason abstractly and to make complex decisions) that my position was the morally correct position, albeit supererogatory, for him to take and that he would have followed my advice.

Late that night, I met with Elaine and three of their children. I told them of the bioethics committee discussion and conclusion, of my disagreement with it, and of my new rationale. I gave them an option that we had not previously discussed. Although I indicated that I could not in good conscience continue to care for Fleet with a DNAR order in place, a colleague was willing to do so. If they preferred, I would transfer responsibility for Fleet's care to my colleague, who would remain his attending physician until Fleet died or until his digoxin level returned to a therapeutic level, at which point he would transfer Fleet's care back to me. After an hour and a half of considering the pros and cons and taking a walk around the block, the patient's family elected this option. For 6 days I visited only socially, but then the digoxin level fell to 2.2 ng/ml, and I resumed Fleet's care.

The wedding was out of town, and though he had improved mentally, Fleet could not have attended unless it had been held at his bedside. One son borrowed a video recorder to tape the wedding for Fleet and me to see. His wife asked me to promise to phone if anything happened to Fleet. The very day of the wedding, Fleet requested last rites. After the wedding but before his family could return, he had an episode of ventricular tachycardia and fibrillation and died, of course without CPR. I phoned.

Although physicians can ill afford to brood or grieve indefinitely, we cannot dismiss a case such as Fleet's. We must ask ourselves whether it was handled satisfactorily. We can ease our conscience that we dealt with the dilemma in good faith and to the best of our ability at the time, but what would we do today? What other options were ethically acceptable? Would any have yielded a better outcome for the patient, for the patient's loved ones, for the health care team, or for the physician? In this case, was my final justification for rescinding the DNAR order (that the patient would himself have wished to do so or that he would have done so on my request) sufficient? Was it authentic, or was it simply rationalization? Was the request to be relieved of responsibility for the patient's care, even though temporary, inappropriately coercive?

Withdrawing Dialysis

One may forgo treatment either by withholding it (as discussed earlier in this section) or by withdrawing it. I will provide some further ethical comparisons of withholding and withdrawing, but I will start with reflection on the more general issue of forgoing treatment. **Ethically, one may forgo treatment if it is (1) ineffective, (2) dangerous (i.e., if the risks of the treatment greatly outweigh the likely benefits—a decision to be made primarily by the physician), (3) disproportionate (i.e., if the burdens outweigh the benefits—a decision to be made by the patient), or (4) refused (by the patient or, if incompetent, by the proxy).** Forgoing treatment is less difficult when the treatment is complex, expensive, risky, or of marginal benefit or if an alternative treatment is available. It is much more difficult if the treatment is simple, inexpensive, safe, effective, or life saving or if there is no alternative treatment. Forgoing therapy is less difficult if the patient is elderly and demented, more difficult if the patient is young and sentient. Forgoing therapy is less difficult if the patient's disease or condition is irreversible and spontaneous, more difficult if reversible and iatrogenic.

Except in an emergency or when third parties would be endangered, a competent adult may refuse any treatment, at any time, at any place, for any reason. Under the law, competent adults need not be informed if they waive the right to be informed, although ethically one would certainly wish patients to make decisions knowledgeably. They need not be rational with regard to the matter to be decided, although they must be competent. They need not even have a reason or be willing to explain or justify it, although physicians understandably are much more accepting when treatment is refused if the reason is understandable and seems appropriate for the patient.

Our discussion of withdrawal from dialysis is restricted for the most part to long-term (as opposed to acute) dialysis and to purposeful discontinuation of dialysis with the intent that death ensue. This practice accounts for approximately 20% of deaths of adults undergoing long-term dialysis and fewer than 10% of deaths of pediatric patients. Approximately 20% of dialyzed patients die each year, thus approximately 4% of dialyzed patients die each year because dialysis is withdrawn. Withdrawal occurs three to four times as often among patients older than 65 years as among those 20 to 45 years of age, and it occurs one and one-half to two times as often in white patients as in those of racial minorities (Native Americans, African-Americans, and Asians, in decreasing order of frequency). Withdrawal from dialysis is more common among patients who have serious conditions in addition to renal failure at the time they start dialysis. This is particularly true of type I diabetic patients and those with a malignancy. Withdrawal is also more common among patients who reside in nursing homes and patients who are incompetent. This was particularly true in the 1970s, when treatment was discontinued at least half of the time for dementia (which then was much more often due to aluminum encephalopathy) and when recommendations to withdraw dialysis were commonly initiated by nephrologists.

Withdrawal from dialysis accounts for approximately a third as many deaths as cardiovascular disease, for approximately the same number of deaths as infection, and approximately four times as many deaths as malignancy (the next most common cause of death). **The frequency of withdrawal from dialysis reflects the fact that dialysis sometimes fails to restore or sustain adequate health. For three reasons, however, withdrawal has increased in recent years despite substantially improved dialysis** (e.g., bicarbonate dialysate, improved ultrafiltration techniques) and ancillary care (e.g., erythropoietin). The first reason is that acceptance of patients with ESRD for dialysis has been liberalized. In the United States, capacity is virtually unlimited and the success of dialysis for elderly patients and for those with comorbidities such as diabetes and cardiovascular disease is better than initially anticipated. A second reason is that the difficulty of predicting which patients will benefit substantially from dialysis and which will not is more widely appreciated, and thus more frequent purposeful trials of dialysis are carried out for borderline or marginal cases, with the intention that treatment will be withdrawn for patients who fail to respond. The third reason is that more nephrologists are more willing to stop dialysis than in the past, when it was commonly thought unethical to stop a life-sustaining treatment even though it was thought ethical never to start one.

The 1996 Annual Data Report of the U.S. Renal Data System indicated that 17.6% of dialyzed patients withdrew from dialysis before death in 1991 to 1993.[14] The death rate from withdrawal per 1000 patient-years at risk was 233. Of withdrawal deaths, 42% were for chronic failure to thrive, 35% for acute medical complications, 5% for access failure, 2% for transplant failure, and the remaining 16% for various other reasons or no reason reported.

Two illustrative cases are presented before returning to practical cautions and proposed guidelines for the care of patients who may benefit from withdrawal of dialysis.

PATIENT NUMBER 8

Theodore Phoenix was a single unemployed man who lived alone, was apparently happy, and seemed content with his lot. At age 40, when injured in an altercation, he was discovered to have hypertension but neither proteinuria nor renal dysfunction. At age 43, when hypertension was very severe, an IVP revealed a decrease in renal size but no cysts. His internist referred him to a urologist, who performed an open needle renal biopsy. Again cysts were not apparent at biopsy or at heminephrectomy for hemorrhage complicating the biopsy. The specimen revealed nephrosclerosis, according to one pathologist, and glomerulonephritis, according to another. At age 45, despite a protein-restricted diet, Theodore had to begin long-term hemodialysis. At age 47, he underwent an unsuccessful cadaveric renal transplant and had to resume center hemodialysis. At age 51, recurrent passage of blood per urethra led to discovery of a large left kidney with innumerable cysts and a tumor blush on angiography. The 750-g nephrectomy specimen had the typical appearance of a polycystic kidney, save for its relatively small size. Although the kidney was sectioned every 0.5 cm, a renal tumor could not be seen, but a renal cell carcinoma with invasion of the renal vein was noted microscopically.

At age 52, in 1978, Theodore had an acute psychotic episode and attempted suicide. For the first time, his relatives were contacted. Aunts living in backwoods Arkansas had not seen the patient in many years, did not have the resources to visit him, and believed it would be inappropriate to serve as proxy decision makers for Theodore despite his incapacitating mental illness. A daughter, Candice, who lived in Chicago, came to visit the patient despite their estrangement (when she was *in utero*, our patient had abandoned her mother). Although she had sympathy for Theodore's circumstances, Candice understandably elected not to serve as his surrogate either. Thus, I found myself in the position of having to make decisions for the patient, without the affirmation of a surrogate.

The patient failed to improve despite inpatient psychotherapy and medication. I arranged for residence in a locked nursing home, where Theodore was doomed to live for the rest of his life. He was transported to the renal center for dialysis three times weekly. It gradually became apparent that the patient was not simply psychotic but was demented, and he was presumed to have the dialysis dementia syndrome, which we later came to believe was due to aluminum excess in brain tissue. Although modest fluctuations occurred in the course of his illness, his condition gradually and progressively deteriorated. He ate poorly, lost weight, and failed physically. He became nearly noncommunicative. He had masklike facies, except for a continuous frown, and he began to drool. We could not discern his mood, but his appearance as well as his inability to interact (in his previously friendly and engaging fashion) greatly upset the nurses and other patients. Although he was generally cooperative with the dialysis staff, he did not seem to recognize even those who had attended him for nearly a decade. In previous years, he enjoyed talking about fishing trips and exploits, but now he sat silent, staring but without eye contact, drooling and smacking his lips but speechless. He seemed to have no meaningful interaction with people or his environment. The nurses believed I should discontinue dialysis and allow Theodore "death with dignity." I suspected they were correct in that improvement seemed extremely unlikely, albeit not impossible. There was no evidence of a reversible cause of the dementia. I again contacted the patient's aunts and daughter, none of whom was willing to participate in a decision to terminate dialysis even though I recommended it. Remember that the year was 1979, and my position was that I must not play God and discontinue dialysis without the concurrence of a patient or surrogate.

This morally outraged two excellent dialysis nurses. Perhaps I would have stopped dialysis if I had been convinced that the patient was suffering, but I saw suffering only in dialysis nurses and other patients. Furthermore, I had never discussed with the patient what to do under such circumstances, and thus I thought I could not discontinue dialysis in the absence of surrogate consent or unequivocal suffering of the patient himself.

The nurses and I, together with my nephrology colleagues, a social worker, and chaplain, requested a meeting with Corrine Bayley, a hospital administrator who had just returned from a 2-year leave of absence during which she obtained a master's degree in bioethics. We discussed the many ethical concerns we had in caring for patients with ESRD but repeatedly returned to the patient then upsetting us all, Theodore Phoenix. The bioethicist asked, Socratically, if there were a significant ethical difference between withdrawing therapy and withholding it. I was certain there was, but when informed bioethicists believed there was no

difference ethically, only emotionally, I was unable to define an ethical difference. When asked if this same patient with no willing surrogate and with the same neuropsychiatric disorder were to present with ESRD, would I initiate dialysis, I said, "No, touché," realizing my intellectual fencing partner had won.

For years, this question of whether or not there is a morally relevant or significant difference between withdrawing and withholding has been a true conundrum for me (i.e., not just a difficult question but one whose only answer was conjectural). In the earlier section on withholding therapy, it was already noted that if the nephrologist or the patient believed it would be wrong to stop a life-sustaining treatment, then the patient might be forced to make a decision whether or not to undergo the treatment (e.g., chronic hemodialysis) without having the opportunity for a trial of the treatment. It was pointed out that if a treatment were withheld surreptitiously, the patient might not know of it and be able to object, whereas if a treatment is withdrawn, the patient or family realizes it and can object. On this ground, it is argued, for didactic purposes, that it is preferable to withdraw than to withhold. Surely, to withdraw feels like an active decision whereas to withhold seems passive (i.e., withdrawal a commission, withholding an omission). I would now teach, as Corrine Bayley tried to convince me in 1979, that if a patient's condition and circumstances are such that it is appropriate to withhold therapy, the same condition and circumstances justify withdrawing the therapy. This is not invariably the case, however. Consider circumstances in which no dialysis opening is available for a new patient. Even if patient Y, who has an excellent prognosis and who could unquestionably benefit from dialysis, comes along, we would not withdraw therapy from patient X, who was already on dialysis and who had a less favorable prognosis and a lesser chance of benefiting from dialysis. The reason we would not is our established relationship with the patient X and our human commitment to him or her.

Consider a slightly different scenario. Suppose we saw and evaluated patient X yesterday morning and we planned to accept him for dialysis. We phoned him repeatedly yesterday, but the line was always busy. Before we had a chance to phone X this morning, patient Y presented for evaluation. We judge Y to be a better candidate. What should we do?

PATIENT NUMBER 9

Heather was a 55-year-old homemaker who had had mild hypertension for 22 years. Her devoted husband, Ryan, was a salesman with the gift of gab. Her only son, Thomas, was discovered to have hypertension on a school physical examination at age 12. In January 1978, Heather's hypertension accelerated and destroyed her kidneys: BUN and creatinine values were 23 and 1.4 mg/dl, respectively, in early February and 152 and 14.3 mg/dl in late March when she began long-term hemodialysis. An open renal biopsy confirmed extremely severe arterial and arteriolar nephrosclerosis.

Four days after starting hemodialysis, Heather forebodingly had an acute organic brain syndrome, which we postulated might be related to rapid changes in the physicochemical composition of body fluids and perhaps dysequilibrium phenomena. Indeed, mentation improved (temporarily), but Heather's condition did not. She was inexplicably catabolic, and in the first 4 months on dialysis her weight declined from 135 to 100 pounds. Although her hypertension was reasonably controlled on minoxidil, we recommended bilateral renal ablation (medical nephrectomy) for hyperreninemia and nocturnal tube feedings because Heather was unable to force herself to drink the nutritional supplements that were prescribed. She refused the latter, tried the tube feedings, and decided the nasogastric tube was intolerable. She became anxious and depressed. After 4 months on dialysis, she again developed an organic brain syndrome, which was to persist intermittently for the rest of her life, although it fluctuated both in manifestations and in severity to an extraordinary degree. At first impaired memory and disturbed speech with perseveration were noted. She was at times flagrantly psychotic and had hallucinations and delusions. She at other times had a flat affect and a blank stare and became obtunded. On some days she seemed herself, but on others she was anxious, tremulous, and depressed and cried a great deal. She had diffusely abnormal electroencephalographic findings, and CT revealed cortical atrophy. Her condition confounded neurologists and psychiatrists alike and failed to respond to innumerable changes in her therapeutic regimen, including antihypertensive medications, antidepressants, anticonvulsants, nutritional supplements, vitamins, and the hemodialysis prescription. Charcoal hemoperfusion was tried for a time. She was even switched to peritoneal dialysis for 2 months, without evident benefit, although the apparently spontaneous fluctuations in her course made the effect of any therapeutic alteration difficult to judge.

It was hoped that a successful renal transplant might ameliorate if not eradicate the encephalopathy, but a donor kidney did not become available. Her catabolic state persisted, and her weight declined to 80 pounds.

Heather was intermittently hospitalized. Whether in the hospital or out, she received the concerned and concerted attention of the entire dialysis staff, most particularly that of the dietitian, the social worker, and the chaplain. We had innumerable conversations and a number of conferences with her husband and son and—when she was lucid—with her. When she was lucid, Heather often told her husband, Ryan, that she wanted to depart this tormented life and to relieve him and their son, Tom, of the burden and worry of caring for her. Heather and Ryan initially kept this conversation to themselves because they thought that their religion would not allow discontinuation of dialysis and would interpret it as suicide. One day, however, the chaplain mentioned another patient who had decided to forgo dialysis. When Heather and Ryan noted that the chaplain was not critical of the patient who had terminated dialysis and died, they asked the appropriate questions. They were relieved to learn that their religion allowed one to refuse even life-sustaining therapy when the burdens of illness and treatment outweighed the benefits.

The nephrologists, neurologists, psychiatrists, endocrinologist, and cardiologist who had consulted and assisted in Heather's care all were as frustrated and felt as helpless as I in contending with her incapacitating, devastating systemic illness. We found it painful to observe her fluctuating but overall deteriorating course and could only imagine what it must be like for her, Ryan, and Tom. Thus, when we heard of her decision to stop dialysis, although we were sad and felt we had failed her, we also were relieved. Needless to say, we wished a neurologist and psychiatrist to confirm that her decision was informed and that she was competent to make it, although we had no doubt ourselves because we had observed Heather to be as lucid and rational and coherent on many occasions as she was psychotic or demented on other occasions. In our personal conversations with Heather, we found that her major concern, as typical of her, was the emotional response of her husband and son. She was enormously relieved to find they would support her in her decision, whether it was to continue fighting and hope for a transplant (or a miracle) or to yield to her overpowering disease that medical science did not understand.

Perhaps as mysterious as her disease was its intermittent, virtually complete albeit temporary remissions, particularly notable in the last 2 weeks of life, when Heather and Ryan struggled with the decision and found their son, the chaplain, and all of us on the dialysis team supportive. Whereas previously Heather might have minutes, even hours of lucidity, after her decision she had no relapse. She remained in the hospital but had daily visits from relatives and friends, whom she bravely bid farewell. Two days after her decision, she celebrated her birthday with her family and with hospital and dialysis staff. A sad, expected event was transformed into a celebration of her life, and Heather died in the presence of her family only 5 days after her last dialysis.

In terms of withdrawals from dialysis, this one was as appropriate and as well accepted and went as smoothly as any I have witnessed. The decision was clearly the patient's, not her family's, and not her physician's. This is a distinctly unusual situation for the nearly half of all patients for whom dialysis is forgone because of dementia or encephalopathy. Such patients are usually incompetent, and unless they have anticipated such a circumstance and executed an advance treatment directive to withdraw dialysis, the decisions are usually made by the family in conjunction with the patient's primary nephrologist, who will often have recommended it. The 5-day interval between discontinuation of dialysis and death was 3 days shorter than the mean. Follow-up discussions with the husband and son both a week later and a year later indicated acceptance of (if not appreciation for) both the process and the outcome. Acceptance by the family is very important because it is the family who survive and must carry on—and who are appreciative of or burdened by the memories. In this case, the hurdle for the patient and her spouse was their church's acceptance of withdrawal of life-supporting treatment. In all cases there are sensitive issues, whether psychologic, familial, social, cultural, religious, ethical, or legal.

Patients with intolerable chronic illnesses such as cancer or AIDS might even say that patients on dialysis are "lucky" because they have a socially, culturally, religiously, ethically, and legally acceptable way out of this world: If they stop treatment (i.e., if they withdraw consent to continue treatment), they will die.

Lest we become complacent, we should consider whether aspects of this case might have been better managed. Heather had not only devastating accelerated hypertension and malignant nephrosclerosis (which might have been interrupted with effective antihypertensive therapy early in its course) but also an incapacitating neuropsychiatric disorder (yet to be understood and effectively treated). We are in one sense disquieted by the observation that the encephalopathic symptoms virtually remitted once Heather

had made the decision—perhaps coincidentally, but if they could remit for 2 weeks, why not for 2 months, or 2 years, or indefinitely? Were we premature in accepting the patient's request to discontinue dialysis? Even if this terminal clearing of the encephalopathy had been just one more temporary event, was there anything we might have studied that would have assisted this or another patient? Shouldn't we have anticipated how onerous Heather's illness was for her and her family, and shouldn't we ourselves have initiated discussion to inquire whether there might be circumstances for which she would wish to discontinue dialysis? Many nephrologists fear that such leading questions may be frightening to patients or suggest inappropriate behavior to them. In fact, by the time we nephrologists think of such matters, most patients have probably been concerned by the same thoughts for a long time already. Many say they appreciate our raising such matters for discussion. After discussions of discontinuation of treatment, patients were found to feel they had better control of their treatment (71%) and to be relieved and feel better (53%); however, some felt nervous (22%), sad (16%), or like giving up (6%).[15]

CAUTIONS: QUESTIONS TO BE ASKED ABOUT PATIENTS WHO REQUEST DISCONTINUATION OF DIALYSIS

For patients who request discontinuation of dialysis (or when families or health care professionals suggest consideration of withdrawal of dialysis, Moss recommends a series of questions,[16] and we have supplemented these questions with a few of our own:

- Does the patient have decision-making capacity? We must be careful to detect depression (which is grossly underdetected, especially in the elderly) or encephalopathy (which may be subtle and which may result from underdialysis).
- Why does the patient want to stop? Would changes in the dialysis and treatment regimen make a significant difference? Does the patient have life stressors (family or work concerns) that could be relieved?
- Does the patient mean what he or she says, or is this a plea for attention and help?
- Can changes be made to improve the situation?
- Has the patient discussed the request with family and friends? The dialysis team should seek their evaluation and counsel.
- Would the patient be willing to continue dial

ysis while these matters are investigated and while factors responsible for his or her request are addressed?

- If the patient lacks decision-making capacity, is there an advance treatment directive (regarding circumstances for which the patient would wish dialysis withdrawn) or has the patient indicated who should make decisions of this sort?

RECOMMENDED GUIDELINES FOR WITHDRAWAL OF DIALYSIS

Just as guidelines may be helpful in selecting patients for ESRD therapy (or for identifying patients for whom the burdens of treatment are likely to outweigh the benefits), so too may they be helpful in consideration of withdrawal of treatment and in the care of patients and families after a decision to discontinue dialysis. Such guidelines may support nephrologists, patients, and families in making emotionally difficult decisions by indicating the current professional and societal consensus, thereby lessening ethical discomfort and fear of litigation. A possible disadvantage of guidelines is their potential for discouraging idiosyncratic decisions that may be appropriate for an individual patient.

Procedural guidelines for withdrawal of dialysis (or consideration thereof) may be categorized according to whether or not the patient is competent and whether or not there is disagreement about withdrawal.

Procedural Guidelines for Competent Patients

- Patients' values, goals, beliefs, and preferences are determinative, although not absolutely. Quality of life determinations are to be made only by the patient.
- In exploring reasons why patients wish to discontinue dialysis, ask not only about their dissatisfactions with dialysis but also their goals for dialysis and how and why they are not being met.
- In excluding treatable depression or dementia, seeking neuropsychiatric consultation is wise, as is asking family and friends their impression of the patient's mood and whether they believe his or her requests are authentic.
- Look for undue influences that may account for the patient's request: misinformation or coercion.
- In exploring changes in regimen that might make continued dialysis acceptable, ask "What would . . . ?" and "What if . . . ?" and propose a further trial of dialysis. When patients elect a

trial of therapy, they may set the criteria by which it is to be judged a success or a failure.
- Recommend advance directives and periodic review of them.
- Dialysis centers may wish to offer educational meetings for patients and families; frank discussion of the limitations of dialysis and of the acceptability of discontinuing dialysis may be helpful. It may also be helpful to clarify that it is the responsibility of nephrologists and the right of dialysis team members to provide information to patients, the responsibility of physicians to make recommendations, and the right of patients to make decisions about their treatment and limitation of it.
- Dialysis centers may also find it helpful to post notices of patients' deaths and of memorial services rather than leave patients to wonder about the disappearance of others.
- One should inform patients who have decided to discontinue dialysis that they may change their mind and resume treatment at any time.

Procedural Guidelines for Incompetent Patients Who Are Not Expected to Recover Decision-Making Capacity

- Ascertain and analyze the reasons why family members or dialysis professionals have recommended that dialysis be discontinued.
- Review advance directives or their equivalent (e.g., the discussions between the patient and the nephrologist or other members of the dialysis team that were held before, at, or after the start of dialysis).
- If it is the dialysis team that has raised consideration of withdrawal of dialysis, discussion should always be held with the patient's proxy and family. Rather than asking what they believe should be done, ask what they believe the patient would want to have done.
- If it is not clear what the patient would want to have done but it seems that the patient's best interests would be served by discontinuing dialysis, the nephrologist may recommend doing so but should not try to elicit such a suggestion from the patient's family (because that often engenders long-standing guilt on their part, whereas accepting the nephrologist's firm recommendation is much less likely to do so).
- Beware of stating that dialysis is futile unless it will not control uremic wastes (e.g., because of failed access and inability to construct another). Rather, state what goals cannot be achieved by continued dialysis and why further dialysis is inappropriate.
- Unless they are thought to be making decisions contrary to the patient's wishes or best inter-

ests, the decisions of morally valid surrogates should be followed.

Procedural Guidelines to Be Used When Physicians Disagree with Patients or Their Proxies

- Assuming that repeated discussion in good faith fails to resolve differences of opinion about the appropriateness of discontinuing dialysis, patients have the right to continue dialysis while seeking to transfer care to another nephrologist or dialysis unit. They also have the right to appeal the conflict to the dialysis unit's or hospital's dispute resolution mechanism. The latter might be an ethics committee or consultant, an ombudsman, or a mediator.
- **Mediation is usually preferable to arbitration, and arbitration to adjudication in a court of law.**
- In general, when good faith discussion and mediation have failed to resolve a patient's or family's desire for continued treatment and a physician's recommendation that dialysis be withdrawn, dialysis should be continued. Not to do so would suggest a less flexible, less compassionate, and more callous health system than we wish to have. This approach may be appropriate, for example, for patients who are benefiting only minimally or marginally or for those who are not suffering (e.g., those in a persistent vegetative state). If patients are suffering, however, and particularly if they previously indicated that under such circumstances they would wish dialysis be discontinued, the nephrologist and dialysis unit have a moral obligation to do so and to override the objection of the family. Such assertive action has rarely been reported.[17]

Substantive Guidelines

- Dialysis may be withdrawn if it is no longer necessary to sustain the health of a patient. This most commonly occurs because of an error in this determination initially or because of unexpected improvement of renal function, as in some patients with malignant hypertension, lupus erythematosus, or mulitple myeloma.
- If societal or institutional decisions are made not to reimburse or provide continued dialysis for patients who have developed permanent unconsciousness, imminently terminal illness, or severe dementia with inability to relate to others, these decisions must be made known to patients or potential patients.

Guidelines for the Care of Patients and Families Who Have Already Decided to Forgo Dialysis

The following are recommendations of Valdez and Rosenblum[18]:

- Remind patients that they may change their mind and have dialysis reinstituted.
- Reassure patients that they will continue to receive individualized care, especially treatment to sustain their comfort.
- Allow patients to decide when to discontinue dialysis.
- Allow patients to decide where they will spend their final days: at home with or without hospice service, in an intermediate care facility, or—if their condition or health care plan will allow it—in the hospital.
- Consider social service, pastoral care, and hospice.
- Assist with legal arrangements.
- Help the patient and the family to say goodbye.
- If the patient is at home, make a home visit and daily telephone calls.
- After the patient's death, recommend that the family come to the office to review the patient's dialysis care, the decision to stop dialysis, and the treatment and support provided thereafter.

CONCLUDING COMMENTS

This chapter discussed the contributions of nephrology to the genesis of bioethics and the extraordinary impact that bioethics has had on the practice of nephrology and the care of, and caring for, the renal patient. The principles, concepts, and methods of clinical bioethics and some of the ethical issues in chronic renal failure, ESRD, and dialysis were reviewed. Many other ethical issues in nephrology are worthy of discussion but are beyond the scope of this chapter.

The discussion of patients in this chapter (using fictitious names, omitting record numbers, and without the need for obtaining informed consent from surviving patients or relatives) was approved by the Institutional Review Board of St. Joseph Hospital, Orange, California, and by the Human Subjects Review Committee of the University of California, Irvine.

Acknowledgments

I wish to express my gratitude to Spectra Laboratories for providing the opportunity to write this chapter and to David Z. Levine for his encouragement and extraordinary accommodation of my other commitments. I am also grateful to my mentors in nephrology (Roger Bulger, Norman Levinsky, Robert Loeb, and Arnold Relman) and in biomedical ethics at the St. Joseph Health System Center for Health Care Ethics (Corrine Bayley, Jack Glaser, and Judith Wilson Ross) and at the MacLean Center for Clinical Medical Ethics of the University of Chicago (Christine Cassel, John Lantos, Steven Miles, Alvin Moss, Robert Orr, Mark Siegler, and Carol Stocking), where I was supported by the Pew Charitable Trusts and the Henry J. Kaiser Family Foundation. Most of all, I thank the many patients, family members, nurses, social workers, chaplains, and physicians who engaged me in the trenches of clinical nephrology and ethics, where I had to translate theoretic knowledge and personal and parental values into practical experience.

REFERENCES

1. Peabody FW: The care of the patient. JAMA 88:877–882, 1927.
2. Beauchamp TL, Childress JF: Principles of Biomedical Ethics, 4th ed. New York, Oxford University Press, 1994.
2a. Brody B: Life and Death Decision Making. New York, Oxford University Press, 1988.
3. Emanuel LL: The health care directive: Learning how to draft advance care documents. J Am Geriatr Soc 39:1221–1228, 1991.
3a. Emanuel LL, Emanuel EJ: The medical directive: A new comprehensive advance care document. JAMA 261:3288, 1989.
3b. Emanuel LL, Emanuel EJ: Decisions at the end of life: Guides by communities of patients. Hastings Center Report 23(5):6–14, 1993.
4. Sehgal A, Galbraith A, Chesney M, et al: How strictly do dialysis patients want their advance directives followed? JAMA 267:59–63, 1992.
4a. Wolf SM, Boyle P, Callahan D, et al: Sources of concern about the Patient Self Determination Act. N Engl J Med 325(23):1666–1671, 1991.
4b. National Kidney Foundation: Advance Directives: A Guide for Patients and Their Families. Washington, DC, National Kidney Foundation, 1993.
4c. National Kidney Foundation: Implementing Advance Directives: Suggested Guidelines for Dialysis Facilities. Washington, DC, National Kidney Foundation, 1993.
4d. National Kidney Foundation: Initiation or withdrawal of dialysis in end-stage renal disease: Guidelines for the healthcare team. Washington, DC, National Kidney Foundation, 1996.
4e. National Kidney Foundation: If you choose not to start dialysis treatment. Washington, DC, National Kidney Foundation, 1996.
4f. National Kidney Foundation: When stopping dialysis treatment is your choice. Washington, DC, National Kidney Foundation, 1996.
5. Gibson JM: National values history project. Generations 14:51–64, (Suppl) 1990.
6. Hirsch DJ, West ML, Cohen AD, Jindal KK: Experience with not offering dialysis to patients with a poor prognosis. Am J Kidney Dis 23(3):463–466, 1994.
7. Moss AH: To use dialysis appropriately: The emerging consensus on patient selection guidelines. Adv Ren Replace Ther 2(2):175–182, 1995.
8. Fletcher J: Morals and Medicine. Princeton, Princeton University Press, 1954.
8a. Rothman D: Strangers at the Bedside: A History of How Law and Bioethics Transformed Medical Decision Making. New York, Basic Books, 1991.
9. Rettig RA, Levinsky NG (eds): Institute of Medicine Committee for the Study of the Medicare End-Stage Renal Disease Program. Kidney Failure and the Federal Government. Washington, DC, National Academy Press, 1991.
10. Miller RB: Selection of patients for chronic dialysis: Let society decide whether rationing is needed. Nephrol News Issues 6(2):36, 40, 41, 43, 1992.
11. Moss AH, Stocking CB, Sachs GA, Siegler M: Variation in the attitudes of dialysis unit medical directors toward decisions to withhold and withdraw dialysis. J Am Soc Nephrol 4:229–234, 1993.
12. Cotran RS, Hull A, Latos DL: Joint statement of principles relating to practice guideline development. J Am Soc Nephrol 7(3):519–520, 1996.
13. Tomlinson T, Brody H: Ethics and communication in do-not-resuscitate orders. N Engl J Med 318(1):43, 1988.
14. U.S. Renal Data System: USRDS 1996 Annual Data Report. Bethesda, MD, National Institutes of Health, National Institute of Diabetes and Digestive and Kidney Diseases, 1996.
15. Lo B, McLeod GA, Saika MA: Patient attitudes to discussing life-sustaining treatment. Arch Intern Med 146:1613–1615, 1986.
16. Moss AH: Dialysis decisions and the elderly. Clin Geriatr Med 10(3):463, 1994.
17. Keating RF, Moss AH, Sorkin MI, Paris JJ: Stopping dialysis of an incompetent patient over the family's objection: Is it ever ethical and legal? J Am Soc Nephrol 4:1879–1883, 1994.
18. Valdez R, Rosenblum A: Voluntary termination of dialysis: When your patient says, "Enough is enough." Dial Transplant 23:566–570, 1994.

SUGGESTED READINGS

Battin MP: The Least Worst Death. Essays in Bioethics on the End of Life. New York, Oxford University Press, 1994.
Beauchamp TL, McCullough LB: Medical Ethics: The Moral Responsibilities of Physicians. New York, Prentice-Hall, 1984.
Brody H: The Healer's Power. New Haven, Yale University Press, 1992.
Bulger RE, Heitman E, Reiser SJ: The Ethical Dimensions of the Biological Sciences. Cambridge, England, Cambridge University Press, 1993.
Cummings NB, Schoenfeld P, Miller RB: Ethical considerations in end-stage renal disease. In Schrier RW, Gottschalk CW (eds): Diseases of the Kidney, 5th ed. Boston, Little, Brown & Co, 1992, pp 3097–3128.
Faden RR, Beauchamp TL: A History and Theory of Informed Consent. New York, Oxford University Press, 1986.
Fox RC, Swazey JP: The Courage to Fail: A Social View of Organ Transplants and Dialysis, 2nd ed. Chicago, University of Chicago Press, 1978.
Friedman EA: End-stage renal disease therapy: An American success story. JAMA 275(14):1118–1122, 1996.
Hackler C, Mosely R, Vawter DE: Advance Directives in Medicine. Eastbourne, East Sussex, England, Praeger, 1989.
Howell JH, Sale WF: Life Choices: A Hastings Center Introduction to Bioethics. Washington, DC, Georgetown University Press, 1995.
Jonsen AR, Toulmin SE: The Abuse of Casuistry. Berkeley, CA, University of California Press, 1988.
Jonsen AR, Siegler M, Winslade WJ: Clinical Ethics: A Practical Approach to Ethical Decisions in Clinical Medicine, 3rd ed. New York, Macmillan, 1992.
Katz J: The Silent World of Doctor and Patient. New York, The Free Press (Macmillan), 1984.
Levine DZ, Bell RC: Eliciting advance directives from in-centre hemodialysis patients: A 3-year follow-up. J Am Soc Nephrol 5(3):433 (97P), 1994.
Levinsky NG, Rettig RA: The Medicare end-stage renal disease program: A report from the Institute of Medicine. N Engl J Med 324:1143–1148, 1991.
Lo B: Resolving Ethical Dilemmas: A Guide for Clinicians. Baltimore, Williams & Wilkins, 1995.
Lowance DC: Factors and guidelines to be considered in offering treatment to patients with end-stage renal disease: A personal opinion. Am J Kidney Dis 21(6):679–683, 1993.

Lynn J: Why I don't have a living will. Law, Medicine, and Health Care 19(1–2):101–104, 1991.

McKenzie J, Moss A, Stocking C, Siegler M: American and Canadian nephrologists differ on decisions to offer and stop dialysis. J Am Soc Nephrol 5:465, 1994.

Mendelsohn DC, Singer PA: Advance directives in dialysis. Adv Ren Replace Ther 3:240–250, 1994.

Mid-Atlantic Renal Coalition: Working with non-compliant and abusive patients. Mid-Atlantic Renal Coalition (ESRD Network 5), 1994.

Miller RB: Dialysis should be withdrawn when the burdens outweigh the benefits. Nephrol News Issues 7(10):33, 34, 38, 1993.

Miller RB: Treating the disruptive patient: Summary of a panel discussion "The Abusive Patient: Ethical, Legal and Moral Responsibilities of the Health Care Team," 4th Annual Spring Clinical Nephrology Meeting of the National Kidney Foundation, Washington, DC, March 23–24, 1995. Nephrol News Issues 9(6):39–40, 1995.

Moss AH, Behnam MB: Outcomes of intensive care unit patients who receive dialysis. J Am Soc Nephrol 4:371, 1993.

Moss AH, Holley JL, Upton MB: Outcomes of cardiopulmonary resuscitation in dialysis patients. J Am Soc Nephrol 2:340, 1991.

Moss AH, Rettig RA, Cassel CK: A proposal for guidelines for patient acceptance to and withdrawal from dialysis: A follow-up to the 10M report. ANNA J 20(5):557–561, 617, 1993.

Novello AC: Ethical, social and financial aspects of end-stage renal disease. In Brenner BM, Rector FC Jr (eds): The Kidney, 4th ed. Philadelphia, WB Saunders, 1991, pp 2424–2443.

Oreopoulos DG: Is there a right time to say no to life? Dial Int 14:205–208, 1994.

Pence GE: Classic Cases in Medical Ethics: Accounts of Cases That Have Shaped Medical Ethics, with Philosophical, Legal, and Historical Backgrounds, 2nd ed. New York, McGraw-Hill, 1995.

Rettig RA: The social contract and the treatment of permanent kidney failure. JAMA 275(14):1123–1126, 1996.

Siegler M, Singer PA: Clinical ethics in the practice of medicine. In Wyngaarden LH, Smith LH Jr, Bennett JC (eds): Cecil's Textbook of Medicine, 19th ed. Philadelphia, WB Saunders, 1992, pp 11–14.

Singer PA: ESRD Network of New England. Nephrologists' experience with and attitudes towards decisions to forgo dialysis. J Am Soc Nephrol 2:1235–1240, 1992.

Swartz RD, Perry E, Schneider C, et al: The option to withdraw from chronic dialysis treatment. Adv Ren Replace Ther 1:264–272, 1994.

Swenson MD, Miller RB: Ethics case review in health care institutions: Committees, consultants, or teams? Arch Intern Med 152:694–697, 1992.

Tobe SW, Senn JS (for the End-Stage Renal Group): Forgoing renal dialysis: A case study and review of ethical issues. Am J Kidney Dis 28:147–153, 1996.

Tulsky JA, Alpers A, Lo B: A middle ground on physician-assisted suicide. Camb Q Health Ethics 5(1):33–43, 1996.

University of New Mexico Center for Health Law and Ethics: Values history form. Caring Magazine, June 1992, pp 30, 31.

Valdez R, Rosenblum A: Suggested steps for dismissal of the problematic patient. Dial Transplant 22:610–613, 1993.

18 | THE ROLE OF THE NURSE IN CARING FOR THE RENAL PATIENT

Linda Panther

The nursing process is the foundation of the role of nurses caring for renal patients. The key elements in the nursing process are assessment, establishing a nursing diagnosis, developing a plan of care, implementing the nursing interventions, and evaluating a patient's response. The types of nursing assessment used are an initial in-depth assessment, ongoing assessment, and selective assessments. Using the case model approach, these types of assessments and patient management are demonstrated in three cases.

INTRODUCING NEW PATIENTS TO DIALYSIS; ASSESSMENT AND CARE PLANNING

PATIENT NUMBER 1

Ian is 47 years old and works in the high-technology industry as a computer programmer. He has had diabetes since he was 20 years old and has been monitored in the renal clinic for the past 10 years. Ian is now approaching end-stage renal failure and will soon require maintenance dialysis.

The initial nursing assessment consists of a multisystem approach incorporating biopsychosocial components. Renal units often have their own specific assessment tool. An example of one kind is shown next.

Demographic Data. Ian lives close to the renal unit, drives his own car, and has a good job with health benefits and an employer who has been accommodating of Ian's need for medical appointments. Referral to a renal social worker is beneficial if an assessment of financial need is required and to evaluate family and community support. The initial assessment continues by evaluating Ian's physical status and establishing a nursing diagnosis.

Activity Level. Focus on questions related to functional mobility, use of mobility aids, energy level, and sleep pattern.

Ian has no physical impairments. He does not use any mobility aids. He says he has noticed he has been more fatigued for the past year and has less energy to play with his children. His sleep habits have changed in the past few months: He has difficulty falling asleep and often wakes up early. The nursing diagnoses of fatigue and sleep pattern disturbance have been identified.

Skin Care and Nutrition. Focus on questions related to healing, condition of the skin, and nutritional status.

Ian gives a history of skin healing problems. A leg injury took a long time to heal. He attributes this to his diabetes. He complains that his skin is dry and itchy. On physical examination, he has no current wounds or abrasions on his body, and his skin is noted to be dry and flaky. From a nutritional standpoint, he has adhered to a diabetic diet for 20 years. Ian says his insulin requirements have been decreasing in the past few months. His appetite is fair, and he suffers from intermittent nausea. His body weight is unchanged. The nursing diagnosis of potential for altered skin integrity and the collaborative problem of nausea have been identified.

Elimination. Ian complains of bouts of diarrhea that have occurred during the past 2 to 3 years. His bowel habits are now normal.

Fluid Balance. Focus on questions related to functioning of the urinary system and fluid balance.

Ian reports no change in urinary habits. He maintains that he still passes significant quantities of urine. He has been experiencing nocturia for many years. He suffers from increased thirst, and his fluid intake is greater than normal. On physical examination, mild edema is noted in his feet and ankles, and no adventitious chest sounds are heard.

Respiratory System. Focus on questions related to the respiratory and circulatory system.

Respiratory rate and rhythm are regular. Ian is a nonsmoker. His pulse is regular, and he has no history of chest pain. His color is normal to pale, with no signs of jaundice. Peripheral pulses are reduced in both the left and right arteriae dorsalis pedis. Collaborative diagnosis of impaired peripheral circulation has been identified.

Sensory and Perceptual System. Focus on questions related to vision, hearing, and the neurologic system.

Ian has been seeing an eye specialist for some time in conjunction with his diabetic care. His last appointment was 2 months ago, and he visits every 6 months. His vision is satisfactory with glasses. His hearing is normal. Neurologically, Ian is alert and oriented. He responds to questions readily and pertinently. Physical examination of his pupils shows that they react to light briskly. Medical examination of reflexes shows slow or impaired reflexes in the lower limbs. Collaborative diagnosis of impaired neurologic status is identified.

Self-Concept. After the physiologic assessment is completed, evaluate the effect that this illness has had on the patient's self-concept. Focus on questions related to self-esteem. Does the patient maintain eye contact during the interview? Is the patient easily distracted or depressed? Are there signs of suffering, such as sadness, anger, or frustration? Does the patient have a living will or an advance directive or has he or she at any time considered the desirable extent of medical intervention?

Ian indicates that he had thought about the use of life-prolonging measures after he had witnessed his father's loss of independence following a stroke. He said he found it hard to talk about it, and so he had not made out a living will or an advance directive for his medical care. The collaborative plan of lack of preparation for the future was identified. Ian was asked how he saw his present situation, and he described it as hopeless. He was greatly disturbed by his renal failure and saw no future for himself. He felt he would

have to leave his job even though his employer was supportive. The nursing diagnosis of hopelessness is therefore identified.

Roles in the Family. Next evaluate the effect this illness has had on the roles in the family.

Ian has been married for 20 years and has two sons, ages 15 and 17. He is afraid that this illness will change his status in the family. As he has become increasingly tired, his wife has had to take on more of the household responsibilities. He has dropped his hobby of model aircraft assembly because of lack of energy. He describes his family as being supportive, but he perceives he is a burden to them. A nursing diagnosis of altered family processes is therefore identified.

DEVELOPING THE PLAN OF NURSING CARE

What is our next step? The initial nursing assessment has identified five nursing diagnoses: fatigue; sleep pattern disturbance; potential for altered skin integrity; hopelessness; and altered family processes. Also identified are the collaborative problems of nausea, impaired peripheral circulation, impaired neurologic status, and lack of preparation for the future. As you can see, this number of nursing diagnoses was easily identified. The next role of the nurse is to develop a plan of care, in conjunction with Ian, that will respond to these nursing diagnoses. Mutual goals, with their accompanying interventions, are set along with target dates for review. At the completion of the target dates, the evaluation process occurs and the goals are reviewed. If the goal has been reached, the nursing diagnosis is probably resolved. If the goal has not been reached, the plan of care needs to be changed; either a new strategy is required, or the goal has become unrealistic or unachievable and should be changed.

Ian begins maintenance dialysis with a plan of care developed from the initial assessment. The identified nursing problems can be managed in the following ways:

Fatigue

- Correct any physiologic factors such as anemia. Ian's physician initiated weekly subcutaneous erythropoietin therapy.
- Refer to an occupational therapist who can give assistance on how to perform activities of daily living that will conserve energy.
- Encourage Ian to exercise regularly by walk-

ing, gradually increasing the time and endurance level.

Sleep Pattern Disturbance

- Teach Ian that a balance between sleep and activity can be achieved by setting routines.
- Physical activity enhances sleep. A walk before bedtime is preferable to pharmacologic agents.
- Relaxation techniques, such as listening to audiotapes that are available at bookstores, are helpful in relaxing before sleep.
- Avoid coffee, chocolate, and cola at bedtime.

Potential for Altered Skin Integrity

- Teach Ian preventive skin care—for example, how to examine his skin regularly.
- Teach good foot care, including appropriate socks and shoes. Diabetic teaching programs have excellent information on foot care, such as how to cut the toenails.
- Special attention needs to be given to care of the blood access. Healing is delayed, and it is critical that needle sites be rotated between treatments.
- Ian must immediately report all injuries.

Hopelessness

- Ian's belief that renal failure will be accompanied by a deteriorating physical condition has led to his feeling of hopelessness. This can be helped by involving Ian in making decisions about his treatments, thereby giving him control.
- Increasing self-care skills can lead to mastery over illness or an acceptance of living with chronic illness instead of being overwhelmed by it.
- Encourage Ian to express his feelings and accept them unconditionally.
- Some patients have found it helpful to meet other patients who have successfully dealt with living with chronic illness. The local chapter of the Kidney Foundation may provide peer resource individuals.

Altered Family Processes

- The transition of Ian's role as father, husband, and friend to one of a person with a chronic illness is tied to his view of his life as hopeless.
- Family members can receive support from the renal unit by being welcomed into the department. After all, this is a disease that affects them also.
- Keep them involved, validate their feelings, and acknowledge their experiences.
- Ian and his wife might be referred for family counseling.

PATIENT NUMBER 1 (continued)

Ian has now been on dialysis for 4 months and has had some encouraging resolution of his initial assessment findings. As indicated earlier, nursing assessments can also be ongoing and selective. These kinds of assessments are used to evaluate the treatment or to monitor Ian's response to treatment. Strategies are implemented if the care deviates from the renal unit's standards. Ongoing issues related to Ian's concerns and the nurse's role in his assessment follow.

Predialysis and Postdialysis Assessment

This is a routine assessment performed at every treatment. It usually consists of measurement of weight, blood pressure, pulse, and temperature and assessment of the vascular access. The role of the nurse is to evaluate and interpret these data. Simply recording weight and vital signs is inadequate. A patient's general well-being is reviewed as well. The nurse can bring important issues to the physician for changes in therapy.

Assessment of the Dialysis Process

The role of the nurse is to monitor intradialytic symptoms that could require a change in prescription. Hypotension may be due to an incorrect weight or may be an indication for a trial of variable sodium. The various parameters that are monitored are discussed later.

Adequacy of Dialysis

This is usually assessed by the physician through urea kinetic modeling. The role of the nurse is to ensure that the patient receives dialysis as ordered, such as actual time on dialysis and maintaining blood flow and dialysate flow rates.

Assessment of the Blood Access

Adequacy of dialysis is affected by the performance of the blood access. The role of the nurse is to be alert to the changes in venous pressures and inform the physician when significant changes occur. One method of the assessment of access performance is by recirculation studies. **The nurse has a critical role in maintaining the life of the access by ensuring correct technique during needle placement and the**

rotation of sites. Teaching the patient postdialysis care of puncture wounds is also necessary.

INTEGRATING A PSYCHOSOCIAL APPROACH TO THE PATIENT

Nursing theory recognizes four universal concepts, those of nursing, person, health, and environment. The next case presentation shows how these four concepts can direct the care of patients with end-stage renal disease. These concepts can be considered in the context of a problem-based setting that is familiar to nephrology nurses.

PATIENT NUMBER 2

Alan is 23 years old and lives with his mother and two sisters in Ontario. The family are new immigrants, having moved to Canada from South America so Alan and his sisters could go to school. Their father remained in Colombia. Alan's mother supports the family by working for a company that cleans houses. They are a deeply religious family. Alan has been seen in the renal clinic only twice because he has missed many follow-up appointments. He does not believe he has anything wrong with his kidneys but instead thinks this is some kind of plot. At this last visit, the physician tried hard to inform Alan of his illness by showing him ultrasound and laboratory results, and Alan has reluctantly agreed to visit the dialysis unit.

Nursing recognizes that every person has rights and responsibilities. One of these is the right of decision making in one's own care. However, the first question is, how can Alan be helped to understand his need for dialysis and to make an informed decision? An informed decision—one that is made voluntarily after the risks and benefits of the procedure have been explained and alternative therapies discussed—is the basis of valid consent. A prediction of events that are likely to occur if no treatment is given should also be discussed.

A number of measures were taken to orient Alan to dialysis. He was taken to the unit and was given a tour; he met with a patient undergoing dialysis, and the procedures were explained to him. Alan was polite and appeared to understand the dialysis process, but he did not alter his belief that dialysis was unnecessary. The dialysis

nursing staff were concerned that Alan still did not appreciate the consequences of accepting or refusing dialysis. If Alan agrees with the physician's request to start dialysis, even though he does not believe he needs it, the nursing staff would likely have to cope with a noncompliant patient. Along with an individual's right to make treatment decisions is the obligation to accept the responsibilities that accompany those decisions.

The physician referred Alan for predialysis education. Here he learned about signs and symptoms of renal failure, different types of dialysis, and which type might suit him better. Finally, he was encouraged to accept support from his family. Predialysis education is an essential component of the successful adaptation of a patient and his or her family to maintenance dialysis, no matter which method of treatment is chosen. These programs are available in most renal centers and vary in their content, but the overall goals are usually consistent with patient autonomy. A nephrology nurse is an essential member of the team. Representatives from home dialysis, self-care dialysis, in-center dialysis, and peritoneal dialysis programs are present.

PATIENT NUMBER 2 (continued)

Alan attended the treatment option session with his mother and sister. They listened politely to the presentations, but Alan continued to insist that he did not need dialysis. He denied that he was ill and continued to believe that this encouragement for dialysis was a plot. He said he came to the presentation because he promised his physician that he would. Alan's mother supported his decisions. She expressed her faith in their religious beliefs and that this faith would take care of them. His sister expressed concern for him but would not oppose her mother.

The nursing role is to recognize and interpret the family dynamics and use them in the best interests of the patient. It is not in nursing's or patients' best interest to challenge patients' beliefs, especially in the absence of psychiatric illness. In this case, our patient Alan has strong personal and religious beliefs, and our role is to coexist with them.

It was thought that continuous ambulatory peritoneal dialysis, a home-based therapy, would not be successful. Failure in following the treatment plan and lack of family support were to be expected. It was recommended that Alan be directed toward dialysis treatment in a hospital-based setting where both he and the nursing staff would have access to support. Although home-based therapies are judged to be superior in quality-of-life studies, the environmental influence has to be considered in a nursing and patient context. Alan's home life would not help to support the goals of the health care team and may, in fact, work against them. In-center dialysis can provide a stable environment and has been found to be beneficial to some patients, providing a social milieu and an extended family. The relationship between the staff and the patients is more relaxed, and some form of bonding takes place. Nonetheless, we were not sure how Alan would tolerate in-center dialysis. He was quiet and withdrawn, whereas a dialysis unit can at times be crowded, noisy, and stressful. Patients may witness unusual and frightening events such as hypotension, seizures, and cardiac arrest; they can overhear inappropriate conversations and suffer loss of privacy.

Preparations for Alan's eventual appearance for dialysis continued. A primary care nurse was included. The primary care nurse has a privileged position as Alan's advocate. He would have one person with whom he could communicate, to share his beliefs and act as his go-between among the team members. The nurse would act as his representative to promote his best interests. Together they would develop a plan of care.

PATIENT NUMBER 2 (continued)

Alan subsequently presented to the emergency department with severe uremia. He gave consent for a temporary access and dialysis. The first dialysis went smoothly, but Alan refused to return. After many discussions and arguments back and forth, the central line catheter was removed and Alan was permitted to leave. This scenario was to happen twice before Alan agreed to attend on a regular basis. He and the primary care nurse developed a schedule for his treatments, and their relationship developed. This one-on-one relationship of trust between the patient and the nurse allowed for the sharing of information that in other circumstances may have taken a long time to elicit. Still, Alan continued to believe that dialysis was harmful to him, that it made him weak.

A person's health is specific to that individual. The maximum achievable level of health depends not only on one's physical functioning but also on how one sees oneself, as healthy or sick, and how one acts in that role. Alan, with dialysis, did not see himself as healthy. Further, he viewed the dialysis process as evidence of sickness rather than a means to achieve health. The nurse's goal was to reverse that view. Alan may never become integrated into the dialysis milieu in the conventional sense, but by means of a caring nursing relationship, he may reach his maximum achiev-

able level of health. Then, nursing will have met its goal.

THE ROLE OF THE NURSE IN ASSESSMENT AND MONITORING DURING HEMODIALYSIS

Nephrology nurses are responsible for assessment and monitoring of patients undergoing hemodialysis. An experienced nurse is expected to synthesize and analyze data from various sources—for example, the health record, the patient's presentation, the patient's past history, and the nurse's own knowledge base.

PATIENT NUMBER 3

Pamela is a 45-year-old single mother with a daughter age 17 years. Before starting dialysis, Pamela worked as a clerk in a department store, but she stopped working 1 year after the initiation of maintenance hemodialysis. Pamela has had a difficult time raising her daughter alone, and she has reported to the staff that her daughter resents discipline. Pamela was recently admitted to the hospital with pneumonia. However, she left without the physician's agreement because she didn't want her daughter to be home alone.

Pamela presents herself to the unit 24 hours before her next scheduled dialysis because of acute shortness of breath. **The predialysis assessment** reveals a weight gain of only 1 kg since her last treatment, elevated blood pressure of 160/100 mm Hg, and a rapid heart rate of 120. Evaluation of her respiratory system reveals abnormal breath sounds, rales, a rapid respiratory rate of 35, and pronounced use of accessory muscles. Oxygen is being delivered by mask, and an oxygen saturation monitor is in use. Pamela is extremely anxious. The physician is told of the abnormal findings of relative low weight gain for her symptoms, high blood pressure, rapid pulse, and compromised respiratory status.

Assessment

A marked increase in weight would account for the sudden onset of shortness of breath. However, Pamela is only 1 kg above her ideal weight. The nurse is aware that Pamela was recently admitted to the hospital and suggests that she has probably lost true body weight and that her ideal weight is actually lower. If the acute shortness of breath was not due to a change in weight, other reasons should be explored. These may include acute medical conditions, such as those involving the cardiac and respiratory systems. Depending on the cause, the nursing response will vary. Fluid overload may also be due to nonadherence to diet. Noncompliance is not always a simple lack of information but may be a cry for help from a patient.

PATIENT NUMBER 3 (continued)

The physician agrees with the nursing assessment, and Pamela's urgent dialysis is adjusted to decrease her ideal weight by 1 to 2 kg, depending on blood pressure. Sequential dialysis/ultrafiltration is started for the first hour to produce rapid fluid removal and improve pulmonary function.

Patient monitoring during dialysis varies according to unit policies. It should consist of the following:

Blood Pressure. Monitor blood pressure frequently until Pamela's condition stabilizes. In this case, her blood pressure is high but is expected to fall as fluid is removed. Hypotension may occur as the cardiovascular space is reduced owing to rapid fluid removal. The blood pressure can be supported in a number of ways, and the choice seems to depend on the individual dialysis unit: saline boluses, increasing the sodium concentration in the dialysate, and administering volume expanders such as mannitol or serum albumin. In this case, sequential dialysis (ultrafiltration without dialysis) was chosen because it can remove fluid rapidly without hypotension. A drawback of this technique is that extra dialysis time is needed, and this may be difficult in a unit where schedules are tightly managed.

Arterial Pressure. Prepump arterial monitoring measures the effort required by the blood pump to achieve the ordered blood flow from the access. It is usually a negative reading, and the greater effort required by the blood pump makes it more negative. Trying to achieve a blood pump speed greater than what the access can deliver elicits continuing alarms and an interruption in the dialysis. Constant stopping of the blood pump increases the likelihood of clotting in the artificial kidney, reducing clearance. Pamela has fluid overload, and thus the arterial pressure will be less negative at the start, indicating increased vascular volume. As dialysis progresses, the arterial pressure will diminish.

Ultrafiltration and Transmembrane Pressure. The ultrafiltration rate is a calculation derived from the total amount of fluid to be removed divided by the actual dialysis time. A maximum rate of ultrafiltration during dialysis is usually established for each patient. This is determined by dialysis unit policies, individual patients' responses, or calculated methods based on a patient's body weight. Transmembrane pressure is the force required to maintain the ultrafiltration rate. A rise of transmembrane pressure during dialysis indicates a loss of membrane surface area, requiring extra force to achieve the prescribed ultrafiltration rate. This could indicate clotting of the dialyzer. Pamela was prescribed sequential dialysis for the first hour, and the ultrafiltration rate was set at 1800 ml/hr. Thereafter she was weighed, and a new ultrafiltration rate was calculated to achieve target weight.

Venous Pressure. Venous pressure is the resistance of the blood as it is returning to the patient. It is always a positive pressure. A sudden increase in venous pressure may signal a venous hematoma, a kinked line, or clotting in the venous drip chamber. An increase in venous pressure over a few weeks usually reflects an access problem, such as venous stenosis, which requires attention before the access clots.

Blood Flow. Maximum blood flow is usually ordered to achieve the most efficient dialysis. In cases of first dialysis treatments, the blood flow is often reduced to avoid the complication of dialysis dysequilibrium.

Heparinization. Heparin is administered throughout the treatment, usually in a continuous form. Heparin delivery is ordered as full heparinization, low-dose, or no heparin. The dialysis nurse should be aware of the indications for each method of heparin delivery. Low-dose or no heparinization is indicated if the patient is at risk for bleeding. Various techniques for successful no-heparin dialysis include normal saline flushes of 100 to 200 ml every 20 minutes, using maximum blood pump speed, and reducing the dialysis time to 3 hours. All of these measures are aimed at reducing blood clotting in the artificial kidney. Sequential dialysis causes cooling of the blood because no dialysate is flowing through the artificial kidney, and thus the likelihood of clotting in the kidney is increased. This can be avoided by periodically (i.e., every 15 minutes) flushing fresh dialysate into the dialysate compartment.

Complications. The patient is monitored for intradialytic symptoms such as hypotension, cramping, and access problems such as hematoma and blood loss.

PATIENT NUMBER 3 (continued)

Postdialysis Assessment. At the end of dialysis, Pamela reached a new ideal weight and is stable for discharge home. Her new ideal weight is entered onto the patient care plan. The renal social worker was consulted to provide individual and family counseling to Pamela and her daughter.

SUMMARY

Three patients have been presented to highlight a nurse's role in managing patients with renal disease. Ian, a computer programmer, requires nursing assessment of signs and symptoms of uremia and plans for dialysis. Alan, an immigrant, denies his need for dialysis, even to the point of refusing dialysis life support. His bonding with his primary nurse made all the difference. Pamela, a 45-year-old single mother on dialysis, presents with shortness of breath without weight gain—an enigma resolved by meticulous monitoring of dialysis parameters by her nurse.

SUGGESTED READINGS

Gutch CF, Stoner MH, Corea AL: Review of Hemodialysis for Nurses and Dialysis Personnel, 5th ed. St Louis, CV Mosby, 1993.

Lancaster LE (ed): A.N.N.A. Core Curriculum for Nephrology Nurses, 3rd ed. Pitman, NJ, A.N.N.A., 1995.

Richard CJ: Comprehensive Nephrology Nursing Boston, Little, Brown & Co, 1986.

Uldall R: Renal Nursing, 3rd ed. Cambridge, MA, Blackwell Scientific Publications, 1988.

19 | PERITONEAL

DIALYSIS

Nicholas V. Dombros, George E. Digenis,
and Dimitrios G. Oreopoulos

The principal objective of this chapter is to provide to medicine and nephrology trainees a simplified yet up-to-date view of peritoneal dialysis
that emphasizes the assessment and treatment of
patients with renal failure.

CHRONIC PERITONEAL DIALYSIS

PATIENT NUMBER 1

Martha, a pleasant 50-year-old gravida 2, para
2 woman, has been monitored regularly for the
past 3 years in the outpatient nephrology clinic
for chronic renal failure secondary to IgA
glomerulonephritis associated with hypertension.
Her initial creatinine clearance was 30 ml/min/
1.73 m². During the follow-up period, her renal
function deteriorated gradually and she started
complaining of nausea, fatigue, weakness, mild
pruritus, and 1+ ankle edema. Medications
included calcium antagonists, beta blockers,
calcium carbonate, and furosemide, but there
was considerable doubt about her compliance.
Her body weight was 54 kg and height was 155
cm. Her blood pressure was 160/95 mm Hg in
both the sitting and lying positions. Laboratory
results showed hematocrit 27%, serum creatinine
8 mg/dl, BUN 85 mg/dl, uric acid 7.2 mg/dl,
potassium 4.8 mmol/L, sodium 138 mmol/L,
calcium 7.6, phosphorus 6.3 mg/dl, serum
albumin 4g/dl, total protein 7.3 g/dl, 24-hour
urine output 1400 ml, and creatinine clearance
6.5 ml/min/1.73m². How should this patient be
treated?

Martha obviously was approaching the end
stage of chronic renal failure and soon would

need continuous renal replacement therapy. The
attending physician explained to her the situation
and the options of dialysis, and the renal coordi-
nator nurse took the patient to visit a hemodialysis unit and a peritoneal dialysis unit. Martha
discussed the two methods in detail with nurses
and other renal patients undergoing dialysis. She
became frightened by the sight of needles, the
idea of blood being pumped out of her body, and
the need for coming to the hospital three times
a week. She instead chose long-term peritoneal
dialysis because it was more compatible with her
lifestyle. The home dialysis training nurse found
that Martha was competent to perform continuous peritoneal dialysis, and she was scheduled
for a permanent peritoneal catheter implantation
2 days later.

Long-Term Peritoneal Access

The most fundamental requirement for continuous peritoneal dialysis is successful long-term
peritoneal access.

The device most widely used for this purpose
is the Tenckhoff catheter, but the Toronto Western Hospital (TWH), the swan neck, and the
Cruz catheters (Fig. 19–1) also are commonly
used. Long-term catheters are implanted by a
surgeon in the operating room or by a nephrologist at the bedside (see Appendix 2).

Attentive postoperative care of a peritoneal
dialysis catheter is essential to the success of this
treatment. The following are the basic guidelines:

1. Keep handling of the catheter and exit site
to a minimum until healing is complete.
2. To avoid leakage of fluid, do not instill large
volumes of dialysate soon after implantation.

The peritoneal cavity is usually flushed with

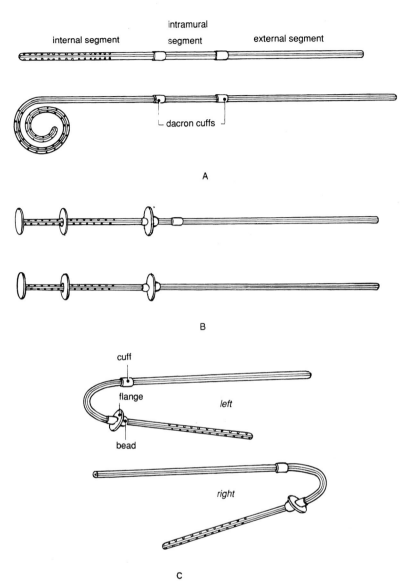

Figure 19–1. The Tenckhoff *(A)*, Toronto Western Hospital *(B)*, and swan neck Missouri *(C)* catheters. (From Khanna R, Nolph KD, Oreopoulos DG: The Essentials of Peritoneal Dialysis. Dordrecht, The Netherlands, Kluwer Academic, 1993, p 20. Reprinted by permission of Kluwer Academic Publishers.)

500 to 1500 ml of dialysate until the effluent becomes clear. Thereafter, the catheter is capped and left for up to 2 weeks before the initiation of continuous ambulatory peritoneal dialysis (CAPD) or other form of peritoneal dialysis.

If dialysis becomes necessary after catheter implantation in a uremic patient, it is performed in the supine position with exchange volumes of 500 to 1500 ml. Volumes are gradually increased to minimize the risk of leakage, and 24 to 48 hours of intermittent peritoneal dialysis (IPD) is followed by a dialysis-free period of the same duration.

If the peritoneal catheter is not used, its patency and function should be checked by infu-

sion and drainage of 1000 ml of dialysate once a week.

Exit Site Care

After catheter implantation, the skin incision and the exit site are covered with sterile gauze and a nonocclusive dressing, which are not changed for several days. One should avoid any movement of the catheter at the exit site, and after the first week, the catheter is immobilized.

If possible, the peritoneal catheter should be inserted several weeks before it is needed for treatment. During this time, the catheter is in-

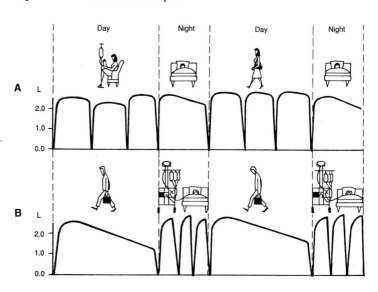

Figure 19–2. Continuous regimens of dialysis. The dialysis exchanges are performed at convenient times, and the dialysis solution is in the peritoneal cavity all the time to provide continuous dialysis. *A:* CAPD. *B:* CCPD. (From Khanna R, Nolph KD, Oreopoulos DG: The Essentials of Peritoneal Dialysis. Dordrecht, The Netherlands, Kluwer Academic, 1993, p 38. Reprinted by permission of Kluwer Academic Publishers.)

fused on various schedules that have been designed to diminish intraperitoneal pressure and minimize pericatheter leaking. One of these schedules is as follows:

- Infuse with sterile heparinized saline or dialysate in a volume of 50 to 2000 ml, once or three times a week. Larger volumes are drained off.
- Control cough and limit the patient's activity.
- The abdominal cavity is left "dry."
- In an active patient, continuous dialysis is usually delayed for 2 to 4 weeks.

Subsequent catheter care includes weekly dressing changes after cleansing with povidone-iodine scrub and rinsing with sterile water. Dressing changes are continued until complete healing takes place, a process that usually requires as long as 6 weeks. During this period, the catheter is protected to avoid pulling or twisting. Specific measures to immobilize the catheter depend on the location of the exit site and the shape of the abdomen.

After the surgical wound heals, meticulous exit site care is essential to prevent infection, which is a major cause of morbidity among patients undergoing CAPD.

Long-term exit site care may be based on cleansing with hydrogen peroxide in combination with soap or povidone-iodine scrub, cleansing with povidone-iodine alone, or cleansing with soap and water.

Patients can start daily showering and cleaning of the exit site 2 to 8 weeks after catheter implantation. They are allowed to swim in the ocean or in a chlorinated swimming pool 4 to 8 weeks after implantation.

PATIENT NUMBER 1 (continued)

After preparation according to the protocol, Martha was taken to the operating room, where a permanent TWH peritoneal catheter was inserted surgically through a paramedian incision. She had no catheter-related complications except for mild pain over the incision; this responded to oral analgesics. She was discharged to her home after 3 days. The volume of peritoneal dialysis solution was increased gradually, and by the 17th day after implantation, she was able to accommodate 2000 ml without discomfort.

REGIMENS OF CHRONIC PERITONEAL DIALYSIS

Several regimens of continuous peritoneal dialysis are in common use. Most of the patients undergoing peritoneal dialysis worldwide have the classic CAPD (Fig. 19–2) as it was modified by Buonchristiani (Y-set twin bag). Other forms of long-term peritoneal dialysis that use a peritoneal dialysis machine (cycler) are classified as automated peritoneal dialysis (APD), either continuous or intermittent. The most common form of APD is continuous cycling peritoneal dialysis (CCPD). Regimens of intermittent cycler-assisted peritoneal dialysis include IPD, nightly peritoneal dialysis (NPD), and its variations of nightly intermittent peritoneal dialysis (NIPD) and nightly tidal peritoneal dialysis (NTPD) (Fig. 19–3).

Continuous Ambulatory Peritoneal Dialysis

CAPD, a form of home dialysis, is used as long-term renal replacement mainly in patients with end-stage renal disease (ESRD). It also may be used in acute renal failure. At least in terms of ultrafiltration, it is less efficient than IPD. However, 7 days of CAPD offers better dialysis than two 20-hour sessions of IPD. After a period of training, a typical adult patient (or helper) would make four 2-L exchanges every 4 to 8 hours, 7 days a week. The time of a complete cycle is divided into inflow (5 min/L), dwell time (4 to 8 hours) and outflow (7 to 12 min/L). Bags would commonly be exchanged at 7, 13, 19, and 23 hours. The inflow and outflow of solutions is by means of gravity alone. During the dwell time, fluid and solute are exchanged (dialysis) between the intraperitoneal solution and the patient's blood.

The bag exchange should be performed only by a trained person.

Transfer Sets

The dialysis solution for CAPD is carried in plastic bags that are connected to a titanium adapter, which is attached to the permanent catheter, through a system of connecting tubing, which is specific for each brand of bag.

Many types of bags, connecting tubes, connectors, and auxiliary devices are available throughout the world, and new modifications are constantly being introduced into the market by the manufacturing companies. Described next are the basic principles and main points of the two most frequently used types.

In general, there are two types of tubing systems: the straight transfer set and the most frequently used Y-shaped transfer set and its modification—the twin bag.

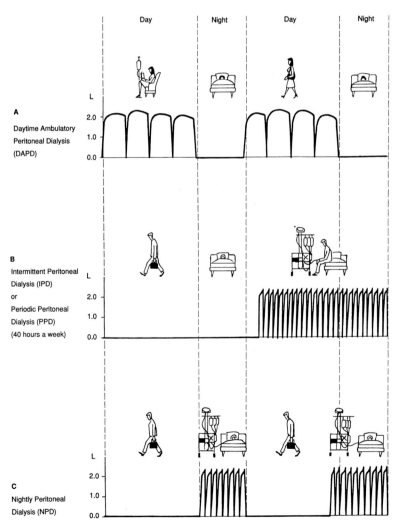

Figure 19–3. Intermittent regimens of peritoneal dialysis. These regimens allow the patient to be free of dialysis for a specified period in between the dialysis treatments. The exchanges are done manually as in DAPD or with the help of a cycler as in IPD or NPD. *A:* DAPD. *B:* IPD. *C:* NPD. (From Khanna R, Nolph KD, Oreopoulos DG: The Essentials of Peritoneal Dialysis. Dordrecht, The Netherlands, Kluwer Academic, 1993, p 37. Reprinted by permission of Kluwer Academic Publishers.)

STRAIGHT TRANSFER SET

At the initiation of CAPD and under strict aseptic conditions, a fresh bag is connected to the peripheral end of the straight transfer set through a spike or Luer-Lock, depending on the brand of bag. The system is primed, and then the other end of the straight transfer set is connected to the catheter via the titanium adapter (Luer-Lock).

The roller clamp on the tubing is then opened, and the fluid is allowed to flow into the peritoneal cavity. At the end of inflow, the clamp is closed and the patient wears the empty bag comfortably under his or her clothing.

Basic Steps of Dialysis Solution Exchange (Bag Exchange) (Fig. 19–4). At the time of dialysis fluid replacement (bag exchange), the following steps are taken. A mask is donned, and hands are washed. The empty bag from under the patient's clothes is placed on the floor or lowered to a level below the patient's abdomen, and the roller clamp on the transfer set is opened (drain position). After the new bag has been checked for clarity and leaks, it is suspended on a pole beside the bed.

After drainage is complete, the roller clamp is closed and the used bag is hung up beside the new one. The spike is removed from the used bag, paying careful attention not to contaminate it, and this spike is immediately inserted into the new bag. The roller clamp is opened and filling begins. When filling is over, the roller clamp is closed and the empty bag is folded and, once again, worn under the clothing.

Y-SHAPED TRANSFER SET

This transfer set is formed into a Y shape in which a full bag and an empty bag are connected to each of the upper limbs of the Y and the lower limb of the Y is connected to the patient's catheter via a short straight transfer set (Fig. 19–5).

The Y-Set Exchange Procedure. The basic step is that before fresh dialysis solution is run into the patient (the fill), dialysate from the new bag and the patient's abdomen (flush) is drained into the empty bag, carrying with it any bacteria introduced by touch contamination during the connection with the bag and the catheter (see Fig. 19–5).

The bag exchange consists of the following steps:

1. Attach the empty (drainage) bag to one of the upper limbs of the Y set.
2. Spike the new solution bag to the other upper limb.
3. Connect the lower limb with the short transfer set attached to the patient.
4. Allow a small volume of fresh dialysis solution to run from the new bag into the empty bag (flush).
5. Drain the dialysis solution from the patient into the drainage bag.
6. Infuse the fresh dialysis solution into the patient.
7. Disconnect the Y set and close the short straight transfer set with an antiseptic-containing cap.

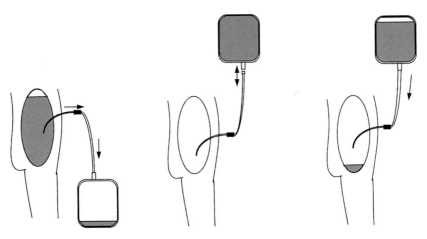

Figure 19–4. The Toronto Western Hospital technique for CAPD. The steps of the technique are described in the text. (From Ziroyanis PN, Agrafiotis A, Dombros N, Tsakiris D: Peritoneal Dialysis. Proceedings of the 2nd Symposium, March 22–23, 1995. Athens, Technogramma/ Hellenic Society of Nephrology, 1995, p 173.)

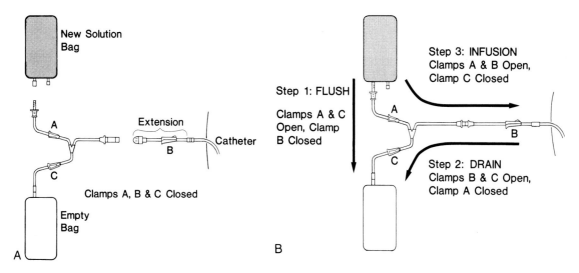

Figure 19–5. Y-set system for solution exchange for CAPD. *A:* Setup before exchange. *B:* Steps during exchange.

DOUBLE- OR TWIN-BAG SYSTEMS

In these systems, the original Y set and antiseptic in line has been replaced with a sterile, disposable, completely integrated system, which includes an empty bag and a bag containing a fresh dialysis solution. The double-bag system still uses the flush-before-fill technique, but no antiseptic is necessary (Fig. 19–6).

Choice of Dialysis Solution

The rate of fluid removal in CAPD varies between individual patients and depends on mem-

brane permeability. In those with average peritoneal transport (discussed later), the common practice is four 2-L exchanges per day. The dextrose concentration depends on body weight and on blood pressure measured in supine and standing positions. If the patient is at his or her target weight (± 0.5 kg), 1.5% solution should be used. If a patient's weight is 0.5 to 1.5 kg above the target weight, a 2.5% solution should be used. If the patient has gained more than 1.5 kg, a 4.25% solution should be used. The 0.5% solution (if available) should be used in patients with a body weight less than the determined dry weight. Rapid ultrafiltration by instillation of hypertonic

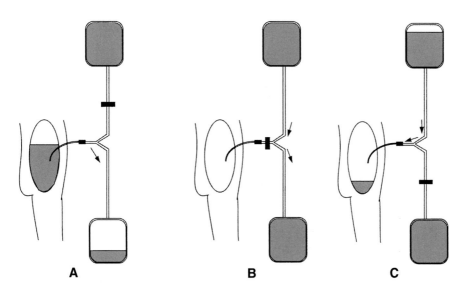

Figure 19–6. The Y-set. The various steps are described in the text. (From Ziroyanis PN, Agrafiotis A, Dombros N, Tsakiris D: Peritoneal Dialysis. Proceedings of the 2nd Symposium, March 22–23, 1995. Athens, Technogramma/Hellenic Society of Nephrology, 1995, p 175.)

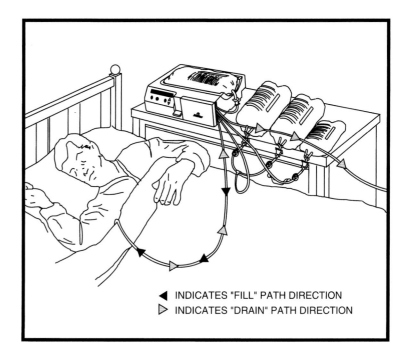

Figure 19–7. APD Baxter (home choice).

INDICATES "FILL" PATH DIRECTION
INDICATES "DRAIN" PATH DIRECTION

solutions may not be well tolerated by diabetic patients (because of autonomic dysfunction) or by patients with poor cardiac function. Patients with large polycystic kidneys, hernias, or a small peritoneal cavity may not be able to tolerate 2 L. In these cases, smaller volumes may be used. Larger patients may tolerate volumes as great as 3 L, which are required for higher solute removal.

Patients without any residual kidney function or large patients (heavier than 70 kg) require daily volumes larger than the standard CAPD dose (four 2-L exchanges per day) in order to achieve adequate dialysis (discussed later). In these patients, the dialysis dose could be increased by increasing either the volume (4 × 3 L/day) or the frequency of dialysis solution exchanges (5 × 2 L/day). An alternative approach is to switch patients with adequate porosity (i.e., creatinine dialysate-to-plasma [D/P] ratio > .55) from CAPD to APD.

Automated Peritoneal Dialysis

In APD, the delivery and drainage of the dialysate are assisted by a mechanical device.

The advantages of APD are that it eliminates manual involvement and patients can perform home dialysis during the hours of sleep. This enables patients or their helpers to be free during the daytime. In APD, the peritonitis rate is lower because connections and disconnections are fewer and probably also because, in intermittent regimens, the peritoneal cavity remains empty for long periods, during which the peritoneal defense mechanisms can act. Finally, APD provides increased volumes of dialysis solution for those patients who require higher clearances. For these reasons, during the past few years, APD has been the fastest-growing renal replacement modality in the United States.

Technique

APD may be used with any type of peritoneal dialysis catheter. The main requirement for its use is an automated cycler able to deliver various preset volumes at a preset time (Fig. 19–7). For CCPD, the cycler is attached to the catheter through an appropriate connector before the patient retires at night; it is programmed to deliver three or more cycles of a volume that the patient can tolerate well during the night. Recumbency helps the individual to tolerate larger volumes and thus increases the efficiency of dialysis.

With the use of 5-L dialysate bags, only two or three spikings are necessary for an individual treatment. Before disconnecting in the morning, the patient instills 1 to 2 L, preferably of hypertonic solution; this remains in the peritoneal cavity during the day. In NIPD, the peritoneal cavity remains empty during the day. Finally, in tidal peritoneal dialysis (TPD), the cycler is programmed to leave a reserve volume in the peritoneal cavity at the end of the exchange and to cycle a tidal volume (i.e., an additional volume on top of it) with the next exchange. In this way, dialysis that is interrupted at the end of the exchange with the intermittent regimens, continues uninterrupted.

PERITONEAL EQUILIBRATION TEST

To provide adequate long-term peritoneal dialysis, one should consider the specific characteristics of each patient's peritoneal membrane, in terms of solute and water transport. The adequacy of dialysis in each patient also depends on the sum of dialysis (water and solute removal) offered by the peritoneum and the residual renal function.

The peritoneal equilibration test (PET) is a simple way to assess the transport characteristics of the peritoneal membrane. This test is used to study the rate of equilibration of small solutes such as creatinine, urea, and glucose between blood and dialysate using the D/P ratio at 2 and 4 hours after instillation of 2 L of 2.5% glucose dialysate. Using data from 101 patients undergoing CAPD, Twardowski classified peritoneal permeability into four groups: high, high average, low average, and low (Fig. 19–8).

A PET performed shortly after initiation of peritoneal dialysis gives information from which the attending physician can choose the optimal dialysis prescription.

A PET is performed as follows:

1. After an 8- to 12-hour overnight exchange, the fluid is drained completely with the patient in the sitting position.

2. The patient assumes the supine position, and 2 L of 2.5% glucose dialysate is infused into the abdomen at a rate of 200 ml/min.

3. At the end of infusion (0 dwell time), 200 ml of dialysis solution is drained into the bag and mixed well. A 10-ml sample is taken for measurement of urea, creatinine and glucose, and the rest is reinfused.

4. After 2 hours, during which the patient is ambulatory, another sample of dialysis solution (as in step 3) and a blood sample are drawn.

5. At the end of the fourth hour, the dialysis solution is drained out completely while the patient is in the sitting position, total volume is measured, and a sample is taken again for urea, creatinine and glucose measurement.

6. The concentration of creatinine in the effluent should be corrected, because glucose interferes with the Jaffé reaction used for creatinine measurement (1 mg/dl of glucose overestimates creatinine concentration by 0.0005 mg/dl).

7. The D/P ratios of effluent dialysate to plasma creatinine, urea, and glucose at 2 and 4 hours are calculated. For glucose, we calculate

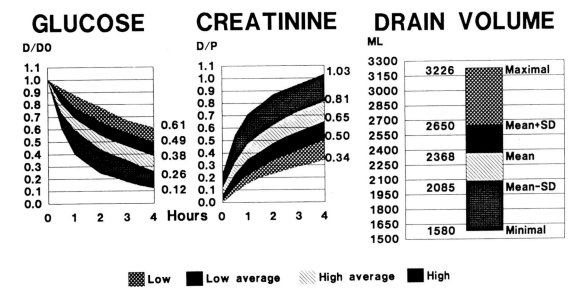

Figure 19–8. The equilibration test results in a study population. The area shaded in different patterns depicts results representing high, high average, average, low average, and low peritoneal transport rates. The bar graph depicts the drain volumes after 4-hour study in the same study population. Patients with high solute transport rates usually have low drain volumes and vice versa.

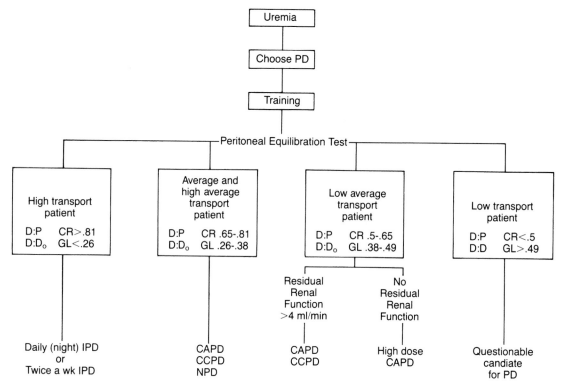

Figure 19–9. Decision-making algorithm for choosing an appropriate dialysis regimen based on the peritoneal equilibration test. CAPD, continuous ambulatory peritoneal dialysis; CCPD, continuous cycling peritoneal dialysis; CR, creatinine; D:P, dialysate to plasma ratio; D:D$_o$, dialysate effluent glucose to dialysate glucose concentration at zero time; GL, glucose; IPD, intermittent peritoneal dialysis; NPD, nightly peritoneal dialysis.

the concentration at time 0 (D$_0$) and 4 hours (D) (D/D$_0$).

In clinical practice, we simplify the previous PET by taking samples only at the end of 4 hours.

PATIENT NUMBER 1 (continued)

Our patient Martha had a PET; the results at the end of 4 hours were a creatinine D/P ratio of 0.66 and a glucose D/D$_0$ ratio of 0.32. Figures 19–8 and 19–9 show that this patient belongs to a high average group. Her daily urine output was 1250 ml, and her creatinine clearance was 5 ml/min.

Patients with high average peritoneal transport are ideal for standard CAPD. Martha was shown how to perform CAPD using four 2-L exchanges of 1.5% solution every day. She was given training on (1) the twin-bag exchange procedure, (2) the injection of antibiotics and heparin into the bag, (3) the diagnosis and treatment of peritonitis, and (4) exit site care. After training, Martha was discharged home with adequate supplies of bags, antibiotics, heparin, povidone-iodine, and so on, with strict instructions to contact the unit if she has any difficulty at home. She was given an appointment to attend the outpatient CAPD clinic in 4 weeks.

PATIENT NUMBER 2

Janet, a fairly independent 70-year-old woman who lived with her husband, developed ESRD of unknown cause and chose CAPD for her treatment. At the end of 4 hours, the results of a PET were as follows: creatinine D/P ratio, 0.97; glucose D/D$_0$ ratio, 0.12.

These values indicate that she was a high transporter (see Fig. 19–8); this means that because of fast glucose absorption, she would have a poor ultrafiltration rate even with a hypertonic solution. She would fare better on an APD schedule because short dwell exchanges lead to better net ultrafiltration (see Fig. 19–9).

We advised Janet to switch from standard CAPD to APD; however, because this change would require her husband to sleep in a separate bed on a permanent basis, she insisted on remaining on CAPD. After 1 month, Janet's body weight increased by 14 kg mainly because of fluid retention. Four 2-L, 4.25% glucose exchanges did not generate any net ultrafiltration. Her catheter was functioning well, and there was no leakage. The patient and her husband then agreed to change to APD with four 2-L exchanges over 8 hours every night. Ultrafiltration was about

1200 ml per session. Two weeks later, Janet reached her dry body weight.

Patients who weigh up to 70 kg and have low average transport characteristics also are good candidates for standard CAPD; they achieve good ultrafiltration using moderate glucose concentrations. However, patients with a high body surface area need a larger volume of dialysis solution. These difficulties are more apparent in patients with low transport characteristics, especially if they have negligible residual renal function. We repeat PETs in the following circumstances:

- To document changes in membrane characteristics
- To help in the diagnosis of leaks in the subcutaneous tissue of the abdominal wall
- To evaluate a patient's compliance with a specific peritoneal dialysis schedule
- To predict membrane failure

PATIENT NUMBER 3

Ken, an active 35-year-old businessman with chronic glomerulonephritis, was maintained on standard CAPD (four 2-L exchanges per day). An initial PET had shown creatinine D/P ratio of 0.71 and glucose D/D_0 ratio of 0.36. Seven months later, he had gained 5 kg in weight, was short of breath, and had nausea and weakness. His peritoneal catheter was functioning well, and there was no evidence of dialysis leak. The results of a second PET were similar to the initial results. His serum creatinine and BUN values were elevated. Residual renal function (renal creatinine clearance) had not decreased significantly.

We consider a weekly total (peritoneal dialysis + renal) creatinine clearance of at least 50 L/1.73m^2 of body surface area adequate for patients on CAPD or CCPD. On further questioning, Ken admitted that for the past 2 weeks, because he had to complete an important business assignment, he had skipped several bag exchanges. His difficulties resolved when he complied with the standard CAPD regimen.

COMPLICATIONS OF CHRONIC PERITONEAL DIALYSIS
Catheter-Related Complications

Catheter-related complications that occur during training are discussed in the chapter on acute peritoneal dialysis. Here we discuss the late (chronic) catheter-related complications.

Exit Site and Tunnel Infection

A noninfected (normal) exit site should be clean, dry, painless, and free of evidence of inflammation. We do not yet have a universally accepted definition of exit site infection (ESI). Most workers define ESI by redness or skin induration or purulent discharge from the exit site with or without exuberant granulation tissue (proud flesh). The presence of a crust around the exit site may not indicate infection. A positive culture in the absence of inflammation does not indicate infection, and we do not recommend routine cultures in the absence of signs of infection.

ESI is encountered with all types of catheters, is unpredictable, may develop at any time during long-term peritoneal dialysis, and tends to be prolonged, chronic, or recurrent. ESI and tunnel infections are major causes of morbidity among patients undergoing peritoneal dialysis because they lead to recurrent peritonitis, catheter failure, and prolonged hospitalization. With the reduction in peritonitis after the introduction of the various forms of the disconnect system, ESI and tunnel infections have become the primary infectious complications of peritoneal dialysis.

Factors that may predispose to ESI include peritoneal dialysate leak, excessive movement of the catheter such as pulling and twisting during bag exchange, a tight tunnel, and pressure necrosis caused by constricting sutures. In addition, a patient's nasal carriage of *Staphylococcus aureus* is associated with a higher incidence of ESI with this organism.

S. aureus alone is responsible for 50% (25% to 85%) of ESI and tunnel infections; on the other hand, various organisms, including *S. aureus,* are isolated from the skin of 16% to 35% of the patients. Such microorganisms include enteric gram-negative bacteria (7% to 14%), *Staphylococcus epidermidis* (5% to 14%), *Pseudomonas aeruginosa* (8% to 12%), and fungi (1% to 3%). Seven to 11% of patients with ESI have negative exit site cultures. ESI rates vary widely, from 0.05 to 1.02 episodes per patient-year. This discrepancy reflects mainly disagreements about the correct definition of ESI. The management of ESI is outlined in Figure 19–10. A traumatized exit site is prone to infection, and in such a situation, the use of a prophylactic antibiotic may prevent serious infection. We routinely perform Gram stains and cultures of the purulent exudate obtained from the exit site. A culture of an erythematous exit site in the absence of

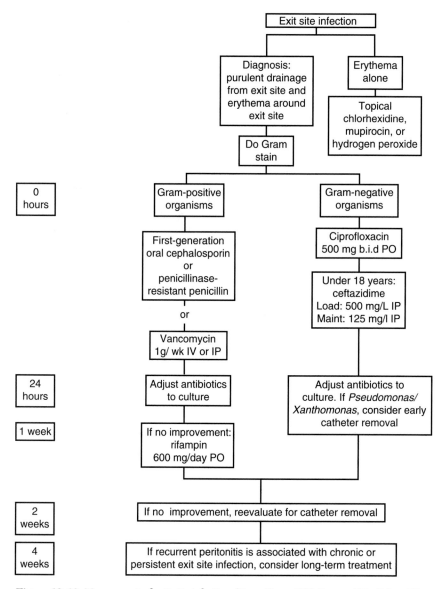

Figure 19–10. Management of exit site infection. (From Keane WF, Everett ED, Golper TA, et al: Peritoneal dialysis-related peritonitis treatment recommendations. 1993 update. Perit Dial Int 13:25, 1993.)

purulent discharge may give misleading results, and we do not recommend this practice as a routine.

TUNNEL INFECTION

The term *tunnel* refers to the catheter's path from the skin through the subcutaneous fat and muscle to the peritoneal cuff. In double-cuff catheters, the tunnel is the area between the two cuffs. The signs of infection in the tunnel include induration or redness, tenderness, and pain, with or without an obvious abscess. Actual tunnel infection without ESI is rare. Although ESI can be treated successfully by antibiotics, rarely can one cure deep cuff infections, and management usually requires catheter removal.

Cuff Extrusion

An important cause of subcutaneous (peripheral) cuff extrusion is placement of the cuff close under the skin, or local infection. Another cause is the resilience of the silicon rubber, which forces the catheter to assume its original shape.

Dialysate Leakage (Late)

Late dialysis leakage may present as a discharge of clear fluid around the catheter, as a localized swelling of the subcutaneous tissue of the anterior abdominal wall, or as swelling of the genitalia. When the site of leakage is unknown, computed tomography (CT) after infusion of 2 L of dialysate containing a radiocontrast material (diatrizoate meglumine, 100 ml), may identify the source. Also, scintigraphy of the lower abdominal and genital area after intraperitoneal instillation of radioisotope (technetium Tc 99m sulfate colloid, 3.5 to 5.0 mCi/2 L dialysate) may demonstrate an inguinal or umbilical hernia). In the management of such leakage, temporary discontinuation of CAPD, substitution with IPD or NIPD, with small volumes in the supine position or temporary hemodialysis for 3 to 4 weeks may be helpful. However, most late leakages defy conservative treatment and require surgical repair.

Various Abdominal Events in Chronic Peritoneal Dialysis

In addition to catheter-related complications and those related to the presence of dialysate in the peritoneal cavity, patients undergoing chronic peritoneal dialysis are subject to the same abdominal events as the general population. Some clues to a surgical emergency in a patient undergoing peritoneal dialysis are localized tenderness and abdominal pain, bowel loop dilatation, an unusual increase in free intraperitoneal air on a plain radiograph, especially under the right diaphragm, mixed flora on Gram stain or culture of dialysate, refractory peritonitis, high peritoneal fluid level of amylase, and hemoperitoneum with measurable hematocrit.

Dialysate-Related Complications

Intraabdominal pressure is determined by the volume of peritoneal dialysis solution as well as by body weight, abdominal girth, body mass index, and age. Coughing, straining, walking, and the sitting position increase intraperitoneal pressure. Many believe the presence of the intraperitoneal solution may contribute to hernias, abdominal wall and genital edema, hemoperitoneum, hydrothorax, and back pain. These complications are less frequent in APD because in this mode the intraabdominal pressure is **lower** during recumbency.

Hernias

It has been estimated that 10% to 25% of the CAPD population develop hernias. Predisposing factors are female sex, old age, obesity, multiparity, early pericatheter dialysate leakage, and previous hernia repair. Of the several types of hernias that occur, the most common are inguinal, umbilical, and those related to catheter incisions. Unlike a midline incision, paramedian entry through the rectus muscle decreases the possibility of local herniation. Because bowel incarceration and strangulation is a risk, especially in small hernias, these should be corrected on an elective basis.

Patients can start CAPD 2 to 4 weeks after a hernia repair. During this period, they are treated by IPD using small volumes or by hemodialysis using subclavian or jugular vein catheters.

Abdominal Wall and Genital Edema

Abdominal wall and genital edema develops in about 10% of patients on CAPD. One should suspect abdominal wall edema in patients with a sudden decrease in effluent volume, increased abdominal girth or body weight, and no evidence of edema elsewhere. A CT scan after contrast medium has been instilled into the peritoneal cavity along with 2 L of dialysate is highly sensitive in identifying peritoneal leaks. Small leaks are initially treated with bed rest and with forms of peritoneal dialysis associated with lower intraabdominal pressure (APD). When this fails, CAPD is discontinued and the patient undergoes hemodialysis for 4 to 6 weeks. In persistent cases, surgical repair is necessary.

Hemoperitoneum

Hemoperitoneum is a transient complication of CAPD that may occur at any time. In women of childbearing age, hemoperitoneum may be associated with menses, ovulation, or endometriosis. Other causes include colonoscopy, ischemic bowel, catheter repositioning, abdominal trauma, pancytopenia, thrombocytopenic purpura, and increased physical activity.

Abdominal bleeding may follow a lesion of an adjacent extraperitoneal structure (e.g., polycystic kidneys, polycystic liver with intracystic bleeding, femoral hematoma, cholecystitis, or pancreatitis). Severe bleeding such as that from a ruptured spleen requires immediate surgical intervention.

Hydrothorax

Hydrothorax, which occurs in 1% to 2% of patients on CAPD, may present early or late as an asymptomatic pleural effusion or as acute respiratory failure. Approximately 90% of hydrothoraces occur on the right side, probably because the heart and pericardium cover left-sided defects in the diaphragm.

Pleural fluid is a transudate with a low concentration of lactate dehydrogenase and high concentration of glucose, much higher than that of blood. Radioactive albumin added to dialysate can be detected in the thorax. The attending physician must rule out other causes of hydrothorax such as cardiac failure and inflammatory and malignant diseases. In more than half of these patients, the hydrothorax can be managed by discontinuing CAPD alone or in combination with pleurodesis; the remaining patients are transferred to hemodialysis permanently.

Back Pain

The factors predisposing to low back pain in patients on CAPD are degenerative or metabolic bone disease of the spine, poor muscle tone, low exercise tolerance, arthritis of the hip, neuropathy, and myopathy. Dialysis fluid in the abdomen pulls forward the center of gravity and changes spinal mechanics by increasing lumbar lordosis. A special abdominal support and an individualized exercise program may control the low back pain. If these are not effective, the patient is converted to NIPD.

Peritonitis

The incidence of peritonitis, which is a common complication during CAPD, varies from center to center. During the 1980s, an overall average incidence was 1.3 episodes per patient per year. With the introduction of disconnect systems (Y-set, double bag), the average incidence of CAPD peritonitis has fallen to 0.75 to 0.5 episodes per patient per year.

Patients undergoing IPD have a low incidence of peritonitis—one episode per 3 to 5 patient-years, and the incidence in the various forms of APD is between that of CAPD and that of IPD.

About 75% of the responsible pathogens are gram-positive organisms derived from normal

TABLE 19–1. Relative Frequency of Organisms Causing Peritonitis

Organism	Frequency (%)
Coagulase-negative *Staphylococcus*	30–40
Staphylococcus aureus	15–20
Streptococcus spp.	10–15
Neisseria spp.	1–2
Diphtheroid spp.	1–2
Escherichia coli	5–10
Pseudomonas spp.	5–10
Enterococcus	3–6
Klebsiella spp.	1–3
Proteus spp.	3–6
Acinetobacter spp.	2–5
Anaerobic organisms	2–5
Fungi	2–10
Other (mycobacteria, etc.)	2–5
Culture negative	0–30

From Vas SI: Treatment of peritonitis. Perit Dial Int 14(Suppl 3):S49, 1994.

skin and nasal flora (i.e., *S. aureus* and *S. epidermidis* (Table 19–1). However, patients using the Y-set systems, who have a lower incidence of gram-positive peritonitis, have a relative increase in gram-negative peritonitis. Table 19–2 shows the route of entry and the common pathogens.

The most common cause of peritonitis is contamination at the connection site of the transfer set and the bag during the exchange procedure; another common source is ESI or tunnel infection.

Peritonitis due to *S. epidermidis* is usually mild and resolves quickly with treatment. In contrast, peritonitis due to *S. aureus* has a more severe and prolonged course and exhibits a tendency to abscess formation. Patients with *S. aureus* perito-

TABLE 19–2. Routes of Infections in CAPD Patients

Route	Organism	%
Transluminal	*S. epidermidis*	
	Acinetobacter	30–40
Periluminal	*S. epidermidis*	
	S. aureus	
	Pseudomonas	20–30
Transmural	Yeast	
	Enteric gram negative	
	Anaerobes	25–30
Hematogenous	*Streptococcus*	
	M. tuberculosis	5–10
Ascending	Yeast	
	Lactobacillus	2–5

From Keane WF, Vas SI: Peritonitis. In Gokal R, Nolph KD: The Textbook of Peritoneal Dialysis. Dordrecht, The Netherlands, Kluwer Academic, 1994, p 476. Reprinted by permission of Kluwer Academic Publishers.

nitis may occasionally present with the septic shock syndrome, and under these circumstances, the peritoneal space should be lavaged with dialysis solution containing appropriate antibiotics for 24 to 48 hours. *Streptococcus viridans* produces severe peritonitis with marked constitutional symptoms, but the infection resolves easily with appropriate treatment. Peritonitis due to *Pseudomonas* often is refractory to antibiotics and produces abscesses in the peritoneal cavity. The peritoneal catheter usually has to be removed for cure. Catheter removal is also indicated in peritonitis caused by gut flora (multiple organisms) or fungi or if the peritonitis is associated with ESI by the same organism.

If the culture of spent dialysate is negative, despite good culture techniques, the condition is called aseptic or culture-negative peritonitis; this usually represents a reaction to chemicals, plasticizers, endotoxin, or antibiotics (vancomycin). Eosinophilic peritonitis, another culture-negative peritonitis of unknown cause, is asymptomatic and is associated with cloudy dialysate, consisting mainly of eosinophils (>20%). This variant usually develops during the first month after catheter implantation and subsides within 1 to 3 months without specific treatment.

Diagnosis of Peritonitis

A clinical diagnosis of peritonitis requires any two of these three:

1. Signs and symptoms of peritoneal inflammation such as abdominal pain, rebound tenderness, and, in children, an elevated temperature
2. Cloudy dialysate (cell count 100 cells/mm^3 with 50% polymorphonuclear cells)
3. Presence of organisms on Gram stain or on subsequent culture of dialysate

Sampling and Culturing the Peritoneal Dialysis Effluent

Ideally, the effluent should be analyzed promptly after peritonitis is suspected. Alternatively, the bag may be stored at room temperature or in a refrigerator and examined within 6 hours.

Initially, a 10- to 50-ml aliquot is centrifuged and the sediment examined by Gram stain.

Use the following techniques for the culture of peritoneal dialysis effluent:

1. Centrifuge 10 to 50 ml of effluent and resuspend in 1 ml of nutrient broth or normal saline. Inoculate a portion of it in blood and McConkey agar. Observe for growth for at least 72 hours (7 days may be preferable).

2. Alternatively, one may use semiautomated blood culture systems such as Septi-Chek, BACTEC, Isolator, or Signal systems.

The addition of antiphagocyte substances, such as polyanethol sulfonate (SPS), and antibiotic-binding resins may increase the yield of positive cultures.

Total WBC counts and differential cell counts are performed on a noncentrifuged aliquot of effluent. A WBC count can be obtained by automated instruments or in a standard hemocytometer counting chamber. The differential cell count should be performed on a cytocentrifuge preparation stained with a supravital dye such as Wright's stain.

Gram stain results are positive in 9% to 40% of peritonitis episodes and, when positive, predict the species of organism in about 85% of cases. A Gram stain may be helpful in the detection of fungal peritonitis. Because the results of dialysate culture will delay treatment for 1 to 2 days, one should rely on Gram stain to initiate therapy (discussed later) (Fig. 19–11).

General Rules in Treating CAPD Peritonitis

- Although initial treatment should be blind—that is, started immediately before isolation of organisms—all treatment should eventually be guided by the antibiotic sensitivity of the causative organism.
- If no clinical improvement or no decrease in cell count of dialysis fluid occurs in 2 to 3 days, repeat the culture.
- If, after 5 days, cultures are consistently positive and the effluent remains cloudy, consider catheter removal, especially in the presence of ESI with the same organism.
- Gram-positive peritonitis is treated for 14 days (three weekly doses of vancomycin); for gram-negative peritonitis, treatment lasts 21 days, and for *Pseudomonas/Xanthomonas* peritonitis 28 days.
- One can attempt to treat fungal peritonitis. If no improvement occurs in clinical course, cell count, or cultures, the catheter should promptly be removed.

Initiation of Peritonitis Therapy Based on Gram Stain (Fig. 19–12)

Table 19–3 shows the pharmacokinetics of the antibiotics commonly used in the regimens proposed for the treatment of CAPD peritonitis.

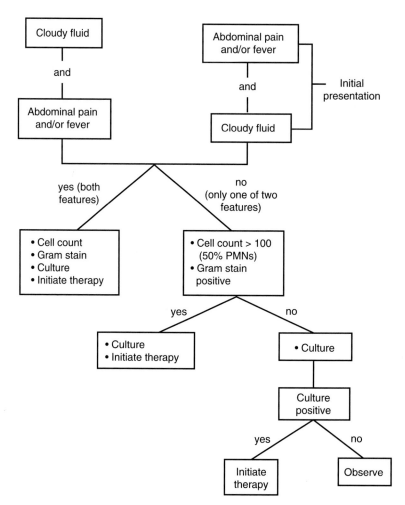

Figure 19–11. Initial clinical and laboratory assessment in CAPD peritonitis. (From Keane WF, Everett ED, Golper TA, et al: Peritoneal dialysis-related peritonitis treatment recommendations. 1993 update. Perit Dial Int 13:16, 1993.)

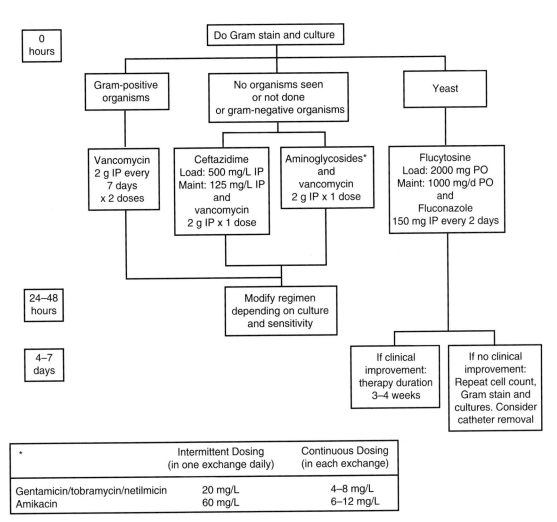

Figure 19–12. On clinical presentation with peritonitis. (From Keane WF, Everett ED, Golper TA, et al: Peritoneal dialysis-related peritonitis treatment recommendations. 1993 update. Perit Dial Int 13:18, 1993.)

TABLE 19–3. Pharmacokinetics of Antibiotics in CAPD Patients and Proposed Regimens for the Treatment of CAPD Peritonitis[*]

| | Half-Life (H) | | | Dose (per 70-kg Adult)[*] | | Maintenance Dose |
	Normal	ESRD	CAPD	Initial Dose (mg/2-L bag)	Intermittent mg/2-L Bag per Dosing Interval	Continuous (mg/2 L-bag)
Aminoglycosides						
Amikacin	1.6	39	40	500	120/d	12–24
Gentamicin	2.2	53	32	70–140	40/d	8–16
Netilmicin	2.1	42	18	70–140	40/d	8–16
Tobramycin	2.5	58	36	70–140	40/d	8–16
Cephalosporins						
First generation						
Cefazolin	2.2	28	30	500–1000	1000/d	250–500
Cefonicid	4.0	68	50	250	ND	50
Cephalothin	0.2	3.7	ND	1000	ND	200
Cephradine	0.9	12	ND	500	ND	250
Cephalexin	0.8	19	9	1000 PO	500/q.i.d. PO	NA
Second generation						
Cefamandole	1.0	10	8.0	1000	1000/d	500
Cefmenoxime	1.3	11.3	8.0	2000	1000/d	100
Cefoxitin	0.8	20	15	1000	ND	200
Cefuroxime	1.3	18	15	1000	400/d IV/PO	150–400
Third generation						
Cefixime	3.2	11.5	15	400 PO	400/d PO	NA
Cefoperazone	1.8	2.3	2.2	2000	ND	400–1000
Cefotaxime	0.9	2.5	2.4	2000	2000/d	500
Cefsulodin	1.8	11	11	1000	500/d	50
Ceftazidime	1.8	26	13	1000	1000/d	250
Ceftizoxime	1.6	28	11	1000	1000/d	250
Ceftriaxone	8.0	15	12	1000	1000/d	250–500
Moxalactam	2.2	20	16	1000	1000/d	350
Penicillins						
Azlocillin	0.9	5.1	ND	500	ND	500
Mezlocillin	1.0	4.3	ND	3000 IV	3000/b.i.d. IV	500
Piperacillin	1.2	3.9	2.4	4000 IV	4000/b.i.d. IV	500
Ticarcillin	1.2	15	ND	1000–2000	2000/b.i.d.	250
Quinolones						
Ciprofloxacin	4.0	8.0	11	500 PO	500/t.i.d. PO	50
Fleroxacin	13	27	27	800 PO	400/d PO	NA
Ofloxacin	7.0	30	25	400 PO	200/d PO	NA
Vancomycin and others						
Vancomycin	6.9	161	92	1000–2000	1–2000/7 d	30–50
Teicoplanin	50	260	260	400	400/b.i.d.	40†
Aztreonam	2.0	7.0	9.3	1000	1000/d	500
Clindamycin	2.8	2.8	ND	300	ND	300
Erythromycin	2.1	4.0	ND	ND	500/q.i.d. PO	150
Metronidazole	7.9	7.7	11	500 PO/IV	500/t.i.d. PO/IV	ND
Minocycline	15.5	20	ND	NA	100/b.i.d. PO	NA
Rifampin	4.0	8.0	ND	600 PO	600/d PO	NA
Antifungal agents						
Amphotericin B	360	360	ND	NA	20–30/d IV	2.8
Flucytosine	4.2	115	ND	2000–3000 PO	1000/d PO	NA
Fluconazole	22	125	72	NA	150 mg q 2 d	ND
Ketoconazole	2.0	1.8	2.4	400 PO	200–800/d PO	NA
Miconazole	24	25	ND	200	ND	100–200
Combinations						
Amphicillin	1.3	15	9.3	1000–2000	1000/b.i.d.	100
Sulbactam	1.0	19	9.7	1000–2000	1000/b.i.d.	100
Imipenem	0.9	3.0	6.4	1000	500/b.i.d.	200
Cilastatin	0.8	15	19	500–1000	500/b.i.d.	100–200
Sulfamethoxazole	10	13	14	1600 PO	1600/1–2 d PO	400
Trimethoprim	14	33	34	320 PO	320/1–2 d PO	80

From Keane WF, Everett ED, Golper TA, et al: Peritoneal dialysis-related peritonitis treatment recommendations. 1993 update. Perit Dial Int 13:14, 1993.

[*]The route of administration is intraperitoneal unless otherwise specified. The pharmacokinetic data and proposed dosage regimens presented here are based on published literature reviewed through April 1992. There is no evidence that mixing different antibiotics in dialysis fluid (except for aminoglycosides and penicillins) is deleterious for the drugs or patients. Do not use the same syringe to mix antibiotics.

†This is in each bag × 7 days, then in 2 bags/day × 7 days, and then in 1 bag/day × 7 days.

ESRD, creatinine clearance < 10 ml/min, patient not on dialysis; NA, not applicable; ND, no data; IV, intravenous; PO, oral; d, once a day; b.i.d., twice a day; t.i.d., three times a day; q.i.d., four times a day.

If a gram-positive organism is seen on Gram stain, treat with vancomycin.

If the stain reveals a gram-negative organism (rarely), treat with one dose of either ceftazidime or an aminoglycoside *plus* vancomycin, 2 g intraperitoneally. Vancomycin can be given continuously in each of the four daily exchanges at a dose of 30 to 50 mg/2 L. Aminoglycosides can be given either intermittently (one dose per day) or continuously (one dose in each exchange). The finding of a mixed infection (gram-positive and gram-negative bacteria or two or more gram-negative organisms) indicates bowel perforation and calls for prompt surgical evaluation.

If the Gram stain reveals no organism, as in most episodes of peritonitis, or the result is not available at the time of decision, we recommend the combination of ceftazidime or an aminoglycoside plus vancomycin, as mentioned earlier. When the results of culture and sensitivity tests become available, usually in 24 to 48 hours, the regimen should be modified according to the new information (discussed later).

If Gram stain reveals yeast, administer flucytosine and fluconazole.

Because prompt initiation of therapy for peritonitis is critical, patients are instructed to report immediately their symptoms to the center. They should be given an adequate supply of antimicrobials and should be trained on the treatment of peritonitis.

For patients on CCPD or NIPD, antibiotics are given into the peritoneal cavity during the daytime exchange and retained there for the whole day. However, because the absorption is complete, they are given half the recommended dose of vancomycin for 6 hours' dwell.

Modification of Peritonitis Therapy Based on Culture and Sensitivity Results (Figs. 19–13 to 19–15)

About 70% to 90% of appropriately cultured dialysate samples yield at least one specific microorganism, usually within 24 to 48 hours.

GRAM-POSITIVE ORGANISMS CULTURED (Fig. 19–13)

If the culture identifies S. aureus, S. epidermidis, or streptococci, we had recommended therapy

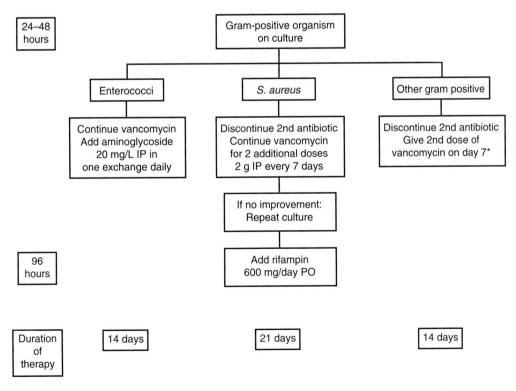

*Choice of treatment should be guided by antibiotic sensitivity patterns

Figure 19–13. Gram-positive organism cultured. (From Keane WF, Everett ED, Golper TA, et al: Peritoneal dialysis-related peritonitis treatment recommendations. 1993 update. Perit Dial Int 13:20, 1993.)

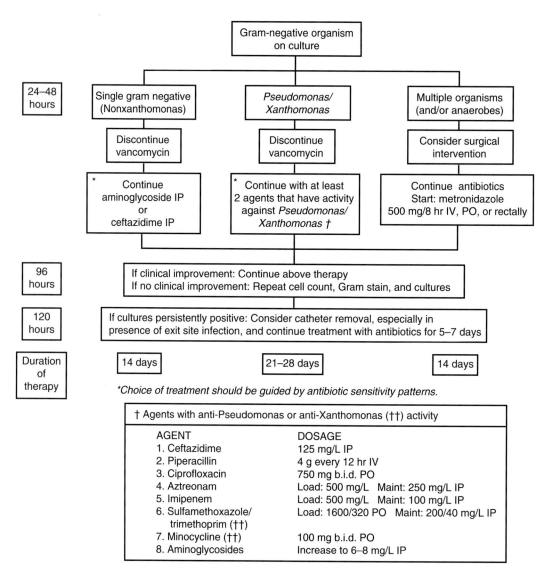

Figure 19–14. Gram-negative organism cultured. (From Keane WF, Everett ED, Golper TA, et al: Peritoneal dialysis-related peritonitis treatment recommendations. 1993 update. Perit Dial Int 13:21, 1993.)

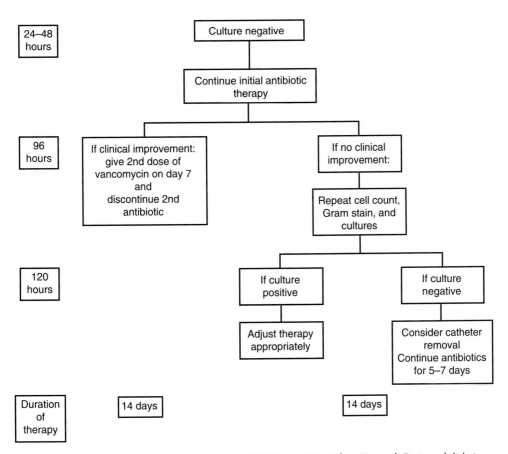

Figure 19–15. No organism cultured. (From Keane WF, Everett ED, Golper TA, et al: Peritoneal dialysis-related peritonitis treatment recommendations. 1993 update. Perit Dial Int 13:22, 1993.)

with vancomycin alone, but new recommendations have just emerged: please see addendum. In *S. aureus* peritonitis, rifampin (600 mg po/day, in three divided doses) should be added and treatment continued for 3 weeks.

If an enterococcus is identified, one should add an aminoglycoside (20 mg/L intraperitoneally in one exchange per day). The choice of antibiotic should be based on sensitivity. Patients should also be carefully evaluated for evidence of intraabdominal pathology.

Addendum

Due to concerns about the increasing prevalence of vancomycin-resistant microorganisms, the Advisory Committee on Peritonitis Management of the International Society of Peritoneal Dialysis has recently changed its recommendations for the treatment of peritonitis in PD patients.

According to the 1996 update, it is recommended that a first-generation cephalosporin (e.g., cefazolin or cephalothin) along with an aminoglycoside be used instead of vancomycin.

The loading dose for either cefazolin or cephalothin is 500 mg/L and the maintenance dose is 125 mg/L. For gentamicin, tobramycin, or netilmicin the dose is 0.6 mg/kg of body weight in only one exchange per day. The dose of amikacin is 2 mg/kg of body weight, also in only one exchange per day.

Detailed recommendations can be found in Peritoneal Dialysis International, Volume 16, 1996.

ISOLATION OF GRAM-NEGATIVE ORGANISMS (Fig. 19–14)

If gram-negative organisms are found, it is imperative to assess the patient for evidence of superadded intraabdominal pathology. If only a single gram-negative organism is identified (*Escherichia coli, Klebsiella, Proteus, Pseudomonas*), the second dose of vancomycin is not necessary. Based on sensitivity results, one should use an aminoglycoside alone or ceftazidine alone.

If anaerobic bacteria are isolated, either alone or in combination with other gram-negative organisms, bowel perforation is very likely and early surgical intervention should be considered. In such cases, add metronidazole (500 mg IV, PO, or rectally every 8 hours) to the combination of vancomycin and ceftazidine (see Fig. 19–12).

If culture reveals *P. aeruginosa* or *Xanthomo-*

nas, one should administer at least two antibiotics that have demonstrable *in vitro* activity against these organisms (see Fig. 19–14). In patients undergoing CAPD, *Pseudomonas* peritonitis, particularly that related to catheter infection, is extremely resistant to treatment and catheter removal should be considered. If the patient is improving clinically, therapy of *Pseudomonas/Xanthomonas* peritonitis should be continued for 3 to 4 weeks. If no improvement is noted, we recommend early catheter removal to avoid loss of peritoneal function.

NO ORGANISMS ISOLATED (Fig. 19–15)

If no organisms are isolated and if the patient is improving clinically with the initial combination regimen (see Fig. 19–12), continue therapy for 4 to 5 days and then stop the second antibiotic (ceftazidime or aminoglycoside). Therapy with vancomycin alone is continued for a total of 2 weeks. If, on the other hand, no clinical improvement occurs, the patient should be reevaluated and catheter removal considered.

FUNGAL ORGANISMS CULTURED

It is reasonable to continue antifungal therapy with flucytosine and fluconazole (or amphotericin B alone) for 4 to 7 days. If, however, no clinical improvement occurs in this time, one should remove the catheter and continue oral therapy with flucytosine 1000 mg and fluconazole 100 mg daily for an additional 10 days. If, on the other hand, clinical improvement is satisfactory, continue antifungal therapy for a total of 4 to 6 weeks.

Adjunctive Therapy of CAPD Peritonitis

A common practice is to perform two to three rapid exchanges of isotonic (1.5% dextrose) dialysate, without antibiotics, every 20 minutes, immediately after the diagnosis of peritonitis. This lavage relieves abdominal pain by removing the mediators of inflammation, but it may also reduce peritoneal defenses and remove valuable phagocytic cells. After these rapid exchanges, one continues the regular CAPD or APD regimen with added antibiotics. We also add heparin (1000 U/L IP) to inhibit fibrin formation due to the large quantities of fibrinogen that appear in the inflamed peritoneal cavity. Some workers have used fibrinolytics such as streptokinase or urokinase in cases of persistent peritonitis or when catheters are blocked by fibrin, but their efficacy has not been proved. The connection tube is changed during the first 24 hours after the initiation of therapy.

Side Effects of Antibiotic Therapy

The use of antibiotics in the treatment of peritonitis in patients undergoing CAPD is associated with side effects such as hypersensitivity reactions, eosinophilia in the peritoneal fluid, skin rash, nephrotoxicity, ototoxicity, and others. In the past, some workers reported chemical peritonitis after the use of intraperitoneal vancomycin, but this side effect is now disappearing.

When prescribing potentially nephrotoxic agents such as aminoglycosides, one should bear in mind that preservation of residual renal function is of the utmost importance in patients undergoing dialysis, because the loss of such function may make necessary one extra bag exchange per day. In the concentrations recommended here, evidence of nephrotoxicity has not been reported. Ototoxicity in patients on CAPD has been attributed to gentamicin but not to tobramycin, netilmicin, or amikacin.

Rifampin may cause nausea or elevation of liver enzyme values, and it may be necessary to decrease the dose or to discontinue the drug. Rifampin also may interfere with the action of oral contraceptives. Finally, some workers have reported pseudomembranous enterocolitis in CAPD recipients undergoing treatment for peritonitis.

Antibiotic Prophylaxis

No solid evidence shows that prophylactic antibiotics prevent peritonitis. Also, no prospective studies have demonstrated that prophylactic antibiotics at the time of catheter insertion decrease catheter-related infections or peritonitis. However, based on other surgical experience, many workers consider its use acceptable.

As has been shown, dental work and gastrointestinal or genitourinary instrumentation may lead to peritonitis in patients on CAPD. Therefore, administration of antibiotic prophylaxis (as in cardiac patients) may be prudent, although its efficacy is not proved (Table 19–4).

We treat accidental contaminations with a tubing change followed by a course of cephalosporin or a single intravenous injection of 1 g of vancomycin.

Consequences of CAPD Peritonitis

During peritonitis, peritoneal clearances of large and small molecules increase and glucose absorption also increases, probably because of the inflammation. This inflammation may result in hypoproteinemia and decreased ultrafiltration. Peritonitis may lead to the formation of extensive adhesions within the peritoneal cavity, particularly if it is due to enteric bacteria, *S. aureus*, or *Pseudomonas*. In such cases, the peritoneum may lose its capacity for ultrafiltration.

Loss of ultrafiltration also is an early sign of sclerosing encapsulating peritonitis, a rare condition characterized by the formation of a dense layer of fibroconnective tissue on the membrane. Other symptoms of this complication include recurrent abdominal pain, vomiting, and bowel obstruction.

PATIENT NUMBER 4

One morning, Charlotte, a 67-year-old widow who had been on CAPD for 26 months (her primary renal lesion was nephrosclerosis), called the peritoneal dialysis unit (PDU) and reported that the effluent of her morning bag exchange was cloudy. In addition, she was nauseated and had mild diffuse abdominal tenderness. Because Charlotte had not had peritonitis in the past and did not know how to perform the peritonitis protocol, the PDU nurse instructed her to come immediately to the hospital with her morning bag. Within 2 hours, Charlotte arrived in the unit, carrying a moderately cloudy bag.

On examination, her temperature was 37.5°C, her blood pressure was 132/76 mm Hg, and her body weight was 71.5 kg (usually 70.0 kg). She had moderate diffuse abdominal pain and rebound tenderness. The exit site was clear. When the effluent of the second bag exchange was grossly cloudy, we made the diagnosis of peritonitis. We immediately performed three exchanges of dialysate, 1.5% dextrose, without antibiotics, every 20 minutes. In the meantime, the bag with the cloudy effluent was sent for Gram stain, cell count/differential, and cultures. A 30-ml aliquot was centrifuged, and the sediment, examined by Gram stain, revealed no organisms. A noncentrifuged aliquot of the cloudy effluent examined in a standard hemocytometer chamber revealed 600 WBCs/mm³, and a cytocentrifuged preparation of the effluent, stained with Wright's stain, showed 75% polymorphonuclear cells. Because the Gram stain revealed no organism, her initial treatment consisted of a combination of aminoglycoside and vancomycin. The specific orders were as follows:

1. After the three rapid exchanges with isotonic dialysate, start regular CAPD
2. To the first 2-L bag add
   a. Tobramycin, 140 mg
   b. Heparin, 2000 U

TABLE 19–4. Antibiotic Prophylaxis for CAPD Patients

For Dental and Upper Respiratory Tract Procedures	

Oral prophylaxis
  Amoxicillin 3 g single dose PO 1 hour before procedure
  followed by 1.5 g PO 6 hours after initial dose
	Parenteral prophylaxis
	  2 g ampicillin IM or IV 30 min before procedure; 1 g of
	  ampicillin IM or IV 6 hours after initial dose

For patients allergic to penicillin or ampicillin
Oral prophylaxis
  Erythromycin stearate 1.0 g PO 1 hour before procedure
  followed by 0.5 g PO 6 hours after initial dose
            or
  Erythromycin ethylsuccinate 800 mg PO 1 hour before
  procedure followed by 400 mg 6 hours after initial dose
            or
  Clindamycin 300 mg PO 1 hour before procedure followed
  by 150 mg PO 6 hours after initial dose
	Parenteral prophylaxis
	  Vancomycin 1 g IV 1 hour before procedure

For Gastrointestinal or Genitourinary Procedures	

Oral prophylaxis
  Amoxicillin 3 g PO 1 hour before procedure followed by
  amoxicillin 1.5 g 6 hours after the initial dose
	Parenteral prophylaxis
	  Ampicillin 2 g IV or IM and 1.5 mg/kg tobramycin 30 min
	  before procedure followed by ampicillin 1 g IV or IM 6
	  hours after the initial dose

For patients allergic to penicillin or ampicillin
Oral prophylaxis
  None
	Parenteral prophylaxis
	  Vancomycin 1 g IV and tobramycin 1.5 mg/kg IV 1 hour
	  before procedure

From Vas SI: Treatment of peritonitis. Perit Dial Int 14(Suppl 3):S53, 1994.

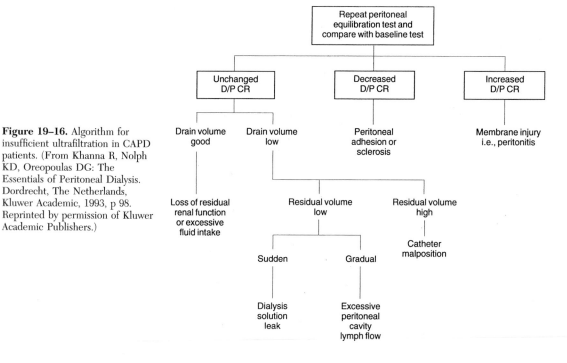

Figure 19–16. Algorithm for insufficient ultrafiltration in CAPD patients. (From Khanna R, Nolph KD, Oreopoulas DG: The Essentials of Peritoneal Dialysis. Dordrecht, The Netherlands, Kluwer Academic, 1993, p 98. Reprinted by permission of Kluwer Academic Publishers.)

3. To each subsequent bag add
   a. Tobramycin, 16 mg
   b. Heparin, 2000 U
4. Vancomycin, 1 g in 250 ml of normal saline, is immediately given IV over 30 minutes
5. Change the connecting tube in the evening

The next day, Charlotte showed considerable improvement. Her abdominal pain had subsided, and she had no rebound tenderness: She had only mild abdominal tenderness on deep palpation. Her vital signs were stable, and she was afebrile. The effluent was only slightly cloudy.

On the third day (48 hours after admission), cultures from both bags revealed *S. viridans* sensitive to vancomycin. Tobramycin was discontinued, and orders were given that the intravenous vancomycin dose be repeated every 7 days for two additional doses.

The patient had no symptoms, her effluent was clear, and she was discharged home with instructions to add heparin to each bag and to visit the PDU for her vancomycin dose (on days 7 and 14).

ULTRAFILTRATION FAILURE IN CAPD

We have no clear quantitative definition of ultrafiltration failure in CAPD. However, for practical reasons, we can agree that a patient on CAPD has ultrafiltration failure when he or she requires more than two hypertonic (3.86% dextrose) exchanges daily to maintain water balance in the absence of edema and of excess fluid intake.

Inadequate ultrafiltration is one of the most common problems encountered in patients receiving long-term peritoneal dialysis. After catheter-related problems, inadequate ultrafiltration is the second leading cause of transfer of CAPD patients to hemodialysis.

Ultrafiltration failure is chiefly encountered during peritonitis and after long-term CAPD.

Based on the postulated pathogenic mechanism, we may classify ultrafiltration failure into the following groups:

Type 1 failure—due to excessive absorption of glucose, secondary to a hyperpermeable peritoneal membrane

Type 2 failure—characterized by poor permeability usually associated with sclerosing peritonitis

Type 3 failure—excessive lymphatic absorption from the peritoneal cavity

Other types of fluid overload without any change in peritoneal transport, usually due to mechanical factors

Finally, it should be kept in mind that one of the most common causes of fluid overload is excessive oral intake.

Figure 19–16 outlines the differential diagnosis of ultrafiltration failure, and Table 19–5 gives the treatment options.

ACUTE PERITONEAL DIALYSIS

PATIENT NUMBER 5

Tony, a 35-year-old divorced man, had been admitted 3 days earlier to a surgical clinic with complicated fractures of the left upper arm and both lower limbs and open wounds on his back. After an earthquake, he had been found by a search team under the debris of his fallen house. After emergency surgical management, his vital signs were stabilized but he became progressively oliguric and edematous. He did not respond to the administration of large doses of furosemide. Since admission, his BUN had risen to 150 mg/dl and serum creatinine to 8 mg/dl. His serum potassium level was 7.2mmol/l, and his levels of serum amino transferases and creatinine kinase were high. A nephrology consultation led to the diagnosis of acute renal failure secondary to rhabdomyolysis. How would you treat this patient?

TABLE 19–5. Management of Reduced Ultrafiltration

Type 1 Failure	Type 2 Failure	Type 3 Failure
Increased permeability	*Sclerosing peritonitis*	*Increased lymphatic absorption*
Use short dwell times only 4 × 6 hr	? Use tidal peritoneal dialysis	No treatment available
	Furosemide	
High-dose furosemide if there is residual renal function	Transfer to hemodialysis	
Use solutions with Icodextrin		
Hemodialysis		

The management of mechanical causes such as hernias, dialysate leakage, catheter malposition, peritoneal adhesions, and so on is discussed under complications of CAPD.

The main indications for acute peritoneal dialysis in uremic patients are

1. Acute renal failure in which recovery of renal function is anticipated
2. Initial dialysis in patients with ESRD. The nonuremic indications for acute peritoneal dialysis are discussed later.

In an emergency, acute peritoneal dialysis can be performed through a semirigid peritoneal catheter. The bedside insertion technique (see Appendix 2) is easy and quickly accomplished.

In patients with acute renal failure who require peritoneal dialysis for only a week or two, most centers use semirigid straight plastic catheters that have multiple side holes (Fig. 19–17). However some centers prefer to insert a soft Tenckhoff-type catheter (see Fig. 19–1) at the bedside because the semirigid one requires frequent manipulation to maintain good function and is associated with an increased risk of peritonitis after 3 or 4 days of use.

Possible Complications After Acute Catheter Implantation

Bleeding and Wound Hematoma. This is rare if hemostasis is carefully performed.

Visceral Trauma or Perforation. Perforation or injury of the large and small bowel, aorta, mesenteric vessels, bladder, and other abdominal viscera has been reported during blind catheter insertion. One should not persist with forceful insertion against intraabdominal resistance.

Bloody Effluent. Such effluent is due to incomplete hemostasis, and the bleeding is usually from the anterior abdominal wall. Several in-and-out exchanges of unwarmed dialysis solution usually clear the dialysate of blood. A patient with a bleeding disorder may require transfusion of fresh blood. On rare occasions, bleeding from a pierced small artery requires surgical exploration.

Abdominal Pain. Diffuse or local pain and tenderness around the incision after catheter implantation are of minor significance and can be controlled with simple analgesics. A few patients have pain over the perineal area, in the rectum, or in the urinary bladder. This subsides spontaneously within a few days. If the pain is severe or lasts longer, the attending physician should obtain radiologic verification of the position of the catheter and should relocate it using a trocar or peritoneoscopy (in the case of a Tenckhoff straight catheter). Localized outflow pain usually indicates catheter entrapment by the omentum. Low or high dialysate temperatures may induce abdominal pain; hence, we recommend a temperature of 37°C. Inflow pain may be controlled by decreasing flow rate or, in case of a stylet catheter, by pulling it out slightly.

Dialysate Leakage (Early). One usually encounters early pericatheter leakage in obese or diabetic patients; aged, multiparous women; and patients who have been on steroids for long periods. Clinically, such leakage presents as a discharge of clear dialysate around the catheter at its exit site, as a localized swelling secondary to infiltration of the subcutaneous tissue of the anterior abdominal wall, or as swelling of the genitalia. In many cases, the leakage stops after temporary discontinuation of peritoneal dialysis.

Surgical Wound Infection. Although now rare, this is a serious complication. The responsible organisms are usually *S. aureus* and *Pseudomo-*

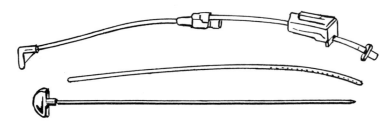

Figure 19–17. A semirigid plastic catheter with its steel stylet and connecting tube. (From Khanna R, Nolph KD, Oreopoulos DG: The Essentials of Peritoneal Dialysis. Dordrecht, The Netherlands, Kluwer Academic, 1993, p 54. Reprinted by permission of Kluwer Academic Publishers.)

nas species. Prevention of contamination is based on strict sterile technique, control of bleeding, and the use of prophylactic antibiotics.

Catheter Malfunction. This complication presents as a one- or two-way obstruction. In the former, peritoneal dialysis fluid flows easily into the peritoneal cavity, but its outflow is slow (partial obstruction) or absent. In two-way obstruction, dialysate does not flow in or out of the cavity (complete obstruction). The main causes of such malfunction are obstruction, dislodgment, and kinking.

Catheter obstruction early after its implantation usually is due to blood or fibrin clots within the lumen. Omentum wrapped around the intraperitoneal segment may cause obstruction and *dislodgment.*

Kinking at the intramural segment of the soft (Tenckhoff) catheter usually is due to poor insertion technique.

To manage these malfunctions, one should rule out a functional cause of obstruction (constipation or bowel loop distention) before looking for a mechanical cause. Catheter position should be checked on a plain film of the abdomen. If the catheter is in a good position, a cannulogram is useful to determine the cause of malfunction. Clots can be dislodged by forceful irrigation with a syringe containing 20 ml of normal saline with 500 to 1000 units of heparin, or they may be dissolved by fibrinolytic agents such as streptokinase (75,000 units) or urokinase (5000 units) in 20 ml of saline left in the catheter lumen for 2 hours.

Finally, medical complications of acute peritoneal dialysis are usually due to rapid alteration of the hemodynamic state brought about by dialysis. These include hypervolemia or hypovolemia, tachyarrhythmias, basal atelectasis, hypoxia, hyperglycemia, hypernatremia, respiratory or metabolic alkalosis, and so on.

PATIENT NUMBER 5 (continued)

After we explained the situation to our patient Tony, who was anxious and restless, he agreed to undergo acute peritoneal dialysis. The nephrology fellow inserted an acute stylet catheter at the bedside and wrote the following peritoneal dialysis orders:

1. Manual peritoneal dialysis for 24 hours with dialysis solution containing 1.5% glucose. No potassium added.

2. Volume I L (inflow time 5 minutes), dwell time 20 minutes, outflow time (if complete) 10 minutes. If inflow and outflow are satisfactory after 24 hours, continue exchanges as follows: Exchange

volume 2 L (inflow time 10 minutes), dwell time 30 minutes, outflow time 20 minutes.

3. Use 1.5% alternating with 2.5% dextrose solutions. No potassium added. Keep fluid balance by measuring the effluent volumes and subtracting these from the infused ones. Weigh the patient every 8 hours and plan a 2-kg weight loss in 24 hours. If this is not achieved, use 2.5% solutions more frequently. After the desired weight loss has been achieved, use only 1.5% dialysis solutions, and increase dwell time to 3 hours. (Hypercatabolic or large patients [> 70 kg] need higher flow rates [2 L, dwell time 15 minutes]).

4. Check serum electrolyte values 4 hours after the initiation of dialysis and every 12 hours thereafter. If serum potassium level is less than 3.5 mmol/L, add 2 mmol of potassium per liter of dialysis solution.

COMMENTS

The prescription of acute peritoneal dialysis should be tailored to each patient's specific needs. The method of exchange (manual or cycler) depends primarily on the availability of cyclers and personnel.

The excess fluid should be removed gradually over 2 to 3 days. If a patient has pulmonary edema, use 4.25 g/L glucose solution. Most patients with acute renal failure need a potassium-free solution. In specific cases, however (e.g., digoxin treatment), in the presence of normal serum concentrations of potassium, potassium should be added to the dialysate to avoid hypokalemia-induced myocardial irritability in the presence of digoxin. The amount needed usually is up to 3 to 4 mmol/L of potassium chloride. Dialysis orders should be for 24 hours only. After this, the patient should be reassessed, and a new order should be written based on the most recent data. In case of unstable vital signs, the patient may need more frequent reevaluation.

PATIENT NUMBER 5 (continued)

Tony reached his dry weight after 4 days of acute peritoneal dialysis. His biochemistry had improved considerably within 7 days. In the meantime, diuresis was reestablished. One week after the initiation of acute dialysis, his serum levels of creatinine were 2.8 mg/dl, BUN 50 mg/dl, and potassium 4.0 mmol/L. His vital signs were stable. Tony was in no distress, was no longer anxious, and showed interest in his own rehabilitation. The acute catheter was removed after a period of prolonged drainage (1 hour). Povidone-iodine cream was applied to the wound, and it was covered with a sterile dry dressing.

PERITONEAL DIALYSIS IN DIABETIC PATIENTS

PATIENT NUMBER 6

Adam, a 34-year-old man with insulin-dependent diabetes mellitus for 20 years, had severe visual impairment. His renal function had undergone progressive deterioration, and he reached ESRD. He needed 20 units of regular insulin daily to maintain satisfactory fasting and 1-hour postprandial blood glucose levels. A peritoneal dialysis Tenckhoff catheter was inserted surgically through a paramedian incision. During the catheter break-in period, he required 20 to 24 units of regular insulin daily. Two weeks later, Adam started CAPD training.

Intraperitoneal Administration of Insulin

When approaching the end stage of renal failure, diabetic patients usually have evidence of the consequences of their disease in many organs such as the heart, eyes, stomach, nerves, and peripheral arteries. CAPD offers many advantages to diabetic patients needing dialysis (Table 19–6).

Selected diabetic patients benefit from nightly IPD during which insulin is given subcutaneously during the daytime hours and intraperitoneally at night. CCPD may achieve excellent glycemic control in most diabetic patients. The average intraperitoneal insulin dose for good glycemic control is about three times the total subcutaneous dose. In most cases, half of the dose is used for the long-dwell daytime exchange and the other half is equally divided among the nocturnal exchanges.

The main indications for CCPP are in young diabetic patients awaiting a renal transplant or in older, blind and dependent diabetic patients who

TABLE 19–6. CAPD in Diabetic Patients

---
1. Slow hemodynamic alterations
2. Slow continuous dialysis process
3. Stable biochemical status
4. Control of hypertension and fluid volume
5. Easy control of blood sugar
6. Reduced cardiovascular stress
7. No need for vascular access
8. Advantages of dialysis at home

---

need a helper to perform dialysis. Those with increased intraabdominal pressure or those complaining of low back pain on CAPD need a low-volume daytime exchange.

Commercial bags containing the dialysis solution or their connecting tube provide an injection port. CAPD exchanges with intraperitoneal insulin are performed before meals in order to control the impending hyperglycemia. The aim of therapy is to maintain a fasting blood glucose level of no more than 140 mg/dl and 2-hour postprandial glycemia less than 180 mg/dl. We recommend self-monitoring of blood glucose levels by the finger-stick technique.

Insulin administered intraperitoneally is absorbed in part by diffusion through the visceral peritoneum to the portal vein and in part across the capsule of the liver, simulating the physiologic secretion of insulin by the pancreas. Slow absorption by the peritoneal lymphatics takes insulin directly to the systemic circulation. Insulin is absorbed with glucose continuously during the dwell period. About 40% to 50% of the intraperitoneal insulin is absorbed after an 8-hour dwell time. During peritonitis, insulin requirements vary depending on the balance between the decreased carbohydrate intake due to anorexia and the increased glucose absorption. The blood glucose level in diabetic patients can be controlled by subcutaneous insulin administration alone or in combination with intraperitoneal instillation. Subcutaneous insulin administration requires multiple injections of regular insulin before meals and before daytime exchanges. Before the night exchange, we recommend a mixture of regular and intermediate-acting insulin.

Finally, oral hypoglycemic agents with or without insulin or specific diets have also been recommended.

PATIENT NUMBER 6 (continued)

During Adam's first day on CAPD, four 2-L exchanges were performed using 1.5% alternating with 2.5% dialysis solution to lower body weight by 1 kg.
The doctor's orders were as follows:

Time of exchanges: 8:00 A.M., 12:30 P.M., 6:00 P.M., 10:00 P.M.
Diet: 1500-calorie diabetic diet.
Breakfast and meal times: 8:15 A.M., 12:45 P.M., 6:15 P.M. A snack may be taken at 10:15 P.M.

By aseptic technique, add regular insulin into the bag using a long needle through the injection port in the following doses:

1.5% solution: 6 units
2.5% solution: 8 units

Mix the bag thoroughly after injection.

Before each exchange, check blood glucose level by finger stick.

During the first day, Adam had the following blood glucose levels:

8:00 A.M.: 82 mg/dl	6:00 P.M.: 296 mg/dl
12:00 noon: 284 mg/dl	10:00 P.M.: 267 mg/dl

On the second CAPD day, the following insulin doses were prescribed: Add regular insulin to each bag of peritoneal dialysis solution (except 10:00 P.M.) as follows:

1.5% solution, 8 units
2.5% solution, 10 units

For the 10:00 P.M. exchange, add insulin as follows:

1.5% solution, 5 units
2.5% solution, 6 units

For the second CAPD day, Adam had the following blood glucose levels:

8:00 A.M.: 109 mg/dl	6:00 P.M.: 286 mg/dl
12:00 noon: 146 mg/dl	10:00 P.M.: 278 mg/dl

The dose of insulin for the 12:00 noon bag was increased by 2 units, and on the subsequent days Adam's blood glucose levels were satisfactory.

In diabetic patients, the peritoneal transport characteristics (estimated by PET) are similar to those of nondiabetics. (Both groups have the same CAPD complications, chiefly due to catheter malfunction or to increased intraabdominal pressure). Diabetic patients on CAPD may suffer irreversible loss of ultrafiltration as a result of severe peritonitis. Ocular function may stabilize or even improve. The main causes of death in diabetic patients on peritoneal dialysis are microangiopathy and atherosclerotic heart disease. Diabetic patients require hospitalization more often than do nondiabetic patients because of medical illness related to the progression of diabetic complications, especially in the aged. During the first few years on CAPD, preservation of residual renal function is valuable because it is associated with beneficial fluid, sodium, and potassium balance. Some workers have alleged a possible increase in peritonitis risk associated with intraperitoneal insulin administration, but this has not been confirmed by others.

In summary, peritoneal dialysis is a reliable mode of dialysis for diabetic patients with ESRD. It gives satisfactory blood pressure, glycemic, and metabolic control. However, the mortality rate is significantly higher in diabetic than in nondiabetic patients, mainly because of cardiovascular complications.

PERITONEAL DIALYSIS IN PATIENTS WITH ACQUIRED IMMUNODEFICIENCY SYNDROME

PATIENT NUMBER 7

George, a 36-year-old black homosexual man, was found to have human immunodeficiency virus (HIV) infection 3 years ago after the appearance of fever and generalized lymphadenopathy. One year previously, the patient presented with proteinuria in the nephrotic range and a kidney biopsy revealed focal glomerulosclerosis. He also had hypertension. His renal function, which had deteriorated, declined further after *Klebsiella pneumoniae* infection, for which gentamicin was used.

George came to the emergency room short of breath and edematous. His pulse rate was 100 and his blood pressure was 170/110 mm Hg. His blood values were as follows: pH, 7.25; PCO_2, 30 mm Hg; HCO_3, 12 mmol/L; hematocrit 23%; and WBC, 8000/mm^3. His BUN was 180 mg/dl and serum potassium level was 7.2 mmol/L. His serum levels of sodium were 135 mmol/L; calcium, 7.5 mg/dl; phosphorus, 6.7 mg/dL; and creatinine, 11.5 mg/dl.

Patients with acquired immunodeficiency syndrome (AIDS) and ESRD have a poor outcome. The prognosis is better for HIV-positive patients who develop renal failure for other reasons than for patients on dialysis who become HIV positive. In these patients, peritoneal dialysis offers some advantages over hemodialysis—namely, a higher hematocrit, home dialysis, caloric supplementation by the dialysate, and reduced risk of exposure for health care personnel. The disadvantages are dialysate protein losses in otherwise nutritionally compromised or nephrotic patients and a tendency to an increased incidence of peritonitis.

In clinical practice, more than half of peritonitis episodes in patients who have HIV infection and who are treated with CAPD are due to gram-positive organisms, predominantly staphylococci.

The peritonitis rate in HIV-positive patients is almost twice that of the HIV-negative CAPD population. Those who are HIV positive more often have gram-negative infections, particularly *Pseudomonas* and fungal peritonitis. Their peritoneal effluent contains the HIV antigen, and this is a potential source of contamination. For these patients, the staff must observe universal precautions. The effluent can be emptied into a toilet after it is treated with sodium hypochlorite. Empty bags should be double bagged before disposal, and the needles used at home should be taken to the hospital center for disposal.

PATIENT NUMBER 7 (continued)

After a Tenckhoff catheter was inserted into the intraperitoneal space, George was treated with acute peritoneal dialysis using small dialysate volumes. Three days later, his clinical status improved. The peritoneal catheter was then capped for a few days but was irrigated daily with heparinized saline.

Because of his relatively good physical and intellectual status, George was trained for CAPD. On the third monthly follow-up visit after the initiation of CAPD, he had an ESI. S. aureus was isolated, and he was treated with vancomycin, 1 g IV in three consecutive weekly doses. At the sixth month, he presented with peritonitis due to Pseudomonas, which was treated successfully with intraperitoneal antibiotics. Because of neurologic HIV involvement, he could no longer cope with CAPD and, helped by his partner, switched to APD. He died of septic shock 9 months after initiation of peritoneal dialysis.

NONUREMIC INDICATIONS FOR PERITONEAL DIALYSIS

Except for renal failure, the two most common indications for peritoneal dialysis are congestive heart failure and pancreatitis.

Congestive Heart Failure

In advanced forms of congestive heart failure, salt and water retention no longer responds to classic therapy with diuretics and digitalis. IPD effectively controls volume overload, and in many cases, it may restore diuretic responsiveness. This improvement, even if transient, permits patients who have correctable lesions to undergo cardiac surgery.

Long-term IPD also has been used in refractory congestive heart failure and gives these patients an improved quality of life with relief of anasarca or pulmonary edema. Their survival is short, however, because of the severity of the heart disease.

By controlling hypervolemia, CAPD has also been used to support patients with severe heart failure, whether or not it is accompanied by renal impairment. The other benefits of this mode of dialysis include improved renal function and decline of plasma levels of renin, aldosterone, and the atrial natriuretic factor.

The prognosis for these patients remains poor, however, if the cardiac dysfunction cannot be treated by operation or is not self-limited.

Acute Pancreatitis

Theoretically, peritoneal lavage with dialysate eliminates potentially harmful mediators, such as trypsin, lipase, kallikrein, kinin, and so on, that originate from the inflamed pancreas in acute pancreatitis.

Clinical experience gives conflicting results, however, presumably because of the multisystem deterioration that accompanies severe acute pancreatitis. In other words, these patients are so ill that any treatment is unlikely to change the outcome. However, current management of acute pancreatitis offers peritoneal dialysis to patients who fail to improve during the first 2 days despite intensive supportive care.

Other nonuremic indications for peritoneal dialysis include psoriasis, acute hepatic failure, hypothermia and hyperthermia, poisoning, multiple myeloma, and inborn errors of metabolism such as urea cycle defects, neonatal hyperammonemia, organic acidemias, and disorders of amino acid and carbohydrate metabolism.

Moreover, one should consider intraperitoneal chemotherapy as alternative to intravenous chemotherapy, especially when the neoplasia is limited to the peritoneal cavity or to the adjacent tissues.

ADEQUACY OF PERITONEAL DIALYSIS—IMPORTANCE OF RESIDUAL RENAL FUNCTION

The principal approach to the concept of adequacy of peritoneal dialysis is by clinical criteria, but several workers have attempted to quantitate it objectively. The criteria for adequate peritoneal dialysis include sufficient removal of metabolic waste products, maintenance of a stable dry body weight, and sustained electrolyte and acid-base balance that rehabilitate the patient and lower the risk of morbidity and mortality over a long period.

A thorough clinical evaluation of a patient undergoing peritoneal dialysis helps to assess the adequacy of dialysis, which is characterized by (1) absence of clinical signs of uremia—weakness, nausea, insomnia, and so on; (2) well-controlled blood pressure; (3) a hematocrit higher than 25%; and (4) stable nerve conduction velocities.

Such clinical evaluation requires a well-trained, observant clinician and frequent examinations. The quantitation of peritoneal dialysis delivery usually uses indices related to small solute (urea or creatinine) removal. The observer should also keep in mind that purification of a patient's blood is based on the sum of dialysis via the peritoneum and the residual renal function.

Peritoneal dialysis preserves residual renal function better than does hemodialysis and is more effective for middle molecule clearance. A residual GFR of 1 ml/min is equivalent to a weekly clearance of 10 L.

Residual creatinine clearance is 1.7 times the residual urea clearance. In patients with ESRD, the average of the residual urea and creatinine clearances approximates residual GFR.

Estimation of dialysis efficiency in CAPD is usually based on the weekly creatinine clearance and urea clearance (KT/V urea).

Weekly Creatinine Clearance

Weekly creatinine clearance is the sum of the renal and the peritoneal component.

$$K = Kr + Kp$$
$$K_r = U/T \times UCr/PCr$$
$$K_p = V/T \times DCr/PCr$$

where U is the volume of the urine, V is the volume of the dialysate (outflow), T is 1440 minutes, UCr is urine creatinine concentration, DCr is dialysate creatinine concentration, and PCr is plasma creatinine concentration.

In order to make a comparison between patients, one needs normalization of the weekly creatinine clearance to a body surface area of 1.73m^2. Creatinine clearances greater than 55 L/wk/1.73m^2 are generally considered adequate.

Urea Clearance

KT/V urea is also an index of adequacy of CAPD. K represents the sum of peritoneal (Kp) *plus* renal urea (Kr) clearance. Kp and Kr can be measured directly. Twenty-four-hour effluent is collected and pooled. Its volume is measured, and an aliquot is analyzed for dialysate urea nitrogen concentration (DUN). During the same 24-hour period, BUN is measured.

$$Kp = \text{total drainage volume (L/day)}$$
$$\times DUN/BUN$$

During this period, a 24-hour urine volume is collected and Kr urea is calculated. V is the volume distribution of urea (i.e., the total body water). In patients on CAPD, a total KT/V of 1.7 and greater per week is considered adequate. Studies indicate that KT/V values of 1.9 to 2.1 per week are associated with a better survival. These measurements should be repeated every 3 to 6 months.

Typical values for the components of KT/V in CAPD are Kp of 9.5 L/day (8 L of dialysate inflow + 1.5 L of ultrafiltration) and Kr of 4.32 L/day (3 ml/min of residual urea clearance expressed in L/day). In a patient with standard body weight of 70 kg, V would be 70 × 0.58, or 40.6 L. The KT/V would be (9.5 + 4.32): 40.6 = 0.341

In this example, residual renal function contributes 31% of the total dialysis (4.32 L/day of the total urea clearance of 13.82 L/day).

A significant reduction in Kr usually occurs after the second year on CAPD; therefore, Kp should be adjusted upward to maintain a satisfactory solute clearance.

APD alone or in combination with CAPD can achieve adequate dialysis in terms of both weekly creatinine clearance and KT/V urea, by using higher volumes of dialysate as long as the D/P creatinine (from the PET) is > 0.55.

In a patient who consumes the necessary amount of protein (i.e., 1.2 g/kg/day), adequate dialysis maintains a constant BUN value (i.e., 70 mg/dl). Reduced protein intake can result in negative nitrogen balance.

APPENDIX 1

ANATOMY AND PHYSIOLOGY

Anatomy of the Peritoneal Membrane

The peritoneum is a continuous serous membrane that covers the peritoneal cavity. Its surface is made up of mesothelial cells that lie on a thin layer of connective tissue. The peritoneal membrane covers the abdominal viscera (visceral peritoneum) and the internal surface of the abdominal wall (parietal peritoneum). A small volume of fluid (100 ml), containing the surfactant phosphatidylcholine, which is secreted by the mesothelial cells, provides lubrication and free movement of the viscera. Many cytoplasmic extensions (microvilli) project from the luminal surface of the mesothelial cells, and a continuous basement membrane underlies the mesothelial cell layer. Beneath this membrane, the interstitium that consists of collagen bundles and proteoglycan filaments slows the flow of the fluid considerably. This fluid is essential to the transport of water, solutes, oxygen, and carbon dioxide.

The *blood supply* of the visceral peritoneum comes mainly from the superior mesenteric artery, whereas the parietal peritoneum is supplied from the intercostal, epigastric, and lumbar arteries. The visceral *venous drainage* is to the portal vein, and the parietal part of the peritoneum drains to the caval vein; this means that intraperitoneal medications are handled partially by the liver. *Peritoneal capillaries* are characterized by continuous endothelium and continuous basement membrane.

The main *lymphatic drainage* of the peritoneal cavity is through specific openings (stomata) in the subdiaphragmatic peritoneum. From the subdiaphragmatic area, lymphatics lead to the anterior mediastinal lymph nodes and to the right lymphatic duct, which drains into the venous circulation. Also in the parietal and visceral interstitium are many lymphatic vessels, which drain mainly into the thoracic lymph duct. Lymphatic flow rate is influenced by diaphragmatic movements, intrathoracic pressure, intraperitoneal hydrostatic pressure, body posture, and peritonitis.

The lymphatics, which drain the peritoneal cavity, may absorb inert particles, proteins, cells and iso-osmotic fluid. Moreover, they contribute to the local host defenses by removing bacteria.

Physiologically, excess intraperitoneal fluid and proteins are drained through the peritoneal lymphatics into the systemic circulation.

Physiology of Peritoneal Dialysis

Excess water and solutes that accumulate in the blood of uremic patients, such as urea, creatinine, phosphate, potassium, and so on, may be removed by peritoneal dialysis. In addition, acidosis may be corrected by a buffer in the dialysis solution, usually in the form of lactate. Peritoneal dialysis takes place through the peritoneal membrane between the blood in the capillaries of the peritoneal interstitium and the solution infused into the peritoneal cavity.

The peritoneal membrane acts as an imperfect semipermeable membrane that allows small molecules and water to pass through faster than large molecules. Solutes are transported to and from the peritoneal microcirculation mainly by *diffusion* and to a lesser degree by *convective flow* (solute drag with ultrafiltrate).

Water transport across the peritoneum is governed by hydrostatic and colloid osmotic pressures in the capillaries and the interstitium, but the main mechanism of fluid removal (*ultrafiltration*) is the osmotic pressure gradient created by the osmotic agent (usually glucose) in the dialysis solution.

Solute Transport Across the Peritoneum

Solutes are transported across the peritoneal membrane by diffusion and convective flow. *Diffusion* is a spontaneous process by which molecules or other particles in liquids reach uniform concentration via random movement throughout the solvent.

The net diffusion rate of a substance between the capillary and peritoneal cavity correlates positively with the solute concentration difference, the pressure difference across the membrane, the effective membrane area, and the temperature of the solution. The diffusion rate correlates negatively with the square root of the solute molecular weight and the thickness of the peritoneal membrane. Diffusion also is affected by the electrical charge of the membrane.

Convective flow (or bulk flow) refers to a transport mechanism by which solutes are transported with osmotically removed water during peritoneal dialysis. During such flow, large numbers of molecules move in the same direction, streaming through the pores as part of the total fluid, as opposed to random movement in pure diffusion. Solutes, as well as water and ions, easily pass through membrane pores and intercellular clefts by diffusion and convection. The exact structure of these pores and clefts is unknown. Colloid particles (proteins) diffuse more slowly than do small molecular substances. These macromolecules also are transported through the cells by *pinocytosis* (vesicular transport). Substances soluble in both water and lipids, such as oxygen, carbon dioxide, alcohols, and fatty acids, are transported more rapidly because they diffuse more easily through the cellular membranes.

Water Transport Across the Peritoneum

Physiologically, water transport across the peritoneum is governed by hydrostatic and colloid osmotic pressures in the capillaries and the interstitium. During peritoneal dialysis, the osmotic pressure within the peritoneal cavity is greatly increased by the presence of the osmotic agent added to the dialysis solution, and it becomes the main force controlling water transport. Glucose is the most common osmotic agent used today in peritoneal dialysis, but other osmotic agents such as amino acids and glucose polymers are undergoing clinical trials.

Solute Equilibration and Net Water Ultrafiltration

The end result of dialysis is the tendency for equilibration of solutes between blood and dialysis solution and net water ultrafiltration.

After the instillation of a solution into the peritoneal cavity there is a slow equilibration of solutes between blood and dialysis solution, and this becomes the main force controlling solute transport. Equilibration rates vary among patients, and by using a specific test, the peritoneal equilibration test (PET), we can estimate the functional characteristics of the peritoneal membrane of a specific patient (discussed earlier). The clearance of a substance through the peritoneal membrane can be increased by increasing the number of dialysis solution exchanges. Peritoneal clearance increases as dialysis solution flow rate increases up to 6 L/hr. Further incre-

ment in flow rate does not augment clearance. For example, urea clearance cannot exceed 40 ml/min even with more rapid exchanges. It should be emphasized, however, that in patients with small pores (low peritoneal equilibration), peritoneal clearance does not increase with flow rate.

Net water ultrafiltration is the algebraic sum of water peritoneal ultrafiltration and cumulative lymphatic absorption of water. Studies of patients undergoing CAPD have shown that instillation of 2 L of 4.25 g/dl glucose dialysis solution for 4 hours produces 800 to 1200 ml of ultrafiltrate. During the same period, cumulative lymphatic absorption is about 250 to 350 ml. Therefore, net measurable ultrafiltration would be 550 to 850 ml.

The net transcapillary ultrafiltration rate is maximum at the beginning of an exchange, and ultrafiltration volume peaks at about 2 to 3 hours when transcapillary ultrafiltration equals reabsorption; intraperitoneal volume begins to decrease thereafter because of glucose absorption, which decreases the osmotic gradient, and because of continued lymphatic absorption of water (Fig. 19–18).

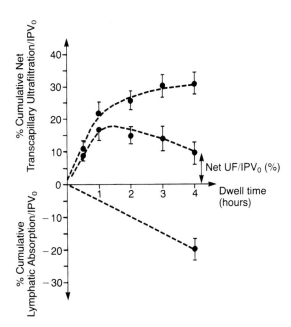

Figure 19–18. Cumulative lymphatic absorption, net ultrafiltration, and cumulative net transcapillary ultrafiltration (mean + SEM) during 4-hour exchanges in 18 CAPD patients using 2 L of 2.5% dextrose dialysis solution. IPV_o, intraperitoneal volume at zero time. (Reproduced with permission from Mactier RA, Khanna R, Twardowski ZJ, et al: Contribution of lymphatic absorption to loss of ultrafiltration and solution clearances in CAPD. J Clin Invest 80:311, 1987.)

APPENDIX 2

PERITONEAL CATHETER INSERTION TECHNIQUES

Bedside Catheter Insertion

Such insertion is usually done by an internist or nephrologist for the treatment of a patient with acute renal failure. The patient should preferably be cooperative, not obese, and without any previous major abdominal surgery.

1. The bladder and rectum should be empty.
2. The hair on the lower abdomen is clipped, and the skin is usually prepared with povidone-iodine.
3. A single dose of prophylactic antibiotic (vancomycin, 1 g) is given intravenously during the 24 hours before implantation.
4. All persons in the immediate area, including the patient, wear surgical masks, and a nurse is present to assist.
5. The area of the linea alba 2 to 3 cm below the umbilicus is anesthetized with a subcutaneous infiltration of 1% or 2% lidocaine without epinephrine. Using a larger needle, anesthesia is extended to deeper tissues.

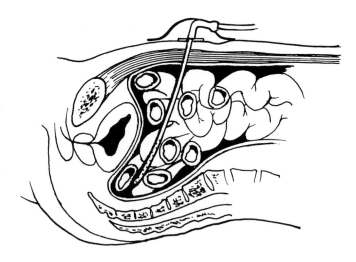

Figure 19–19. The position of a rigid catheter after insertion in relation to the abdominal wall and internal organs in the peritoneal cavity. (From Khanna R, Nolph KD, Oreopoulos DG: The Essentials of Peritoneal Dialysis. Dordrecht, The Netherlands, Kluwer Academic, 1993, p 56. Reprinted by permission of Kluwer Academic Publishers.)

Semirigid (Stylet) Catheter

Under strict sterile technique, a stab wound (2 to 3 mm) is made in the anesthetized area. To facilitate catheter insertion, some workers prefer to fill the peritoneal cavity with 2 L of dialysis solution using a 16-gauge angiocatheter. With the patient distending the abdominal wall, the catheter, with the stylet in place, is forced through the wall by a short thrust or rotating motion. The catheter tip should be directed toward the coccyx. Once the operator recognizes entry into the peritoneal cavity, the stylet tip is withdrawn a little inside the catheter lumen to avoid injury to the viscera. The catheter is advanced deep into the pelvis in the direction of the coccyx. The stylet is withdrawn completely, the catheter is connected to the sterile infusion tubing, and its patency is checked with an exchange of 500 to 1000 ml. After its patency is ensured, the catheter is secured to the skin with the metal or plastic disk (provided with the catheter) or with sutures (Fig. 19–19). A dry sterile dressing is applied over the incision.

It should be emphasized that instead of the stylet catheter, one may use a Tenckhoff catheter, which is introduced through a trocar or over a guide wire.

Permanent Catheter Implantation

The three types of catheter implantation techniques in use are the percutaneous or blind, the surgical, and the peritoneoscopic insertion. The most common method, surgical placement, is described next. Peritoneoscopic insertion is performed under continuous visualization of the catheter course into the peritoneal cavity.

Catheter insertion technique varies from center to center, but it must be emphasized that a vital element is a dedicated, competent, and experienced surgeon or a nephrologist with special interest in catheter implantation.

A competent staff person must conduct a careful clinical evaluation of the patient before catheter implantation. Any active peritonitis from previous acute dialysis should be treated completely before implanting a permanent catheter. Abdominal hernias should be repaired, preferably at the time of catheter insertion. Intraabdominal adhesions from previous operations may interfere with the catheter insertion and its subsequent function. Although they do not constitute an absolute contraindication, abdominal stomata (colostomy, ureterostomy, ileal conduit, nephrostomy) increase the risk of infection.

It is imperative that a trained and experienced staff member describe to patients and family members the whole CAPD/APD protocol and the associated technical procedures. Persons unable or unwilling to perform the treatment should be excluded from the program.

Preimplantation Patient Preparation

Day −1

Day −1 preimplantation preparation includes an enema, hair clipping of the abdomen, shower, a signed consent form, and fasting overnight.

To determine the catheter exit position, examine the patient in an upright (sitting) position. The exit site needs to be away from (above or below) the belt line or any other areas where pressure may produce trauma. It should be on the crest of rolls of fat rather than between them, to avoid a selective environment for bacterial growth. The catheter exit site also should be distant from any stoma.

The catheter exit site should be predetermined and marked on the abdomen before going to the operating room.

Day 0

Most centers advocate prophylactic antibiotics, such as vancomycin, 1 g slowly IV 24 hours before surgery, or cefamandole, 1 g administered 30 to 60 minutes before operation.

Blind Catheter Insertion

Blind catheter insertion includes the trocar and the guide-wire techniques.

Insertion of a Tenckhoff Catheter Through a Trocar (Figs. 19–20 and 19–21)

After patient preparation, the operator performs a blunt dissection with a curved hemostat through a skin incision 2 to 3 cm below the umbilicus on the linea alba. Acceptable alternative sites are the lateral margins of either rectus muscle. With an angiocatheter or a semirigid catheter, the peritoneal cavity is filled with 2 L of dialysis solution, especially in an unconscious patient. A pursestring is inserted in the fascia (to later anchor the catheter).

During instillation of the dialysis solution, the Tenckhoff catheter and its cuffs are prepared by wetting them with normal saline. A wet stylet is inserted into the catheter to assist it into the trocar and into the correct intraabdominal position.

A specially designed trocar surrounded by a metallic barrel (see Fig. 19–20) is introduced with firm and gentle pressure into the peritoneal cavity. While it is being advanced, the trocar should be directed toward the coccyx to ensure pelvic placement (see Fig. 19–21). After the peritoneal cavity is entered, the trocar is removed, and the dialysis solution should then well up into the barrel of the trocar. The catheter with the stylet in it is then introduced through the barrel into the peritoneal cavity and placed in the pelvis. The patient may report a feeling of rectal or bladder pressure, which indicates that the catheter is in the pelvis.

The trocar barrel is then removed, and the split side pieces remain in place until the final positioning. Next the catheter stylet is removed and the two longitudinal sections of the trocar are withdrawn, leaving the catheter in its proper position. The operator must ensure that the inner cuff is at the preperitoneal level. The infusion set is connected to the catheter, and its patency is tested. If patency is satisfactory, the catheter is secured in place (with the inner cuff at the posterior rectus fascia) by tightening the preprositioned anchoring pursestring suture at the inner cuff level. After the site of the subcutaneous

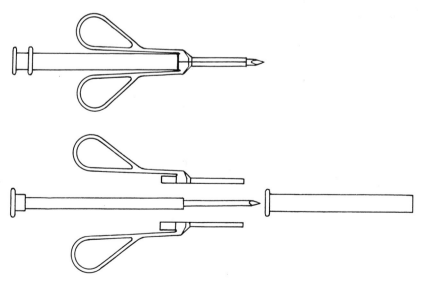

Figure 19–20. The Tenckhoff catheter introducer fully assembled (above) and with parts separated (below). (From Khanna R, Nolph KD, Oreopoulos DG: The Essentials of Peritoneal Dialysis. Dordrecht, The Netherlands, Kluwer Academic, 1993, p 57. Reprinted by permission of Kluwer Academic Publishers.)

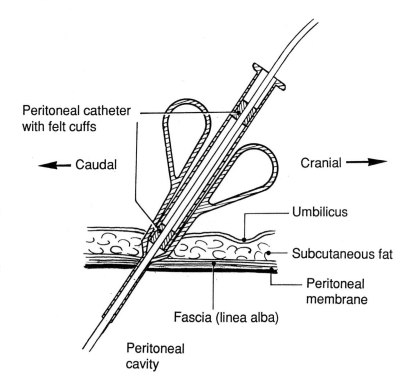

Figure 19–21. The position and direction of the trocar during the catheter insertion. Only the thin sharp tip of the fully assembled trocar penetrates the peritoneum. The thick tubular body is halted at the peritoneal level for positioning the internal cuff. (From Khanna R, Nolph KD, Oreopoulos DG: The Essentials of Peritoneal Dialysis. Dordrecht, The Netherlands, Kluwer Academic, 1993, p 58. Reprinted by permission of Kluwer Academic Publishers.)

tunnel has been chosen, the exit site is made by a stab wound using a blade just the size of the catheter. The subcutaneous tunnel is created using a piercing trocar (e.g., the Faller trocar) with an external diameter similar to that of the catheter tubing. The external cuff must be placed at least 2 cm below the skin (Fig. 19–22).

Insertion of a Tenckhoff Catheter Through a Guide Wire (Fig. 19–23)

This technique requires a guide needle attached to a syringe, a Seldinger guide wire, and a ta-

pered dilator with a scored peel-away sheath. The initial steps are similar to those of trocar insertion. After the peritoneal cavity is filled with 1 to 2 L of dialysis solution, the Seldinger guide wire is inserted into the peritoneal cavity through the needle that is used for the fluid infusion. The needle is then removed, leaving the guide wire in place.

First, the hole through the abdominal wall is enlarged with the tapered dilator. Then the cylindrical peel-away sheath is inserted into the abdomen over an internal dilator. The guide wire and dilator are removed, and the Tenckhoff cath-

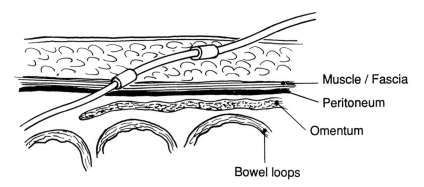

Figure 19–22. A peritoneal catheter in the abdominal wall and adjacent tissues. (From Khanna R, Nolph KD, Oreopoulos DG: The Essentials of Peritoneal Dialysis. Dordrecht, The Netherlands, Kluwer Academic, 1993, p 58. Reprinted by permission of Kluwer Academic Publishers.)

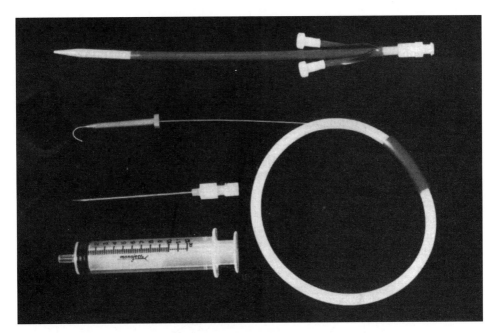

Figure 19–23. Equipment for guide-wire insertion method. *From the top:* Peel-away sheath with dilator, guide wire, needle, and syringe. (From Gokal R, Nolph KD [eds]: The Textbook of Peritoneal Dialysis. Dordrecht, The Netherlands, Kluwer Academic, 1994, p 290. Reprinted by permission of Kluwer Academic Publishers.)

eter with its flexible metal rod is introduced into the peritoneal cavity through the plastic sheath. As the cuff enters the sheath, the sheath splits and allows the cuff to advance until it stops at the outer rectus fascia. At this time, the sheath is withdrawn by peeling. The previously positioned pursestring suture is tightened around the inner cuff. The final steps are similar to those of the trocar technique.

Surgical Insertion of a Peritoneal Catheter (Fig. 19–24)

The preferred approach is at the medial or lateral border of the rectus muscle. After general or local anesthesia with 1% lidocaine and after skin preparation, a 3- to 4-cm transverse paramedian incision is made. Perfect hemostasis, which is crucial, is best achieved by electrocautery. After blunt and sharp dissection, a 2- to 3-cm incision is made in the anterior rectus sheath, and muscle fibers are separated by blunt dissection. A pursestring suture (1.5 cm diameter) is placed in the posterior rectus fascia. A small incision is made through this fascia and the peritoneum, with specific care to avoid bowel injury. The edges of the fascia and the peritoneum are ele-

vated to create a space between them and the underlying viscera. A stiffening stylet that earlier was prepared by soaking in sterile saline is inserted into the catheter, leaving 1 cm of soft catheter beyond the stylet tip. By feel, the catheter is inserted caudally into the pelvis to its correct position in the pouch of Douglas. The inner cuff should be on the posterior rectus fascia, and the peritoneum is closed tightly by tying the pursestring suture. The TWH catheter requires a larger incision, which should be closed carefully. At this point, the catheter is tested with an infusion of 500 ml to check patency and to exclude leakage. The inner cuff is laid longitudinally parallel to the rectus muscle. A stab wound is made in the anterior rectus fascia 1 to 2 cm cephalad to the transverse incision. The external part of the catheter is pulled carefully through, and the inner cuff is placed deep in the rectus muscle. Then a subcutaneous tunnel is made to the previously marked exit site, using a tunneler or other instrument. The external cuff should be at least 2 cm from the skin exit site, whose diameter should match that of the catheter. The external portion of the catheter is brought through the exit site and attached to a connector and sterile tubing to allow infusion and drainage of dialysate.

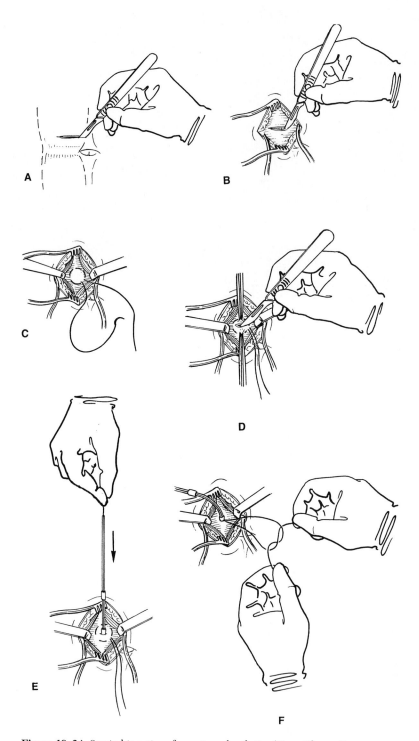

Figure 19–24. Surgical insertion of a peritoneal catheter. (From Khanna R, Nolph KD, Oreopoulos DG: The Essentials of Peritoneal Dialysis. Dordrecht, The Netherlands, Kluwer Academic, 1993, pp 26, 27. Reprinted by permission of Kluwer Academic Publishers.)

Illustration continued on opposite page

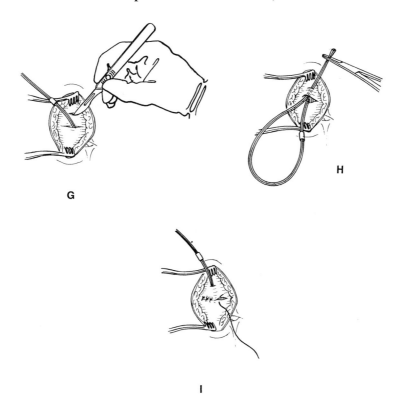

G

H

I

Figure 19–24. *Continued*

Peritoneoscopic Catheter Insertion
(Fig. 19–25)

The necessary instruments include a peritoneo-scope (15-cm-long Y-TEC with a 2.2-mm diameter), a 2.5-mm steel cannula with trocar, and a catheter guide surrounding the cannula (spiral-wound Quill).

After careful surgical preparation of the skin, the cannula with the trocar is inserted into the abdomen through a puncture in the medial or lateral border of the rectus muscle. After the trocar is removed, the scope is inserted through the cannula. The intraperitoneal position is ensured by observing glistening surfaces. With the patient in a Trendelenburg position, the scope is

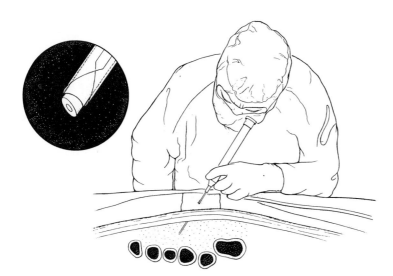

Figure 19–25. The peritoneal space is being viewed under direct vision through a Y-TEC Scope. (From Khanna R, Nolph KD, Oreopoulos DG: The Essentials of Peritoneal Dialysis. Dordrecht, The Netherlands, Kluwer Academic, 1993, p 21. Figure provided by and reproduced with permission of Medigroup, Inc., North Aurora, IL.)

removed and 600 ml of air is inflated into the intraperitoneal space. The scope is inserted again and advanced with the catheter guide and the cannula. After this, the scope and cannula are removed.

The Quill catheter guide, which has been left in place, is dilated along with the musculature to approximately 0.5 cm to allow the catheter to be inserted and the cuff to be advanced into the rectus muscle. Through the Quill guide in place, the catheter is advanced on a stylet and dilates its way until the cuff stops at the muscular layer. Advancing the cuff within the Quill guide with a pair of hemostats buries the cuff in the muscle. The Quill guide is then removed, and the function of the catheter is checked. Finally, using a trocar, the subcutaneous tunnel is made and the catheter is brought out through the exit site in a manner similar to that used in the surgical technique.

General Comments on Peritoneal Catheter Insertion

Irrespective of the technique, one must consider the following points:

1. Before catheter implantation, the exit site should be identified and marked clearly with a skin marker. A good place for it is laterally on either flank, especially in sexually active persons. If a swan neck catheter is used, a stencil can be applied to indicate the tunnel and the exit site.
2. The deep cuff should be in the musculature of the anterior abdominal wall. Nevertheless, a direct attachment to the peritoneum is equally correct. The subcutaneous cuff should be near the skin, at least 2 cm from the exit site, and should not be under mechanical stress.
3. The exit site should be directed downward or laterally. An exit site that is directed upward should be avoided.
4. The intraperitoneal part of the catheter should be between the visceral and the parietal peritoneum. It should not be between bowel loops or just below the omentum.

Catheter Removal

The four main indications for peritoneal catheter removal are (1) recurrent peritonitis, (2) persistent exit or tunnel infection or abscess, (3) outflow failure, and (4) successful renal transplantation.

It occasionally becomes necessary to remove the catheter because of unusual peritonitis (tuberculous or fungal), bowel perforation (multiple organism peritonitis), accidental catheter break, late dialysis solution leak around the catheter, and other rare reasons.

20 | HEMODIALYSIS

Nuhad Ismail and Raymond Hakim

End-stage renal disease (ESRD) in the 1990s is characterized by tremendous challenges and efforts to accommodate an ever increasing patient population. Estimates of ESRD prevalence based on 1990 data from the United States Renal Data System (USRDS) suggest that ESRD now affects more than 220,000 patients in the United States, with an increase in incidence (number of new patients) of approximately 9.0% annually and an increase of prevalence (number of treated patients) of more than 12% annually. These data reflect an increased acceptance, a decrease in the untreated number of patients with chronic renal failure (CRF), and improvements in the care of patients with ESRD. These trends also suggest that comorbid conditions that influence early mortality in patients with renal failure are now more readily treated, thus allowing ESRD to be manifested. This factor certainly affects the larger number of 65- to 74-year-old patients in the United States (680 treated per million) and patients older than 74 (566 treated per million) diagnosed and treated for ESRD. According to a Health Care Financing Administration (HCFA) publication (1993), the percent of dialysis patients age 65 and older in 1990 was 40.1%. The percent of patients age 75 and older for the same year was 14.1%. Similar trends of increased incidence rates of ESRD are also apparent in all countries with renal data bases.

Hemodialysis is by far the most prevalent treatment modality for ESRD. Approximately 60% of U.S. patients with ESRD undergo in-center hemodialysis, compared with 10% receiving peritoneal dialysis (chronic ambulatory peritoneal dialysis [CAPD] and/or continuous cycling peritoneal dialysis [CCPD]. A much smaller fraction, about 2% to 2.5%, elect home hemodialysis. The rest, about 25%, have functioning renal allografts.

During the past decade, hemodialysis has undergone tremendous evolution. Advances in dialysis technology as well as recent economic pressures on dialysis units, coupled with patient preference for shorter dialysis treatment times, have led to the introduction of "high-flux" and "high-efficiency" dialysis. Successful application of these treatment modalities has been already demonstrated, and the majority of patients undergoing long-term hemodialysis have proved to be candidates for this mode of therapy.

Despite the fact that our knowledge of the molecular basis of uremia is still incomplete and we still have not defined all toxic solutes, the delivery of safer and more "optimal" dialysis has steadily progressed and our understanding of blood-dialyzer membrane interactions has led to the manufacture and use of safer "biocompatible" membranes. In addition, because of several advances in the treatment of uremic complications, including treatment of anemia of ESRD with recombinant human erythropoietin (EPO), more specific attention to the nutritional requirements of patients undergoing hemodialysis, implementation of urea kinetic modeling, prescription of adequate dose of dialysis, and avoidance (and treatment) of aluminum-related bone disease and aluminum encephalopathy) with deferoxamine (DFO), hemodialysis is likely to improve the quality of life (and possibly the survival) of dialyzed patients more than it did in the past.

An important element in the management of ESRD is to identify and treat patients before the ravaging complications of uremia set in. In addition to timing initiation of dialysis therapy, this chapter discusses the factors (medical and nonmedical) that affect the choice of dialysis treatment modality and the timing and choice of hemodialysis vascular access. The more important clinical aspects of dialyzers and dialysates and the most common medical complications on dialysis are briefly discussed. How to dialyze a patient optimally is outlined, and the chapter concludes with a brief overview of high-flux and high-efficiency dialysis.

INITIATION OF DIALYSIS

PATIENT NUMBER 1

Concetta, a 40-year old white woman of Italian origin, has ESRD secondary to analgesic-associated nephropathy. She presents to the emergency room with a 1-week history of nausea and vomiting. Three weeks ago she was seen in the outpatient clinic on a routine visit. At that time, she was asymptomatic, with a BUN of 96 mg/dl, a serum creatinine level of 7.8 mg/dl, and hematocrit of 26%. Results of the SMA-6 follow: serum Na 136 mEq/L, K 5.6 mEq/L, Cl 110 mEq/L, and a CO_2 content of 15 mEq/L. Her serum albumin level was 3.7 g/dl. On a 24-hour urine collection, she had 2 g of proteinuria. She was instructed on continuation of a low-protein diet (0.6 g/kg/day), with potassium restriction to less than 40 mEq/day, and was started on sodium bicarbonate, 650 mg t.i.d. Concetta's weight was 60 kg, and physical examination disclosed no abnormalities, although she looked older than her chronologic age. In the emergency room, physical examination disclosed the patient to be in no acute distress. She weighed 60 kg, her blood pressure was 150/96 mm Hg, her heart rate was 112, and her temperature was 98.6°F. She was oriented as to time, place, and person. Her neck veins were not distended. Cardiac examination disclosed a soft systolic ejection murmur at the left sternal border but no friction rubs. Her chest was clear. On abdominal examination, her epigastrium was mildly tender but otherwise unremarkable. Extremities showed 2+ pretibial edema bilaterally. Results of neurologic examination were unremarkable. Laboratory evaluation now disclosed the following results: hematocrit 24%, BUN 80 mg/dl, Cr 7.6 mg/dl, Na 132 mEq/L, K 5.4 mEq/L, Cl 110 mEq/L, CO_2 content 18 mEq/L, serum albumin 3.5 g/dl and cholesterol 120 mg/dl. Stool guaiac results are trace positive.

Concetta has ESRD with mild proteinuria and a borderline nutritional status, as reflected by a serum albumin value of 3.7 g/dl. She has a recent history of nausea and vomiting, which may reflect symptoms of uremia or an organic disease of the upper gastrointestinal (GI) tract (peptic ulcer disease or gastritis) related to use of nonsteroidal antiinflammatory drugs (NSAIDs).

PATIENT NUMBER 1 (continued)

On her return visit, her serum albumin (3.5 g/dl) as well as cholesterol (120 mg/dl) values are lower. Though her weight has remained stable, Concetta now has evidence of peripheral edema, suggesting a decrease in lean body mass in the presence of extracellular volume expansion. These features attest to further undernutrition. Although her BUN and serum creatinine levels are, by laboratory assessment, better than on her previous visit, they are further evidence of poor dietary protein intake rather than an improvement in renal function.

Concetta's nausea and vomiting should be further evaluated by appropriate studies to rule out organic disease of the upper GI tract, especially with a positive guaiac test result. However, initiation of hemodialysis may be particularly indicated in this patient because of evidence of progressive malnutrition. In absence of such evidence, Concetta could continue on conservative measures, if the intent is to ameliorate her symptoms (e.g., treatment of organic GI disease, if found on evaluation) or biochemical abnormalities (hyperkalemia, metabolic acidosis, and so on).

Absolute indications to start dialysis in a patient with ESRD include the development of pericarditis, fluid overload or pulmonary edema refractory to diuretics, accelerated hypertension poorly responsive to antihypertensive medications, and clinically significant bleeding diathesis. In addition, persistent nausea and vomiting and other advanced manifestations of other CNS toxicity of uremia, such as seizures, constitute formal indications for initiation of dialysis (Table 20–1).

Because these indications are life threatening and reflect far advanced degrees of uremia, most nephrologists agree that delaying initiation of dialysis until these complications appear jeopardizes the life of the patient unnecessarily. Because the basic principle of initiation of dialysis is to enhance the quality of life and not just prolong survival, it is important to seek less acute indications for dialysis. These **relative indica-**

TABLE 20–1. Absolute Indications for Initiation of Dialysis

- Pericarditis
- Progressive uremic encephalopathy or neuropathy
- Seizures, disorientation, confusion, asterixis, myoclonus, wristdrop or footdrop
- Volume overload or pulmonary edema unresponsive to ceiling doses of loop diuretics
- Bleeding diathesis attributed to uremia (platelet dysfunction, ↑ bleeding time)
- Hypertension unresponsive to treatment
- Persistent nausea/vomiting
- Serum creatinine level > 12 mg/dl and BUN > 100 mg/dl

tions for initiation of dialysis include symptoms of anorexia progressing to nausea and vomiting, decreased attentiveness and cognitive functioning, depression, severe anemia, persistent pruritus, or the restless leg syndrome. However, the expressions of these signs and symptoms in patients with slowly progressive renal disease are variable and patients may accommodate to these symptoms and downgrade their sense of well-being and habits as renal failure progresses. Further, many of the medications that patients with chronic renal failure require as part of their therapy may have side effects that mimic uremic symptoms. For example, oral iron therapy often leads to nausea and centrally acting blood pressure medications may lead to drowsiness independent of the degree of renal failure. Conversely, partial correction of anemia by EPO may improve a patient's sense of well-being without affecting the extent of uremia. Thus, more objective findings of renal failure must be identified to lessen the subjective component of the decision to initiate dialysis.

Measures of renal function in patients with CRF are an obvious standard for timing the beginning of renal replacement therapy. Many nephrologists have already implemented such target levels of renal function—for example, serum creatinine level (S_{Cr}) 10 mg/dl or reciprocal S_{Cr} 0.1. However, these standards have many inherent difficulties. Marked changes occur in the generation and elimination of creatinine in patients with progressive renal disease. Inadequate diet, increased tubular secretion of creatinine in patients with CRF, and low muscle mass often invalidate S_{Cr} as a measure of renal function. Similarly, creatinine clearance (C_{Cr}) often overestimates actual GFR in patients with renal failure. Indeed, it has been shown that patients may have "normal" S_{Cr} values (< 1.5 mg/dl) yet may have an actual GFR determined by inulin clearance of 20 to 25 ml/min/1.73 m².

> **Creatinine clearance is unreliable for estimating actual GFR in patients with CRF.**

One study demonstrated this finding in 80 patients with a mean GFR of 22 ml/min. In this study population, the ratio of C_{Cr} to inulin clearance (true GFR) ratio was nearly 2. For these reasons, many investigators believe that other markers of GFR such as ^{125}I iothalamate, chromium-51 ethylenediamine tetraacetic acid (^{51}Cr-EDTA), inulin, or technetium-99m diethylenetriamine pentaacetic acid (^{99m}Tc-DTPA) will prove to be better determinants of true renal function in patients with CRF. BUN and urea clearance (C_{urea}) are poor surrogates of GFR. However, when GFR is less than 15 ml/min/1.73 m², the mean of the C_{Cr} and C_{urea} approximates the GFR, which may be because C_{urea} underestimates GFR (owing to tubular reabsorption) to about the same degree as C_{Cr} overestimates GFR at this level of renal function.

Better benchmarks for dialysis initiation might improve quality of life and rehabilitation potential and might possibly even prolong life in patients with ESRD. One standard that may serve well in this capacity is nutritional status. **Many**

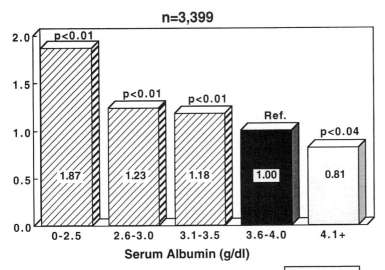

Figure 20–1. Relative mortality risk (Cox) in new hemodialysis patients according to *serum albumin* concentration at time of *initiation* of dialysis. The risk of death in patients starting hemodialysis with low serum albumin concentrations is strikingly greater than in patients with normal serum albumin concentrations (3.6–4.0 g/dL). Note that relative mortality risk of patients with serum albumin > 4 g/dL is even better (relative mortality risk = 0.81) than that of the reference range of serum albumin.

studies have shown the increased mortality risk associated with malnutrition in patients undergoing hemodialysis. The risk of death in patients on hemodialysis actually seems to increase exponentially as serum albumin concentrations decrease. The USRDS extended this observation by examining serum albumin concentrations in patients at the time of *initiation* of dialysis (Fig. 20–1). The risk of death in patients starting hemodialysis with low serum albumin concentrations is strikingly greater than in patients with normal serum albumin concentrations (3.6 to 4.0 g/dl). This applies even when diabetic patients, who may have significant proteinuria and low serum albumin levels, are excluded from the analysis. It should be noted that the significance of low serum albumin levels in patients with the nephrotic syndrome (other than diabetes) and ESRD is undetermined at present.

Another marker of nutritional status at the time of dialysis initiation is S_{Cr}. This marker reflects not only renal function but also muscle mass. Data from the USRDS show an inverse correlation between low S_{Cr} values at the time of initiation and subsequent mortality. For S_{Cr} values less than 10 to 12 mg/dl at the start of hemodialysis, mortality rates increased significantly. Notably, BUN did not show a correlation with mortality risk. These data strongly suggest that malnutrition, determined by serum albumin concentrations less than 4 g/dl, and/or decreased muscle mass, reflected by S_{Cr} less than 10 to 12 mg/dl at the time of initiation of dialysis for symptomatic uremia, are important prognostic variables when deciding to initiate dialysis in patients with CRF.

The focus for primary caregivers of patients with ESRD is to identify and treat patients as early as possible before the ravaging complications of uremia set in. Delaying initiation of dialysis until absolute indications arise jeopardizes the life of patients unnecessarily.

Other markers of malnutrition ultimately might prove to be as useful as serum levels of albumin and creatinine. Candidates include determinations of serum transferrin, somatomedin C (IGF-1), prealbumin, and cholesterol. Interestingly, in patients on CAPD as well as hemodialysis, low serum prealbumin levels (< 30 mg/dl) have also been associated with increased mortality risk. One study found an increased risk of death with low serum prealbumin levels in pa-

tients on hemodialysis. (The relative risk of mortality was 4.4 when serum prealbumin was < 15 mg/dl.)

Recommendations

Our current guidelines for initiation of dialysis are as follows:

1. Dialysis should be initiated whenever indices of malnutrition develop in patients with CRF.
   - Serum albumin < 4 g/dl
   - Dietary protein intake (protein catabolic rate) < 0.8 g/kg/day on unrestricted protein intake (see Table 20–2 for calculation of protein catabolic rate)
   - Serum prealbumin levels < 30 mg/dl, total serum cholesterol levels < 150 mg/dl, and transferrin concentration < 200 mg/dl

2. Dialysis should be initiated when S_{Cr} exceeds 10 to 12 mg/dl.

3. Patients with CRF should be monitored by one of the more accurate and current measurements of GFR (iothalamate GFR, ^{51}Cr-EDTA, ^{99m}Tc-DTPA). If these measures are not available, we suggest serial determinations of C_{Cr} (or the average clearance of urea and creatinine) and strong consideration of dialysis when "true" GFR is < 10 ml/min or C_{Cr} is < 10 ml/min (< 15 ml/min in diabetics).

Dialysis should be initiated whenever indices of malnutrition develop in patients with CRF.

HOW TO INITIATE DIALYSIS

During initiation of dialysis, patients with ESRD may develop the **dialysis disequilibrium syndrome (DDS).** Symptoms may include head-

TABLE 20–2. Estimating Nitrogen Intake in Stable Noncatabolic Patients with Chronic Renal Failure

Dietary protein intake (DPI) or protein catabolic rate (PCR)
 = [(UUN g/day) + (0.031 × body weight kg)] × 6.25
UUN = urine urea nitrogen [g/L × urine volume (L)]
NUN° = nonurea nitrogen [0.031 × body weight (kg)]
 6.25 = conversion factor [nitrogen to protein]
  (nitrogen = 16% of protein weight)
If proteinuria > 5 g/day, add amount of g/24 hr of protein to PCR formula.
[PCR = (UUN + NUN) × 6.25 + g/24 hr of protein]

°NUN is independent of DPI.

aches, restlessness, nausea, emesis, blurring of vision, muscle twitching, disorientation, hypertension, tremor, and seizures. Patients with pre-existing neurologic disorders (head trauma, recent stroke, brain tumor, subdural hematoma) and patients with cerebral edema (hyponatremia, malignant hypertension, hepatic encephalopathy) or severe acidosis, diabetic ketoacidosis, volume overload, and advanced azotemia are at particular risk for development of DDS.

Prevention and management of this syndrome include (1) slow initiation of dialysis (using low blood flow rates (e.g., 150 to 200 ml/min), short dialysis (e.g., 2 hours), a small surface area dialyzer (e.g., 0.9 to 1.2 m^2), and cocurrent rather than countercurrent blood and dialysate flows. The intensity of dialysis is then gradually increased during the subsequent 3 days to reach blood flows of 400 ml/min with a duration of dialysis of 4 hours. Use of bicarbonate dialysis, high dialysate sodium (> 140 mEq/L) if hyponatremia prevails, and a dialysate glucose of 200 mg/dl in diabetic patients with high blood glucose levels may also aid in prevention of DDS. For patients with advanced azotemia (BUN > 150 to 200 mg/dl) or altered mental status, we recommend giving prophylactic Dilantin (1000 mg loading dose, then 300 mg/day) until uremia is controlled.

In the absence of such advanced uremic symptoms, a useful rule of thumb is to calculate the dose of dialysis on the first day to be equivalent to a Kt/V (K = dialyzer urea clearance, t = dialysis time, V = total body water) of 0.3, increasing by 0.3 every treatment until the goal of Kt/V of greater than 1.2 is achieved.

Once uremia is controlled, patients are discharged with an initial hemodialysis prescription of 4 hours of dialysis thrice weekly. A urea kinetic modeling is performed once a month, and time on dialysis is adjusted accordingly. We find that patients are happier when time is shortened rather than when it increased.

CHOICE OF TREATMENT MODALITY

Planning a treatment modality for patients with ESRD should ideally include a patient's wishes and real-life circumstances. In this regard, physicians have the responsibility of not only discussing the therapeutic options available but also offering their advice and recommendations about the choices, based on the patient's age, renal diagnosis, and associated medical conditions. In general, renal transplantation should be recom-

mended as the preferred mode of renal replacement therapy for most patients who have ESRD and for whom surgery and subsequent immunosuppression are safe and feasible. The amount of renal function provided by a well-functioning allograft exceeds that provided by any type of dialysis; even with cyclosporine therapy, C$_{Cr}$ levels between 50 and 100 ml/min are achieved. Transplantation benefits also include the normalization of bone metabolism, resolution of anemia, and work rehabilitation. Conception and childbearing become possible, and growth in children is improved. On the other hand, the most efficient hemodialysis technique used today provides only 15% of the small solute removal of normal kidneys and considerably less for large solutes. Peritoneal dialysis offers less small-solute clearance but by contrast has the advantage of increased clearance of larger solutes.

A unique problem is persistently noncompliant patients who have already lost one renal allograft because of failure to take medications but who wish to pursue cadaveric transplantation. **In such cases, it is reasonable to request that the patient demonstrate long-term compliance with acceptable goals (e.g., blood pressure control, serum phosphorus levels, dialysis time) before being placed on the transplant list.**

Hemodialysis Versus Peritoneal Dialysis

The major choice in long-term dialysis treatment is between hemodialysis and peritoneal dialysis. These very different therapies now are recognized by most nephrologists as equivalent and complementary. However, some important medical considerations can influence the choice of one over the other. Factors such as lifestyle, age, social and family support, occupation, physical ability, and psychologic and emotional health also may make one treatment preferable. Renal diagnosis is an element that needs to be integrated into the selection of treatment options. Patients with autosomal dominant polycystic kidney disease and patients who have had previous abdominal surgery make the choice of peritoneal dialysis less than optimal, whereas patients with severe cardiomyopathy may render the choice of hemodialysis less advisable. When both dialysis modalities are equally possible from a medical point of view, practical issues such as a supportive family environment, work habits, economic factors (e.g., availability of transportation, apartment dwelling, and distance from dialysis centers) often favor one modality over another.

Finally, in many countries that have government health care systems, the incentive is to choose the modality costing the least. At times, education deficits and physician's bias also have an important role in the selection.

Advocates of peritoneal dialysis have recommended this modality of renal replacement therapy (RRT) for patients with ESRD for various reasons, including (1) avoidance of DDS, (2) reduced cardiovascular instability and risk of arrhythmias, (3) better control of hypertension, (4) better maintenance of residual kidney function, (5) improvement of anemia, (6) no need for vascular access, (7) efficacy of intraperitoneal insulin therapy, and (8) removal of β_2-microglobulin and "middle molecules" (compared with cellulosic hemodialysis membranes). However, there are absolute and relative (major and minor) contraindications to the successful application of peritoneal dialysis. Reduced peritoneal surface due to adhesions from previous extensive abdominal operations is an absolute contraindication to CAPD, whereas long-term ostomies, fresh aortic prosthesis, blindness, quadriplegia, and other physical handicaps are major relative contraindications. In our opinion, a hernia is a contraindication to CAPD until it is repaired. Peripheral vascular disease, diverticulosis, polycystic kidneys, obesity, and low back problems are relative minor contraindications to peritoneal dialysis.

Age is probably the most important factor that affects the choice of modality. For infants and children, transplantation, particularly from donor siblings or parents, offers them the modality that allows the best growth potential and a more normal life. Elderly and diabetic patients are special cases (in whom no one form of RRT has been ascertained to be superior to the other).

Once the impact of any form of RRT on survival and cost-effectiveness of treatment become well established, these variables may become the most vital factors in the choice of treatment modality of ESRD in a well-informed patient. One study analyzed in a simple comparison the costs of transplantation and dialysis and confirmed the widely held belief that kidney transplantation is, over time, a less costly alternative to maintenance dialysis. The high initial cost of transplantation is recovered in about 4½ years, with a net discounted savings of about $42,000 over a 10-year time frame. This cost advantage is by no means a fixed matter but depends on a number of factors, one of the most obvious being the transplant graft survival rate. Almost half of the costs associated with transplantation after the first year are the maintenance costs of a failed transplant (e.g., expensive immunosuppressive therapy and significant hospitalization rate).

Comparison of Treatment Outcomes

Survival and an acceptable quality of life are the most fundamental outcomes for patients receiving RRT. Although survival is easier to measure, the definition as well as the actual measurement of the quality of life is not as straightforward. In the past decade, several reports have compared morbidity, mortality, and the quality of life of patients with ESRD treated by dialysis or transplantation, but the results remain difficult to interpret. Available evidence suggests the following: (1) Living-related transplant is associated with better survival than cadaveric renal transplant (CRT); (2) in age groups younger than 65 years, CRT may be associated with better patient survival rates than dialysis, especially in diabetic patients; (3) the improved survival rate with CRT is noted only in the late transplant period; and (4) mortality associated with hemodialysis or peritoneal dialysis depends on pretreatment status and generally appears to be the same for either form of dialysis after correction for comorbid conditions.

PERMANENT VASCULAR ACCESS FOR HEMODIALYSIS

One of the most important aspects in the total treatment of patients with ESRD is planning and creating a permanent vascular access for hemodialysis. A skillful and meticulous operative procedure is the most critical determinant of outcome for this lifeline for patients with ESRD. Clotting, stenosis, and low flow not only cause inefficient dialysis and poor control of uremia but together with access site infection constitute the most common causes of morbidity and hospitalization of patients undergoing dialysis. Planning of vascular access must start with strong emphasis on preservation of extremity veins, particularly those of the forearms and especially those of the nondominant arm, where initial access is inserted. Early placement of the permanent vascular access prevents loss of forearm veins and allows time for proper fistula maturation. Primary arteriovenous (AV) fistulas require as long as 4 months of maturation before being suitable for use. This significant lead time means it must be placed at least 4 months before a patient requires hemodialysis or an alternate form of hemodialysis access is needed while the fistula is maturing. **This generally should occur when the S_{Cr} is approximately 6 to 8 mg/dl or when the C_{Cr} is less than 15 ml/min.**

In access planning, two basic rules should be observed:

1. The *most distal* site available should be used first to keep maximal vessel length for future revisions.
2. An endogenous AV fistula is always preferable to a synthetic AV shunt because of its longer patency rate and low infectious and thrombotic complications. A vein of adequate size must be found preoperatively for creation of an AV fistula. If a patient has small, thin-walled veins lying deep in the subcutaneous fat, fistulas are impractical and prosthetic grafts should then be the first choice. Likewise, older debilitated patients, diabetic patients, and patients with arteriosclerosis may not have suitable vessels for a successful AV fistula.

Only about 20% of American patients on hemodialysis have primary AV fistulas, and more than 80% of hemodialysis vascular access is composed of synthetic fistulas (bridge grafts) composed of polytetrafluoroethylene (PTFE).

Complications of Permanent Vascular Assess and their Treatment

Thrombosis is the most common complication of permanent vascular access. Thrombosis in the first month after access placement is due to technical error in fistula construction or premature use of the access. The most common cause of late fistula thrombosis is venous stenosis (80% of cases). Fewer than 20% of thromboses occur in absence of a documented anatomic lesion. Nonstenosis-associated access thrombosis may result from periods of decreased fistula blood flow such as hypotension, hypovolemia, or prolonged compression of the fistula during sleep or excessive fistula compression by patients or dialysis staff when achieving hemostasis after dialysis. Hypercoagulable states, though rare, also can cause nonstenotic fistula thrombosis.

Methods to detect venous stenosis before thrombosis are essential for access salvage. The two most commonly used methods of screening for venous stenosis that have been rigorously tested are monitoring of the venous dialysis pressures and urea recirculation. Duplex Doppler–color flow ultrasonography is also becoming popular and is proposed as a suitable screening technique. In the presence of high venous pressures (> 100 mm Hg) at blood flow of 200 ml/min on three consecutive dialysis sessions, plus a high urea recirculation value (> 10%), one should proceed with a fistulogram for further assessment of the fistula function.

> **Methods to detect venous stenosis before thrombosis are essential for access salvage. The two most commonly used screening methods for venous stenosis that have been rigorously tested are (1) high dialysis venous pressure (> 100 to 150 mm Hg on blood flow rates of 200 ml/min) and (2) high recirculation (> 10%).**

Treatment of Vascular Access Thrombosis

Percutaneous angioplasty is an excellent means of correcting venous stenosis in both native and synthetic fistulas. Its principal drawback is a high recurrence rate (25% to 50% in 1 year). Surgical revision, in contrast, has a low recurrence rate but extends the fistula up in the involved extremity, thereby minimizing future vascular access sites. Endovascular stents have been explored by some groups, who found them of little use.

Fistula thrombosis is treated by either surgical thrombectomy or thrombolytic therapy (urokinase or streptokinase) with clot maceration. After either procedure, a fistulogram is performed. If a stenosis is identified, it should be repaired (surgical revision with jump graft or angioplasty). At present, the role of platelet inhibitors and coumarin anticoagulation in preventing access thrombosis is unclear.

> ### PATIENT NUMBER 2
>
> Oscar, a 50-year-old man, was referred to the nephrology service in March 1990 because of deteriorating renal function. His S_{Cr} concentration was 9.6 mg/dl. He had a history of long-standing severe hypertension and trifascicular heart block. The heart block began in 1982 and necessitated multiple transvenous pacemakers. In April 1990, his S_{Cr} level had risen to 10.8 mg/dl. An AV fistula was created in his left forearm with an end-to-side anastomosis (cephalic vein to radial artery). He was discharged the next day without

complaints. When seen in the clinic 2 weeks later, the patient was noted to have swelling of the arm. There had been no swelling in his arm before placement of the fistula. The sutures were removed from the wrist incision, and Oscar was instructed to elevate his arm and start arm exercises to aid in fistula maturation. One week later, the swelling had not improved, and Oscar had anorexia, recurrent episodes of vomiting, and poor appetite. His S_{Cr} level was now 12.8 mg/dl and serum albumin 3.7 g/dl. He was admitted to the hospital, and dialysis was initiated via a left subclavian catheter. After stabilization, the patient was discharged to resume maintenance hemodialysis therapy at a long-term dialysis facility. In the subsequent 4 months, Oscar was very compliant with the dialysis prescription, dialyzing three times weekly on a high-flux membrane, with blood flow rates (Q_B) of 350 ml/min, dialysate flow rate (Q_D) 500 ml/min. The duration of each dialysis session was 3 hours and 15 minutes. Urea kinetic modeling in June showed a Kt/V of 1.26. In July, the fistula matured well, thus allowing dialysis through this access and discontinuation of the subclavian catheter. At that time, the Kt/V was 1.04. The blood flow rate was increased to 400 ml/min, and the dialysate flow rate to 800 ml/min. Oscar continued to dialyze three times per week. In August, the Kt/V had remained at 1.00 and the time on dialysis was increased to 4 hours. In September, marked swelling of the left upper extremity was noted. No pain, inflammation, tenderness, increased warmth, or sensory or motor deficits were noted in the extremity. The patient was frankly uremic, and despite no change in the dialysis prescription, the Kt/V was 0.76, and his protein catabolic rate (PCR) was 0.9 g/kg/day. A chest radiograph showed a broken pacemaker wire in the left subclavian vein and a functioning pacemaker on the right. The venous dialysis pressures in the recent five hemodialysis treatments were > 250 mm Hg (250 to 280 range) on blood flow rates of 300 mm Hg. A recirculation test revealed a urea recirculation of 38%. A fistulogram was performed and showed a stenosis at the venous anastomosis in the fistula, complete occlusion of the left subclavian vein, but a patent venous system on the right. The left forearm fistula was ligated, and another was created in the right arm.

Oscar illustrates several features of vascular access dysfunction. He became uremic and malnourished with progressive decrease in dialysis efficiency (measured Kt/V) without change in prescription (in fact the decreasing Kt/V occurred despite attempts at increasing Q_B, Q_D, and time on dialysis—the maneuvers known to

enhance dialyzer solute clearances). His malnutrition was undoubtedly due to uremia. The increased venous pressures and high percentages of recirculation further attest to his access dysfunction. The arm edema after creation of an AV fistula should have alerted the physicians to a central venous occlusion, especially with a history of several previous pacemakers and repeated catheterization of the subclavian vessels. Of note, Oscar also has a history of placement of a subclavian catheter ipsilateral to the site of the fistula (left).

There is an association between central venous cannulation and the development of central vein stenosis. This complication appears to occur more often with subclavian (40% to 50% of cases in some studies) than internal jugular insertions (rare). It has been proposed that central venous cannulation creates a nidus of vascular injury and fibrosis. The rapid blood flow, associated with the hemodialysis access, creates turbulence around the catheter that can accelerate endothelial proliferation, eventually leading to venous stenosis. This sequence is more likely with subclavian catheterization, because curving of the catheter between the clavicle and first rib as the catheter enters the superior vena cava creates pressure points on the vascular wall. In comparison, internal jugular catheters have a relatively straight course in the superior vena cava, thereby minimizing vascular irritation.

Most central venous stenoses are initially asymptomatic. Symptoms consist of edema and raised venous dialysis pressures and primarily occur after a peripheral access has been created in the ipsilateral arm. In this setting, the high blood flow through the access (sometimes as high as 800 ml/min) exceeds the rate at which blood can flow at normal pressure across the stenotic lesion. Central venous thrombosis, if detected early, responds well to directly applied thrombolytic therapy or to percutaneous transluminal angioplasty. Highly stenotic lesions that recur after angioplasty may be treated with metallic stents or surgical revision.

In summary, the long-term stricture rate of subclavian catheters is unacceptably high (50%). We recommend that the internal jugular vein be preferentially used for acute hemodialysis vascular access occlusion. Placement of an ipsilateral (to fistula) central venous catheter should be discouraged. Finally, in patients with progressive azotemia despite no changes in dialysis prescription, an investigation for access stenosis and/or thrombosis (e.g., fistulogram) should be initiated.

> Early planning of permanent vascular access avoids the need for acute subclavian vascular access. Placement of acute vascular access on the same side of the fistula is contraindicated. If an acute access is necessary, the internal jugular vein is preferable to the subclavian vein.

Double-Lumen Catheters for Permanent Hemodialysis Access

A double-lumen central venous catheter made of silicone rubber has been developed as a vascular access device. This device is particularly useful in patients who have exhausted other vascular access sites or who have severe cardiovascular disease (when a native fistula or an AV graft worsens congestive heart failure). Children, elderly patients, morbidly obese patients, and diabetic patients benefit from such access as well. In the operating room, the catheter is placed through a subcutaneous tunnel into the external or internal jugular vein. Such catheters may function for as long as 6 months, and some have functioned for longer than 1 to 2 years. They have the advantage of immediate access to the circulation after placement, high blood flow rate, no repetitive venipuncture, lack of vascular "steal" syndrome, and no effect on cardiac function.

PHYSIOLOGIC PRINCIPLES OF HEMODIALYSIS

The process of hemodialysis is simply the interaction of a patient's blood with a balanced solution (the dialysate) across a semipermeable membrane (the hemodialyzer). During hemodialysis, two physical processes operate simultaneously: diffusion and ultrafiltration.

Diffusion

Diffusion across a semipermeable membrane is the primary mechanism for toxin removal by hemodialysis. The driving force for this movement is the *concentration gradient* across the membrane. Solutes, such as urea, with concentrations higher in blood than in the dialysis fluid, diffuse across the concentration gradient from the blood to the dialysate, whereas bicarbonate (or acetate), with a concentration higher in the dialysate than

in blood, diffuses in the opposite direction. The rate of diffuse transport increases with an increase in the concentration difference across the membrane, an increase in the membrane surface area available for transport, and an increase in the mass transfer coefficient of the membrane (Ko). The Ko of a membrane is a function of the porosity and thickness of the membrane, the molecular size of the toxin, and the conditions of flow perfusing the two faces of the membrane (Q_B and Q_D). The Ko increases with thinner, more porous membranes, with decreasing molecular size, and with increased Q_B and Q_D. The contribution of charge of solute to clearance is exemplified by phosphate, in which the charge and water of hydration surrounding the molecule may decrease its clearance. Phosphate has a lower molecular weight than creatinine, yet it has an effective clearance approximately two thirds that of creatinine.

Clearance (or diffusion) of small molecules (e.g., urea) is *flow* dependent. As evident from Figure 20–2, for a small solute such as urea, clearance increases with flow rate (blood or dialysate), reaching a plateau beyond which no further increases occur with increasing flow. However, for a middle molecule or large solute such as vitamin B_{12}, the plateau occurs at much lower flow rates, and clearance is relatively insensitive to flow rates exceeding this plateau limit. In other words, the diffusion of small solutes is *flow limited* and large solutes are *membrane-limited*, with the limiting clearance being the mass-transfer times area coefficient (KoA). KoA (and hence clearance) can be increased by either increasing the effective surface area of the dialyzer membrane (A) or by increasing Ko as described earlier.

Applying this to clinical practice, the most effective way to increase small solute clearance would be to increase blood flow rates (e.g., from 250 ml/min to 400 ml/min or higher) and dialysate flow rates from 500 ml/min to 800 ml/min. However, when increases in Q_B and Q_D are no longer effective, a larger surface area dialyzer or a thinner membrane should be used to achieve higher clearances. For increasing large solute clearance, the choices would be to use a more porous membrane, a higher surface area, a thinner dialyzer membrane, or some combination of these three approaches.

Ultrafiltration

Ultrafiltration (or convective transport) involves bulk movement of solvent across the membrane.

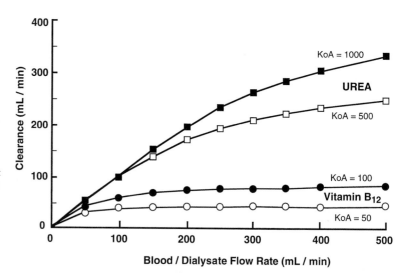

Figure 20–2. Dialyzer clearance of substances of different molecular weights as a function of blood/dialysate flow rate and the mass-transfer coefficient areas product [KoA]. The clearance of large molecules (vitamin B_{12}) is not so flow dependent as the clearance of small molecules.

In this process, solutes are "dragged" or "convected" across the membrane by fluid transport. The driving force in this circumstance is the hydrostatic pressure gradient across the dialysis membrane (called the *transmembrane pressure* [TMP]). To establish ultrafiltration, one applies a pressure gradient across the dialyzer membrane either by pressurizing the blood compartment of the dialyzer (positive pressure) or by applying suction (negative pressure) to the dialysate compartment. Usually, both the positive (venous pressure [VP]) and the negative (dialysate pressure [DP]) contribute to the transmembrane pressure in the following relationship:

TMP equals the pressure difference across the dialysis membrane and is the algebraic difference of the blood compartment pressure and dialysate compartment pressure: TMP = VP − DP (e.g., VP = 75 mm Hg and DP = −200 mm Hg, then TMP = 75 − (−200) = 275 mm Hg).

The ultrafiltration coefficient (K_{uf}) reflects the permeability of a particular membrane to water and is defined as the number of milliliters of fluid that can be transferred across the membrane per 1 mm Hg in 1 hour (i.e., If the K_{uf} of a dialyzer is 4 ml/mm Hg per hour, then at the above TMP, this dialyzer will result in net ultrafiltration of 4 × 275 = 1100 ml/hr).

In clinical practice, a particular TMP required for a given rate of fluid removal is based on the manufacturer's specifications of the K_{uf}. However, significant underestimation or overestimation of fluid removal can occur with this technique, with consequent cardiovascular sequelae. Manufacturing technology has allowed the introduction of hardware modules that can control the rate of ultrafiltration directly (rather than relying indirectly on TMP monitoring). As a re-

sult of this technologic advancement, flow sensor schemes of ultrafiltration control allow accurate measurements of rates of ultrafiltration that match the desired rates. For accomplishing this, appropriate microprocessor circuitry adjusts the TMP to match difference between dialysate outflow and inflow rates (the rate of ultrafiltration).

DIALYZERS

An optimal dialyzer should satisfy two fundamental characteristics: (1) *biofunctionality* (with the greatest possible approximation to the elimination characteristics of the natural kidneys and (2) *biocompatibility* (no release of toxic substances and low interaction of blood components with the membrane and dialyzer components).

Dialyzer Types

Two forms of dialyzers have been used for hemodialysis. Plate dialyzers consist of a number of sheets of membranes separated by a space in rectangular compartments placed in parallel alignment, and hollow-fiber dialyzers consist of several thousand (10,000 to 15,000) hollow fibers wrapped in a bundle inside a plastic jacket. Hollow-fiber dialyzers are easy to use and provide low blood flow resistance, excellent mass transfer, low compliance, and controllable ultrafiltration. These dialyzers are easier to reuse than are the other types of dialyzers.

Large surface area dialyzers generally using synthetic membranes with high permeability are a subset of hollow-fiber dialyzers. These so-called high-flux dialyzers have greater surface area than their hollow-fiber counterparts with similar low

TABLE 20–3. Representative Listing of Commonly Used Hollow-Fiber Dialyzers

Model	Membrane	K_{uf}	In vitro KoA (urea)	Surface Area (m^2)	Urea Clearance ($Q_B = 200$)
Cobe 400	Cellulose	5.3	520	0.9	173
Terumo C-101	Cellulose	3.5	520	1.0	171
Fresenius F-80	Polysulfone	60	945	1.8	192
Toray B1-1.6-H	PMMA	12	720	1.6	186
Gambro/Hospal Biospn-1800-S	AN69	18	270	0.6	137

priming volumes. Their utility obviously lies in their provision of increased clearance for certain solutes; however, their marked permeability requires special devices and monitoring to control the rate of ultrafiltration.

A multitude of dialyzers are currently available (Table 20–3). As mentioned, most are hollow-fiber dialyzers. Each dialyzer includes a specification sheet that describes the pertinent operating information for the dialyzer: the ultrafiltration coefficient (K_{uf}); the clearance of certain molecules such as creatinine, phosphate, vitamin B_{12}, and urea; the membrane surface area; the priming volume; and fiber thickness and length.

Obviously, dialyzer specification sheets provide useful information about the function and efficiency of membranes, but their data cannot be completely extrapolated to the *in vivo* dialysis setting. Such information is best used as a guide for choosing a specific dialyzer and determining the general effectiveness of the dialysis delivered with this membrane.

In addition to their structural differences, dialyzers also vary in the *composition of the membrane* material and can be made from cellulose that is derived from cotton fibers (regenerated cellulose, e.g., cuprophane), substituted cellulose (cellulose acetate), or cellulosynthetic (e.g., hemophane). Alternatively, they may be noncellulose synthetic membranes such as polysulfone (PS), polyacrilonitrile (PAN), polymethylmethacrylate (PMMA), polycarbonate, and polyamide.

The cellulose polymer of cuprophane membranes has a large number of *free* hydroxyl groups at its surface. In the cellulose acetate membranes, a substantial number of these hydroxyl groups are chemically bonded to acetate. In manufacturing a cellulosynthetic membrane, a synthetic material (a tertiary amino compound) is added to liquefied cellulose. As a result, the surface of the membrane is altered and biocompatibility (discussed later) is greatly increased. During dialysis using membranes from unsubstituted cellulose, the free hydroxyl groups on the membrane surface are believed to activate the complement system in the blood flowing through the dialyzer. In substituted cellulose (or semisynthetic), a substantial number of the hydroxyl groups are chemically bonded and complement activation occurs to a much lesser extent. As discussed later, synthetic membranes are generally associated with a very low degree of complement activation, although some are more prone to activate complement than others.

A typical dialysis setup starting from the arterial needle in the vascular access of the patient and back to the venous needle is schematically shown in Figure 20–3. Pertinent parameters of the dialysis procedure are described below the figure. An important aspect of the hemodialysis machine is its monitoring function. The segment between the arterial access and blood pump is the high-risk segment and is the only source of passive entry of air into the circuit. In addition to the arterial and venous pressure monitors, the overall purpose of which is to stop the roller blood pump, the air-foam detector not only stops the roller pump but also clamps the venous line, preventing further return of blood to the patient.

The dialysate circuit monitors assure the safety of dialysis against improperly mixed dialysate concentrates, overheated dialysate, or blood leaks. Dialysate monitors include the conductivity, pH, temperature, dialysate pressure, and blood leak monitors.

PATIENT NUMBER 3

Patrisha, a 48-year-old woman, had been on long-term hemodialysis and had a 3-year history of ESRD secondary to polycystic kidney disease. Her medical history also included chronic reversible airway disease in childhood. While vacationing in Hawaii, she went to a local dialysis unit for routine treatment. The unit did not have a reuse program, and all dialyzers were new. Approximately 7 minutes after the start of dialysis, she began to experience moderate to severe dyspnea, chest tightness, and back pain. Dialyzer blood flow was immediately stopped, and on examination she was found to have a change in blood pressure from 132/74 mm Hg after initiation of treatment to 82/50 mm Hg. Her pulse had increased from 76 to 136, and the respiratory examination showed marked tachypnea and labored breathing at a rate of 32 per minute. The auscultatory examination revealed poor air entry bilaterally, diffuse midinspiratory and expiratory wheezing, cough without sputum production, tachypnea, and tachycardia. A regular rhythm with no evidence of friction rub was noted on cardiac examination. Patrisha's skin was cold and clammy but showed no evidence of cyanosis or ecchymosis.

The dialyzer circuit was examined. All monitors and alarms were appropriately set. The air level foam detector was appropriately set and had not been activated. A sample of dialysate was obtained. It was found to have normal conductivity and showed no evidence of hemolysis; the temperature was 37°C. Blood samples were drawn from the patient for complete blood count (CBC) and to determine complement factors, and an additional serum sample was obtained for IgE analysis. There was no visual evidence of hemolysis in these samples.

The patient was given 400 ml of 0.9% saline solution, and dialysis was discontinued without return of blood from the extracorporeal circuit. The circuit was maintained by recirculation. Oxygen was given at 4 L/min by nasal cannula, and symptoms gradually subsided after 30 minutes from the start of treatment. Dialysis was restarted with slow increase in blood flow, and symptoms did not recur for the remainder of the treatment. Patrisha told the dialysis nurse that she had similar but less severe symptoms during several treatments when she first started dialysis 2 years earlier but had noticed that these symptoms had subsided when the dialysis unit changed to a different type of dialyzer.

An ECG was obtained and showed a sinus rhythm, with no evidence of ischemia or infarction, normal voltages across all leads, and no evidence of pericarditis-induced changes.

Laboratory and Radiologic Studies: Subsequent blood tests found a WBC count of 900 cells/mm^3, 80% of the cells being lymphocytes. Complement levels were C3a 7832 ng/ml and C5a 198 ng/ml. Both of these should be undetectable in normal persons. The serum IgE level was normal. A chest radiograph was subsequently obtained and showed no evidence of air space disease or vascular redistribution.

The differential diagnosis for a patient with these symptoms includes the first-use syndrome (FUS) from use of nonbiocompatible membranes, anaphylactic reactions from contact of blood with the membrane or from the sterilant

ethylene oxide (ETO), formaldehyde reactions, air embolus, and acute hemolysis due to either overheated dialysate or incorrect water-dialysate mixtures leading to hypo-osmolar dialysate. Less likely was the consideration of pyrogenic reactions. A more extensive differential diagnosis would include diagnoses unrelated to the dialysis procedure, such as myocardial infarction, pulmonary embolus, arrhythmias leading to hypotension, acute intracranial bleed, and acute pericardial tamponade. If a subclavian catheter is in place, complications related to the catheter, such as rupture of the vein, creation of a traumatic AV fistula, or acute perforation of the vein wall and protrusion of the catheter into the thorax or pericardium, should also be considered.

The course of the problem and subsequent analysis of data obtained at the time of the event indicated that the most likely explanation was Patrisha's reaction to the dialyzer circuit.

BIOCOMPATIBILITY

Biocompatibility is best defined as the sum of the interactions between blood and the hemodialysis circuit. The artificial components of hemodialysis are "foreign." Therefore, when blood encounters these materials, it initiates an "inflammatory response." These reactions are often minimal, and the membrane can be termed "biocompatible." On other occasions, however, severe reactions can lead to patient morbidity and even the risk of death. The importance of this concept for patients on hemodialysis lies in their repetitive exposure to the nonself structures of the dialysis circuit. Thus, the chronicity of contact may transform even mild interactions to deleterious and detrimental clinical sequelae in the long term.

When blood encounters the hemodialysis membrane, several reactions are triggered, including the complement cascade, the coagulation cascade, and the contact-phase reaction. In addition, evidence suggests that neutrophils, monocytes, and platelets that directly contact membranes become activated, leading to up-regulation of adhesion receptors, cytokine release, and generation of cyclooxygenase metabolites.

The **acute effects** of these events can be profound. Dialysis-related neutropenia, hypoxemia, and anaphylaxis all have been described. The finding that complement activation occurs during hemodialysis via the alternative pathway provides the pathophysiology for these phenomena. It is noteworthy that cellulose-based membranes generally result in far greater activation

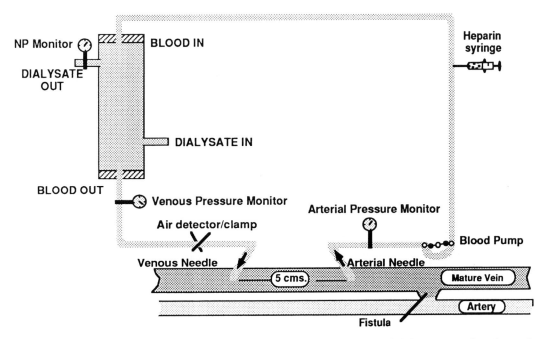

Figure 20–3. Important aspects of the dialysis treatment. The hemodialysis blood and dialyzer circuits show the usual location of the pressure monitors. The pressure monitor proximal to the blood pump is placed here to guard against excessive suction of the vascular access site by the blood pump. The venous pressure monitor (distal to the dialyzer) guards against excessive resistance to return of blood. It is also used to estimate the dialyzer blood compartment pressure. Either of these monitors can be adjusted to give off an alarm or shut off the blood pump when the desired pressure limits are exceeded. The dialyzer outflow pressure monitor (negative pressure usually) can be used in conjunction with the venous pressure to calculate TMP (TMP = VP + DP). Note the usual *countercurrent* flow of blood and dialysate into the dialyzer. Both arterial and venous needles stick into the mature vein of the fistula. To lessen recirculation, the tips of the cannulating needles should be separated by at least 5 cm. Recirculation is defined as:

$$R = \frac{P - A}{P - V} \times 100\%$$

where
P = BUN concentration in systemic circulation
A = BUN concentration at dialyzer blood inlet (arterial)
V = BUN concentration at dialyzer blood outlet (venous)

of complement than noncellulose-derived membranes.

The products of complement activation, C3a and C5a, have been termed *anaphylatoxins*. These proteins produce intense vasoconstriction and anaphylaxis in some animal models, hence, their designation. **Blood exposed to cellulose membranes has been experimentally infused into animals, with resulting ischemic ECG changes, elevations in pulmonary artery pressure, histamine release, and increased vascular permeability.** When C5a was introduced in a similar manner, many similar findings were noted, suggesting that C5a was the primary mediator of these complement-induced effects.

The clinical relevance of this has been well examined in the context of patient exposure to new cellulosic dialyzers. Many studies have documented a significant difference in the incidence of symptoms (e.g., chest pain or dyspnea) in patients dialyzed with new cellulosic membranes compared with reprocessed membranes, which do not activate complement as extensively. Another study also has demonstrated elevated levels of C3a and C5a in patients experiencing adverse symptoms compared with other patients dialyzing with the same membrane surface. It has been postulated that this difference may be responsible for FUS. This syndrome affects patients early in their dialysis session and has been subdivided based on the extent of their symptoms. Type A is manifested usually very early in the dialysis treatment as dyspnea, cramping, angioedema, and pruritus. Its incidence approximates 5 in

100,000. Type B often occurs after about 1 hour of hemodialysis, with the onset of back pain or chest pain. Both forms of FUS can be prevented by instituting an appropriate reuse program for dialyzers or switching to more biocompatible membranes. Interestingly, a similar syndrome has been associated with the use of PAN membranes in hemodialysis recipients given angiotensin-converting enzyme inhibitors. This reaction is believed to be secondary to the bradykinin-generating effects of the membrane in combination with converting enzyme inhibitors, which also inhibit the kininase enzymes, resulting in high concentrations of bradykinin in the circulation, profound hypotension, and cardiopulmonary arrest.

Complement proteins, generated on exposure to hemodialysis membranes, also induce neutrophil and monocyte activation. Neutrophils thus stimulated produce reactive oxygen species, which may be involved in various pathogenetic pathways in dialyzed patients, including progressive pulmonary fibrosis, atherogenesis, and potentially carcinogenesis. Neutrophil activation also results in up-regulation of adhesion receptors and consequently granulocyte adherence to the vasculature, primarily the pulmonary vasculature. Cell aggregates can lead to thromboembolic events or decreases in peak expiratory flow rates and PaO_2, two events observed in patients dialyzed with new cellulosic membranes.

In contrast to the aforementioned acute syndromes, the chronic sequelae associated with bioincompatibility are less dramatic but no less potent in their deleterious effects. The accumulation of amyloid fibrils, consisting of β_2-microglobulin fibrils, has been recognized in long-term hemodialysis since the mid-1980s. **This form of amyloidosis is manifested as patients develop carpal tunnel syndrome, arthropathy, lytic bone lesions, and pathologic fractures.** Available evidence suggests that membrane bioincompatibility may be directly involved in the evolution of this process. Several studies have shown an increased incidence of β_2-microglobulin-related amyloidosis in patients dialyzed with cellulosic membranes. The pathogenesis of β_2-microglobulin-related amyloidosis appears to be multifactorial and is associated with an increase in mononuclear cell synthesis and release of β_2-microglobulin after contact with cellulosic membranes. In addition, cellulosic membranes may enhance the polymerization of β_2-microglobulin fibrils by stimulating the release of proteases from WBCs. Furthermore, these membranes do not adsorb or clear β_2-microglobulin readily from the circulation.

Membrane bioincompatibility also appears to affect recovery from acute renal failure. Conger and colleagues as well as Solez and co-workers initially advanced the notion that dialysis may alter the pace of recovery in acute renal failure. Both studies examined renal histopathology in individuals who had acute renal failure and who required lengthy courses of hemodialysis. Fresh areas of acute tubular necrosis were evident despite the fact that the initial injury was remote. Certain investigators have implicated infiltrating WBCs in this ongoing injury, accompanying acute renal failure. It appears therefore that cellulosic membranes, because they activate complement and WBCs, may contribute significantly to this injury, thereby delaying recovery in acute renal failure. Studies of animals with reversible acute renal failure have shown that renal recovery is slower when animals have been exposed to cellulosic membranes than when they have been exposed to biocompatible membranes.

Biocompatible membranes also appear to reduce the incidence of infections in patients on hemodialysis. This may be partly because of alterations in cellular immunity. Long-term dialysis with cellulosic membranes further depresses T-cell function and decreases the expression of high-affinity interleukin-2 receptors on mononuclear cells. Changing to a more biocompatible membrane, PMMA, allows these receptors to increase in number to near normal levels. Other investigators have also found decreased natural killer function in patients dialyzed with bioincompatible membranes, as well as decreased IL-2 generation and a decreased proliferative response.

Several studies have also suggested the possibility that bioincompatibility may be a catabolic stimulus in patients on long-term hemodialysis. Exposure to cellulosic membranes appears to increase net protein catabolism, whereas PS or PAN membranes do not affect protein catabolism. Moreover, patients dialyzed with biocompatible membranes appear to have greater protein intake than do patients dialyzed with cellulosic membranes. Although further studies are necessary to establish the extent to which bioincompatibility alone accounts for these findings, these observations support the contention that biocompatibility directly affects the catabolic nature of hemodialysis.

Clearly then, biocompatibility is very important for understanding and optimizing membrane use. In addition to the foregoing list, biocompatibility may affect residual renal function, long-term pulmonary changes, and RBC survival. Perhaps most important is the view that biocompatibility appears to reduce morbidity and mortality. Retrospective analyses suggest that patients dialyzed with cuprophane membranes experience more in-hospital days and greater annual mortality than patients dialyzed with PAN membranes. **Biocompatibility therefore should be a consideration, along with membrane clearance, K_{uf}, and KoA, when choosing a dialyzer for a patient.**

DIALYSATE COMPOSITION

The composition of the dialysis solution has undergone substantial changes since the inception of hemodialysis. One of the major aims of hemodialysis is restoration of normal ion concentrations (via diffusional transfer between dialysis fluid and blood). To accomplish this the level of individual ions in the dialysate can be set to approximate the desired levels in plasma water. For calcium and magnesium, dialysate levels are set for the *diffusible* fraction found in plasma water.

A discussion of the principles governing the concentrations of each major dialysate component follows.

Dialysate Glucose

Contemporary dialysis fluids range from glucose free to isoglycemia (5 to 5.5 mmol/L [90 to 100 mg/dl]) or slightly hyperglycemic (5.5 to 11.0 mmol/L [100 to 200 mg/dl]). Most non–insulin-dependent patients tolerate dialysis with glucose-free dialysate without ill effects despite losing 25 to 30 g of glucose across the dialyzer. A few studies, however, have shown that this glucose loss may adversely affect intermediary metabolism of carbohydrates and proteins. The adverse effects of glucose-free dialysate include a reduction in plasma glucose, a corresponding decrease in plasma insulin levels, and a marked decrease in lactate and pyruvate levels. Although these biochemical measures often are sufficient to maintain serum glucose levels in the physiologic range, hypoglycemia may develop during the use of glucose-free dialysate, especially in the presence of cachexia, sepsis, diabetes mellitus, or drugs such as aspirin or propranolol. Available data also indicate that dialysate glucose does not have a significant role in determining total cholesterol levels in non–insulin-dependent hemodialyzed patients.

Dialysate Sodium

The pivotal role that plasma osmolality has in maintaining hemodynamic stability during hemodialysis is now well established. Hyposmolality impairs peripheral vasoconstriction during volume removal and exacerbates autonomic insufficiency. This decline in P_{osm} is more apparent when solute removal is rapid and is not counteracted by diffusion of sodium from the dialysate to the blood. Use of low-sodium dialysate (< 135 mEq/L) favors this intracellular fluid shift as plasma becomes more hypo-osmolar consequent to sodium movement from plasma to dialysate. On the other hand, by maintaining a relatively constant plasma osmolality, high dialysate sodium (140 to 145 mEq/L) minimizes water movement intracellularly during dialysis, therefore better preserving plasma volume, which is clinically paralleled by an increased tolerance to hemodialysis—namely, a reduction in cramping, nausea, vomiting, and headaches. Therefore, the use of lower dialysate sodium in routine maintenance hemodialysis has now been abandoned.

Dialysate Buffer

Bicarbonate dialysis is considered the dialytic treatment of choice for critically ill patients, conferring many benefits over acetate dialysis in these patients, including a lower incidence of arterial hypotension, less hypoxemia, and improved left ventricular stroke work. Hakim and colleagues have also found less hypoxemia and fewer hypotensive episodes with bicarbonate dialysis in patients undergoing long-term dialysis.

The mechanisms by which acetate buffer results in hemodynamic instability include direct vasodilation, stimulating the release of interleukin-1, a vasodilatory compound, and arterial hypoxemia, which results from the transfer of carbon dioxide across the dialysis membrane, from blood to dialysate, with consequent reflex hypoventilation. Finally, acetate dialysate may have a myocardial depressant effect.

In conclusion, bicarbonate dialysis is the dialysate buffer of choice and confers advantages in critically ill patients. Stable patients on long-term hemodialysis, patients who are unable to metabolize acetate well, elderly patients, patients with reduced muscle mass, malnourished patients, and possibly females tolerate bicarbonate dialysate better. These patients may be particularly intolerant of acetate with the use of high-flux dialysis,

because of the high influx of acetate with these dialyzers.

Dialysate Calcium

Because dialysate calcium equilibrates with the diffusible (ionized) fraction of calcium in the plasma, a dialysate calcium of 2.5 mEq/L is equivalent to serum calcium level of 10 mg/dl. The use of high dialysate calcium (3.5 mEq/L) or low dialysate calcium ($\leq$ 2.5 mEq/L) entails separate advantages and risks. Numerous studies have shown a beneficial effect of high dialysate calcium on the indices of metabolic bone disease as well as a reduction in parathyroid hormone (PTH) levels. High dialysate calcium has also been shown to improve hemodynamic stability during dialysis by augmenting stroke volume and cardiac output without changing peripheral vascular resistance (PVR). One complication of high dialysate calcium is the development of hypercalcemia with concurrent use of calcium-based phosphate binders and oral or intravenous 1,25-dihydroxyvitamin D_3.

In summary, in a hemodynamically stable patient and particularly those prone to hypercalcemia during treatment with vitamin D and calcium salts, a dialysate calcium concentration of 2.5 mEq/L is recommended.

Dialysate Potassium

Typically, 50 to 80 mEq of potassium is removed with each dialysis treatment. Because internal [K^+] transfer is affected by many factors, the acid-base status of a hemodialyzed patient must be considered when choosing a dialysate [K^+]. Extracellular acidosis promotes [K^+] egress from cells, whereas alkalosis causes cellular [K^+] uptake. Because plasma tonicity favors [K^+] removal, hypertonic saline or mannitol, used in the treatment of hypotension or muscle cramps during dialysis, can increase [K^+] dialysance. Glucose-free dialysate also promotes [K^+] removal.

Low dialysate [K^+] can precipitate ventricular ectopia. This is most pronounced in patients with left ventricular hypertrophy or impaired left ventricular function or in patients taking digoxin. Therefore, for patients at risk for arrhythmias, the use of dialysate [K^+] < 2 mEq/L should be avoided. Finally, before instituting digoxin therapy for a patient on hemodialysis, the potential risk versus benefit of such therapy should be carefully assessed because patients on hemodialysis experience considerable variability in [K^+].

ADEQUACY OF HEMODIALYSIS

Until recently, the prescription of dialysis has remained empirical, and the length of dialysis was determined primarily by the clinical judgment of the attending nephrologist. Although several proposals were made to guide clinicians, these suffered from a lack of correlation between the prescription and patient outcome. An earlier multicenter study to investigate this issue was completed in the United States in the early 1980s, and the results have allowed the quantitation of dialysis prescription.

The National Cooperative Dialysis Study (NCDS) was designed to investigate the effect of altering dialysis prescription to change either the ambient *urea level* or the *dialysis time*. Because there was no universal agreement about the timing of the urea measurement (before or after dialysis, at the beginning of the week or at the end of the week), the concept of a *time-averaged concentration (TAC)* of urea was developed to represent the surrogate parameter for small molecules, whereas time on dialysis was used as a surrogate parameter of the middle molecules. TAC_{urea} can be defined as

$$TAC_{urea} = \frac{(C_1 + C_2) \times td + (C_2 + C_3) \times Id}{2(td + Id)}$$

where td = time on dialysis, Id = interdialytic time, C_1 = predialysis BUN, C_2 = postdialysis BUN, and C_3 = next predialysis BUN.

The patients participating in the NCDS were divided into four groups:

Group 1: Long dialysis time (4½ to 5 hours) + TAC = 50 mg/dl
Group 2: Long dialysis time (4½ to 5 hours) + TAC = 100 mg/dl
Group 3: Short dialysis time (2½ to 3 hours) + TAC = 50 mg/dl
Group 4: Short dialysis time (2½ to 3 hours) + TAC = 100 mg/dl

No difference in mortality was found among the four groups during the study period; however, withdrawal from the study for medical reasons was significantly greater in patients in the high-BUN groups than in the low-BUN groups. Hospitalization rate was also greater in the high-BUN groups. Although time on dialysis was not a statistically significant parameter, it nevertheless was an important parameter. Similarly, although no difference in mortality between different groups was noted during the study, the

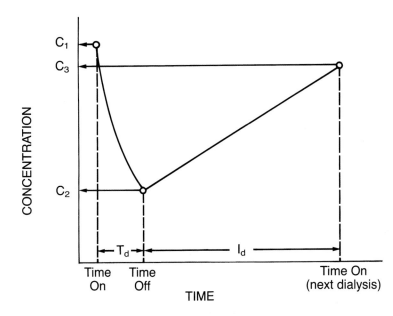

Figure 20–4. Change in solute concentration during and between dialysis. (From Sargent JA: Kinetic modeling in the guidance of dialysis therapy. Dial Transplant 8:1101, 1979.)

mortality rate in the high-BUN groups was higher after termination of the study.

This prospective study therefore indicated that the dialysis prescription had an effect on the occurrence of medical complications and hospitalization rates and that TAC_{urea} was a useful target for monitoring and prescribing dialysis.

One possible definition of adequate dialysis is a treatment prescription that ameliorates and prevents complications of uremia. Although there may be no single measure of the adequacy of dialysis treatment, patients who are adequately dialyzed must have satisfactory blood pressure control and achieve reasonable overall rehabilitation. Patients must have adequate nutritional status, with improvement in the degree of platelet function, cardiovascular status, musculoskeletal function, and neurobehavioral status.

Another index that was partly derived from the results of the NCDS is generally labeled the *Kt/V parameter.* To understand this, it is important to recollect that the cycle of changes of blood urea and nitrogen in a patient on long-term hemodialysis (Fig. 20–4) indicates a sharp decrease during the dialytic treatment and a gradual increase during the interdialytic period.

During dialysis, BUN concentration decreases as a function of three parameters: dialyzer urea clearance (K_0), dialysis treatment time (td), and the volume of distribution of urea (V).

> **Despite having the same BUN as a smaller patient, a large patient requires more dialysis because of larger total body urea content and urea volume of distribution.**

On the other hand, the increase in BUN during the interdialytic period depends on the following:

1. The rate of generation of urea. This is a function of the protein catabolic rate, which in a stable noncatabolic patient reflects dietary protein intake.
2. The volume of distribution of urea.
3. Residual renal function.

> **Kt/V is the most accepted index for determining adequacy of dialysis.**

The amount of plasma cleared of urea during dialysis is reflected by the ratio of the postdialysis to the predialysis (post/pre) urea nitrogen (UN) levels: R = post/pre plasma UN. A urea reduction ratio (URR) is simply $1 - R$. For example, if the predialysis UN is 100 mg/dl and the postdialysis value is 40 mg/dl, then

$$R = 40/100 = 0.40 \text{ and}$$
$$URR = 1 - 0.40 = 0.60 \text{ or } 60\%$$

In other words, the lower the R, the greater is the amount of urea clearance. A Kt/V of 1.4 is approximately equal to a URR of 65% to 70%.

Target Kt/V

Optimal dialysis can be defined as the dose of dialysis above which no further improvement in the morbidity and mortality of dialysis can be expected. The target Kt/V that should be delivered for optimal dialysis is not exactly defined. We have learned from the mechanistic analysis of the NCDS to strive for a Kt/V more than 1.0, because levels of Kt/V less than 1.0 predict a high rate of failure. However, it should be emphasized that on the basis of the NCDS entry criteria, such recommendations apply to nondiabetic patients between the ages of 18 and 70 years. Further, it should also be recalled that Kt/V was not the primary variable on which randomization was performed in the NCDS. Despite this, Kt/V has become a common basis for reporting and assessing the adequacy of dialysis treatment. The American Association of Kidney Patients Advisory released its recommendations on adequate dialysis: a target dose of dialysis of a URR more than 60% (equivalent to a Kt/V of 1.2). The Renal Physicians Association recently had set a Kt/V of 1.0 as "adequate" and 1.2 as "ideal." Reports also associate dialysis treatment duration with mortality.

Although no similar prospective studies addressing optimal dialysis are yet available, several reports suggest that **more dialysis leads to better survival.** In one study at Vanderbilt University, the effects on mortality of gradually increasing doses of dialysis were investigated in 130 patients by increasing the Kt/V from 0.82 ± 0.32 in 1988 to 1.33 ± 0.23 in 1991. Gross annual mortality declined, from 22.8% in 1988 to 9.1% in 1991 concurrent with this dosage increase. To account for potential differences in patients' characteristics during those years, the ratio of observed to expected deaths, based on data from the USRDS, was also calculated. This ratio (expected/observed deaths) decreased from 1.3 in 1988 to 0.61 in 1991. In addition, the number of hospital days per patient in a year decreased from 15.2 to less than 10.

The importance of the actual duration of dialysis as an independent factor and as a determinant of optimal dialysis needs further clarification. The currently available limited data support the contention that the relative mortality risk correlates inversely with treatment time. Compared with patients dialyzed for more than 4 hours, one report found a relative mortality risk of 1.17 to 2.18 in patients dialyzed for less than 3.5 hours. In the same report, dialysis for less than 3.5 hours was also associated with more intradialytic symptoms and lower S_{Cr} levels (possibly reflecting poorer nutritional status). Although dialysis time did not reach statistical significance in the NCDS, reanalysis of the data for patients randomized to the lower time-averaged

urea concentration group suggested that longer dialysis time might benefit long-term outcome. Although these studies may incriminate time on dialysis as an independent variable affecting mortality and morbidity in patients on hemodialysis, it should be recalled that most of these data are based on conventional cellulosic membrane dialysis, and the impact of time on dialysis with dialysis using more biocompatible membranes remains to be clarified. A single-center 10-year patient survival analysis suggests that hemodialysis with a biocompatible membrane (PAN/AN/69) may be an important explanation for improved patient survival.

> The National Institutes of Health (Bethesda, Maryland) has launched a landmark clinical trial multicenter, prospective, randomized, 7-year study to investigate the role of the dose of dialysis and type of dialysis membranes on morbidity and mortality of 1600 to 1800 patients on hemodialysis. In this 2 × 2 factorial clinical trial, standard [Kt/V = 1.0 (double pool, and 1.2 (single pool)] and high [(Kt/V = 1.4 (double pool) and 1.6 (single pool)] and membrane flux (low versus high flux) are the primary focus. The effects of maintenance of adequate nutrition and of time on dialysis on morbidity and mortality of hemodialysis patients will also be explored in this study.

Until the results of this randomized multicenter prospective study examining the impact of the dialysis dose, the dialysis membrane, and the duration of dialysis on patient morbidity and mortality become available, we recommend an optimal dialysis prescription as outlined in Table 20–4. In addition to Kt/V, optimal dialysis should strive to achieve a functionally rehabilitated, well-nourished, and normotensive patient.

MEDICAL COMPLICATIONS ON HEMODIALYSIS

The most common complications of hemodialysis are

- Intradialytic hypotension
- Malnutrition
- Infections
- GI bleeding
- β_2-microglobulin amyloidosis
- Muscle cramps
- Nausea and vomiting
- Pruritus

TABLE 20–4. Guidelines for Optimal Dialysis

- Target Kt/V ≥ 1.4
  (equivalent to urea reduction ratio ≥ 65–70%)
- Target PCR ≥ 1.0 g/kg/day
- Target serum albumin ≥ 4.0 g/dl
- Rigorously monitor amount of "delivered" dialysis
  dose to ensure delivered dose equals prescribed
  dose
- Use biocompatible membrane
- Avoid ultrafiltration rates in excess of 0.3
  ml/min/kg (1.3 L/hr in a 70-kg adult)

Certain other medical conditions commonly afflict dialyzed patients and require special attention by physicians caring for renal patients. These conditions include anemia, secondary hyperparathyroidism and aluminum-related bone disease, uremic bleeding, acquired cystic kidney disease, seizures, and arrhythmias during dialysis. It is beyond the scope of this chapter to discuss all systemic conditions and diseases occurring in patients who have ESRD and are on dialysis.

Hypotension

Hypotension is the most frequent complication during dialysis, occurring in 20% to 30% of dialysis treatments. The sequelae of this hypotension are protean and include nausea and vomiting, decreased mental status (particularly in the elderly), and postdialysis malaise and fatigue. The sequelae of hypotension, however, may not be necessarily benign and may be accompanied by neurologic complications such as stroke; cardiac ischemia manifesting as angina, myocardial infarction, or arrhythmias; aspiration pneumonia; or vascular access clotting. To understand the etiology and management of dialysis-associated hypotension, a brief review of the determinants of mean arterial blood pressure on dialysis follows.

Mean arterial pressure is determined by PVR and cardiac output. Cardiac output is a function of stroke volume and heart rate, and stroke volume in turn depends on plasma volume and myocardial contractility. During hemodialysis, reduction of plasma volume results in hypotension if the compensatory changes in heart rate, PVR, or myocardial contractility do not occur. The major problem underlying the development of dialysis-induced hypotension is more rapid removal of fluid from the intravascular space than can be replaced, coupled with an inability to increase PVR adequately. Generally, ultrafiltration rates in excess of 0.3 ml/min/kg (e.g., > 1.2

L/hr in a 70-kg patient) are associated with a steep increase in the incidence of hypotension on dialysis.

The rate of ultrafiltration required during dialysis is determined by the interdialytic weight gain and duration of dialysis. Greater weight gains and shorter treatment times often cause hypotension. Patients should restrict interdialytic weight gains to 5% of their body weight. An estimated dry weight that is too low also results in ultrafiltration rates that can exceed the rate of plasma refilling. The first measure of patients on long-term dialysis who were previously stable and who develop recurrent hypotension, particularly toward the end of dialysis, is reassessment of their dry weight. If a patient has a good appetite and no manifestations of fluid overload such as peripheral edema or predialysis hypertension, it is possible that muscle mass has increased. This type of hypotension would be particularly evident toward the end of dialysis as the patient nears his or her estimated dry weight. Evaluation of dry weight should be gradual only (0.5 to 1 kg at a time).

The major problem underlying the development of dialysis-associated hypotension is more rapid removal of fluid from the intravascular space than can be replaced, coupled with an inability to increase PVR adequately. Generally, ultrafiltration rates in excess of 0.3 ml/min/kg (e.g., > 1.2 L/hr in a 70-kg patient) are associated with a steep increase in the incidence of hypotension on dialysis.

The etiology of dialysis-associated hypotension is multifactorial. The most common causes of dialysis hypotension are listed in Table 20–5. The interplay of ultrafiltration rate and dialysate composition on the determinants of mean arterial pressure in patients on dialysis is depicted in Figure 20–5. Dialysate sodium appears to be the major factor determining blood pressure stability. The roles of dialysate sodium and dialysate buffer have already been discussed in the section on dialysate composition. The effect of dialysate sodium is most pronounced during the early part of dialysis, when plasma sodium is decreasing most abruptly. The role of acetate buffer in cardiovascular instability is most notable in elderly dialyzed patients who metabolize acetate slowly. Autonomic nervous system dysfunction remains a common finding in patients on long-term dialysis, especially those who are diabetic and those with severe secondary hyperparathyroidism.

TABLE 20–5. Causes of Hypotension
During Dialysis

Excessive or rapid removal of fluid greater than
  plasma refilling rate
  High ultrafiltration rates, large interdialysis weight
    gain, and short treatment time
  Low estimated dry weight
  Low dialysate sodium concentration
  Low plasma protein level
Dialysate buffer
  Sodium acetate
Autonomic nervous system dysfunction
Antihypertensive medications
Cardiac factors
  Hypertension
  Pericardial effusion
  Coronary artery disease
  Cardiomyopathy
  Negative inotropic agents
  Anemia and arteriovenous fistula
  Calcification of conduction system
  Aortic stenosis
Warm dialysate solution
Hypoxemia
Blood-membrane interactions
Miscellaneous: low dialysate calcium, eating during
  dialysis

Antihypertensive Medications. Many antihypertensive medications impair vasoconstriction (e.g., hydralazine hydrochloride). Beta blockers decrease cardiac contractility and limit the increase in heart rate in response to sympathetic influences. Because hypotension caused by these medications is associated with predialysis hypertension, a therapeutic dilemma often arises. Hypertensive patients are often advised not to ingest these medications until after dialysis. Most antihypertensive medications, long-acting nitrates, and narcotics/anxiolytics should be withheld 4 hours before dialysis. A specific family of drugs that do not seem to predispose to hypotension during dialysis, even if ingested before dialysis, are the converting enzyme inhibitors, which are effective in the absence of renal function.

Cardiac Factors. The heart's ability to maintain or increase cardiac output in response to volume depletion has a major role in preventing hypotension. Hypertrophy and dilatation of the left ventricle, increased age and atherosclerosis, and coronary artery disease all can limit this response. Decreased cardiac reserve may also be caused by the chronic high-output state secondary to the anemia and the presence of an AV fistula. Pericardial effusions are usually small and not clinically significant. In the presence of congestive heart failure or pericarditis, which may be clinically silent, the pericardial effusions may increase and thus impair ventricular filling. Long-standing calcium and phosphorus abnormalities may predispose to ectopic calcification in the myocardium or conduction system, leading to decreased contractility or arrhythmias.

Warm Dialysate Solution. During hemodialysis, blood comes in contact with warmed dialysate and returns to the patient at a slightly increased temperature. Vasodilation and hypotension may occur.

Dialysate Calcium. Several studies have examined the effect of dialysate calcium on myocardial performance during dialysis. An increase in the velocity of circumferential fiber shortening (an index of contractility) is noted, in association with an increased ionized calcium concentration during dialysis.

Miscellaneous Causes. Postprandial hypotension is common and may aggravate the risk of hypotension during dialysis. Other causes include dialysate pyrogens, which may cause monocyte activation, increase interleukin-1 levels, and promote hypotension. Refractory hypotensive episodes have also occurred with severe hypermagnesemia. The management of *frequent* dialysis hypotension is summarized in Table 20–6.

TABLE 20–6. Strategies to Minimize
Dialysis-Induced Hypotension

- Frequent assessment of dry weight
- Avoid excessive interdialytic weight gain (<5% body weight)
- Avoid antihypertensive drugs before dialysis or altogether
- Reduce intake of narcotic analgesics and sedative-hypnotics
- No heavy meals during or just before dialysis
- Increase hematocrit to 33%
- Evaluate for silent pericardial effusion
- Use dialysate sodium of ≥ 140 mEq/L
- High dialysate calcium concentration (?)
- Use bicarbonate dialysis (especially with high blood flow)
- Administer prophylactic oxygen, especially in elderly patients with cardiac or respiratory disease and a predialysis PaO$_2$ < 80 mm Hg
- Use biocompatible membrane
- In selected patients, use a cool dialysate (34°C)
- Use dialysis machines with UF controls
- Use sequential UF dialysis; occasionally necessary when high UF rates are required
- Ameliorate risk factors for left ventricular hypertrophy (anemia, hyperparathyroidism, aluminum overload)
- Improve nutritional status and hypoalbuminemia if present

UF, ultrafiltration.

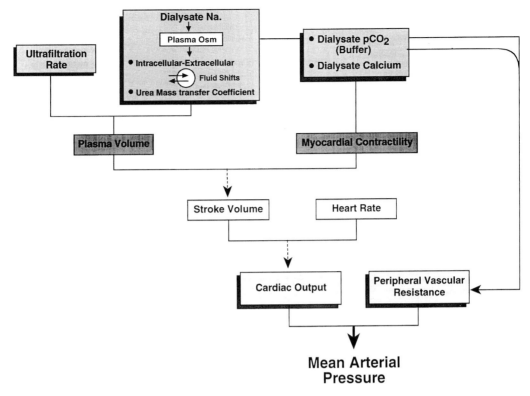

Figure 20–5. Determinants of systemic blood pressure and effects of dialysis composition on systemic hemodynamics. During ultrafiltration and/or dialysis, reduction of plasma volume will result in hypotension if compensatory changes in myocardial contractility, heart rate, or peripheral vascular resistance do not occur. During conventional dialysis, the reduction in plasma osmolality favors fluid shift from ECF to ICF, exacerbating the volume-depleting effects of dialysis. This is further augmented by using low dialysate sodium (< 130–135 mEq/L) and in patients with reduced urea mass transfer coefficients. Low dialysate calcium and/or hypoventilation/hypoxemia due to low PCO_2 reduce myocardial contractility. Low dialysate sodium and IL-2 impair compensatory peripheral vasoconstriction. The role of acetate on myocardial contractility is controversial.

Muscle Cramps

Muscle cramps occur in approximately 5% to 15% of dialysis treatments. Cramps tend to occur more frequently after large amounts of ultrafiltration and most commonly occur in the last hour of dialysis and in association with hypotension.

Prevention of muscle cramps is best achieved by reduction of interdialytic weight gains and hence the consequent need for rapid ultrafiltration. In general, weight reductions of less than 5% of estimated dry weight can be easily tolerated. Higher interdialytic weight gain is also associated with more pronounced hyponatremia before dialysis, and thus osmolality changes during dialysis are also accentuated. Treatment of muscle cramps includes (1) temporary decrease of ultrafiltration rate; (2) intermittent administration of normal saline in 100-ml boluses or hypertonic sodium chloride, 10 ml of 23% solution

(repetitive use of hypertonic sodium chloride, particularly when given toward the end of dialysis, may lead to hyperosmolarity and increased thirst and weight gain in the interdialytic period); (3) 10 to 20 ml of 50% hypertonic glucose or 10 to 20 ml of 25 percent mannitol, both of which are equally effective as hypertonic sodium chloride; (4) dialysate sodium, 140 mEq/L; and (5) stretching muscles and standing up.

For patients with modest interdialytic weight gains and frequent cramping during dialysis, quinine sulfate may be beneficial. A 325-mg dose given ½ to 1 hour before initiation of dialysis can decrease the frequency of intradialytic cramps.

PATIENT NUMBER 4

Eric, 35 years old, frequently misses dialysis treatments. He abuses fluids and gains 7 to 8 kg

> between treatments. He demonstrates volume-sensitive hypertension with predialysis seated blood pressures of 180/100 to 200/115 mmHg. His 3-hour treatments are often complicated by leg cramps during the last hour, occasionally associated with hypotension. He periodically demands to quit dialysis early because of cramps.

Painful intradialytic muscle cramps can be a strong disincentive to dialyze. As a result, missed treatments by patients with large fluid gains can perpetuate vicious cycles of missed treatments and larger fluid gains, which exacerbate cramping and noncompliance. Prevention is important. Because the prevalence of muscle cramps correlates best with large fluid gains, behavioral changes to reduce fluid intake are most effective long term. Scheduling extra dialysis treatments to optimize volume removal seems only to encourage more fluid intake. Because of frequent earlier termination of dialysis, as well as frequent missed treatments, these patients have inadequate dialysis. It is important for these patients to extend their treatment times to reduce the ultrafiltration rate and optimize Kt/V. This may be difficult with tight dialysis schedules, but these patients can dialyze at times when the schedule is more flexible (e.g., the last or third shift).

> **Scheduling extra dialysis treatments encourages more fluid intake in patients who gain large amounts of fluid between dialysis sessions.**

Hypertonic solutions and reduction in ultrafiltration rates should be the cornerstone of therapy (as described earlier). Quinine sulfate is effective but not without complications (thrombocytopenic purpura and cinchonism). Although rare (quinine undergoes hepatic metabolism), cinchonism may progress to deafness, optic atrophy, and severe GI symptoms. It is usually safe at doses of 325 mg during or just before dialysis. However, it should not be used routinely or, in larger doses, between dialysis sessions. A controlled, randomized, double-blind study compared quinine with vitamin E (400 IU daily orally) and found both drugs to be equally efficacious for treating leg cramps in patients with ESRD. Verapamil, in addition to blood pressure control, perhaps specifically reduces cramps as well. L-carnitine (20 mg/kg IV after hemodialysis) may also reduce

the incidence of intradialytic hypotension and muscle cramps.

Malnutrition

Protein-calorie malnutrition is common in patients on maintenance dialysis. Malnutrition is mild to moderate in approximately 30% of patients on maintenance dialysis and severe in approximately 6% to 8%. Protein-calorie malnutrition in dialysis patients on maintenance has many causes (Table 20–7), the major causes being the dialysis procedure itself, intercurrent or underlying illnesses, membrane bioincompatibility, and socioeconomic factors. Once malnutrition is established, parenteral nutrition may reverse the objective evidence of malnutrition, but its effects on survival have not yet been documented.

Several clinical and biochemical indices of malnutrition in patients on hemodialysis have been suggested (Table 20–8). Nonfluid weight loss, serum albumin level (< 4.0 g/dl), protein catabolic rate (< 0.8/kg/day), and BUN (< 50

TABLE 20–7. Causes of Malnutrition in Patients on Dialysis

Dialysis factors
- Kt/V < 1.0
- Bioincompatible membranes (catabolic effects of blood-membrane interactions)
- Loss of amino acids and peptides in dialysate
- Protein losses (peritoneal dialysis)
- Use of acetate and high-calcium dialysate

Dietary restrictions
- Continuation of long-term low-protein diet
- Intern-resident admission orders for "renal diet"

Biochemical/metabolic and endocrine disturbances
- Metabolic acidosis
- Catabolic effects of high PTH levels?
- Low IGF-1; resistance to IGF-1
- Insulin resistance, increased gluconeogenesis, and decreased glycogen stores
- Altered amino acid metabolism

Gastrointestinal
- Gastroparesis
- Malabsorption
- Pancreatitis
- Esophagitis, gastritis, ulcer disease
- Anorexia
- Constipation

Miscellaneous
- Depression
- Low socioeconomic status
- Multiple medications, especially sedatives
- Underlying illness
- Recurrent hospitalizations
- Lack of partner

TABLE 20–8. Indices of Malnutrition in Hemodialysis Patients

- Serum albumin < 4.0 g/dl
- Continuous decline of estimated dry weight
- PCR < 0.8 g/kg/day
- Body weight < 80% of ideal weight
- Low serum creatinine and urea° concentration in patients without residual renal function
- Marked reduction in anthropometric measurements
- Cholesterol concentration < 180 mg/dl
- Transferring concentration < 200 mg/dl
- IGF-1 (somatomedin C) concentration < 300 μg/L
- Low predialysis serum potassium (and possibly serum phosphorus)
- Serum prealbumin < 30 mg/dl

°BUN <50 mg/dl in a patient with residual renal function < 3 ml/min.

mg/dl) are the most commonly measured parameters currently used to assess nutritional status of patients undergoing dialysis.

Several studies, though not all, suggest that optimal dialysis improves the nutritional states of patients on dialysis. Such optimal dialysis now must include the use of biocompatible membranes to deliver Kt/V > 1.4 (equivalent to urea reduction ratio > 65%). Additional interventions can include the use of enteral or intravenous hyperalimentation, as well as recombinant growth hormone. The use of EPO has also been shown to have an impact on protein nutrition, as documented by urea kinetic analysis. Antinausea medications (metoclopramide) stimulate the motility of the upper GI tract and are particularly effective in diabetic patients. Recommended dietary protein and energy intake for patients undergoing maintenance hemodialysis are indicated in Table 20–9.

> Nonfluid weight loss, serum albumin level (< 4.0 g/dl), cholesterol level (< 180 mg/dL), and transferrin (< 200 mg/dl) are the most commonly measured parameters currently used to assess nutritional status of patients undergoing dialysis.

β₂-Microglobulin Amyloidosis

β_2-microglobulin amyloidosis has emerged during the past 10 years as a major complication of long-term hemodialysis. Pathologically, it is characterized by Congo red–positive deposits exhibiting the typical birefringence of amyloid deposit. Because its clearance depends exclusively on the kidneys, β_2-microglobulin tends to accumulate during renal insufficiency. The clinical manifestations of β_2-microglobulin amyloidosis are related to the propensity of β_2-microglobulin amyloid to accumulate in the tenosynovial tissue. **The first symptoms involve the wrist in the so-called carpal tunnel syndrome.** They are related to a thickening of the carpal ligaments with an attendant compression of the median nerve with or without hand tenosynovitis. They are characterized by paresthesias and eventually pain in the first three fingers, exacerbated at night, elicited by percussion of the median nerve at the carpal tunnel level (Tinel's sign) or by forced flexion of the wrist for 1 minute (Phalen's sign). Further progression leads to atrophy of the thenar muscles and retraction of the fingers. Electrophysiologic studies are required to confirm the diagnosis. Early surgical release of the nerve may correct the symptoms. In two thirds of cases, the removed material contains β_2-microglobulin amyloid in addition to a dense fibrous tissue. The carpal tunnel syndrome may appear as early as a few years after the onset of hemodialysis. Its prevalence progressively increases thereafter and may reach 80% to 100% after 15 years of dialysis.

The second series of symptoms involves the joints. They develop around 5 years after the carpal tunnel syndrome and may be present in 80% to 100% after 15 years of dialysis. Symptoms result from the deposition of β_2-microglobulin amyloid in the cartilage, capsules, and synovia of large joints: the shoulders, hips, knees, and the wrists. It is also observed in the spine.

The main clinical symptom is **arthralgia**, exacerbated at night, sometimes incapacitating, involving the shoulders, hips, and occasionally the

TABLE 20–9. Recommended Dietary Protein and Energy Intake for Patients on Maintenance Hemodialysis

• Protein	1.2 g/kg/day
	≥ 50–60% high-biologic-value protein
• Energy	≥ 35 kcal/kg/day unless patient's relative body weight is > 120%
	≥ 30 kcal/kg/day for patients older than 60 years
• Fat (percent of total energy intake)	30–40%
• Polyunsaturated-saturated fatty acid ratio	1.0:1.0
• Carbohydrates	Rest of nonprotein calories should be primarily complex carbohydrates

knees. Ultrasonography of the joints may evidence a thickening of the tendons (supraspinatus) in the shoulders and of the capsule of the hip preceding the onset of clinical symptoms. Herniation of amyloid substance through fragile cartilages or at the insertion site of tendons creates erosions and cysts within the bones. The radiologic characteristics of the latter cystic lesions have been delineated and provide a specific tool to diagnose β_2-microglobulin amyloid osteoarthropathy. Cyst expansion, especially at the level of the femoral neck, may occasionally lead to pathologic fractures. Massive deposits in the spine may lead to spondylarthropathy and sometimes to medullary compression. The most sensitive joint for pathologic demonstration of β_2-microglobulin amyloid is the sternoclavicular joint.

In addition to ultrasonography and radiology, scintigraphy with labeled β_2-microglobulin or P component (a protein always associated with amyloid deposits) may offer early diagnostic identification of β_2-microglobulin amyloidosis.

The third series of symptoms is related to organ deposition of β_2-microglobulin amyloid. Organ involvement is rare. Small deposits may be observed after more than 10 years of dialysis and are usually asymptomatic. In the gut it has been associated with GI hemorrhage.

The prevention of β_2-microglobulin amyloidosis remains disputed. Clinical studies have demonstrated that the onset of β_2-microglobulin amyloidosis, established by surgery for carpal tunnel syndrome or the appearance of amyloid bone cysts, is postponed in patients treated by high-flux biocompatible membranes such as polyacrilonitrile (AN69) when compared with patients given dialysis with cuprophane, a low-flux, poorly biocompatible membrane. Both cross-sectional and longitudinal studies have supported this conclusion. The preventive effect of high-flux biocompatible membrane on the development of β_2-microglobulin amyloidosis is multifactorial. In vitro evidence suggests that poorly biocompatible membranes stimulate β_2-microglobulin production by monocytes. Alternatively, high-flux membrane, unlike low-flux membranes such as cuprophane, clear β_2-microglobulin to a significant extent. Whatever the β_2-microglobulin clearing capacity of the membrane, it always fails to clear the daily endogenous β_2-microglobulin production, eventually leading to an unabated accumulation of β_2-microglobulin. A slower accumulation of β_2-microglobulin might account for the postponement of clinical evidence of amyloidosis in patients treated with high-flux biocompatible membranes such as AN69.

It is noteworthy that β_2-microglobulin amyloidosis has also been reported in patients undergoing long-term peritoneal dialysis.

Treatment of β_2-Microglobulin Amyloidosis. In symptomatic patients, various therapeutic strategies have been proposed, including surgical release of the median nerve in the presence of the carpal tunnel syndrome, endoscopic section of the coracoacromial ligament of the shoulder, or surgery on the capsula of symptomatic shoulders to relieve articular hypertension. The reported experience of surgery on large symptomatic joints remains limited.

Effect of Renal Transplantation on β_2-Microglobulin Amyloidosis. The best form of treatment for β_2-microglobulin amyloidosis is a successful renal graft. Arthralgias disappear almost immediately, a response taken to indicate the beneficial role of the concomitant high-dose steroid treatment. However, pain does not recur when steroids are tapered.

Radiologic evidence suggests that after transplantation, growth of the bone cysts is arrested; however, despite the return of normal β_2-microglobulin clearance, they do not regress even after 10 years. Histologic evidence of β_2-microglobulin amyloidosis has been obtained in joints more than 10 years after a successful graft.

PATIENT NUMBER 5

Herb, a 66-year-old man with ESRD secondary to hypertension, on maintenance hemodialysis for 15 years, was hospitalized for evaluation of neck and bilateral shoulder pain.

The patient had been in good health until 10 years before admission, when he developed left wrist pain and underwent carpal tunnel release, with improvement in the symptoms. Three years later, he began to experience pain and paresthesias in both hands. Nerve conduction studies revealed bilateral median nerve entrapment. He underwent bilateral carpal tunnel release shortly afterward. Staining of the surgical specimens with Congo red yielded positive results for amyloid. A postoperative skeletal survey revealed numerous periarticular lytic lesions in both humeral heads, the right acetabulum, and the right scaphoid. In addition, diffuse osteopenia, "rugger jersey" spine, erosions of the distal clavicles, and subperiosteal erosion of the medial aspects of the middle phalanges of the hand were noted.

One year later, Herb experienced progressive bilateral shoulder pain, with symptoms worsening at night. He had had no fever or swelling of the joints. He failed to respond to multiple courses of NSAIDs. He was admitted for evaluation of joint symptoms. During this admission, his intact serum PTH level was 410 pg/ml (normal 10 to 65). His baseline serum aluminum level was 48 μg/L and rose to 156 μg/L after a DFO challenge. A bone biopsy specimen from the right iliac crest revealed lamellar bone with no evidence of increased osteoid, and negative aluminum and Congo red staining. Herb received intraarticular corticosteroids, which relieved the shoulder pain partially, and he continued to require oral analgesics with acetaminophen/codeine. A few months later, he was readmitted because of persistent neck and shoulder pain.

On physical examination, decreased range of motion was noted in both shoulders, as well as tenderness on palpation of the left shoulder. Results of an EMG suggested a C8–T1 radiculopathy. Cervical spine radiographs revealed an old C5–C6 compression fracture and widening of the disk space between C6 and C7. Shoulder films revealed no fractures, dislocations, or bone erosions. An arthrogram of the right shoulder ruled out a rotator cuff tear. An MRI scan of the cervical region and shoulder area revealed compression fractures at C4, C5, and C6. Areas of infiltrate were noted in the left humeral head and soft tissues of the left shoulder.

The major features of illness in Herb, who was undergoing long-term hemodialysis, are a polyarthropathy involving both peripheral joints and the axial skeleton, compression fractures, lytic lesions in the bone, and amyloid-related carpal tunnel syndrome. He did not fit the picture of typical axial arthritides such as ankylosing spondylitis, Reiter's syndrome, psoriatic arthritis, or arthritis of inflammatory bowel disease, some of which are associated with AA (reactive systemic) amyloid. AL (immunocyte derived) amyloidosis wear involves bone, but it is an unusual feature of this disease. Neoplastic involvement of the skeleton is always a consideration in older patients, but Herb had no evidence of a malignancy. Renal osteodystrophy due to secondary hyperparathyroidism may cause many of the foregoing findings, with the exception of amyloid and carpal tunnel syndrome, although the destructive skeletal lesions due to PTH hormone excess may mimic a polyarthritis. However, the foregoing combination of clinical findings is almost diagnostic of β₂-microglobulin amyloidosis. Undoubtedly, this is the major problem, although some element of hyperparathyroidism or aluminum-related bone disease (osteomalacia) may also be present. An aluminum stain would have

been helpful in establishing (or precluding) the latter possibility. Finding a low rate of bone formation would establish the diagnosis of aluminum-related bone disease (ARBD).

Secondary Hyperparathyroidism
(see also Chapter 14)

The pathogenesis of secondary hyperparathyroidism is clearly more complicated than originally thought (Fig. 20–6). Hyperphosphatemia has a key role in causing PTH hypersecretion in CRF. The mechanisms are much more complex than the induction of hypocalcemia or modification of 1,25-dihydroxyvitamin D_3 (calcitriol) metabolism. Studies of experimental renal failure have shown that reduction of dietary phosphate in proportion to the decrease in GFR can substantially prevent secondary hyperparathyroidism. Similar results have also been obtained in uremic human subjects. In humans, phosphate (P_1) restriction has also been shown to lower PTH levels in patients with severe renal failure independent of calcitriol or calcium levels. These studies suggest that P_1 may affect PTH secretion through mechanisms that have yet to be clarified.

In CRF, calcitriol levels fall because of high phosphate levels (suppressing 1α-hydroxylase) and the loss of renal mass. Because one of the main actions of calcitriol is to promote intestinal transport of calcium, advanced renal failure is associated with calcium malabsorption. Although phosphorus restriction increases calcitriol levels in early renal failure, this has no effect on calcitriol levels in patients with advanced disease. Hence, without calcium or vitamin D supplementation, patients with severe renal failure are in negative calcium balance. Calcitriol treatment normalizes PTH secretion in patients with CRF by several mechanistic actions; mainly by suppression of pre-pro-PTH synthesis, calcitriol decreases PTH secretion.

In uremia, bone resistance to the calcemic action of PTH results in further aggravation of hyperparathyroidism. This resistance has clinical implications. During therapeutic interventions at reversal of hyperparathyroidism, the intact PTH level need not be normalized strictly to 10 to 65 pg/ml.

In uremic patients, normal bone formation rates are associated with intact PTH levels of 165 to 200 pg/ml.

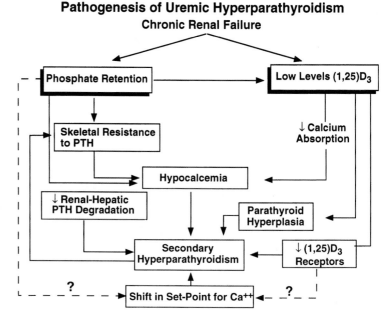

Figure 20–6. Pathogenesis of uremic hyperparathyroidism.

Hyperphosphatemia plays a key role, as do low levels of 1,25-dihydroxy-vitamin D₃ (calcitriol). Note that normalization of serum calcium and phosphorus levels is not enough for suppression of parathormone (PTH) hypersecretion. Calcitriol treatment normalizes PTH secretion in patients with CRF by several mechanistic actions. Directly, calcitriol suppresses the secretion of PTH independent of serum calcium (decreased gene transcription of pre-pro-PTH-mRNA).

The concept of a higher calcium set-point in secondary hyperparathyroidism is controversial. *In vitro* experiments have clearly demonstrated that parathyroid glands obtained from uremic subjects are relatively insensitive to the suppressive effects of calcium. Because parathyroid glands contain calcitriol nuclear receptors, deficiency of this hormone in renal failure may be responsible for the abnormal regulation of PTH secretion. We now know that calcitriol directly suppresses the secretion of PTH independently of calcium (decreased gene transcription of pre-pro-PTH-mRNA). Several studies have shown that calcitriol increases the sensitivity of parathyroid glands to suppression by calcium in patients with CRF. Guidelines for the management of secondary hyperparathyroidism are summarized in Table 20–10.

Aluminum-Related Bone Disease (Low-Turnover Osteomalacia)

(see also Chapter 14)

ARBD manifests clinically as proximal muscle pain and weakness (often severe), bone pain, multiple or recurrent skeletal fractures, spontaneous or iatrogenic hypercalcemia, low to normal serum alkaline phosphatase levels, and frequently (90%) low to normal serum PTH levels. Other features include microcytic anemia, encephalopathy with typical EEG pattern, and decreased myocardial contractility. **Prior parathyroidec-** **tomy, diabetes mellitus, and ingestion of aluminum-based PO₄ binders are risk factors for ARBD.** The gold standard for the diagnosis of ARBD is a transiliac bone biopsy and demonstration of 20% to 25% aluminum stain on the mineralization front.

Dialysis Encephalopathy (Dialysis Dementia)

Dialysis encephalopathy is a neurologic condition that occurs primarily in patients undergoing maintenance hemodialysis for many years. It is largely accepted now that the disease is **caused by aluminum intoxication.** Its earliest manifestations are stuttering and stammering speech. Other features include myoclonus, seizures, personality changes, and progressive dementia. The EEG characteristically shows multiple bursts of delta or theta activity, at times accompanied by spikes, which may precede any clinical features of the disease by 4 to 6 months and may persist through its course. Other associated evidence of aluminum intoxication may be found, such as microcytic-hypochromic anemia without iron deficiency and ARBD. Baseline plasma aluminum levels exceeding 200 mg/L are strongly suspicious of high aluminum burden. It is uncommon, however, when baseline levels are less than 50 mg/L. A rise in plasma aluminum of 200 mg/L after DFO challenge test is very suggestive of increased tissue burden of aluminum, and a rise

TABLE 20–10. Management of Secondary Hyperparathyroidism

- Restrict dietary phosphate. Avoid milk and milk products.
- PO_4–binders (either $CaCO_3$ or Ca-acetate should be given to target serum P_i at 4–5.5 mg/dl (< 6.0 mg/dl).
- Abandon aluminum gels; if absolutely necessary, use minimum doses for shortest time.
- Phosphate binders should be given *with* meals. Adjust dose in proportion to the amount of phosphorus in meals (e.g., largest dose with largest meal).
- Target "supernormal" serum calcium (10.0–11.5 mg/dl).
- "Corrected" serum calcium = "measured" serum Ca (mg/dl) + 0.8 × [4.5 − measured $S_{albumin}$ (g/dl)].
- Routine dialysate calcium = 2.5 mEq/L (unless substantial hypocalcemia; e.g., "corrected" serum Ca < 8.5 mg/dl).
- Target iPTH 1.5–2.5 times upper limits of normal (100–165 pg/ml).[*]
- Avoid Ca × P product > 70.
- Avoid serum calcium levels > 11.5 mg/dl.
- Hold vitamin D and/or Ca supplements for 2–4 days, then restart at lower doses if serum Ca > 11.5 mg/dl.
- Monitor serum calcium levels more rigorously and avoid hypercalcemia in patients on digitalis.
- For treatment of hypocalcemia
    Oral Rocaltrol, 0.25–0.5 µg once to twice daily.
- Pulse calcitriol (oral or intravenous)
    Reserve for patients whose PTH levels continue to rise while on daily oral calcitriol dose that causes hypercalcemia on dialysate Ca = 2.5 mEq/L.
- Pulse calcitriol also indicated for "refractory" hyperparathyroidism.

---

[*]iPTH = serum intact PTH level.

of more than 400 mg/L is very highly predictive of the diagnosis. If the baseline aluminum level is 150 mg/L or greater, the DFO challenge should be done with caution and a lower challenge dose used (1 g) because of the risk of precipitating an encephalopathy. A bone biopsy specimen of the iliac crest for aluminum stain is diagnostic. Dialysis frequently exacerbates the symptoms of dialysis dementia, especially seizures. When seizures occur, they respond well to diazepam. The disease is no longer necessarily debilitating and fatal if early diagnosis is made and chelation therapy with DFO initiated. The best treatment of the disease is preventive. Substituting calcium-containing for aluminum-containing phosphate binders and ensuring aluminum-free dialysate are the most important preventive aspects. Chelation therapy with DFO should be continued until basal plasma aluminum levels are only slightly elevated and there is

only a small rise of serum aluminum levels (20 to 30 mg/L) after DFO challenge.

Acquired Cystic Kidney Disease

Acquired cystic kidney disease (ACKD) is an almost inevitable accompaniment of long-term dialysis, with an overall prevalence of 50% in patients on dialysis. The proportion of patients with ACKD and the extent of cystic change both steadily increase with duration on dialysis, occurring in as many as 90% of patients treated with dialysis for 10 years or more. Dialyzed patients also have about a fivefold increase in prevalence of renal cell carcinoma as compared with the general population. Patients with CRF not yet on dialysis may also have evidence of ACKD, with a prevalence ranging from 7% to 26%. A reasonable definition of ACKD may be the presence of four or more cysts per failing kidney.

There is no widely held consensus about the need for universal screening for ACKD and renal cell carcinoma. One suggestion is that asymptomatic patients on dialysis for at least 3 years have a renal ultrasound study every 1 to 3 years thereafter. In any case, any dialyzed patient with unexplained hematuria, worsening anemia, abdominal pain, or constitutional symptoms of malignancy should be promptly evaluated. Paradoxically, spontaneous normalization of hematocrit or even frank polycythemia may also be a clue to the possibility of ACKD, especially in patients not receiving EPO.

Follow-up ultrasonography or CT is required to differentiate a hemorrhagic cyst from renal cell carcinoma if the lesion shows internal echoes or other atypical sonographic features. If a hemorrhagic cyst ruptures into the collecting system, it may not be evident on follow-up examination. Lesions that remain indeterminate should be surgically removed, depending on the general medical condition of the patient.

Infections

Septicemia and pulmonary infections are the second leading cause of death in patients on hemodialysis. Infection may be occult; fever and leukocytosis may not be manifested. Urinary tract infections in dialyzed patients may be overlooked, but pyocystitis and retroperitoneal abscess are not uncommon.

Pathogens can be predicted according to site of infection. In vascular access infections, gram-positive and gram-negative bacteria are the usual causative agents. In GI and genitourinary infections, gram-negative organisms predominate. *Escherichia coli* and *Yersinia enterocolitica* infection can develop in iron-overloaded patients and patients receiving DFO therapy (usually for aluminum toxicity).

When a patient on hemodialysis develops fever or signs of infection, multiple cultures (especially blood cultures) should be taken. As the diagnostic workup is in progress, vancomycin (usually 1 g IV in the last 30 to 60 minutes of dialysis) and an aminoglycoside (1.5 mg/kg loading dose, then 1 mg/kg, gentamicin or tobramycin) should be administered while awaiting culture results and results of other diagnostic tests.

Gastrointestinal Bleeding

Uremic gastritis is the most common cause of GI bleeding in patients on hemodialysis. It is often exacerbated by NSAIDs. Blood loss is usually minimal. Angiodysplasias (AV malformations) are the second most common cause, accounting for 20% of upper GI and 30% of lower GI bleeding in dialyzed patients. Other causes include perforation of colonic diverticulosis and rarely carcinoma and perivascular GI amyloidosis. The management of hemorrhagic gastritis includes avoidance of NSAIDs; H_2 blockers, control of uremia (Kt/V > 1.4), and misoprostol (100 to 200 μg at bedtime and with meals).

In some patients with angiodysplasia, bleeding stops spontaneously. RBC-tagged scintigraphy may be helpful in its diagnosis, but endoscopic localization is often required, followed by either laser photocoagulation or electrocautery. Surgery may be necessary if conservative measures fail, together with intraoperative endoscopy to localize lesions beyond the duodenum. Patients are usually dialyzed on tight heparin or citrate anticoagulation. Adequate dialysis (Kt/V > 1.4) is required, and if the bleeding time is prolonged, DDAVP, 0.3 μg/kg in 50 ml saline, is given intravenously over 15 to 30 minutes with or without cryoprecipitate or fresh frozen plasma. Recurrent bleeding can be managed with 2 to 3 months of estrogen-progesterone.

Colonic diverticular perforation may be insidious, and signs of peritonitis may not occur until late. The condition is often worsened by the constipating effects of aluminum-based phosphorus binders. Vague abdominal pain with low-grade fever should be pursued aggressively in dialyzed patients (especially the elderly) to preclude the possibility of colonic perforation.

Uremic Bleeding

Clinical bleeding represents a major complication of acute and chronic renal failure and appears to be most directly related to a functional platelet disorder. It has been suggested that uremic patients have an abnormal platelet–vessel wall interaction. The capability of the vessel wall to generate a potent antiaggregatory substance, prostacyclin, increases in uremia, whereas endothelial cells seem to generate an abnormal factor VIII:vonWillebrand factor (VIII:vWF). The hemorrhagic tendency in uremic patients is also influenced by the presence of anemia. A low hematocrit value negatively influences the rheologic component of platelet–vessel wall interaction. The best laboratory hallmark of clinical bleeding caused by uremia is the bleeding time. Treatment of the uremic platelet dysfunction is outlined in Table 20–11.

Although institution of dialysis corrects the functional platelet disorder in uremic patients, the use of heparin has an additional role in the bleeding complications related to hemodialysis. Patients differ in their sensitivities to the anticoagulant action of heparin as well as their ability to metabolize heparin. **In addition to its effect on clotting parameters (enhancement of antithrombin III effect), heparin may cause bleeding complications due to heparin-induced thrombocytopenia, which has been reported in as many as 25% of patients receiving heparin.** The highest incidence of thrombocytopenia is associated with heparin from bovine lung, whereas that from bovine intestinal mucosa appears to have a lower incidence. Thrombocytopenia during dialysis may also result from blood-membrane interactions,

TABLE 20–11. Treatment of Uremic Platelet Dysfunction

• RBC transfusions Recombinant erythropoietin	Keep hematocrit > 30%
• DDAVP°	0.3 μg/kg IV over 15–30 min (in 50 ml saline)
• Cryoprecipitate†	10 units IV every 12–24 hours
• Conjugated estrogens‡	0.6 mg/kg IV daily for 5 days

°Useful for acute bleeding before surgery; releases factor VIII/vWF from vascular endothelium; onset of action < 1 hour, duration 4–8 hours; tachyphylaxis may develop after 1–2 doses.

†Useful for acute bleeding; risk of viral hepatitis and AIDS; rich in factor VIII/vWF and fibrinogen; onset of action 1–4 hours, duration 24–36 hours.

‡Not useful for acute bleeding; onset of action in 6 hours, with progressive shortening of bleeding time over next 5–7 days; duration of action of about 2 weeks; mechanism of action unknown.

leading to platelet aggregation, and is maximum at 1 hour into dialysis, with platelet counts dropping to less than 100,000 after 1 hour from normal values at the start of dialysis.

> **The laboratory hallmark of uremic bleeding is a prolonged bleeding time.**

Anemia

The primary cause of anemia in dialyzed patients is inadequate production of EPO by the dysfunctional kidneys. In adults, EPO is produced primarily ($> 90\%$) by peritubular capillary endothelial cells of the kidneys. Although the liver also synthesizes some EPO ($< 10\%$), the amount is insufficient to maintain adequate erythropoiesis. EPO circulates in plasma and acts on erythroid progenitor cells in the bone marrow to produce RBCs. EPO acts at several different levels along the erythroid development cascade by stimulating the proliferation and differentiation of burst-forming units and colony-forming units. Farther down the cascade, EPO stimulates the release of bone marrow reticulocytes, which mature into RBCs in the bloodstream.

In addition to inadequate production of EPO by the failed kidneys, shortened RBC survival, which is variable from patient to patient, may contribute to the anemia of CRF. It has been unclear whether there are uremic inhibitors of erythropoiesis. Studies with EPO suggest that if such inhibitors are present, their effect is physiologically insignificant. Blood loss (such as chronic GI bleeding), iron deficiency, suppression of bone marrow by transfusions, aluminum toxicity, osteitis fibrosa cystica, folate deficiency, blood loss in the dialyzer (1.5 to 5 L annually), and routine phlebotomy for blood tests (800 to 1000 ml annually) may aggravate the hypoproliferative anemia of ESRD.

> **The primary cause of anemia in dialysis patients is inadequate production of EPO by the kidneys.**

Before the use of recombinant human EPO, the administration of androgens and RBC transfusions were the only management options available, in addition to optimizing dialysis, to treat anemia in dialyzed patients. The successful use of rHuEPO in the treatment of anemia in patients with CRF and undergoing dialysis made all other therapeutic modalities obsolete. In fact, intermittent blood transfusions are attended by the risk of transmission of viral hepatitis, iron overload, HLA-antigen sensitization, and further erythroid marrow suppression.

Guidelines for Use of rHuEPO in Patients on Dialysis

Most patients feel better when their hematocrit is 30% to 36%, and a hematocrit of 33% to 36% is therefore a reasonable target for dialyzed patients. Either the intravenous or subcutaneous route of administration can be used. With the intravenous route, 50 to 75 units/kg body weight can be administered with each dialysis (i.e., thrice weekly, a total of 150 to 225 units/kg/wk). The rise in hematocrit in response to rHuEPO is dose dependent. The dose is adjusted every 2 to 4 weeks in increments of 500 to 1000 units to achieve the target hematocrit.

Iron deficiency and chronic inflammatory processes are the main reasons for decreased responsiveness to EPO therapy. Iron status is routinely assessed by measurements of serum iron, transferrin saturation, and serum ferritin levels. When transferrin saturation is less than 20% or ferritin level less than 100 ng/ml, the patient needs to be treated with supplemental iron (oral or parenteral). In fact, before commencing EPO therapy, a patient's iron status should be assessed. Chronic inflammatory diseases reduce the release of iron from storage sites (reticuloendothelial blockade), resulting in low serum Fe and transferrin saturation and a high serum ferritin level and refractoriness to oral or parenteral iron supplementation.

> **Low serum iron and transferrin saturation ($< 20\%$) and ferritin levels (< 100 ng/ml) suggest iron deficiency. Low serum iron and transferrin saturation and high serum ferritin levels, on the other hand, suggest reticuloendothelial blockade due to chronic inflammation, folate or B_{12} deficiencies, or drug interactions.**

Other conditions that should be looked for whenever a suboptimal response to EPO therapy occurs include drug interactions, vitamin deficiencies (folate and B_{12}), osteitis fibrosa cystica, aluminum toxicity, and hemolysis.

PATIENT NUMBER 6

Kyle, a 40-year-old African-American man with diabetic nephropathy, has been receiving hemodialysis for 11 years. He has stable angina, peptic ulcer disease, hypertension, and severe psoriasis. Prescribed medications included insulin, extended-release nifedipine (30 mg b.i.d.), EPO (3000 units IV 3 times a week), ferrous sulfate (325 mg t.i.d.,) multivitamins, calcium carbonate (1250 mg t.i.d.), ranitidine (150 mg daily), and methotrexate (20 mg PO once a week).

Although his hematocrit stabilized at 34% to 35% for 12 weeks, it gradually declined to 27% during the next month. On questioning, Kyle said that he had experienced rather severe pain in both knee joints for several weeks. On the advice of a friend, he began taking daily doses of the over-the-counter analgesic naproxen. He also complained of increasing abdominal discomfort, for which he had been taking an antacid (Tums), two tablets as needed. Evaluation of the patient revealed abdominal pain on palpation. His stool guaiac results were positive. Iron studies disclosed a transferrin saturation level of 12% and a serum ferritin level of 65 ng/ml.

The physician discontinued the naproxen and added misoprostol, 200 mcg daily, and the patient was instructed to space ferrous sulfate and Tums. Iron dextran, 200 mg IV, was given with each dialysis session for five sessions. His hematocrit gradually increased to 35%.

Kyle's psoriasis was very difficult to control, and his dermatologist discontinued the methotrexate and added dapsone. After 8 weeks of stability of his hematocrit at 33% to 35%, the hematocrit declined to 24% during the next five dialysis sessions. Iron saturation showed a transferrin saturation of 22% and a serum ferritin level of 120 ng/ml. He had no evidence of blood loss in his stools and no history of recent infection. Examination of the peripheral smear revealed some fragmented RBCs. Kyle's level of unconjugated bilirubin was elevated, and his plasma haptoglobin was reduced.

This case illustrates that at least two factors contributed to the decline in the patient's hematocrit (before the start of dapsone) and hemolysis due to glucose-6-phosphate dehydrogenase (G6PD) deficiency (after the start of dapsone).

Before Starting Dapsone. Kyle's history of peptic ulcer disease, the positive stool guaiac results, and abdominal discomfort strongly suggest gastritis and blood loss caused by the recent consumption of naproxen. Occult blood loss should always be suspected as a cause of suboptimal response to EPO. A second factor is the potential interaction between the prescribed ferrous sulfate and the increased antacid doses (Tums). This drug combination can cause decreased iron absorption. Extra doses of antacids should be discontinued, and if coadministration of $FeSO_4$ and antacids is required, doses should be spaced apart as much as possible (e.g., antacids taken immediately after meals and $FeSO_4$ between meals). If $FeSO_4$ intake is tolerated between meals, its absorption can be maximized when taken on a relatively empty stomach.

Kyle's case thus illustrates the potential hazards of two over-the-counter medications taken without first consulting the physician. The iron studies demonstrate that the patient was significantly iron deficient (transferrin saturation 12%, ferritin 65 ng/ml), apparently because of GI bleeding and reduced iron absorption. Intravenous iron should be instituted in this case to restore the responsiveness to EPO.

After Dapsone Therapy. The subsequent stabilization of the hematocrit and response to EPO were interrupted by the addition of a medication that caused hemolysis (as evidenced by the peripheral smear, increased serum bilirubin [unconjugated], and decreased serum haptoglobin levels). Dapsone is a drug capable of inducing hemolysis. An African-American is at increased risk of G6PD deficiency and of hemolysis in a state of G6PD deficiency when given dapsone. The hemolysis presumably occurred rather quickly after giving dapsone. The absence of stool occult blood, the serum ferritin level of 150 ng/ml, transferin saturation > 20%, and the clinical picture are evidence that hemolysis and not iron deficiency underlies the poor response to EPO at this time.

In conclusion, polypharmacy is common in patients with ESRD, and the potential for drug interactions is great. Many commonly prescribed drugs can alter the therapeutic effectiveness of EPO. These drugs cause aplastic anemia, megaloblastosis, or hemolysis. Physicians can increase the successful treatment with EPO by educating patients about the importance of potential drug interactions.

Seizures on Hemodialysis

Several clinical conditions predispose to seizure activity in patients on dialysis. The seizure activity associated with uremia or dialysis tends to be generalized. The presence of focal seizure activity often indicates localized neurologic disease. Dialysis-associated seizures can occur during hemodialysis or after its termination. Hypotension is a frequent cause of seizures and should be avoided and treated accordingly.

To lessen the risk of seizure activity in patients on dialysis, particularly in predisposed patients, the following measures should be taken:

- Preventive measures against the development of DDS.
- If a patient is known to be taking anticonvulsant drugs, an additional dose should be given after dialysis if the drug is dialyzable.
- In severely hypocalcemic patients, especially in presence of severe metabolic acidosis, calcium treatment should be considered even before dialysis if serum phosphate level is not very high (Ca × P product > 70), and a 3.5 mEq/L of dialysate calcium should be used.
- Rapid correction of uremia and hypertonicity simultaneously should be avoided.
- The doses of drugs that may have untoward CNS effects in uremia should be carefully adjusted. These include penicillins, cephalosporins, nitrofurantoin, isoniazid, meperidine, morphine, cimetidine, phenothiazines, haloperidol, barbiturates, benzodiazepines, antihistamines, hypoglycemic agents, methyldopa, beta-adrenergic antagonists, cyproheptadine, anticoagulants, and neuromuscular blocking agents.

Treatment of acute seizure activity in patients on dialysis is outlined in Table 20–12.

Anticonvulsant Drug Therapy. The following are general guidelines for anticonvulsant drug therapy on dialysis. Nondialyzable drugs include phenytoin and carbamazepine. Valproic acid may be removed by hemodialysis. Dialyzable drugs (supplemental dose needed after dialysis) include phenobarbital, ethosuximide, trimethadione, paraldehyde, and primidone. Primidone should be used with extreme caution. Carbamazepine, ethosuximide, valproic acid, and phenobarbital can

TABLE 20–12. Emergency Treatment of Seizure Activity During Hemodialysis

1. Stop dialysis.
2. Ensure patent airway, give oxygen.
3. Treat hypoglycemia and hypotension accordingly.
4. Give 5–10 mg diazepam IV every 5 minutes to a maximal total dose of 30 mg to terminate seizure.
5. Give a loading dose of phenytoin (10–15 mg/kg) by slow IV infusion and no greater than 50 mg/min and with constant ECG monitoring.

be given in 75% to 100% of the usual dose to patients on dialysis.

With **phenytoin,** 90% is normally protein bound and the volume of distribution is 0.6 L/kg. Its half-life is 24 hours. In ESRD, *protein binding decreases* and half-life decreases to 8 hours. The normal therapeutic range of total drug is 10 to 20 μg/ml. If the fraction unbound is 0.1 (normally), then the free (unbound) fraction that is associated with optimal treatment is 1 to 2 μg/ml. Drugs known to displace phenytoin from plasma protein-binding sites include valproic acid, NSAIDs, and salicylic acid. In uremia, the unbound protein fraction can increase up to 0.3. Thus, the concentration of the *total* drug recommended for patients with ESRD is 5 to 10 μg/ml.

Phenytoin follows dose-dependent kinetics. Any increase in dosing should be small, and sufficient time should be allowed for patients to achieve a new steady state. The altered protein binding and shortened half-life necessitate two adjustments in the dosage schedules of phenytoin in uremia. Give the drug in divided dosage (three times daily). If the unbound fraction determinations are not available, then one half to one third of normal-range total blood levels should be sufficiently therapeutic.

Cardiac Arrhythmias

Patients on hemodialysis are at special risk for arrhythmias owing to factors unique to dialysis. These factors include hypotension, which may impair coronary perfusion, acute shifts in electrolytes (particularly potassium), and cardiovascular instability during acetate dialysis. Patients taking digitalis preparations are particularly at risk. Ischemic and hypertensive cardiovascular disease, pericarditis, and conduction system calcifications are frequently present in dialyzed patients and underlie recurrent and sustained arrhythmias.

Treatment of arrhythmias during the hemodialysis session is much the same as in nondialysis situations, except that in ESRD the altered pharmacokinetics and protein binding of drugs should be taken into account. If a critical coronary perfusion underlies the arrhythmia, transfusion to maintain hematocrit close to 36% is important.

Patients taking digitalis should have their dialysate K concentration between 2 and 3 mEq/L, and their serum K level should not be allowed to drop below 2.0 to 3.5 mEq/L.

In ESRD, the serum half-life of digoxin is prolonged to 80 to 120 hours (normal 40 hours), and the volume of distribution is decreased from

7 L/kg to 4.2 L/kg. For these reasons, the loading dose of digoxin should be reduced by around 40% and the maintenance dose decreased by 50% to 75%. Hemodialysis does not remove digoxin, and thus a supplemental dose is unnecessary. A loading dose of 0.325 to 0.5 mg IV in 24 hours and a maintenance dose of 0.125 mg every other day are appropriate.

Lidocaine half-life (2 hours) is unaltered in dialyzed patients, but the half-life of one of its metabolites (glycine xylide) is increased. Glycine xylide accumulation may cause adverse reactions undetected by standard plasma levels. The major elimination route of lidocaine is hepatic (90%). The loading dose of lidocaine in patients on dialysis is 1 to 3 mg/kg at maximal rate of 7 mg/min, with a maintenance dose of 1 to 4 mg/kg. No postdialysis supplemental dose is necessary because of negligible removal by dialysis.

The decreased protein binding of phenytoin in uremia and increased volume of distribution lead to an increase in the unbound fraction of this drug. A loading dose of 250 mg in normal saline is given over 10 minutes, then 100 mg IV every 5 minutes (maximum 50 mg/min) is recommended. Maintenance doses of 300 mg/day should be followed by measurement of blood levels (the target *total* therapeutic level is 5 to 10 mg/L; an *unbound* level of 1 to 2 mg/L is appropriate). No postdialysis dose is necessary.

It is best to avoid procainamide in dialyzed patients because of the marked increase in the half-life of its metabolite (*N*-acetylated procainamide [NAPA]). If used, procainamide blood levels (4 to 10 mg/ml) and NAPA (10 to 20 mg/ml) should not be exceeded. The loading dose is 100 mg IV every 5 minutes (maximum 1000 mg); 250 to 500 mg every 12 hours is an appropriate maintenance dose.

Quinidine has an increased volume of distribution (2 L/kg, normal 0.6 L/kg), and its protein binding is increased in uremia. Therefore, greater serum concentration in uremia results in same amount of free drug. Increased serum levels (> 2 to 5 mg/L) may be misleading. For effects of toxicity, the QT interval should be frequently checked for prolonged intervals. The loading dose of quinidine is 600 mg PO. Maintenance doses should be reduced to 200 to 324 mg every 8 hours.

The half-life of disopyramide is increased to 30 hours in dialyzed patients (normal 7 hours). The loading dose is 150 mg PO, and the maintenance dose should be reduced by 50% (50 to 100 mg PO every 12 hours).

Bretylium is 80% renally excreted. Its half-life (105 hours) is markedly increased in ESRD

(normal 7 to 8 hours). Approximately one-fifth the normal dose is recommended. Twenty-five percent of the dose is removed during 4 hours of dialysis, and a supplemental postdialysis dose is necessary to ensure continued therapeutic efficacy at this lower dosing regimen. The loading dose is 5 mg/kg IV over 20 minutes, and a maintenance dose of 2 to 6 mg/hour is recommended.

The loading dose of verapamil in dialysis is 5 to 10 mg IV over 3 to 5 minutes; 40 to 80 mg every 6 hours is given as a maintenance dose.

Uremic Pruritus

Pruritus frequently complicates ESRD, occurring in approximately 25% to 50% percent of patients. In some patients, pruritus is only a subjective sensation without any cutaneous lesions. In others, itching and scratching may be associated with the appearance of nodular prurigo, keratotic papules, or lichen simplex. In most cases, elevated PTH and phosphate levels are a common biochemical finding and presumably reflect the deposition of calcium phosphate crystals in the skin. Most commonly, patients become symptomatic coincident with the terminal stages of renal failure and before beginning dialysis. The institution of dialysis, whether hemodialysis or peritoneal dialysis, frequently has little or no impact on itching. Some patients itch mostly during dialysis; others are most symptomatic on days during which they are not on dialysis. Itching may worsen during the summer. Pruritus is often episodic. The cause of uremic pruritus in patients with normal calcium and phosphorus concentrations remains obscure. Evidence suggests that dermal mast cells have a role in its etiology. In a small group of patients, the mast-cell stabilizer *ketotifen fumarate* offered dramatic improvement. Dryness of the skin, allergens such as heparin and ethylene oxide, and histamine release from mast cells all have been implicated in the production of pruritus; with these, itching is usually associated with urticarial manifestations. An early sensory neuropathy might also have a role. The management of severe pruritus is summarized in Table 20–13.

HIGH-FLUX AND HIGH-EFFICIENCY HEMODIALYSIS

Advances in dialysis technology as well as strong patient preference for shorter treatments have led to successful implementation of "short dialysis" to treat uremic patients. Dialysis time

TABLE 20–13. Treatment of Uremic Pruritus

- Control hyperphosphatemia and hyperparathyroidism.
- Topical emollients (triple lanolin).
- Phototherapy with UV-B light twice weekly for 2–6 weeks. Repeat courses may be considered.
- Diphenhydramine, 25–50 mg PO b.i.d.; or hydroxyzine, 10 mg PO t.i.d.
- Oral activated charcoal (6 g/day).
- Cholestyramine, 5 g PO b.i.d.
- Consider subtotal parathyroidectomy for severe itching unresponsive to medical measures.

with such therapy has been reduced to between 6 and 9 hr/wk. It has been convincingly demonstrated in a large number of patients that shortening treatment time need not compromise adequacy of dialysis as long as therapy prescription is such that the Kt/V index is maintained by appropriate increase in (K) to compensate for reduction in (t). Long-term follow-up evaluations in a population with a mean age of 60 years and a large percentage of diabetic patients (30%) has documented stable serum chemistry values (urea, creatinine, phosphorus, potassium, and bicarbonate) with treatment durations as short as 6 to 9 hr/wk. It has also been shown that the incidence of intradialytic complications can be maintained at or below the levels that occur with standard 4-hour acetate dialysis. Achievement of the desired dry weight and adequate blood pressure control have also been documented. The frequency of hospitalization and number of days hospitalized per year have not increased with rapid high-efficiency dialysis.

To achieve a high rate of solute removal during ultrashort dialysis, two approaches have been used. In the first, using high-efficiency dialyzers with a high permeability for small solutes of molecular weight < 1000, diffusion across a concentration gradient is the primary mode of solute transport. Such dialyzers have an ultrafiltration coefficient of 8 to 12 ml/mm Hg/hr. In the second, called "high-flux," dialyzers which have ultrafiltration coefficients of 25 to 60 ml/mm Hg/hr are used. With such dialyzers, the convective contribution to the removal of middle- and large-molecular-weight solutes is significant; hence, much higher clearances of large solutes such as β_2-microglobulin can be achieved. However, it has not been shown that removal of β_2-microglobulin with highly permeable dialyzers ameliorates β_2-microglobulin amyloidosis. The amount of β_2-microglobulin removed by PS dialyzers approaches the daily production only, and therefore, unloading of tissue stores may not be realis-

tic at this time. The impact of such treatment modality on the treatment of carpal tunnel syndrome is unknown. The ability to remove large solutes from blood also poses the potential problem of convective transport of large solutes from dialysate to blood. Such back-filtration, particularly of endotoxins, may limit the usefulness of high-flux dialysis.

Technical requirements for rapid high-efficiency therapies include high blood flow rates, ultrafiltration control systems, and bicarbonate as the buffer source. Strict control of endotoxin/bacterial levels and limited interdialytic weight gain (< 5 to 6 kg) are also required for success of high-efficiency/high-flux dialysis.

The achievement of adequate fluid removal depends not only on the ability to obtain the desired rate of fluid removal in a reliable and predictable manner but also on a patient's ability to tolerate the desired rate of fluid removal without untoward symptoms. The use of a direct ultrafiltration control system rather than the indirect control of TMP greatly facilitates fluid removal with high-efficiency dialysis. One of the principal causes of dialysis-induced hypotension is hypovolemia, which results from imbalance between the rate of ultrafiltration and the rate of vascular refilling. Modeling studies of the dynamics of vascular refilling show large interpatient differences in the hydraulic capillary endothelium permeability. Patients with low permeability are prone to hypovolemia, and such interpatient variability may pose a limiting factor to shortening treatment time.

In delivering bicarbonate dialysate, many technical considerations must be tackled. Producing bicarbonate dialysate requires two concentrates (acid and bicarbonate), two proportionating systems, and two monitoring systems, thus increasing the overall complexity of the dialysis equipment. Serious patient consequences may ensue if the acid and bicarbonate concentrates are switched. Most important of all, however, is the fact that bicarbonate concentrates support the proliferation of halo-tolerant gram-negative organisms that produce a significant amount of endotoxin. As many as 10^5 to 10^6 cfu/ml can develop in liquid bicarbonate in as few as 10 days after preparation; thus, it is essential to avoid prolonged storage of liquid bicarbonate concentrate and to clean and disinfect the dialysate delivery system frequently. These halophilic rods are facultative anaerobes and may be very difficult to culture using standard media recommended for water organisms. These organisms require sodium chloride and, in fact, may require sodium bicarbonate for their growth, making their recovery in standard culture media very difficult.

The long-term success of any program using high-efficiency/high-flux modalities therefore rests on (1) bleaching and sterilization of dialysate containers on a daily basis, (2) control of microbial levels to < 100 colonies/ml in dialysate, and (3) appropriate control of endotoxin level.

Finally, in order to apply high-flux dialysis, a vascular access must be capable of delivering a blood flow rate of about 400 to 450 ml/min without causing > 5% to 10% recirculation, a dialysate flow rate of 500 to 800 ml/min, and variable sodium concentration, especially high dialysate sodium early in dialysis to balance the rapidly changing urea gradients.

The effect of highly permeable membranes on drug removal needs to be explored. Use of PS membranes has been associated with markedly increased vancomycin clearance, necessitating supplemental vancomycin administration (500 mg) after each hemodialysis session to maintain therapeutic vancomycin blood levels. Other drugs with relatively small volume of distribution and minimal protein binding and a molecular weight in the range of 1000 to 1200 may also require postdialysis supplementation.

Acknowledgment

The excellent secretarial assistance of Ms. Jane McLaughlin is greatly appreciated.

SUGGESTED READINGS

Beathard GA: The treatment of vascular access graft dysfunction: A nephrologist view and experience. Advances in Renal Replacement Therapy 1:131–147, 1994.

Conger JD, Robinette JB, Hammond WS: Difference in vascular reactivity in models of ischemic acute renal failure. Kidney Int 39:1087–1097, 1991.

Conlon PJ, Schwab SJ: Optimal hemodialysis: Access. Seminars in Dialysis 7:268–271, 1994.

Depner TA: Techniques for prospective detection of venous stenosis. Advances in Renal Replacement Therapy 1:119–130, 1994.

Depner TA: Assessing adequacy of hemodialysis: Urea modeling. Kidney Int 45:1522–1535, 1994.

Eschbach JW: The anemia of chronic renal failure: Pathophysiology and the effects of recombinant erythropoietin. Kidney Int 35:134–148, 1989.

Hakim RM, Levin N: Malnutrition in hemodialysis patients. Am J Kidney Dis 21:125–137, 1993.

Hakim RM, Breyer J, Ismail N, Schulman G: Effects of dose of dialysis on morbidity and mortality. Am J Kidney Dis 23:661–669, 1994.

Hakim RM: Clinical implications of hemodialysis membrane biocompatibility. Kidney Int 44:484–494, 1993.

Ismail N, Becker B: Treatment options and strategies in uremia: Current trends and future directions. Semin Nephrol 14:282–299, 1994.

Keshaviah P: Technology and clinical application of hemodialysis. *In* Jacobson HR, Striker GE, Klahr S (eds): The Principles and Practice of Nephrology, 2nd ed. St Louis, Mosby/Year Book, 1995, pp 654–664.

Lowrie EG, Lew NL: Death risk in hemodialysis patients: The predictive value of commonly measured variables and an evaluation of death rate differences between facilities. Am J Kidney Dis 15:458–482, 1990.

Solez K, Morel-Moroger L, Sraer JD: The morphology of "acute tubular necrosis in man." Medicine 58:362–376, 1979.

Stivelman JC: Optimization of iron therapy in hemodialysis patients treated with rHuEPO. Seminars in Dialysis 7:288–292, 1994.

Stone WJ, Hakim RM: Beta-2-microglobulin amyloidosis in long-term dialysis patients. Am J Nephrol 9:177–183, 1989.

Van Ypersele de Strihou, Jadoul M, Malghem J, et al: Effect of dialysis membrane and patient's age on signs of dialysis related amyloidosis. Kidney Int 39:1012–1019, 1991.

21 | RENAL TRANSPLANTATION:

APPROACHES TO GRAFT DYSFUNCTION

AND THE CONSEQUENCES

OF IMMUNOSUPPRESSION

Simin Goral and J. Harold Helderman

This chapter presents nine instructive cases that reflect classic problems in renal transplant diagnosis and management. Each case was selected to illustrate a separate and unique problem with real patients. It is hoped that this format of the presentation will humanize and focus the medical problems for the reader.

A chapter such as this runs the risk of highlighting the negative aspects of organ transplantation by the very nature of the style and presentation. As one reads the stories of these nine problem patients, it is important to understand and keep in mind how very successful renal transplantation in the late 1990s truly is. With present immunosuppressive regimens and management skills, 1-year renal transplant graft survivals as reported formally by the United Network of Organ Sharing (UNOS), the mandated repository for such accurate data, is about 83% for all centers in the United States. Through UNOS, many centers report cadaver graft survivals approaching 90% at 1 year, and living related transplantation of any match enjoys more than 95% graft survival at 1 year. Longer-term graft survival is also excellent, although not improving equivalently as the early graft survival. Almost half of all cadaveric renal recipients can be expected to retain allograft function a decade after their surgery. The disparity in graft improvement between early and later periods provides a continuing challenge to the transplantation community. Thus, the nine cases presented here represent the problems facing nephrologists and are not characteristic of the general experience after renal transplantation for the majority.

The case presentations have been divided into four basic areas of concern: (1) pretreatment evaluation, (2) renal transplant dysfunction, (3) infections of immunocompromised renal transplant recipients, and (4) neoplasms in immunocompromised organ recipients. We begin with a case that illustrates the events in preparing a patient with chronic renal failure for receipt of a transplant. Next, four patients with graft excretory dysfunction are presented, each one with a different resolution. A 37-year-old woman presented with fever and pain over the transplant, representing the symptom complex resulting from an acute allograft cellular rejection. Another woman also presented with fever, graft discomfort, and reduced excretory function but was found to have the severest complication of cyclosporine toxicity, the hemolytic-uremic syndrome (HUS) with intravascular coagulopathy and intraglomerular fibrin deposition. A 26-year-old man presented with reduced urine flow, an elevated serum creatinine level, and abdominal discomfort, the consequence of obstruction secondary to distal ureteric scarring. A woman who received her renal allograft to reverse renal failure secondary to systemic lupus erythematosus (SLE) is an example of the diagnostic dilemma facing nephrologists when transplant graft function diminishes without symptoms years after surgery. In this case, the cause of renal dysfunction was recurrent glomerulonephritis, permitting a discussion of the entity of recurrent disease in a transplanted kidney.

Four patients described here represent typical management problems that result from the use of immunosuppression to maintain allografts—infections and neoplasms. We have selected two patients with the most common transplant-related infections for presentation, a 33-year-old woman who presented with fever, cough, dyspnea, and leukopenia as a consequence of acute reactivation of cytomegalovirus (CMV) infection and an older gentleman who presented with fever and mental confusion caused by cryptococcal meningitis 8 years after successful engraftment. These cases allow discussion of these early and late infections that typically characterize the complications of immunosuppression. Also included are two cases of neoplasms particularly related to immunosuppression in general and organ transplantation in particular. One of these patients, an unfortunate 28-year-old diabetic man, succumbed to a very aggressive form of posttransplant lymphoproliferative disease, the range of presentation of which is discussed. The last patient is a 67-year-old woman who presented 9 years after successful transplantation with a breast mass on the background of multiple squamous cell carcinomas of the skin. Skin cancer represents the most common of the posttransplant neoplasms.

As transplantation becomes ever more successful, it is hoped that the number of problem cases continues to dwindle; however, these nine paradigmatic patients represent those issues that will continually need to be addressed in this discipline of nephrology.

PRETRANSPLANT EVALUATION

PATIENT NUMBER 1

Emily is a 36-year-old photographer working for a local newspaper. Three years earlier, she was diagnosed with focal segmental glomerulosclerosis (FSGS). Her kidney function deteriorated slowly. A month before her first transplant clinic visit, she started peritoneal dialysis. She expressed interest in undergoing evaluation for possible renal transplantation.

Transplant evaluation should start with a carefully taken history including a family history. Certain diseases including FSGS can recur in the kidney transplant. Emily had been informed about the risk of recurrence (20% to 30%) and graft loss (30% to 40%) secondary to FSGS. She was also counseled about success rates of transplant using living related and unrelated donors. Her brother and her sister wanted to be evaluated as potential donors. Initial screening started with blood and tissue typing. Emily is 5 feet 6 inches tall and

weighs 115 pounds. Obesity is a well-known risk factor for posttransplant morbidity and mortality and can be an absolute contraindication to transplantation. That was not a problem for Emily! She had no evidence of any current or past cancer. Results of her mammogram and Papanicolaou smear completed 4 months ago were normal. She was HIV negative. Her PPD was negative with negative controls, along with old granulomas in her chest radiograph requiring INH prophylaxis at the time of transplantation. She had not received any blood transfusions. Because monthly blood work revealed no serologic evidence of CMV infection, prophylactic acyclovir or CMV immune globulin should be considered if the donor is CMV positive. Her liver enzymes were normal, and hepatitis C test results were negative. She did not have any history of coronary artery disease, congestive heart failure, thyroid dysfunction, alcoholism, or drug addiction. Although she had had recurrent urinary tract infections in the past, she had not been infected in the past year, and her current urine culture was sterile. Native nephrectomy therefore was not required. Renal ultrasonography was unremarkable except for small kidneys. A voiding cystourethrogram (VCUG) was negative for reflux. Two years ago, she had been treated for anxiety disorder. She was cleared for transplant by the transplant psychiatrist.

Brother Don represented a two-haplotype match because they shared both strands of chromosome inherited from their parents, auguring a greater than 98% 1-year graft survival and a half-life of more than 20 years. Don had a full clinical evaluation including history taking and physical, psychosocial, and laboratory examinations. His renal function was superb, with an isotopically measured GFR of 140 ml/min. Anatomic study of his kidneys by arteriography revealed two arteries supplying the right and one to the left kidney. The transplant surgeon chose the left kidney, and a transplant date was set. Despite the absence of sensitization revealed by testing for the presence of cytotoxic HLA-IgG antibodies directed against a panel of lymphocytes representing a cross section of transplantation antigens from the community, a final antiglobulin crossmatch between Emily and Don was performed and results were negative. Emily eagerly awaited her transplant date, an anticipation tempered by a modicum of trepidation. Two days before planned admission, Emily developed a temperature of 100°F orally, vague abdominal discomfort, and a cloudy peritoneal fluid. Her transplant was postponed, and antibiotics were administered with a good clinical result. Her transplant was rescheduled for 2 weeks after the last antibiotic, with three peritoneal dialysis fluid cultures remaining negative. A repeat crossmatch again yielded negative results. The surgery was finally performed, with removal of the Tenckhoff catheter at the same time. Solu-Medrol and azathioprine were administered during surgery. The graft functioned immediately, and 12 L of urine was produced on the first postoperative day. Anti T-cell antibody induction was begun along with oral prednisone and azathioprine. Cyclosporin A was introduced on the third postoperative day as the microemulsion formulation Neoral when the serum creatinine level fell below 3.0 mg/dl. The antibody overlapped with the cyclosporine for 3 days, when whole blood levels of the latter reached the target therapeutic window of 250 to 300 ng/ml (TDX [monoclonal antibody whole blood] method). She was discharged to the clinic with a creatinine of 0.9 mg/dl on the sixth postoperative day.

ACUTE REJECTION

PATIENT NUMBER 2

Anna is a 37-year-old accountant with a two-antigen matched cadaveric kidney transplant placed 4 months prior to admission because of end-stage renal disease (ESRD) secondary to insulin-dependent diabetes mellitus. She was admitted for a transplant kidney biopsy because of a rise in creatinine level, a low-grade fever, and perigraft tenderness. Her past medical history was also notable for hypertension, diabetic retinopathy, and neuropathy. Her usual posttransplant serum creatinine level of 1.4 to 1.8 mg/dl had increased to 3.4 mg/dl on admission. Her abdomen was diffusely tender, with a mass effect in the right lower quadrant over her graft. Her temperature was 100.5°F. Ultrasonography with Doppler showed no evidence of hydronephrosis or renal artery stenosis. The renal biopsy specimen revealed diffuse interstitial aggregates of lymphocytes, monocytes, and macrophages, with tubular infiltration consistent with acute cellular rejection. She was treated with antithymocyte serum (ATS) for 14 days and four doses of 250 mg IV methylprednisolone pulses. Her serum creatinine level returned to baseline at discharge.

Anna's case represents the diagnosis of renal transplant dysfunction in the first 6 months after surgery. Various conditions including mechanical problems, infection, rejection, and cyclosporine nephrotoxicity need to be differentiated in a patient with renal allograft dysfunction at this point. Posttransplant fever is always significant in a transplant recipient and may indicate either infection or rejection. Infection is usually due to classic opportunistic pathogens during the 6 months after the operation. Viruses of the herpes class, tuberculosis, listeriosis, nontyphoid *Salmonella,* cryptococcal and other fungal infections, *Pneumocystis carinii* pneumonia, and urinary tract infections are the most common infections in this period. The majority of clinically significant CMV infections (primary or reactivation) also occur 1 to 6 months after transplant. Renal dysfunction, fever, and graft tenderness may also be caused by bacterial pyelonephritis, which must be remembered during evaluation of a patient. Although infection is the most common cause of fever in renal transplant recipients, assessment must include the noninfective causes such as rejection, hematomas, and venous thromboses. Transplant recipients with fever must have a full fever workup including chest radiographs and multiple cultures.

Acute rejection, which generally occurs days to weeks after surgery, is a systemic inflammatory disorder that may present with multiple constitutional symptoms, including fever, chills, myalgias, and arthralgias. Perigraft pain and tenderness can occur because of swelling of the graft. Oliguria, hypertension, elevated serum creatinine and BUN values, hyperkalemia, and renal tubular acidosis can be observed. Patients who are taking cyclosporine may have rejection episodes with reduced signs and symptoms, often without any fever or graft tenderness. Acute rejection should be diagnosed immediately in order to start antirejection therapy and prevent irreversible damage. The gold standard diagnostic tool is kidney biopsy. Tubulitis and perivascular infiltration with lymphocytes, natural killer cells, and mononuclear cells on biopsy specimens are defining features of acute rejection. In severe forms, vascular occlusion and interstitial hemorrhage may also develop. Treatment of acute rejection includes high-dose oral corticosteroids, intravenous pulse steroids, and/or various polyclonal or monoclonal antilymphocyte antibodies (Table 21–1).

TABLE 21–1. Treatment of Acute Rejection

Corticosteroids (high-dose pulse intravenous or high-dose oral therapy)
Polyclonal anti–T-cell antibodies
Monoclonal anti-CD3 antibodies

Experimental rescue approaches include a switch from cyclosporin A to FK506 (tacrolimus) or *vice versa* or a switch to mycophenolate mofetil if not part of the primary regimen.

- **In a patient with renal allograft dysfunction, before any intervention, one must perform studies to rule out anatomic and surgical problems.**
- **Renal biopsy remains the mainstay of diagnosis.**

CYCLOSPORINE NEPHROTOXICITY

PATIENT NUMBER 3

Becky is a married 38-year old system analyst from Texas. She has ESRD secondary to medullary cystic disease. She had returned to peritoneal dialysis after losing her first kidney transplant to chronic rejection. Her medical history included steroid-induced insulin-dependent diabetes, frequent urinary tract infections, and CMV disease treated with ganciclovir. After 8 months on the waiting list, she was admitted for a second kidney transplant and received a 1B, 1DR matched cadaver kidney. The graft functioned immediately, and her creatinine level dropped to 1.3 mg/dl after 3 days. On the third posttransplant day, cyclosporine was started. During the first hospital week, she developed fever, graft tenderness, and worsening renal function. A rising serum creatinine level and abnormal results of a radionuclide renogram were noted. Concurrent with this, Becky was noted to have a drop in her hematocrit and platelets. Her serum lactate dehydrogenase level (LDH) was significantly elevated. Renal biopsy showed thrombotic microangiopathy involving both the glomeruli and the arterioles consistent with HUS. Becky had no evidence of rejection, including no tubulitis and no interstitial lymphocytic infiltrate. Cyclosporine was discontinued, and her creatinine level consistently fell from 5.6 mg/dl to 2.0 mg/dl during the next 5 days. The patient was subsequently started on FK506.

Nephrotoxicity is a well-known side effect of cyclosporine. Several forms are described. The drug is associated with reversible acute dose-dependent renal dysfunction in part related to increases in renal vascular resistance, but it may also cause permanent kidney damage. The characteristic features of cyclosporine nephrotoxicity are a reduced creatinine clearance with increased serum creatinine level, hyperkalemia, hypertension, hyperuricemia, and hyperkalemic hyperchloremic type IV renal tubular acidosis. Clinically, it may be difficult to differentiate from acute rejection.

Progressive deterioration of renal function even in the presence of persistently high cyclosporine levels is highly suggestive of acute rejection. A percutaneous kidney biopsy is necessary to differentiate these two entities. In acute cyclosporine toxicity, few structural abnormalities are seen in the kidney biopsy specimen; indeed, the tissue may appear normal. Microcalcification and isometric vacuolation of the proximal tubule, without interstitial lymphocytic infiltration, occasionally may be seen. A pattern of striped interstitial fibrosis along with tubular atrophy and glomerular sclerosis leading to compromised renal function characterizes chronic cyclosporine nephrotoxicity. Experimental data on animal models suggests that chronic cyclosporine-induced vasoconstriction coupled to direct endothelial injury culminates in arteriolopathy and interstitial fibrosis leading to irreversible renal insufficiency. The acute episodic form of cyclosporine toxicity is usually associated with high blood levels of cyclosporine and responds in 24 to 48 hours to decreasing the dose of the drug. The precise mediators for the variant forms of toxicity remain to be elucidated. The precise role of the renin-angiotensin-aldosterone axis is unclear. Early or after acute intravenous boluses, renin generation is stimulated, whereas with long-term use renin is inhibited, leading to low levels of angiotensin and aldosterone. The latter, along with decreased filtered loads associated with constrained GFR, accounts for the often observed hyperkalemia. Endothelin generation is also acutely stimulated, but endothelin receptor blockade fails to prevent the hypertension associated with cyclosporine. Sodium retention beyond that accounted for by the level of GFR, intracellular calcium accumulation, and heightened sensitivity of renal vasculature to catecholamines all are important mediators, an understanding of which can lead to a rational therapeutic approach. Evidence that cyclosporine increases translation of transforming growth factor-β may also explain enhanced matrix formation and interstitial fibrosis after long-standing cyclosporine use.

De novo HUS is a rare complication of cyclosporine use. It results from a direct toxic effect of cyclosporine on vascular endothelium.

HUS is characterized histologically by microvascular hyaline thrombosis composed of primarily platelets and fibrin. Plasma infusion/exchange has been used in several uncontrolled trials, resulting in an overall 60% graft survival rate. The risk of recurrence is greater if cyclosporine use is resumed. In some patients, a reduction in cyclosporine dose or cessation of therapy can resolve HUS. In this case, the absence of fibrous glomerular crescents suggests an element of reversibility borne out by a switch to a different immunophilin-binding immunosuppressant agent. Although HUS can be initiated by FK 506, as well as cyclosporine, a switch from one immunophilin-binding agent can lead to cessation of the problem.

Acute cyclosporine nephrotoxicity is dose dependent and dose responsive. Improvement in GFR must occur in 24 to 48 hours, and a search for an alternate explanation must be made if response has not occurred in this time.

OBSTRUCTION

PATIENT NUMBER 4

Jeremy is a married 26-year-old part-time cashier at a local grocery store in Tennessee. He received his second renal transplant to reverse ESRD secondary to SLE, first diagnosed at the age of 14. A renal biopsy performed to evaluate the nephrotic syndrome revealed World Health Organization (WHO) class-IV lupus nephritis culminating in renal failure at the age of 24. A first attempt at cadaveric renal transplantation was unsuccessful because of thrombosis of the transplant renal vein and artery related to a hypercoagulable state secondary to anticardiolipin antibody. Placed on long-term anticoagulation therapy, he returned to dialysis. Three months before admission, he underwent his second cadaveric kidney transplant surgery, which was complicated by postoperative hematuria and perigraft hematoma formation requiring surgical intervention and prolonged hospitalization. One episode of acute rejection after the transplantation reduced renal function, accounting for a discharge creatinine level between 2.0 and 2.5 mg/dl. Jeremy was maintained on cyclosporin A, prednisone, azathioprine "triple immunosuppression," and Coumadin after transplantation. Three days before admission, he noticed diminished urine output and some abdominal discomfort. He had

---

no history of fever, dysuria, hematuria, or graft tenderness. Laboratory findings revealed increased serum BUN and creatinine levels (66 mg/dl and 6.2 mg/dl, respectively). Ultrasonography showed a markedly dilated collecting system, and the intraureteric stent placed at the time of transplant surgery was out of position. Despite removal of the stent, hydronephrosis remained and his renal function continued to deteriorate. Percutaneous nephrostomy was performed, and an antegrade pyelogram demonstrated the distal ureteral stenosis leading to obstruction. Jeremy's renal function improved significantly. A few days later he underwent surgical repair of distal ureteral stenosis with reimplantation of the distal ureter into the bladder. Jeremy's discharge serum creatinine level was 1.9 mg/dl.

Urinary obstruction is usually diagnosed by worsening renal function and is confirmed by ultrasound examination of the graft. It can occur early or late after transplantation. The common causes of obstruction (Table 21–2) occurring within 3 months of the transplant include edema at the vesicoureteric junction, blood clots, and ureteral compression by a hematoma. Lymphoceles, ureteral stricture, periureteral fibrosis, a fungus ball, or renal calculi can cause obstruction and deterioration of renal function, usually 3 months after transplantation. Other reported causes of obstruction include infection, tumors, or misaligned intraureteric stents. Ureteral stenosis usually occurs at the lower end of the ureter. Knowledge of ureteric blood supply explains the predilection of ischemic injury to the distal ureter. The top third of the ureter receives its blood from the renal pelvis, the lower third from perforating vessels from the perinephric fat, and the middle third from both. The distal ureter therefore is most vulnerable to vascular disruption, ischemic injury, and scar formation with consequent obstruction of the flow of urine. Because a transplanted

TABLE 21–2. Common Causes of Obstruction After Transplantation

Edema at the vesicoureteric junction
Blood clots
Ureteral compression by hematoma or lymphocele
Ureteral stricture
Periureteral fibrosis
Renal calculi
Fungus ball
Donor abnormality: renal calculi or stricture at the pelviureteric junction

kidney is denervated, patients may not experience any pain; decreased urinary output may be the only sign. A renogram with furosemide aids in the diagnosis, with antegrade or retrograde pyelography the gold standard. Increasing experience with endoscopic management allows some cases to be treated nonsurgically.

> **Early postoperative ureteral obstruction is commonly a technical problem that may require immediate surgical exploration, especially when urinary extravasation is suspected.**

RECURRENT GLOMERULONEPHRITIS

PATIENT NUMBER 5

Sarah is a 47-year-old country music songwriter from Nashville. She had a one-antigen matched cadaveric kidney transplant 4 months before admission for ESRD secondary to SLE and presented to the clinic with generalized malaise and diminished urine output. Twelve years before admission, Sarah developed fever, rash, generalized pruritus, and lymphadenopathy. Serologic testing documented a positive ANA (1:180) and a positive anti-DNA (1:160). SLE was diagnosed, and prednisone and azathioprine were started. Two years later, she developed nephrotic syndrome with an active urinary sediment. A percutaneous kidney biopsy demonstrated WHO class V glomerulonephritis, and cyclophosphamide was added to her treatment. Hemodialysis was started 3 years later. She had numerous access problems, including subclavian vein thrombosis with swelling of her left breast and left arm. The course of her illness was also complicated by sepsis, a cerebrovascular accident, and reactivation of her lupus.

Her transplant course had been characterized by immediate postoperative renal function and one easily reversed, biopsy-proven acute cellular rejection. Sarah was otherwise asymptomatic when she presented to the clinic with increased serum BUN and creatinine levels, which accompanied the reduced urine flow rate. She denied any abdominal pain, dysuria, arthritis, arthralgia, skin rash, chest pain, or dyspnea. Renal ultrasound examination was unremarkable, but an isotope renogram showed reduced function. A renal biopsy revealed focal proliferative nephritis with subendothelial immune deposits and diffuse reticular aggregates by electron microscopy consistent with WHO class III SLE nephritis without any evidence of acute rejection. She had serologic evidence of active SLE with positive ANA and anti-DNA antibodies and low serum complement levels. Her kidney function started to improve after cyclophosphamide therapy was added to her maintenance transplant immunosuppression. Her last serum creatinine level was 1.5 mg/dl.

Sarah represents a case of recurrent glomerulonephritis in the renal transplant (Table 21–3). Although all diseases occurring in the native kidney can recur in the transplanted kidney within days to several years after transplantation, the chance of losing the allograft to recurring disease is less than 5%. Some disorders have a high predilection for recurrence, such as HUS, IgA nephropathy, FSGS, membranoproliferative glomerulonephritis (MPGN), and Henoch-Schönlein purpura. Some diseases such as SLE recur uncommonly. Although some have reported approximately 35% histologic recurrence of SLE in the transplant, the risk of clinically significant recurrence is less than 2%, with minimal chance of graft loss. Renal failure is most often associated with dissipation of the autoimmune diathesis that led to SLE. Curiously, restoring normal renal function by a successful transplant does not trigger reactivation. When recurrence has been encountered in SLE, it almost always reflects transplantation into a patient with active autoimmunity at the time of surgery, as in Sarah's case. Most of the patients reported had recurrence 1 to 6 years after transplantation, with typical clinical and laboratory findings including malar rash, Raynaud's phenomenon, proteinuria, and an active urinary sediment, as well as elevated serum creatinine, antinuclear antibody, and anti-DNA titers along with decreased complement levels. There is no known predisposing factor leading to recurrence in patients with SLE. To prevent

TABLE 21–3. Recurrent Diseases in Kidney Allografts

	Recurrence Rate	Graft Loss
Type II MPGN	>80%	10–20%
IgA nephropathy	50%	10%
Type I MPGN	20–30%	30–40%
FSGS	20–30%	30–40%
HUS	13–25%	40–50%
Henoch-Schönlein purpura	10–15%	10–20%
SLE	<2%	Minimal chance

recurrence, it has been recommended that clinical manifestations and serologic parameters of SLE be stable on no or only minimal doses of corticosteroids at the time of transplantation. Treatment regimens include pulse steroids, cyclophosphamide, and a combination of plasmapheresis and chlorambucil.

> **Focal and segmental glomerulosclerosis, IgA nephropathy, Henoch-Schönlein purpura, HUS, and type II MPGN have the highest rates of recurrence.**

CYTOMEGALOVIRUS INFECTION

PATIENT NUMBER 6

Robin, a 33-year-old mother of two boys, is a University of Tennessee biology graduate whose return to the workplace was delayed because of her renal disease. She received a cadaveric renal transplant for ESRD secondary to SLE. She underwent hemodialysis for 2 years. Although the graft functioned well immediately, acute rejection ensued 6 weeks after transplantation. She received 4 doses of 250 mg of methylprednisolone and 14 days of a polyclonal antilymphocyte antibody. Her kidney function improved significantly, and she was discharged with a serum creatinine level of 1.1 mg/dl on a maintenance immunosuppression regimen that included cyclosporine, prednisone, and azathioprine. She was seropositive for CMV before transplantation and received a graft from a CMV-seronegative donor. Three weeks after discharge, she presented to the emergency room with fever (101°F), arthralgia, cough, and exertional dyspnea. Her WBC count was 2.2 thousand per cubic millimeter. Chest radiographs revealed bilateral lower lobe infiltrates. Treatment with broad-spectrum antibiotics and ganciclovir was initiated. Bronchoscopy with bronchoalveolar lavage revealed intranuclear inclusion bodies. CMV early antigen was detected in her urine and blood cultures the next day. Robin responded well to therapy and remained disease free thereafter.

CMV remains a significant cause of posttransplantation morbidity and mortality in kidney recipients. The risk of CMV infection is between 70% and 88% among CMV-seronegative recipients who receive transplants from CMV-seropositive donors. Antilymphocyte antibody (polyclonal

TABLE 21–4. Clinical Syndromes of Cytomegalovirus

Type	CMV Serology		Source
	Donor	Recipient	
Primary	+	−	Transplant
Reactivation	+	+	Recipient
	−	+	
Superinfection	+	+	Transplant

or monoclonal) administration for either induction or rejection increases the incidence of clinical CMV disease at least threefold. Three clinical syndromes are recognized: (1) primary infection, (2) secondary or reactivation, and (3) superinfection (Table 21–4). Patients usually present with fever, myalgia, and lethargy. Syndromes associated with leukopenia or solid organ involvement increase the morbidity. Less common syndromes include hepatitis, splenomegaly, gastrointestinal ulceration with bleeding, myocarditis, retinitis, and encephalitis. Interstitial pneumonitis with gas exchange blockade presenting with tachypnea and dyspnea is the most dreaded CMV syndrome. It is most common after bone marrow or lung transplantation but can complicate the course of renal transplantation as well. The laboratory diagnosis of CMV infection depends on either isolation of the virus or demonstration of a greater than fourfold increase for IgG and twofold increase for IgM titers in the serum after transplantation. CMV cultures on human fibroblast cell cultures may take 1 to 4 weeks. Techniques such as direct CMV antigen detection and polymerase chain reaction lead to rapid diagnosis of CMV in 24 to 48 hours. The virus may be isolated from urine, throat, buffy coat, cervical swabs, or other infected tissues. Ganciclovir, a guanine analogue, inhibits replication of CMV *in vitro* and has been used successfully for the treatment of clinical CMV infection and prophylaxis. Hyperimmune globulin is often added to ganciclovir therapy for patients with serious CMV disease. The major side effect of ganciclovir is bone marrow toxicity, which is dose related. Ganciclovir is excreted by the kidneys; therefore, the standard dose must be reduced in patients with significant renal impairment. Passive immunization with high-titer CMV plasma or immune globulin or standard intravenous immune globulin, Towne strain of attenuated CMV vaccine, and antiviral drugs such as acyclovir have been recommended for prophylaxis in high-risk CMV-seronegative recipients of CMV-seropositive donor organs.

> **The greatest risk of CMV infection occurs when a CMV-seronegative patient receives a kidney from a CMV-seropositive donor ("primary infection").**

FUNGAL INFECTIONS

> ### PATIENT NUMBER 7
>
> David is a 61-year-old retired manager from Alabama. This man who prided himself on his mental sharpness and wit was admitted for fever and confusion. He had a 1A, 1B matched cadaveric kidney transplant for ESRD secondary to autosomal dominant polycystic kidney disease 8 years before his admission. Nine months before admission, he was diagnosed with squamous cell cancer of the right pinna metastatic to the chest wall. He underwent extensive resection of his right mastoid and parotid and a radical neck dissection. Radiotherapy was initiated. His maintenance immunosuppression included cyclosporine and prednisone. His disease course was complicated by ethmoid sinus fracture followed by CSF rhinorrhea. Replacement of a lumboperitoneal shunt resulted in cessation of the CSF leak. Three days before admission, he developed fever, malaise, and confusion. Lumbar puncture revealed 50 lymphocytes in the CSF, with elevated protein levels and a normal glucose concentration. Test for cryptococcal antigen was positive in CSF. Amphotericin B was started. He remains well after 2 months of therapy.

The risk of fungal infections increases 6 weeks after transplantation, with an incidence of about 5% in kidney transplant recipients. Despite newer diagnostic techniques and antifungal agents, morbidity and mortality remain high. *Candida* species, *Cryptococcus neoformans,* and *Aspergillus* are most frequently isolated and account for more than 80% of fungal infections in this patient population. Some mycoses such as histoplasmosis, coccidioidomycosis, and blastomycosis can cause either disseminated primary or reactivation infection in highly endemic areas. The most common site of fungal infections, especially with *Candida*, is the urinary tract in renal transplant recipients. The clinical presentation may also be catheter-related sepsis, esophagitis, meningitis, or pneumonitis. Prolonged hospitalization with long-term central venous catheter placement, antirejection therapy, and underlying

diabetes mellitus are some of the predisposing factors. Clinicians caring for renal transplant recipients should monitor those with specific risk factors with a high index of suspicion. Amphotericin B is still the drug of choice in many conditions. In addition to bone marrow toxicity, nephrotoxicity is a major concern. Newly available azole compounds offer an alternative treatment to amphotericin B against fungal infections in transplant recipients with a less toxic profile.

C. neoformans is an encapsulated yeast that has a worldwide distribution rather than any defined endemic area. The fungus can frequently be found in pigeon droppings. The incidence of cryptococcosis is increased in patients with lymphoreticular malignancies and sarcoidosis, patients receiving corticosteroids, and those with diabetes mellitus and AIDS, as well as transplant recipients. Although the primary route of infection is the respiratory tract, the most common clinical presentation is meningitis. The onset is usually insidious, with a waxing and waning course. Patients are often afebrile or have only a mildly elevated temperature. Complaints may be mild and nonspecific, such as headache, nausea, dizziness, irritability, and somnolence. Impaired memory, behavioral changes, hyperreflexia, and myoclonic jerks may occur. However, focal neurologic findings are rare. Lumbar puncture reveals a high opening pressure, depressed glucose levels in half the cases, increased protein concentration, and 40 to 400 WBCs/mm^3, mainly lymphocytes in CSF. By using India ink preparation, cryptococci can be seen in 50% of patients with cryptococcal meningitis. Confirmation by culture should follow. Both serum and CSF should also be tested for cryptococcal polysaccharide capsular antigen by the latex agglutination procedure, which detects antigen in CSF or serum in more than 90% of patients with meningitis. The treatment of choice for cryptococcal meningitis has been amphotericin B, with or without flucytosine, for at least 6 weeks. However, studies have suggested that oral fluconazole is also effective. Because 20% to 25% of patients suffer a relapse, patients with cryptococcoses should be evaluated every few months for at least 1 year after treatment, even in the absence of the signs or symptoms of infection.

> **Lumbar puncture is frequently an important element of fever evaluation in transplant recipients.**

POSTTRANSPLANT LYMPHOPROLIFERATIVE DISORDER

PATIENT NUMBER 8

Bill is a 28-year-old graduate student in mathematics. He underwent a cadaveric kidney transplantation for ESRD due to insulin-dependent diabetes mellitus. The graft functioned immediately, and his serum creatinine level dropped to 1.4 mg/dl in 8 days. He received 17 days of polyclonal antithymocyte globulin, azathioprine, and glucocorticoids for induction. His maintenance immunosuppression included prednisone, azathioprine, and cyclosporin A. Results of pretransplant serologic studies for CMV and Epstein-Barr virus (EBV) were negative. After 13 months of decent transplant function, he developed dysuria and hematuria. His 24-hour urine protein excretion was 2.3 g; serum creatinine level was stable at 1.7 mg/dl. Transplant biopsy performed 6 weeks before admission showed immune complex glomerulonephritis with widespread immune deposits. Bill had no systemic or laboratory manifestations of SLE. One day before admission, he had two wisdom teeth extracted from the right side, without immediate complications. He received prophylactic antibiotics before and after the procedure. On the day of admission, he developed high fever with chills, as well as pain and swelling of his right jaw. On examination, the right side of his face was tender and showed nonfluctuant swelling. No lymphadenopathy was found. His renal allograft was not tender. CT scan of the maxillofacial region demonstrated opacification of the right maxillary sinus, suggesting an infection. After all cultures were prepared, he was started on broad-spectrum antibiotics. He continued to have high fevers, and on the fourth hospital day, he developed abdominal distention and diffuse pain. CT scan of the abdomen showed a round, 3-cm lesion in the posterior segment of the right lobe of the liver and a small lesion in the inferior pole of the allograft. Fine-needle aspirate of the hepatic mass showed neoplastic cells with vacuolated dark cytoplasm. Immunologic typing studies revealed B-cell markers with IgM kappa on the surface of the neoplastic cells. Bone marrow biopsy confirmed the diagnosis of a posttransplantation lymphoproliferative disorder (PTLD), small noncleaved cell (non-Burkitt's) type malignant lymphoma. EBV serology was strongly positive. Despite tapering cyclosporine and treatment with acyclovir, gamma globulin, and interferon-α, the patient's condition deteriorated rapidly, culminating in death.

PTLD is an uncommon but well-recognized complication of some congenital immunodeficiencies, HIV infection, and solid organ and bone marrow transplantation and is associated with EBV infection in more than 80% of patients. The incidence of PTLD varies in various organ transplants. The overall incidence is 1% for renal, 1.8% for cardiac, 2.2% for liver, and 9.4% for heart-lung transplant recipients. The clinical presentation includes a benign, self-limited disease as well as an aggressive and widely disseminated disease. Since the introduction of cyclosporine and the wider use of antilymphocyte antibodies, PTLD usually presents within a few months after transplantation. Patients may present with an infectious mononucleosis-like syndrome with fever and cervical lymphadenopathy or multiorgan failure leading to death. CNS involvement is common. Although T-cell lesions have been described, PTLD is usually associated with a polyclonal or monoclonal B-cell proliferation. The risk of PTLD is high in patients who receive antilymphocyte antibodies (especially monoclonal antibodies) and in patients with a primary EBV infection. The relative risk of PTLD in EBV-seronegative recipients is more than 20-fold greater than in EBV-seropositive recipients and more than 200-fold greater than in the EBV-seronegative normal population. Cockfield and colleagues reported four cases with PTLD in 162 recipients of cadaveric renal allografts (2.5%). In this patient population, PTLD developed within 2 months of transplantation and was associated with EBV infection in all cases. Of the four cases, three were associated with primary infection. Management consists primarily of reduction or cessation of immunosuppression, especially cyclosporine. Overall response rate is approximately 40%. Patients with CNS disease or monoclonal B-cell proliferation and rapidly progressive disease respond poorly to any treatment. Occasional cases respond to high-dose acyclovir or ganciclovir, interferon-α, or chemotherapy.

TABLE 21–5. Tumors Associated with Organ Transplantation

Skin cancer
Lip cancer
Non-Hodgkin's lymphoma
Kaposi's sarcoma
Carcinoma of vulva and perineum
Hepatobiliary carcinoma
Carcinoma *in situ* of uterine cervix

> **Primary EBV infection poses a higher risk for the development of PTLD than reactivation or reinfection.**

CANCER

PATIENT NUMBER 9

Ellen is a 67-year-old mother of two and grandmother of five who had escaped to the United States from Germany with her family 55 years earlier. She had ESRD secondary to hypertension and started on hemodialysis 10 years ago. She underwent a cadaveric renal transplantation 9 years before evaluation. Her maintenance immunosuppression included cyclosporine, azathioprine, and prednisone. Her renal function remained stable, with a serum creatinine level between 0.8 and 1.0 mg/dl. She had multiple skin cancers, which were treated locally. Biopsy on all occasions revealed squamous cell carcinoma. Eleven years after transplantation, she presented to the clinic with a right axillary mass. Mammography showed a cystic mass in her right breast. Dissection of the breast mass revealed well-differentiated squamous cell carcinoma focally extending from the margin of resection. She also had metastasis in her right axillary lymph nodes. Radiation therapy was initiated.

The incidence of some malignancies after transplantation is significantly increased in renal transplant recipients and ranges from 4% to 18% (Table 21–5). Interestingly, the incidence of particular cancers including squamous and basal cell carcinomas of the skin and lip, non-Hodgkin's lymphoma, Kaposi's sarcoma, carcinomas of the vulva and perineum, hepatobiliary carcinoma, and carcinoma *in situ* of the uterine cervix is more frequent in transplant recipients (10- to 30-fold above expectation) than in the general population. Those malignancies occurring after transplantation often tend to behave more aggressively, with rapid tumor dissemination. Kaposi's sarcomas are the earliest to appear (in an average of 22 months) after transplantation. Non-Hodgkin's lymphomas may involve the brain, (an unusual site), extranodal sites, and the allograft. Several different factors contribute to the increased risk of cancer in allograft recipi-

ents, such as immunosuppressive therapy, especially with polyclonal and monoclonal antibodies, oncogenic viruses such as EBV, herpes simplex, herpes zoster, and polyoma viruses; chronic antigenic stimulation by the graft itself; and genetic differences. Treatment modalities include standard surgery, radiotherapy, or chemotherapy. In addition, reduction or cessation of immunosuppressive therapy may help in some forms of cancers and should be considered on a case-by-case basis for all tumors.

Skin cancers are the most common malignancies in transplant recipients. In the general population, basal cell carcinomas outnumber squamous cell carcinomas. On the other hand, squamous cell cancers are more common (1.8:1) in this patient population, occurring at least 20 times more often than expected. The lesions occur mostly in the areas of sun exposure and tend to be multiple and aggressive. In a review of 6562 transplant recipients, 37% had skin and lip cancers. Lymph node metastases were found in 5.8% of transplant recipients with skin cancers. All transplant recipients should be warned of the dangers of skin cancer and advised of protection from the sun. All skin lesions must be reviewed and treated as early as possible.

> **Close dermatologic monitoring is necessary in renal transplant recipients, especially in those who have had a previous skin cancer.**

SUGGESTED READINGS

Barrett WL, First MR, Aron BS, Penn I: Clinical course of malignancies in renal transplant recipients. Cancer 72:2186–2189, 1993.

Cockfield SM, Preiksaitis JK, Jewell LD, Panfrey NA: Post-transplant lymphoproliferative disorder in renal allograft recipients. Transplantation 56:88–96, 1993.

Helderman JH, Frist WH (eds): Grand Rounds in Transplantation. New York, Chapman & Hall, 1995.

Hibberd PL, Tolkoff-Rubin NE, Conti D, et al: Preemptive ganciclovir therapy to prevent cytomegalovirus disease in cytomegalovirus antibody-positive renal transplant recipients. A randomized controlled trial. Ann Intern Med 123:18–26, 1995.

Kasiske BL, Ramos EL, Gaston RS, et al: The evaluation of renal transplant candidates: Clinical practice guidelines. J Am Soc Nephrol 6:1–34, 1995.

Paya CV: Fungal infections in solid-organ transplantation. Clin Infect Dis 16:677–688, 1993.

Ramos EL: Recurrent diseases in the renal allograft. J Am Soc Nephrol 2:109–121, 1991.

Remuzzi G, Gotti E: The girl with the curl. N Engl J Med 333:928–931, 1995.

Suthanthiran M, Strom TB: Renal transplantation. N Engl J Med 331:365–376, 1994.

Tolkoff-Rubin NE, Rubin RH: Opportunistic fungal and bacterial infection in the renal transplant recipient. J Am Soc Nephrol 2:S264–S269, 1992.

22 | URGENT PROBLEMS IN THE RENAL PATIENT

Kevin D. Burns, Nicholas B. Argent, and Robert C. Bell

This chapter presents problems in renal patients that require urgent decision making. Selected case histories from the Ottawa General Hospital Nephrology service are presented, as appropriate, to illustrate the unique approach to the patient's urgent problem and briefly summarize the management. The emphasis is on rapid recognition and institution of initial therapy for these common disorders. Detailed pathophysiology is not discussed, nor are extensive differential diagnoses or treatment strategies offered. This information is intended to be used as a rapid reference for busy practitioners or house officers, who may encounter similar cases in practice. The initial discussion of fluid, electrolyte, and acid-base disorders is followed by hypertensive crises, urgent problems in hemodialysis patients, and finally urgencies in renal transplantation.

FLUID, ELECTROLYTE, AND ACID-BASE URGENCIES

Hyponatremia

PATIENT NUMBER 1

Mary is a 52-year-old woman admitted to the Ottawa General Hospital because of hyponatremia (serum sodium concentration 97 mEq/L) associated with drowsiness and marked lethargy. The patient lived in a remote community and had a history of alcoholism and hypertension (treated with indapamide and hydrochlorothiazide). She had no other significant past history. On physical examination, Mary was found to have ECF volume contraction. Her serum potassium concentration was also severely reduced, at 1.9 mEq/L. In the emergency room, she received 1 L of normal saline with 40 mEq KCl IV over 2 hours, as well as 80 mEq KCl orally. She was then transferred to the intensive care unit and was seen by the nephrology consultant, who, not knowing whether the hyponatremia was acute or chronic, wished to

correct the hypotonicity at a slow rate to avoid the complication of permanent brain damage. The patient was water restricted and received oral KCl. Serum sodium concentration was monitored hourly, and arginine vasopressin was periodically administered intravenously to finely regulate the rise in serum sodium concentration. With this cautious approach, serum sodium concentration rose to 110 mEq/L during the ensuing 24 hours and to 117 mEq/L after 48 hours. Despite this, Mary developed motor paralysis, associated with brain MRI findings consistent with osmotic demyelination syndrome (ODS). With intensive rehabilitation, the patient had a remarkable neurologic recovery and returned to her home, with minimal deficits. She has had no recurrence of the hyponatremia.

Hyponatremia is present when the serum sodium concentration is less than 135 mEq/L. Symptoms are related to the hypotonicity of body fluids, causing cell swelling. Hypotonicity is not always present with hyponatremia, however. With severe hyperglycemia, a hypertonic hyponatremia ensues. In pseudohyponatremia, the volume of the solid phase of plasma is increased by an excess of lipids or proteins, causing the measured serum sodium concentration to be reduced. The urgency of hyponatremia depends on both the degree of hyponatremia and the rate at which the serum sodium concentration has fallen. Symptoms, primarily related to swelling of cells within the CNS, range from lethargy and confusion to status epilepticus or coma.

Mary's case highlights the difficulties with management of severe hyponatremia. In patients with acute symptomatic hyponatremia, it is desirable to increase the serum sodium concentration by 1 to 2 mEq/L/hr, until serious neurologic symptoms such as seizures subside. This can be achieved with intravenous hypertonic saline (50 mmol/L/hr IV), along with restriction of free-water intake. Administration of a loop diuretic (e.g., furosemide) may be useful to increase free-water excretion in these cases and to prevent

333

fluid overload. This therapy should be monitored by ensuring that the osmolality of the fluid administered is greater than that of the urine. Of course, serum sodium concentration must be measured frequently (hourly) in these seriously ill patients.

Patients with chronic symptomatic hyponatremia are especially problematic, and optimal therapy is controversial. Mary developed ODS despite appropriately slow correction of the hyponatremia. Indeed, she received vasopressin to suppress a rapid rise in serum sodium concentration. Patients who develop cerebral demyelination often do so despite cautious correction of the hyponatremia, suggesting that other factors (e.g., alcoholism, liver disease) may contribute to the pathogenesis. **We continue to recommend that patients presenting with severe symptomatic hyponatremia of unclear duration undergo correction of the serum sodium concentration initially at a rate not exceeding 0.6 mEq/L/hr and not greater than a 20 mEq/L change in the first 24 hours.** Patients who have had severe hyponatremia for longer than 48 hours, who likely have adaptive changes in brain osmole concentrations, stand to benefit from this cautious approach to raising the serum osmolality.

Hypernatremia

Hypernatremia is present when the serum sodium concentration is greater than 145 mEq/L. The vast majority of these cases are due to loss of water in excess of sodium rather than sodium gain. In contrast to hyponatremia, the symptoms of hypernatremia are related to cell shrinkage. Neurologic impairment, due to brain cell shrinkage, generally occurs in proportion to the degree of hypernatremia. Brain hemorrhage may occur owing to traction of venous sinuses, especially when the serum sodium concentration exceeds 155 mEq/L. Infants with hypernatremia are particularly vulnerable, because thirst is not communicated directly. Similarly, elderly patients may not have access to water and their thirst sensation may be impaired.

With hypernatremia, the expected normal renal response is excretion of a minimal volume of maximally concentrated urine. Excretion of hypotonic urine implies renal water loss due to diabetes insipidus (central or nephrogenic) or use of diuretics.

The treatment of severe symptomatic hypernatremia is based on three principles:

1. End ongoing water loss: Antidiuretic hormone (ADH) deficiency can be treated with the synthetic nasal spray 1-desamino-8-D-arginine vasopressin (DDAVP) or other forms of vasopressin. If water loss is due to nephrogenic diabetes insipidus, initial therapy should be directed at the underlying cause. Thus, hypokalemia and hypercalcemia must be corrected and possible causative drugs such as lithium eliminated.

2. Replace the water deficit: Oral water is preferable. Because many of these patients are unable to ingest fluids, however, free water is often given intravenously as a hypotonic solution of 5% dextrose in water (D_5W) at a rate not exceeding 300 ml/hr, to avoid serious hyperglycemia. If the patient is hypovolemic from excess sodium and water loss, intravenous isotonic saline should be given until the patient is hemodynamically stable.

3. Avoid overly rapid correction: In general, the serum sodium concentration should be decreased no faster than 2 mEq/L/hr in the first 24 hours. Rapid correction is associated with development of neurologic complications, such as cerebral edema or seizures.

> In severe hypernatremia, (1) end the water loss (e.g., give vasopressin), (2) replace the water deficit (e.g., oral water or intravenous D_5W), and (3) avoid rapid correction (< 2 mEq/L/hr decrease in serum sodium concentration).

In rare cases of hypernatremia caused by pure sodium gain, a diuretic may be necessary in addition to free-water replacement. Patients who have severely impaired renal function and are unresponsive to diuretics may require dialysis.

Hypokalemia

PATIENT NUMBER 2

Norman is a 32-year-old schoolteacher who came to the hospital because of severe weakness. He had been well up until the day of admission. He was lying on his couch, watching television, and suddenly could not lift his head off the couch. He called out to his wife, who naturally became alarmed and called 911 for an ambulance. Norman had no other medical problems and was taking no medications. In the emergency room, he was hypertensive (blood pressure 160/115 mm Hg) and had generalized weakness of all limbs. His serum potassium concentration was 2.6 mEq/L, with a plasma [HCO_3^-] of 32 mEq/L. Norman was given an intravenous infusion of KCl at 20 mEq/hr, along with oral potassium supplements, after demonstrating intact swallowing ability.

Hypokalemia is present when the serum potassium concentration is less than 3.5 mEq/L. Severe hypokalemia can be defined as a serum potassium concentration less than 3.0 mEq/L, a level at which there is increased risk of cardiac arrhythmias in patients with preexisting heart disease. Arrhythmias are also more frequent when hypokalemia occurs in patients on digoxin therapy. Severe hypokalemia is associated with impaired neuromuscular transmission, leading to muscle weakness or frank paralysis.

PATIENT NUMBER 2 (Continued)

Norman had severe hypokalemia associated with hypertension and metabolic alkalosis. His weakness improved dramatically within hours of receiving potassium supplementation. His urine potassium excretion was later found to be abnormally high. This suggests a state of hyperaldosteronism. Investigations in hospital revealed the presence of bilateral adrenal cortical hyperplasia. He has since been treated with oral amiloride (10 mg/day) and has suffered no further hypokalemia.

Severe hypokalemia can be treated with a combination of intravenous and oral potassium supplements, as in Norman's case. Intravenous KCl, when given at high concentrations (> 40 mEq/L), causes local irritation to peripheral veins and therefore should be administered into a central vein if possible and at a rate not exceeding 20 mEq/hr, to avoid sudden exposure of the myocardium to high potassium levels. Oral potassium supplements are preferable because larger quantities may be given, and provided gut absorption is adequate, the hypokalemia can be readily corrected, at least temporarily.

Hyperkalemia

Hyperkalemia is defined as serum potassium concentration greater than 5.5 mEq/L. This is a common problem in renal patients, who have impaired renal excretion of potassium. When faced with an elevated serum potassium level, however, the physician must rule out pseudohyperkalemia due to hemolysis, thrombocytosis, or leukocytosis.

The urgency of therapy depends on the degree of elevation of serum potassium concentration, the presence of symptoms such as muscle weakness, nausea and vomiting, and the degree of ECG change (progressing from peaked T waves, to widening of the QRS, to loss of the P wave and sine wave formation). Serious elevation of the serum potassium concentration associated with ECG changes is a potentially life-threatening emergency because of the risk of cardiac arrest.

All potassium intake must be stopped. The patient should be given calcium gluconate 10%, 10 ml IV over 10 minutes, to stabilize the myocardium against the proarrhythmic effects of hyperkalemia. Potassium should be shifted into cells with use of glucose and insulin (infused as 500 ml of 10% dextrose in water with 10 units of regular insulin over 20 to 30 minutes). The use of beta-adrenergic agents, such as aerosolized salbutamol, has been shown to be effective in acutely reducing serum potassium concentration. In contrast, intravenous $NaHCO_3$ has a variable effect on serum potassium concentration. With administration of intravenous $NaHCO_3$ (50 to 100 mEq), a decrease in serum potassium concentration can be expected only after several hours.

> **Initial therapy of severe hyperkalemia consists of (1) discontinuation of all potassium intake and (2) administration of intravenous calcium gluconate 10% (10 ml) and intravenous insulin and glucose.**

After this initial therapy, measures should be taken to remove potassium from the body. In renal patients, this often means institution of hemodialysis with a low-potassium dialysate. In patients on peritoneal dialysis, frequent dialysate exchanges (hourly) may be effective. Potassium may also be removed with cation exchange resins (Kayexalate), although these work slowly. In this regard, Kayexalate enemas (100 g) are more effective than use of the oral resin.

Hypocalcemia

PATIENT NUMBER 3

Claire is a 42-year-old woman who came to our hospital after suffering a generalized tonic-clonic seizure at home in her kitchen. This patient had asymptomatic HIV infection for more than 10 years but had recently developed proteinuria and progressive renal failure, presumed to be due to HIV nephropathy. Two months before admission, a decrease in her serum calcium concentration was noted (1.90 mmol/L [3.8 mEq/L, 7.6 mg/dl]). Associated with this was only a mild reduction in serum albumin concentration (32 g/L) and a decrease in ionized calcium level. She was taking no medications other than trimethoprim-sulfamethoxazole for *Pneumocystis carinii* prophylaxis, and she had recently been prescribed an oral vitamin D supplement. Claire had been complaining of paresthesias for a few days before admission. On arrival at the emergency room, she was in a postictal state. Physical examination revealed a positive Chvostek's sign (facial twitching on tapping the facial nerve) and Trousseau's sign (carpal spasm after inflation of the blood pressure cuff above systolic pressure). Her serum calcium concentration was 1.74 mmol/L (3.48 mEq/L, 7.0 mg/dl), associated with a marked reduction in her serum ionized calcium level. Claire received 2 ampules of intravenous calcium gluconate (10%, 4.5 mEq/10 ml [93 mg elemental calcium/10 ml]) over 10 minutes, followed by an intravenous infusion of calcium in normal saline. She was also started on oral calcium carbonate (1 g elemental calcium t.i.d.) and vitamin D derivative (calcitriol, 1.0 μg/day). The ionized calcium concentration rose during the next 24 hours, and Claire's symptoms disappeared.

Hypocalcemia occurs when the serum calcium concentration is less than 2.20 mmol/L (4.4 mEq/L, 8.8 mg/dl). It must be distinguished from the decrease in protein-bound calcium occurring secondary to hypoalbuminemia. Acute hypocalcemia commonly occurs after surgical correction of hyperparathyroidism. Claire developed hypocalcemia associated with a rapid progression of renal failure. Unfortunately, she had brain CT scan findings suggestive of progressive multifocal leukoencephalopathy, and the decrease in serum calcium concentration likely predisposed her to generalized seizures. This contrasts with many patients with advanced renal failure, who tolerate profound hypocalcemia without symptoms. With severe hypocalcemia (serum calcium concentration < 1.7 mmol/L [3.4 mEq/L, 7.0 mg/dl]), the physician should also be alert to the possible development of cardiac arrhythmias, associated with prolongation of the QT interval on ECG.

As in Claire's case, urgent therapy is required to relieve signs of tetany and seizures and to prevent cardiac arrhythmias. Patients should re- ceive intravenous calcium, administered as 10% calcium gluconate or as 10% calcium chloride (18 mEq/10 ml). This may be followed by an infusion of calcium (0.75 mEq/kg over 4 to 6 hours).

Hypomagnesemia must be ruled out as a factor contributing to hypocalcemia (serum magnesium concentration < 0.8 mEq/L [1.0 mg/dl]). If hypomagnesemia is present, treat with parenteral magnesium (8 to 16 mEq magnesium sulfate IV over 10 to 15 minutes).

Long-term treatment requires oral calcium to ensure that at least 1 g of elemental calcium is ingested each day, along with vitamin D preparations, as indicated.

Hypercalcemia

Hypercalcemia is defined as serum calcium concentration greater than 2.60 mmol/L (5.2 mEq/L, 10.5 mg/dl). Patients with severe hypercalcemia (serum calcium concentration > 3.40 mmol/L [6.8 mEq/L, 14 mg/dl]) typically have nausea, vomiting, confusion, and somnolence. Polyuria may result from impaired ability to concentrate the urine. With severe hypercalcemia, patients are at increased risk of nephrocalcinosis, metastatic calcification, and ECG changes characterized by a shortened QT interval, broadening of the T wave, and first-degree heart block. Many patients with hypercalcemia and polyuria present with profound ECF volume contraction and prerenal azotemia.

Patients with severe elevations of the serum calcium concentration require urgent therapy. The ECF volume should be expanded with intravenous isotonic saline (1 to 2 L over 1 hour), then 200 to 300 ml/hr, to increase urinary calcium excretion. Once a patient is volume replete, furosemide may be necessary (20 to 40 mg IV every 4 to 6 hours) to prevent fluid overload. The input and output and serum and urinary electrolytes should be strictly monitored. Ongoing potassium losses should be replaced. In patients with cardiac disease, monitoring of the central venous pressure is recommended.

Control of hypercalcemia by ECF volume expansion is temporary. Other measures are required to decrease calcium efflux from bone (e.g., calcitonin, bisphosphonates, mithramycin, or gallium nitrate). Glucocorticoids are also effective in this regard and may diminish gut calcium absorption. In patients with severe renal failure, acute hemodialysis with a low- or zero-calcium dialysate is effective, although rebound hypercalcemia may occur after the dialysis treatment.

Hypophosphatemia

Hypophosphatemia is defined as serum inorganic phosphorus concentration less than 0.8 mmol/L (2.5 mg/dl). Hypophosphatemia is severe when the phosphorus concentration is less than 0.5 mmol/L (1.5 mg/dl). It may be associated with normal total body phosphate or with phosphate deficiency.

Severe hypophosphatemia is associated with skeletal muscle weakness, ileus, and cardiomyopathy. It may also impair diaphragmatic movements, decreasing effective ventilation. Rhabdomyolysis has been reported. Hemolysis may occur. Severe hypophosphatemia is most frequently observed in alcoholics, during the recovery phase of diabetic ketoacidosis, with excessive use of phosphate binders, and with hyperalimentation.

For acute severe hypophosphatemia, the physician should administer phosphate, 1 mmol/kg IV over 24 hours (as potassium phosphate), if phosphate depletion is identified. If a patient is able to eat, an excellent source of phosphorus is milk, because it contains about 1 g/L (33 mmol) of inorganic phosphorus. Patients may also be given oral phosphorus as Neutra-Phos tablets at a dose up to 3 g/day. Monitor serum calcium, phosphorus, and potassium levels during therapy. Beware of hyperphosphatemia. Stop parenteral treatment when serum phosphorus concentration exceeds 0.5 mmol/L.

Hyperphosphatemia

Hyperphosphatemia is defined as serum phosphorus concentration greater than 1.7 mmol/L (5 mg/dl). Hyperphosphatemia most commonly results from decreased urinary excretion of phosphorus (as in renal failure). It can also be induced by intravenous phosphate infusion, and it is observed in states of increased catabolism and tissue breakdown (e.g., tumor lysis syndrome caused by cytotoxic therapy of malignancies). Hyperphosphatemia can cause hypocalcemia and tetany. Ectopic calcifications may occur.

The physician should decrease gut phosphate absorption with phosphate-binding agents and should expand the ECF volume to increase urinary phosphate excretion, if renal function is adequate. In cases of severe renal failure or tissue breakdown, peritoneal dialysis or hemodialysis may be necessary to remove phosphorus.

Acid-Base Disorders

Metabolic Acidosis

> **PATIENT NUMBER 4**
>
> James is a 47-year-old man who came to the hospital because of fatigue and shortness of breath. He worked at a truck loading dock and had received complaints from his superior for the previous few days because of his inability to keep up the pace of work. The patient had a history of bladder carcinoma requiring resection and creation of an ileal conduit. When seen in the emergency room, James was noted to be dyspneic. Although his respiratory rate was only 18 per minute, increased ventilation was evident on inspection of his chest movements. Physical examination was otherwise unremarkable, except for volume contraction. His serum creatinine concentration was minimally elevated, and his serum potassium concentration was 4.5 mEq/L. Arterial blood gas determination revealed pH 7.00, $PaCO_2$ 12 mm Hg, HCO_3^- 3 mEq/L, and PaO_2 115 mm Hg on room air. The anion gap $(Na - [Cl^- + HCO_3^-])$ was normal. James had no history of medication use or diarrhea. He received 4 ampules of $NaHCO_3$ (50 mEq/ampule) IV over 1 hour, followed by an infusion of D_5W plus 3 ampules $NaHCO_3/L$, at 150 ml/hr. After 24 hours, the plasma $[HCO_3^-]$ was 18 mEq/L, associated with a blood pH of 7.36. James felt considerably better and, indeed, asked about leaving the hospital to get back to work. He was convinced to stay for 2 more days and was sent home on oral $NaHCO_3$ supplements. Results of blood and urine cultures were negative.

Metabolic acidosis is a primary reduction in the plasma $[HCO_3^-]$ below 24 mEq/L. Severe metabolic acidosis is defined as plasma $[HCO_3^-]$ less than 10 mEq/L. Below this level, blood pH is sensitive to small changes in $PaCO_2$ and $[HCO_3^-]$. The physician can expect that for every 1 mEq/L decrease in plasma $[HCO_3^-]$ below 24 mEq/L, $PaCO_2$ will decrease by about 1 mm Hg below 40 mm Hg.

PATIENT NUMBER 4 (Continued)

James had severe metabolic acidosis with a normal anion gap, due to urinary losses of HCO_3^- from the ileal conduit. He was primarily affected by *generalized weakness and dyspnea. The severity of this situation can be appreciated by noting that if his* $Paco_2$ *had risen from 12 mm Hg to 18 mm Hg or if his plasma* $[HCO_3^-]$ *had declined further from 3 mEq/ L to 2 mEq/L, his blood pH would have decreased to approximately 6.8, a level at which myocardial contractility may become seriously impaired.*

We recommend treating metabolic acidosis when the plasma $[HCO_3^-]$ is less than 10 mEq/L, or to increase the blood pH above 7.10. This does not always require HCO_3^- therapy, however. For instance, in severe metabolic acidosis due to type A lactic acidosis, measures to improve tissue perfusion and oxygenation are essential to arrest ongoing acid generation. Indeed, HCO_3^- therapy has not been shown to improve prognosis in these critically ill patients. Similarly, in severe diabetic ketoacidosis, insulin must be provided as initial therapy.

When administering $NaHCO_3$, the amount required (mEq) can be estimated as = (the desired plasma $[HCO_3^-]$ − actual plasma $[HCO_3^-]$ × 50% body weight in kilograms). With increasing acidemia, the volume of distribution of HCO_3^- increases, necessitating higher quantities of $NaHCO_3$. The physician should initially administer $NaHCO_3$ intravenously, with attention to the following potential complications: sodium overload; overshoot alkalosis (especially in patients with organic acidoses, in which the salts are potential HCO_3^- sources); hypokalemia (give potassium supplements if serum potassium concentration is less than 4 mEq/L at the start of therapy; rising $Paco_2$ in mechanically ventilated patients ($NaHCO_3$ is a source of carbon dioxide); and tetany due to a decrease in the serum ionized calcium concentration.

In patients with severe renal failure, dialysis against a HCO_3^- bath (35 mEq/L) is useful because of the danger of fluid overload with intravenous $NaHCO_3$. When combined severe metabolic and respiratory acidosis are present, immediate mechanical ventilation should be instituted to correct the pH.

Metabolic Alkalosis

PATIENT NUMBER 5

Henry, 40 years old, was transferred to our hospital from a chronic care mental health institution. He had been vomiting for several days and was unable to keep food or fluids down. Physical examination revealed profound ECF volume contraction. Tetany was absent.

Abdominal radiographs revealed massive gastric dilatation consistent with pyloric stenosis. Laboratory results were as follows: arterial pH 7.61, $Paco_2$ 49 mm Hg, plasma $[HCO_3^-]$ 49 mEq/L, Na^+ 140 mEq/L, K^+ 2.8 mEq/L, Cl^- 80 mEq/L, serum creatinine level 512 μmol/L (5.8 mg/dl), and urine Cl^- 3 mEq/L. The patient was treated initially with intravenous normal saline with KCl supplementation. On restoration of Henry's ECF volume both his serum creatinine level and plasma $[HCO_3^-]$ normalized.

A primary increase in the plasma $[HCO_3^-]$ greater than 25 mEq/L in association with an elevation in blood pH (> 7.40) signifies metabolic alkalosis. For every 1 mEq rise in $[HCO_3^-]$ above 25 mEq/L, the physician can expect a 0.6 mm Hg increase in $Paco_2$ above 40 mm Hg.

With severe metabolic alkalosis (blood pH > 7.60), a patient may present with mental confusion, paresthesias, cramping, tetany, or seizures. Cardiac arrhythmias may occur. Severe hypokalemia is not uncommon.

PATIENT NUMBER 5 (Continued)

Henry had a severe Cl^- depletion metabolic alkalosis, secondary to gastric losses from vomiting, associated with marked potassium losses. His GFR was severely reduced because of volume contraction, and failure to filter plasma HCO_3^- contributed to the maintenance of the metabolic alkalosis. History taking was difficult in this unfortunate patient, and urgency of therapy was dictated by his abnormal laboratory values. Henry responded with initial therapy to increase GFR, although surgical intervention was ultimately required to correct the problem.

In treating metabolic alkalosis, the physician should remove the underlying stimulus to HCO_3^- generation; for example, discontinue diuretics or prevent vomiting. Factors sustaining alkalosis should also be removed. NaCl and KCl correct saline-responsive alkalosis, whereas saline-resistant forms require therapy directed at the specific cause.

In severe alkalemia, dilute HCl or NH_4Cl infusion can be used to reduce plasma $[HCO_3^-]$. Acetazolamide (250 mg IV every 8 hours) can be given to increase renal HCO_3^- excretion. In patients with irreversible severe renal failure, hemodialysis with a low bath $[HCO_3^-]$ is preferred. In patients on peritoneal dialysis, intravenous solutions lacking lactate may be used as HCO_3^--free dialysate, although these may cause abdominal distress because of the low pH.

Respiratory Acidosis

Increased $PaCO_2$ ($>$ 40 mm Hg) and blood pH $<$ 7.40 signify respiratory acidosis. In acute respiratory acidosis, expect a 1 mEq/L increase in the plasma $[HCO_3^-]$ for every 10 mm Hg increase in the $PaCO_2$. In chronic respiratory acidosis, expect a 3 mEq/L increase in plasma $[HCO_3^-]$ for every 10 mm Hg increase in $PaCO_2$.

Acute respiratory acidosis is associated with CNS dysfunction (anxiety, confusion, or coma). Chronic respiratory acidosis may be well tolerated. The absence of a history of chronic lung disease or illness causing chronic CNS depression suggests that the respiratory acidosis is acute.

Therapy involves improved ventilation. When ventilating patients with chronic respiratory acidosis, the $PaCO_2$ should be corrected to the known chronic $PaCO_2$.

Respiratory Alkalosis

A low $PaCO_2$ ($<$ 40 mm Hg) and high blood pH ($>$ 7.40) signify respiratory alkalosis. In acute respiratory alkalosis, expect a 2 mEq/L decrease in plasma $[HCO_3^-]$ for every 10 mm Hg decrease in $PaCO_2$. In chronic respiratory alkalosis, expect a 5 mEq/L decrease in $[HCO_3^-]$ for every 10 mm Hg reduction in $PaCO_2$.

Symptoms of alkalemia may be present. Acute respiratory alkalosis reduces cerebral blood flow and may cause lightheadedness or even seizures.

Treatment of severe respiratory alkalosis should be directed at the underlying cause. When due to anxiety states, air rebreathing may be useful to relieve symptoms.

HYPERTENSIVE EMERGENCIES AND URGENCIES (HYPERTENSIVE CRISES)

Hypertensive crises are divided into the hypertensive emergencies and urgencies, an important distinction that determines the rapidity with which the blood pressure should be reduced. In hypertensive emergencies, blood pressure is elevated in association with ongoing acute end-organ damage, and blood pressure must be lowered within 1 hour. These situations are not defined solely by the degree of elevation of blood pressure (Table 22–1). Rather, the clinical situation accompanying the rise in blood pressure determines the need for emergent therapy.

In contrast, hypertensive urgency is present when there is marked elevation of blood pressure (diastolic pressure usually $>$ 115 to 120 mm Hg) without signs of acute end-organ dysfunction or grade IV hypertensive neuroretinopathy. Blood pressure should be reduced within 24 hours in these situations, because persistent elevation of pressure may lead to heart failure, stroke, or other serious sequelae.

When evaluating a patient with a hypertensive crisis, the physician should spend the first few minutes obtaining a focused history. Symptoms of end-organ injury such as headache and blurred

TABLE 22–1. Hypertensive Crises

Hypertensive Emergencies	Hypertensive Urgencies
Malignant/accelerated hypertension	Severe elevation in blood pressure ($\geq$120 diastolic) without severe hypertensive neuroretinopathy or acute end-organ dysfunction
Hypertensive encephalopathy	Severe hypertension in patients with a history of congestive heart failure, stable angina, chronic renal failure, or transient ischemic attacks
Severe hypertension accompanied by	Pre- and postoperative hypertension
Acute pulmonary edema	
Angina or myocardial infarction	
Dissecting aortic aneurysm	
Acute renal failure	
Postoperative bleeding	
CNS catastrophes (subarachnoid hemorrhage, intracerebral bleeding, head trauma)	
Extensive burns	
Preeclampsia/eclampsia	
Catecholamine excess states with severe hypertension	
Pheochromocytoma	
MAO inhibitor interactions	
Antihypertensive drug withdrawal syndromes	

vision are common in malignant/accelerated hypertension. Factors predisposing to hypertensive crisis, such as a history of difficult-to-control blood pressure or recent change or cessation of antihypertensive therapy, should be sought. Any underlying illnesses such as angina, heart failure, or cerebrovascular disease that may affect the choice of initial antihypertensive therapy must be determined.

Next, the physician should perform a brief physical examination. Blood pressure should be recorded in both arms, with the patient both supine and sitting. Patients with malignant hypertension may be volume contracted and may therefore demonstrate significant postural decrease in blood pressure. The examination should also determine the degree of target organ involvement, by examination of the optic fundi, cardiovascular system, and CNS. In malignant hypertension, the optic fundi reveal grade IV hypertensive neuroretinopathy, characterized by papilledema, flame-shaped hemorrhages, and cotton-wool exudates.

At the conclusion of the brief physical examination, the physician usually has enough information to decide if the patient has a hypertensive emergency or urgency. Initial laboratory studies should be ordered at this point (Table 22–2) to assist in diagnosis and to assess end-organ injury. **In hypertensive emergencies, therapy should be initiated before return of laboratory results. Hypertensive emergencies generally warrant intravenous antihypertensive therapy (Table 22–3) and admission to an intensive care unit.** A wide selection of parenteral medications is available. Nitroprusside remains the drug of choice for most hypertensive emergencies. In malignant hypertension, hypertensive encephalopathy, or stroke, diastolic pressure should not be initially reduced below 100 mm Hg, in order to avoid further decreases in cerebral perfusion.

For hypertensive urgencies, the blood pressure can be lowered more gradually. Oral antihypertensive therapy may be started in the emergency room and the patient monitored for the first few hours. The patient can then be discharged, with follow-up arranged within 24 hours.

MEDICAL EMERGENCIES IN PATIENTS ON HEMODIALYSIS

During the past 10 to 15 years, dialysis machine technology and associated safety features have become increasingly sophisticated. As a direct consequence, the type and frequency of dialysis-related emergencies have decreased. Indeed, very few potentially life-threatening problems now are truly related to the dialysis procedure itself. For example, the occurrence of hypotonic or overheated dialysate, which has in the past led to lethal hemolysis, is now exceedingly rare. Nevertheless, patients with renal failure requiring dialysis do remain susceptible to common complications that must be managed with care and speed if serious morbidity and mortality are to be avoided.

Dialysis emergencies can be grouped into two broad categories:

1. Problems directly related to the dialysis procedure
2. Common medical problems that arise during dialysis and require special management

The following discussion focuses on the immediate care of urgent medical problems within the dialysis unit.

Problems Directly Related to the Dialysis Procedure

First-Use Reactions

First-use syndromes refer to two different clinical conditions:

TABLE 22–2. Initial Laboratory Evaluation of Severe Hypertension

Test	Significance
Complete blood count	Rule out microangiopathic hemolytic anemia (in malignant/accelerated hypertension)
Electrolytes	Rule out hypokalemic metabolic alkalosis (occurs in malignant/accelerated hypertension due to hyperreninemic hyperaldosteronism)
BUN, creatinine	Helpful to know previous values. If creatinine is elevated and anemia is present (hemoglobin <12.5 g/dL) without microangiopathy, chronic renal disease may be the cause of the hypertensive crisis
Urinalysis	Proteinuria, micro/macroscopic hematuria (+/− RBC casts) in malignant/accelerated hypertension
ECG	Left ventricular hypertrophy suggests longstanding hypertension
Chest radiograph	Rule out heart failure. Check for widened mediastinum (aortic dissection)

TABLE 22–3. Drug Therapy for Hypertensive Crises

Drugs	Route	Dose	Onset	Comments
		Emergencies		
Nitroprusside	IV	0.5–10 µg/kg/min	Instantaneous	Direct areriolar and venous dilator. ICU monitoring needed. Thiocyanate toxicity may occur in patients with renal insufficiency.
Nitroglycerin	IV	3–5 µg/min initially	Minutes	Use in ICU setting. Advantageous in myocardial ischemia.
Diazoxide	IV	Minibolus 50–100 mg over 5–10 min	Minutes	Reflex tachycardia, sustained hypotension may occur.
Labetalol	IV	Minibolus 20 mg, then 40–80 mg over 10 min	Minutes	α_1 and β blocker. Contraindicated in heart block, asthma, congestive heart failure.
Enalaprilat	IV	1.25–5 mg q 6 h	15 min	ACE inhibitor. Active metabolite of enalapril.
Trimethaphan	IV	0.5–5.0 mg/min	Minutes	Ganglionic blocker.
Phentolamine	IV	1–5 mg bolus	Minutes	Useful in catecholamine crises.
Hydralazine	IM	10–50 mg	30 min	Safe in pregnancy. Avoid in angina, aortic dissection, stroke.
	IV	5–10 mg bolus or continuous infusion 50–150 µg/min, after loading dose of 200–300 µg/min for 30–60 min		
		Urgencies		
Clonidine	Oral	0.2 mg, then 0.1 mg q1h	30 min	No reflex tachycardia. May cause sedation.
Captopril	Oral	10–50 mg	30 min	Treatment of choice in scleroderma renal crisis. Hypovolemia leads to increased hypotensive effect.
Minoxidil	Oral	5–20 mg	1–4 hr	Causes Na and H_2O retention. Concomitant use of a diuretic recommended.

1. Immediate hypersensitivity reactions are rare but may be severe and life threatening.

2. Minor reactions are common and consist of a symptom complex of nonspecific chest and back pain that may be associated with nausea and pruritus.

HYPERSENSITIVITY

Severe reactions involving respiratory distress and anaphylaxis are rare and are usually associated with the use of cuprophane membranes. The syndrome typically begins within a few minutes of starting dialysis. It may be due to hypersensitivity to ethylene oxide, which is used to sterilize the dialysis membrane and which can act as a hapten. Intense activation of complement occurs, and serum concentrations of C3a desarginine, the stable metabolite of C3 activation, may rise dramatically. A similar reaction has been observed in patients taking angiotensin-converting enzyme (ACE) inhibitors and being dialyzed with polyacrylonitrile membranes.

Immediate treatment consists of discontinuing dialysis and clamping the blood lines to prevent retransfusion of contaminated blood. Standard therapy for anaphylaxis, including oxygen, epinephrine, antihistamines, and glucocorticoids, may be necessary, depending on the individual response. Dialysis may be subsequently restarted, using an adequately rinsed membrane. The syndrome is extremely rare in programs in which dialyzer reuse is practiced.

PATIENT NUMBER 6

A 56-year-old Vietnamese woman who spoke little English or French repeatedly developed chest pain on dialysis. She had no history of angina, and no similar episodes were thought to occur outside the dialysis unit. ECG during symptoms revealed nonspecific anterolateral T-wave changes on some but not all occasions, and echocardiographic findings were normal. Her symptoms improved inconsistently with sublingual nitrates, but she refused further evaluation or hospital admission because her symptoms resolved before completion of dialysis on each occasion. As part of her transplantation workup, she agreed to cardiologic evaluation and underwent cardiac angiography. Results were entirely normal. With the help of a Vietnamese interpreter, it was subsequently determined that during dialysis, the development of chest pain invariably coincided with the onset of back pain and generalized pruritus. All symptoms resolved before the completion of dialysis. Changing her dialyzer membrane from cuprophane to polysulfone led to complete resolution of her dialytic symptoms.

MINOR FIRST-USE REACTIONS

Mild episodes of chest and back pain are not rare in the first hour of dialysis and usually subside without specific treatment. These are also thought to be related to complement activation and occur less frequently with biocompatible membranes such as those consisting of polysulfone or polyacrylonitrile. These reactions may cause diagnostic confusion with angina or musculoskeletal syndromes. Treatment is supportive, although some patients with recurrent symptoms may benefit from premedication with an antihistamine before dialysis.

Air Embolus

The development of multiple safety alarms on modern dialysis machines has rendered air embolus on dialysis a very rare event. However, insertion of central venous catheters for dialysis access, a common procedure in any dialysis unit, gives rise to opportunities for air to enter the central circulation.

Air can enter a vein only when a communication between the vessel lumen and the atmosphere is formed and when pressure within the vessel is subatmospheric. For this reason, internal jugular and subclavian lines are inserted with the patient in a Trendelenberg position to raise venous pressure to well above atmospheric. Despite this, occasions may arise when pressure falls, particularly in a patient with respiratory distress, in whom large swings of intrathoracic pressure are generated, or in a patient who coughs and then takes a deep inspiration during the procedure. The physician must therefore be constantly alert to the risk of air's entering the vein and must know how to manage this emergency.

CLINICAL FEATURES

As much as 50 to 100 ml of air in the circulation may be tolerated, but as little as 5 ml may be fatal to a patient in whom cardiac or respiratory status is already compromised. The immediate effects of air embolus depend on the position of the patient. If a patient is sitting or is lying with the head up, the air tends to enter the jugular veins, which may cause rapid loss of consciousness, seizures, or a lateralizing neurologic deficit. If a patient is lying flat, the air may foam in the right ventricle, causing a reduction in cardiac output and syncope. Air may also enter the pulmonary artery, causing acute pulmonary hypertension mimicking massive pulmonary embolus.

MANAGEMENT

First and foremost, no further air must be allowed to enter the venous circulation. This requires clamping of the venous line or occluding the introducing needle if the emergency arises during catheter placement. The patient should be immediately placed in Trendelenberg position lying on the left side. This promotes trapping of air at the apex of the right ventricle, thereby minimizing foaming, and keeps the air bubble away from the pulmonary valve. One-hundred percent oxygen should be administered, via an endotracheal tube if the patient is unconscious. It may be possible to aspirate air from the right ventricle if a suitably long catheter can be rapidly placed safely via a central vein. Intracardiac needle aspiration is not recommended because of the risk of coronary artery laceration and arrhythmia generation. If facilities are available, the patient should be placed in a decompression chamber.

Pericardial Tamponade

Severe uremia may result in pericarditis. The presence of a small pericardial effusion may be of no hemodynamic significance. A sudden deterioration in clinical status during dialysis, however, may be a sign of pericardial tamponade. Tamponade may be subtle and undetected before dialysis, in which case hypotension may occur rapidly in a volume-overloaded patient when cardiac filling pressures fall. It may also develop *de novo* in a patient who has hemorrhagic pericarditis and who is anticoagulated for the dialysis procedure.

In general, a patient with severe uremia should be dialyzed frequently for short periods without using heparin to reduce the risk of this serious complication. In patients in whom significant effusion or tamponade is suspected, an urgent echocardiogram and cardiologic opinion should be sought. If tamponade is confirmed, pericardiocentesis or surgical creation of a pericardial window should be done before dialysis.

Other Medical Problems in the Dialysis Unit

Patients with kidney failure frequently have multiple other medical problems. As a result, general medical emergencies often occur in the dialysis unit. Nephrologists are commonly called on to deal with these problems and must be aware of the special circumstances that dialysis imposes on management.

Seizures

Severe uremia may lead to seizure activity. Adequate dialysis prevents seizures from recurring under these circumstances. Conversely, aggressive dialysis in a patient with high serum urea concentrations may trigger seizures due to dialysis disequilibrium syndrome. Seizures may also occur on dialysis in patients with an undetected underlying tendency to seizure activity. Dialysis-related seizures are usually generalized; the presence of focal seizures should prompt a search for structural neurologic disease.

MANAGEMENT

Standard treatment for generalized seizures should be provided. A patent airway and administration of supplemental oxygen are essential. The dialysis procedure should be discontinued to prevent dislodgement of access needles during the seizure. A rapid bedside screen for hypoglycemia should be undertaken, followed by intravenous administration of 50% dextrose if warranted. It is rarely necessary to intervene with drugs to terminate a seizure, because the majority last for less than a minute. The knee-jerk reflex of giving diazepam to a patient with an uncomplicated seizure should be avoided because it may cause respiratory depression. Only if seizure activity lasts for more than 2 or 3 minutes or if recurrent seizures occur without

full recovery should acute treatment be undertaken.

Although some common anticonvulsant drugs such as phenytoin, valproic acid, and carbamazepine are not readily dialyzed, bioavailability may be affected by changes in protein binding in uremic patients. If recurrent seizure activity is a problem, serum free-drug concentrations may help to guide long-term dosing in individual patients.

Arrhythmias

Patients undergoing dialysis are at increased risk of cardiac arrhythmias because of the rapid fluid and electrolyte shifts imposed on them by the dialysis procedure. In addition, many older patients have coronary artery disease, hypertensive cardiomyopathy, or conduction system abnormalities. Patients who are on digoxin are at high risk for the development of tachyarrhythmias on dialysis, because serum potassium concentrations may fall rapidly and promote digoxin toxicity. In our dialysis unit, we routinely dialyze patients on digoxin against a high-potassium dialysate (3 mEq/L) to avoid large decrements in serum potassium during the dialysis procedure.

MANAGEMENT

In the event of a severe arrhythmia, dialysis should be stopped and the patient's blood returned. The dialysis needles should be flushed and left in place to facilitate drug administration. For immediately life-threatening arrhythmias such as ventricular fibrillation, ventricular tachycardia, or complete heart block, treatment should be started without delay according to standard protocols, including DC countershock or an external pacemaker if appropriate. In less urgent circumstances, an ECG should be obtained urgently to diagnose the arrhythmia. The temptation to rush in with antiarrhythmic agents without an accurate diagnosis can confuse subsequent management and must be avoided.

Once a patient has been stabilized and moved to a monitored environment, dialysis may be restarted to correct any remaining fluid or electrolyte disturbance.

Atrial fibrillation frequently occurs on dialysis and may be caused by changes in serum potassium levels or right atrial size. Under these circumstances, the arrhythmia often resolves within a few hours without specific treatment. Long-term treatment with a beta-blocking agent such as sotalol may be required to prevent excessive ventricular response rates even if the atrial fibrillation is transient. Individuals who develop recurrent atrial fibrillation with intervening episodes of normal sinus rhythm should be considered for long-term anticoagulation to reduce the risk of arterial embolism.

Angina

Chest pain on dialysis can be due to a number of causes, including myocardial ischemia and infarction, pericarditis, and first-use syndrome. Diagnosis may be straightforward if a patient is known to have ischemic heart disease, but ECG confirmation should be sought in all cases. Reversible contributing factors such as anemia should be corrected by blood transfusion. Standard treatment with restoration of blood pressure, oxygen administration, and sublingual nitrates should not, however, be delayed while awaiting the ECG.

Dialysis frequently can be continued, but if the episode is severe, prolonged, or of new onset, dialysis should be stopped and the patient stabilized before restarting in a monitored setting.

Hemorrhage

Bleeding episodes on dialysis may be overt and substantial, as when an access needle becomes dislodged or with a brisk upper gastrointestinal hemorrhage. Few events in a dialysis unit are more alarming to patients and staff than accidental or intentional removal of a dialysis needle from a high-flow arteriovenous fistula. More common, however, are insidious bleeds from venipuncture sites or previously asymptomatic gastrointestinal lesions.

MANAGEMENT

External hemorrhage can always be initially controlled with direct pressure, although the bleeding may recur as soon as the pressure is lifted. Traumatic bleeding including vessel puncture for dialysis access may require surgical repair or cautery. If possible, heparin-induced hypocoagulability should be corrected with protamine. Uremic platelet dysfunction is more difficult to manage. DDAVP (0.3 units/kg) infused in a small volume of normal saline may improve platelet function for 12 to 24 hours and may be repeated once. Cryoprecipitate, 10 units IV, is also useful in the management of persistent bleeding.

Conjugated estrogen (0.6 mg/kg daily for 5 days or 25 mg PO for 10 days) has proved to be useful in the management of prolonged bleeding when other agents have been unsuccessful. It is not useful in the management of acute bleeding episodes.

Hypotension

Episodes of hypotension are common on dialysis. The symptoms depend to a large extent on the individual patient. In the elderly, seizures, transient neurologic deficit, and altered mental status are frequent sequelae to a hypotensive event. In younger patients, diaphoresis and a feeling of lightheadedness are more common. Recurrent hypotension may lead to vascular access clotting problems. Rapid volume removal by the ultrafiltration component of dialysis is the most common cause of hypotension, when the capacity to recruit fluid from the interstitial fluid compartment to the vascular space is exceeded. Because water passes more rapidly into the intracellular fluid compartment than urea diffuses out, a solute gradient across the cell membrane arises during dialysis. Water moves into the cell from a region of lower osmolality to a region of higher osmolality, causing a net shift of fluid out of the ECF compartment. For this reason, variable dialysate sodium ramping can be used to minimize the osmotic gradient across the body fluid compartments.

MANAGEMENT

Immediate management consists of placing the patient in a head-down position, reducing or eliminating ultrafiltration, and administering a volume expander through the venous line. The choice of fluid is somewhat controversial. We use normal saline (0.9%) in boluses of 100 to 200 ml initially. Some centers prefer to use 5% or 25% albumin or synthetic colloids such as Pentaspan, because these agents are confined to the vascular space for longer periods. Little evidence suggests improved efficacy of these agents, however, and they are substantially more expensive than crystalloid fluids.

The episode of hypotension usually is short lived, and dialysis can continue. Persistent or severe hypotension should prompt a search for a more serious underlying cause such as myocardial ischemia or pericardial tamponade. Patients who habitually become hypotensive toward the end of dialysis should undergo reassessment of their dry weight, which may need to be increased. Antihypertensive therapy may need to be omitted on the day of dialysis to reduce the incidence of hypotension in some individuals.

URGENCIES IN RENAL TRANSPLANTATION

PATIENT NUMBER 7

Joe is a 34-year-old government employee who underwent his first renal transplantation for renal failure due to IgA nephropathy. His younger brother Ron was found to be one-haplotype identical and was the donor. All went smoothly, Joe's serum creatinine leveled off at 110 to 120 μmol/L (1.2 to 1.4 mg/dL), and he was discharged from hospital 10 days postoperatively taking cyclosporine, prednisone, and azathioprine. He began attending the outpatient clinic for routine monitoring. Fifteen days after transplantation, he and his wife, who gave him a ride that day, were told that Joe's serum creatinine level had risen to 150 μmol/L (1.7 mg/dL). They were both surprised and disappointed, especially because Joe felt "just fine." Physical examination revealed a temperature of 36.9°C, blood pressure of 135/80 mm Hg, and no tenderness over the transplanted kidney. Cyclosporine levels were in the target range. Ultrasound examination did not reveal obstruction. A fine-needle aspiration biopsy of the transplant was performed, showing evidence of acute rejection with no suggestion of cyclosporine toxicity. Intravenous pulse methylprednisolone was started. Joe's serum creatinine level peaked at 174 μmol/L (2.0 mg/dL) and subsequently dropped back to 125 μmol/L (1.4 mg/dL) by the following week. Joe remained asymptomatic the whole time.

Joe's case illustrates that of a patient found to have a rise in serum creatinine level 2 weeks after renal transplantation. The differential diagnosis of a rise in creatinine in a renal transplant recipient is influenced by the **time of the event after transplantation.**

Rise in Creatinine Several Days to 1 Week After Transplantation

At this time, major possibilities include accelerated acute rejection (generally a diagnosis made by renal biopsy), urinary tract obstruction, urinary leak, or thrombosis of a renal vein or artery.

Rise in Creatinine 1 Week to 3 Months After Transplantation (as in Joe's Case)

Likely diagnoses are acute rejection and cyclosporine toxicity. Other problems to consider during this period are urinary tract obstruction, urinary leak, sepsis, and recurrence of primary renal disease.

Longer-Term Rise in Serum Creatinine Level

The differential diagnosis includes acute rejection (especially if immunosuppressive medications are not taken), chronic rejection, acute or chronic cyclosporine toxicity, recurrence of primary renal disease, new renal disease, urinary tract obstruction, and renal artery stenosis.

Delayed Graft Function

Aside from deterioration of a previously functioning transplant, another pattern that may occur is persistence of renal failure after transplantation (delayed graft function). Some causes of this are acute tubular necrosis, accelerated acute rejection, urinary tract obstruction, and occlusion of the transplant artery or vein.

Several of these problems are reviewed in more detail in the sections that follow.

Acute Rejection

With current immunosuppression methods, rejection often presents without fever or transplant graft tenderness. The general approach to this diagnosis is to rule out structural problems (renal ultrasonography and Doppler studies of renal vessels can help to exclude urinary tract obstruction or occlusion of a renal artery or vein). Transplant biopsy remains the gold standard for diagnosis of acute rejection. Some centers use fine-needle aspiration biopsy of the graft, a technique shown to correlate well with full biopsy in differentiating between acute cyclosporine toxicity and acute cellular rejection.

Treatment of acute cellular rejection commonly consists of high-dose pulse corticosteroids. Monoclonal (e.g., OKT3) or polyclonal antibodies are sometimes used as alternative therapy or in the case of failure of corticosteroids.

Cyclosporine Nephrotoxicity

As is the case with acute rejection, it is often difficult to confirm the presence of cyclosporine toxicity by clinical or noninvasive evidence alone. High cyclosporine levels may be helpful in making this diagnosis, but transplant biopsy or fine-needle aspiration biopsy is often necessary. Treatment consists of decreasing the dose of cyclosporine.

Ureteric Obstruction

Ultrasonography of the transplant is quite sensitive in detecting significant urinary tract obstruction. Treatment is aimed at correction of the structural abnormality.

Urinary Leak

Urinary leak may present with a rise in serum creatinine level, graft tenderness, or swelling of the groin area on the side of the transplant. Ultrasound examination and nuclear renal scanning may demonstrate urine collection near the transplant, and a sample of the fluid should have the biochemical properties of urine (fluid creatinine level much higher than serum creatinine level). Surgical consultation is required, because operative treatment may be necessary.

Joe's case demonstrates a presentation of acute rejection. It is often difficult to differentiate between cyclosporine toxicity and rejection by clinical evidence and noninvasive tests alone. A renal biopsy or fine-needle aspirate of the renal transplant is often required.

Infection

PATIENT NUMBER 8

Margaret received her first renal transplant from a cadaveric donor after being on hemodialysis for 2 years for renal failure due to chronic glomerulonephritis. The transplant functioned immediately, and her serum creatinine level was 104 μmol/L (1.2 mg/dL) on the sixth day after transplantation while she was taking cyclosporine, azathioprine, and prednisone. Eight days postoperatively, she developed a temperature of 38.5°C but had no symptoms other than fatigue. Physical examination did not reveal any focus of infection, the transplant kidney was minimally tender in the area of the incision, and no clinical evidence of deep venous thrombosis was found. A Foley catheter had been removed 1 day before development of fever. Margaret's serum creatinine level was 99 μmol/L (1.1 mg/dL), her chest radiograph showed no abnormalities, her WBC count was 5.9 × 10⁹/L, and urinalysis revealed 50 WBCs per high-power field. Blood and urine cultures were obtained. Antibiotics were started for presumed urinary tract infection pending urine culture results. Her serum creatinine level remained stable, and urine cultures grew significant numbers of enterococci. Margaret's fever resolved in 2 days, and her energy has returned.

Fever in a renal transplant recipient often represents infection, although rejection and other processes such as venous thrombosis must be considered. Both the duration and amount of immunosuppression influence the types of infection that occur after transplantation. The degree of immunosuppression is generally highest during the first 3 to 6 months after transplantation.

The kinds of infection that occur vary at different times after renal transplantation.

The First Month

Types of infection at this time tend to parallel those that occur in postsurgical patients not taking immunosuppresives. Examples are wound, catheter, and intravenous line sepsis.

One to 6 Months

This is the period during which opportunistic infections are most likely to happen. Examples are *Pneumocystis* pneumonia, fungal sepsis, herpes simplex and zoster viruses, cytomegalovirus, and tuberculosis. Nonopportunistic infections, especially urinary tract infections, may still occur at this time.

Later Than 6 Months

Infections at this point are more like those in nonimmunosuppressed persons, with some increase in the occurrence of opportunistic infections.

The **workup** of a patient with a fever after transplantation therefore depends on the time after the surgery, the amount of immunosuppression received, and the clinical situation. Basic workup includes clinical evaluation of the patient, cultures, chest radiographs, serum creatinine determination, complete blood count, and any tests that pertain to the particular clinical presentation.

SUGGESTED READINGS

Halperin ML, Goldstein MB (eds): Fluid, Electrolyte and Acid-Base Physiology. A Problem-Based Approach. Philadelphia, WB Saunders, 1994.

Jacobson HR, Striker GE, Klahr S (eds): The Principles and Practice of Nephrology. Philadelphia, BC Decker, 1991.

Reuler JB, Magarian GJ: Hypertensive emergencies and urgencies: Definition, recognition, and management. J Gen Intern Med 3:64, 1988.

Rubin RH: Infectious disease complications of renal transplantation. Kidney Int 44:221, 1993.

INDEX

Page numbers in *italics* refer to illustrations;
page numbers followed by t indicate tables.